Controversies in Neurosurgery

OSSAMA AL-MEFTY, M.D.

Professor and Chairman, Department of Neurosurgery,
University of Arkansas for Medical Sciences

T.C. ORIGITANO, M.D., PH.D.

Associate Professor, Division of Neurological Surgery,
Loyola University Medical Center

H. LOUIS HARKEY, M.D.

Department of Neurosurgery,
University of Mississippi Medical Center

1996
THIEME NEW YORK
GEORG THIEME VERLAG STUTTGART · NEW YORK

Thieme Medical Publishers, Inc.
381 Park Avenue South
New York, New York 10016

CONTROVERSIES IN NEUROSURGERY
Ossama Al-Mefty
T.C. Origitano
H. Louis Harkey

Library of Congress Cataloging-in-Publication Data

Controversies in neurosurgery/[edited by] Ossama Al-Mefty, T.C.
  Origitano, H. Louis Harkey.
     p.   cm.
  Includes bibliographical references and index.
  ISBN 0-86577-538-9 (Thieme Medical Publishers).—ISBN
3-13-102671-5 (Georg Thieme Verlag)
  1. Nervous system—Surgery. 2. Brain—Tumors—Surgery. I. Al-
Mefty, Ossama. II. Origitano, T. C. III. Harkey, H. Louis.
  [DNLM: 1. Nervous System Diseases—surgery.   2. Nervous System
Neoplasms—surgery. WL 368 C764 1995]
  RD593.C597   1995
  617.4′8—dc20
  DNLM/DLC
  for Library of Congress   95-24354
                                                                CIP

Important note: Medicine is an ever-changing science. Research and clinical experience are continually broadening our knowledge, in particular our knowledge of proper treatment and drug therapy. Insofar as this book mentions any dosage or applications, readers may rest assured that the authors, editors, and publishers have made every effort to ensure that such references are strictly in accordance with the state of knowledge at the time of production of the book. Nevertheless, every user is requested to carefully examine the manufacturers' leaflets accompanying each drug to check on his own responsibility whether the dosage schedules recommended therein or the contraindications stated by the manufacturers differ from the statements made in the present book. Such examination is particularly important with drugs that are either rarely used or have been newly released on the market.

Some of the product names, patents, and registered designs referred to in this book are in fact registered trademarks or proprietary names even though specific reference to this fact is not always made in the text. Therefore, the appearance of a name without designation as proprietary is not to be construed as a representation by the publisher that it is in the public domain.

Printed in the United States of America.

5 4 3 2

TMP ISBN 0-86577-538-9
GTV ISBN 3-13-102671-5

Contents

Preface

Controversy. A discussion marked by the expression of opposing views. The connotation of this word is often negative; however, within the realm of neurological surgery, the word represents the sharpening stone by which our art and science are critically tested. It is the nature of the neurological surgeon to be curious and questioning. We are also a diverse group separated by age, location, experience, and resources. These factors contribute to the spectrum of "correct" answers for any particular clinical dilemma.

In keeping with the proverb that "wisdom comes from the counsel of many," this book assembles contributions of over 150 authors from 10 countries. The point-counter point format is structured to be provocative, forcing the authors to substantiate their points of view. Each chapter is moderated to give a balanced response to controversial view points.

One of us, OA, was privileged to work closely with, learn from, and exchange thoughts with Professor M. Gazi Yasargil during this past year at the University of Arkansas for Medical Sciences. Unfortunately, this year came after this book was already in press. I have learned that what many neurosurgeons consider controversial issues actually are not. Professor Yasargil takes clear action based on a sound knowledge and understanding of the anatomy, physiology, and pathophysiology, coupled with a masterful technique. With profound knowledge, deep understanding, and a wealth of experience, many of the controversies just vanish. I am so grateful for the opportunity to work with this living legend.

For the younger neurosurgeon, this book offers a wealth of clinical experience. It exposes the diversity of opinions and a spectrum of approaches to any one clinical problem. To the experienced neurosurgeon, it reflects the rapid changes that are occurring in both the art and science of modern neurosurgery. It serves to remind even the masters that today's answers will be challenged by tomorrow's neurosurgeon.

T.C. Origitano, M.D., Ph.D.
H. Louis Harkey, M.D.
Ossama Al-Mefty, M.D.

Contributors

Arvind Ahuja, M.D.
Division of Neurosurgery
State University of New York
Buffalo, NY

Eben Alexander, III, M.D.
Division of Neurosurgery
Brigham and Women's Hospital
Boston, MA

Ossama Al-Mefty, M.D.
Department of Neurosurgery
University of Arkansas for Medical Sciences
Little Rock, AR

Douglas E. Anderson, M.D.
Division of Neurological Surgery
Loyola University Medical Center
Maywood, IL

Ronald I. Apfelbaum, M.D.
Division of Neurosurgery
University of Utah Medical Center
Salt Lake City, UT

Michael L.J. Apuzzo, M.D.
Department of Neurosurgery
University of Southern California
Los Angeles, CA

James I. Ausman, M.D., Ph.D.
Department of Neurosurgery
Neuropsychiatric Institute
University of Illinois at Chicago College of
  Medicine
Chicago, IL

John R. Austin, M.D.
Head and Neck Surgery
University of Texas
M.D. Anderson Cancer Center
Houston, TX

Philip Azordegan, M.D.
University of Mississippi Medical Center
Jackson, MS

Joanne N. Bacchus, M.D.
London Regional Cancer Center
London, Ontario, Canada

Armando Basso, M.D.
Division of Neurology
University of Buenos Aires
Buenos Aires, Argentina

H. Hunt Batjer, M.D.
Division of Neurological Surgery
Chicago, IL

Donald P. Becker, M.D.
Division of Neurosurgery
UCLA School of Medicine
Los Angeles, CA

Steven E. Benner, M.D.
Division of Hematology/Oncology
University of North Carolina
Chapel Hill, NC

Edward C. Benzel, M.D.
Department of Neurosurgery
University of New Mexico
Albuquerque, NM

Mitchel S. Berger, M.D.
Department of Neurological Surgery
University of Washington Medical Center
Seattle, WA

Rajesh K. Bindal, M.D.
Department of Neurosurgery
University of Texas
M.D. Anderson Cancer Center
Houston, TX

Robert Blacklock, M.D.
Department of Neurosurgery
Baylor College of Medicine
Houston, TX

Frederick A. Boop, M.D.
Department of Neurosurgery
University of Arkansas for Medical Sciences
Little Rock, AR

Alfred P. Bowles, Jr., M.D.
Department of Neurosurgery
University of Mississippi
Jackson, MS

Derald E. Brackmann, M.D.
Division of Otolaryngology
University of Southern California
House Ear Institute
Los Angeles, CA

Fernando M. Braga, M.D.
Department of Neurosurgery
Escola Paulista de Medicina
São Paulo, Brazil

Charles L. Branch, Jr., M.D.
Department of Neurosurgery
Bowman Gray School of Medicine
Wake Forest University
Winston-Salem, NC

Albino Bricolo, M.D.
Department of Neurosurgery
Verona, Italy

Jacques Brotchi, M.D.
Department of Neurosurgery
Hospital Erasme
Free University of Brussels
Brussels, Belgium

Jeffrey A. Brown, M.D.
Department of Neurological Surgery
Medical College of Ohio
Toledo, OH

Jeffrey Bruce, M.D.
Departments of Neurological Surgery and
    Pathology
Columbia University
Neurological Institute
New York, NY

Dennis E. Bullard, M.D.
Neurological Surgery
Raleigh Neurosurgical Clinic
Raleigh, NC

Kim J. Burchiel, M.D.
Division of Neurosurgery
Oregon Health Sciences University
Portland, OR

J. Gregory Cairncross, M.D.
London Regional Cancer Center
London, Ontario, Canada

Antonio Carrizo, M.D.
Division of Neurology
University of Buenos Aires
Buenos Aires, Argentina

Ivan Ciric, M.D.
Division of Neurosurgery
Evanston Hospital
Northwestern University Medical School
Evanston, IL

Mark E. Coggins, M.D.
Department of Orthopaedic Surgery
Carolinas Medical Center
Charlotte, NC

Edward S. Connolly, M.D.
Department of Neurosurgery
Louisiana State University
New Orleans, LA

Paul R. Cooper, M.D.
Division of Neurosurgery
New York University Medical Center
New York, NY

H. Alan Crockard, M.D.
Department of Surgical Neurology
National Hospitals for Neurology and
    Neurosurgery
London, England

John D. Day, M.D.
University of Southern California
Los Angeles, CA

Evandro de Oliveira, M.D.
Department of Neurosurgery
São Paulo Neurological Institute
São Paulo, Brazil

Gerard Debrun, M.D.
Department of Neurosurgery
Neuropsychiatric Institute
University of Illinois at Chicago College of
    Medicine
Chicago, IL

Franco DeMonte, M.D.
Department of Neurosurgery
University of Texas
M.D. Anderson Cancer Center
Houston, TX

Curtis Dickman, M.D.
Division of Neurological Surgery
Barrow Neurological Institute
Phoeniz, AZ

Vinko V. Dolenc, M.D., Ph.D.
Department of Neurosurgery
University Medical Center
Ljubljana, Slovenia

Thomas Ducker, M.D.
Department of Neurosurgery
Johns Hopkins University
Baltimore, MD

Rudolf Fahlbusch, M.D.
Division of Neurosurgery
University of Erlangen-Nurnberg
Erlangen, Germany

Richard G. Fessler, M.D., Ph.D.
Department of Neurosurgery
University of Florida
Gainesville, FL

Gordon Findlay, M.D.
Walton Center for Neurology and Neurosurgery
University of Liverpool
Walton Hospital
Liverpool, England

John C. Flickinger, M.D.
Radiology and Radiation Oncology
University of Pittsburgh
Presbyterian University Hospital
Pittsburgh, PA

Kevin T. Foley, M.D.
Complex Spine Service
Semmes-Murphy Clinic
University of Tennessee
Memphis, TN

John L. Fox, M.D.
Department of Neurosurgery
University of Nebraska Medical Center
Omaha, NE

Masashi Fukui, M.D.
Department of Neurosurgery
Kyushu University Medical Center
Kyushu, Japan

Takanori Fukushima, M.D., D.M.Sc.
Allegheny General Hospital
Pittsburgh, PA

Adam S. Garden, M.D.
Radiation Oncology
University of Texas
M.D. Anderson Cancer Center
Houston, TX

Bernard George, M.D.
University of Paris
Neurochiurgie Hospital de Lariboisiere
Paris, France

Eugene George, M.D.
Department of Neurosurgery
University of Rochester Medical Center
Rochester, NY

Richard George, M.D.
Methodist Neurosurgical Associates
Lubbock, TX

Y. Pierre Gobin, M.D.
Department of Neurosurgery
Barrow Neurological Institute
Phoenix, AZ

John G. Golfinos, M.D.
Department of Neurosurgery
Barrow Neurological Institute
Phoenix, AZ

Deiter Grob, M.D.
Department of Orthopedics
Schulthess Hospital
Zurich, Switzerland

J.M. Gybels, M.D., Ph.D.

Stephen J. Haines, M.D.
Department of Neurosurgery
University of Minnesota
Minneapolis, MN

Sten Håkanson, M.D.
Department of Neurosurgery
Karolinska Sjukhuset
Stockholm, Sweden

Akira Hakuba, M.D.
Department of Neurosurgery
Osaka City University Medical School
Osaka, Japan

Walter A. Hall, M.D.
Department of Neurosurgery
University of Minnesota
Minneapolis, MN

P. Hallacq, M.D.
Department of Neurosurgery
Hospital Neurologique of Lyon
Lyon, France

Edward N. Hanley, Jr., M.D.
Department of Orthopedic Surgery
Carolinas Medical Center
Charlotte, NC

H. Louis Harkey, M.D.
Department of Neurosurgery
University of Mississippi Medical Center
Jackson, MS

Tomasz K. Helenowski, M.D.
Stereotactic Radiosurgery
Chicago Institute of Neurosurgery and
    Neuroresearch
Chicago, IL

Fraser Henderson, M.D.
Department of Neurosurgery
Georgetown University Medical Center
Washington, DC

Roberto C. Heros, M.D.
Department of Neurosurgery
University of Miami
Miami, FL

Harold J. Hoffman, M.D.
Division of Neurosurgery
Hospital for Sick Children
Toronto, Ontario, Canada

Leo N. Hopkins, M.D.
Division of Neurosurgery
State University of New York
Buffalo, NY

John A. Jane, M.D., Ph.D.
Department of Neurological Surgery
University of Virginia
Charlottesville, VA

Iain Kalfas, M.D.
Section of Spinal Surgery
Department of Neurosurgery
Cleveland Clinic Foundation
Cleveland, OH

Takeshi Kawase, M.D.
Department of Neurosurgery
Keio University School of Medicine
Tokyo, Japan

Andrew H. Kaye, M.D.
Division of Neurosurgery
Royal Melbourne Hospital
Melbourne University
Melbourne, Australia

Evren Keles, M.D.
Department of Neurological Surgery
University of Washington Medical Center
Seattle, WA

Mazen H. Khayata, M.D.
Department of Neurosurgery
Barrow Neurological Institute
Phoenix, AZ

Wesley A. King, M.D.
Division of Neurosurgery
UCLA School of Medicine
Los Angeles, CA

Peter M. Klara, M.D., Ph.D.
Complex Spine Service
Semmes-Murphy Clinic
University of Tennessee
Memphis, TN

David G. Kline, M.D.
Department of Neurosurgery
Louisiana State University Medical Center
New Orleans, LA

Shigeaki Kobayashi, M.D.
Department of Neurosurgery
Shinshu University School of Medicine
Matsumoto, Japan

Friedrich W. Kreth, M.D.
Abteilung Stereotaktische Neurochirurgie
Neurochirurgische Universitätsklinik
Freiburg, Germany

Ali F. Krisht, M.D.
Department of Neurosurgery
University of Arkansas for Medical Sciences
Little Rock, AR

David A. Larson, M.D., Ph.D.
Departments of Radiation, Oncology, and
  Neurological Surgery
University of California
San Francisco, CA

Edward R. Laws, Jr., M.D.
Department of Neurosurgery
University of Virginia Health Sciences Center
Charlottesville, VA

Kimberly Livingston, M.D.
Division of Neurosurgery
State University of New York
Buffalo, NY

Jay S. Loeffler, M.D.
Division of Neurosurgery
Brigham and Women's Hospital
Boston, MA

Donlin M. Long, M.D.
Department of Neurosurgery
Johns Hopkins University School of Medicine
Baltimore, MD

L. Dade Lunsford, M.D.
Radiation and Radiation Oncology
University of Pittsburgh
Presbyterian University Hospital
Pittsburgh, PA

Joseph C. Maroon, M.D.
Department of Neurosurgery
Allegheny General Hospital
Pittsburgh, PA

Toshio Matsushima, M.D.
Department of Neurosurgery
Kyushu University Medical Center
Kyushu, Japan

Paul C. McCormick, M.D.
Division of Neurological Surgery
Columbia-Presbyterian Medical Center
Neurological Institute
New York, NY

John E. McGillicuddy, M.D.
Department of Neurosurgery
University of Michigan
Ann Arbor, MI

Robert McGuire, M.D.
Department of Orthopedic Surgery
University of Mississippi Medical Center
Jackson, MS

Gregory K. Meekin, M.D.
Department of Neurological Surgery
University of Virginia
Charlottesville, VA

Arnold H. Menezes, M.D.
Department of Neurosurgery
University of Iowa College of Medicine
Iowa City, IA

Carole A. Miller, M.D.
Division of Neurosurgery
Ohio State University
Columbus, OH

Mark E. Molitch, M.D.
Division of Medicine
Northwestern University Medical School
Chicago, IL

Robert A. Morantz, M.D.
Midwest Neurosurgery
Kansas City, MO

Jules M. Nazzaro, M.D.
Department of Neurosurgery
Boston University Medical Center
Boston, MA

Steven A. Newman, M.D.
Department of Neurological Surgery
University of Virginia
Charlottesville, VA

Edward A. Neuwelt, M.D.
Department of Neurology
Oregon Health Sciences University
Portland, OR

G. Robert Nugent, M.D.
Department of Neurosurgery
West Virginia University Health Sciences Center
Morgantown, WV

Kenji Ohata, M.D.
Department of Neurosurgery
Osaka City University Medical Center
Osaka, Japan

Robert G. Ojemann, M.D.
Division of Surgery
Harvard Medical School
Massachusetts General Hospital
Boston, MA

Sean O'Laoire, M.D.
Department of Neurosurgery
National Neurological Center
Mater Private Hospital
Dublin, Ireland

Gary Onik, M.D.
Department of Neurosurgery
Allegheny General Hospital
Pittsburgh, PA

T.C. Origitano, M.D., Ph.D.
Division of Neurological Surgery
Loyola University Medical Center
Maywood, IL

Christoph B. Ostertag, M.D.
Abteilung Stereotaktische Neurochirurgie
Neurochirurgische Universitätsklinik
Freiburg, Germany

Stephen M. Papadopoulos, M.D.
Department of Neurosurgery
University of Michigan Medical Center
Ann Arbor, MI

Andrew D. Parent, M.D.
Department of Neurosurgery
University of Mississippi
Jackson, MS

David A. Peace, M.S., M.A.
University of Florida School of Medicine
Gainesville, FL

Noel Perin, M.D.
Mayfield Neurological Institute
Cincinnati, OH

Michael Polinsky, M.D.
Department of Neurosurgery
University of Michigan Medical Center
Ann Arbor, MI

Kalmon D. Post, M.D.
Department of Neurosurgery
Mount Sinai School of Medicine
New York, NY

Stephen K. Powers, M.D.
Division of Neurosurgery
Pennsylvania State University Medical Center
Hershey, PA

John Reeves, M.D.
Department of Neurosurgery
Louisiana State University Medical Center
New Orleans, LA

James F. Reibel, M.D.
Department of Neurological Surgery
University of Virginia
Charlottesville, VA

O. Howard Reichman, M.D.
Department of Neurological Surgery
Loyola University Medical Center
Maywood, IL

Albert L. Rhoton, Jr., M.D.
Department of Neurosurgery
University of Florida School of Medicine
Gainesville, FL

Charles J. Riedel, M.D.
Division of Neurological Surgery
The Spine Center
George Washington University Medical Center
Washington, DC

Lewis P. Rowland, M.D.
Department of Neurology
Neurological Institute
Columbia-Presbyterian Medical Center
New York, NY

Oren Sagher, M.D.
Division of Neurosurgery
University of Michigan
Ann Arbor, MI

Michael Salcman, M.D.
Department of Neurosurgery
George Washington University School of
   Medicine
Towson, MD

Madjid Samii, M.D.
Division of Neurosurgery
Neurosurgical Clinic
Nordstadtkrankenhaus
Hannover, Germany

Duke Samson, M.D.
Department of Neurological Surgery
University of Texas Southwestern Medical Center
Dallas, TX

Robert A. Sanford, M.D.
Semmes-Murphy Clinic
Memphis, TN

H. Säveland, M.D.
Department of Neurosurgery
University Hospital of Northern Sweden
Umea, Sweden

Raymond Sawaya, M.D.
Department of Neurosurgery
University of Texas
M.D. Anderson Cancer Center
Houston, TX

John D. Schlegel, M.D.
Division of Orthopedic Surgery
University of Utah
Salt Lake City, UT

Jorge R. Schvarcz, M.D.
Division of Neurosurgery
University of Buenos Aires
Buenos Aires, Argentina

Laligam N. Sekhar, M.D.
George Washington University Hospital
Washington, DC

Chandranath Sen, M.D.
Department of Neurosurgery
Mount Sinai Medical Center
New York, NY

Jatin P. Shah, M.D.
Head and Neck Service
Memorial Sloan-Kettering Cancer Center
New York, NY

Frederick A. Simeone, M.D.
Division of Neurosurgery
University of Pennsylvania School of Medicine
Pennsylvania Hospital
Philadelphia, PA

Marc Sindou, M.D.
Division of Neurosurgery
Hospital Neurologique of Lyon
Lyon, France

Michael B. Sisti, M.D.
Department of Neurosurgery
Neurological Institute
Columbia-Presbyterian Medical Center
New York, NY

Robert R. Smith, M.D.
Department of Neurosurgery
Methodist Hospital
Jackson, MS

Volker K.H. Sonntag, M.D.
Barrow Neurological Institute
Phoenix, AZ

Robert F. Spetzler, M.D.
Department of Neurosurgery
Barrow Neurological Institute
Phoenix, AZ

Bennett M. Stein, M.D.
Department of Neurosurgery
Neurological Institute
Columbia-Presbyterian Medical Center
New York, NY

Kintomo Takakura, M.D.
Division of Neurosurgery
Tokyo Women's Medical College
Tokyo, Japan

Edward Tarlov, M.D.
Lahey Clinic Medical Center
Burlington, MA

Helder Tedeschi, M.D.
Department of Neurosurgery
São Paulo Neurological Institute
São Paulo, Brazil

David G.T. Thomas, M.D.
Institute of Neurology
National Hospitals
London, England

David C. Thomasma, Ph.D.
Medical Humanities Program
Loyola University Medical Center
Maywood, IL

George T. Tindall, M.D.
Department of Neurosurgery
Emory University School of Medicine
Atlanta, GA

Suzie C. Tindall, M.D.
Department of Neurosurgery
Emory University School of Medicine
Atlanta, GA

Vincent Traynelis, M.D.
Department of Surgery
University of Iowa Hospitals and Clinics
Iowa City, IA

Fernando Viñuela, M.D.
Department of Radiological Sciences
UCLA Medical Center
Los Angeles, CA

W. Michael Vise, M.D.
Department of Neurosurgery
University of Mississippi Medical Center
Jackson, MS

Ajay K. Wakhloo, M.D.
Department of Neurosurgery
Barrow Neurological Institute
Phoenix, AZ

Bryce K. Weir, M.D.
Section of Neurosurgery
University of Chicago Medical Center
Chicago, IL

Robert H. Wilkins, M.D.
Department of Neurosurgery
Duke University Medical Center
Durham, NC

Charles B. Wilson, M.D.
Department of Neurological Surgery
University of California
San Francisco, CA

Donald C. Wright, M.D.
Division of Neurosurgery
George Washington University Hospital
Washington, DC

Isao Yamamoto, M.D.
Department of Neurosurgery
Yokohama City University School of Medicine
Yokohama, Japan

M. Gazi Yasargil, M.D.
Department of Neurosurgery
University of Arkansas for Medical Sciences
Little Rock, AR

Daniel Yoshor, M.D.
Department of Neurosurgery
Baylor College of Medicine
Houston, TX

Paul Young, M.D.
Microsurgery Brain Research Institute
St. Louis, MO

S. Zygmunt, M.D., Ph.D.
Department of Neurosurgery
University Hospital of Northern Sweden
Umea, Sweden

Acknowledgment

We are indebted to all contributors who provided excellent chapters and were willing to be bold in their advocacy. Our appreciation goes to Dr. Howard R. Reichman for preparing the vascular case studies. We thank Gina Falco, Amy Keeland, Jill Wallock, and Julie Yamamoto who spent countless hours tracking, editing, and organizing to bring this work to fruition.

Dedication

To John L. Fox, M.D.
great mentor and true friend
by example he taught *"we must unlearn all to learn again."*

1

Medical vs. Surgical Treatment
of Giant Pituitary Prolactinomas

CASE

A 45-year-old, right-handed man came to medical attention with headaches and a noted decrease in peripheral vision. A formal examination of the visual field showed bitemporal hemianopsia. The patient's serum prolactin level was 20,000 IU.

PARTICIPANTS

Medical Treatment of Giant Pituitary Prolactinomas–Mark E. Molitch, M.D.

Surgical Treatment of Giant Pituitary Prolactinomas–Ivan Ciric, M.D.

Moderator–Rudolf Fahlbusch, M.D.

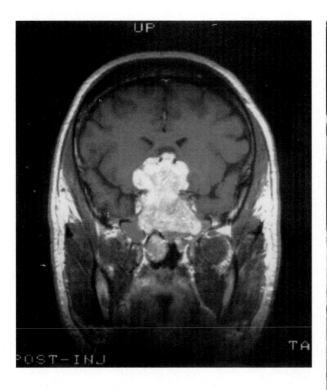 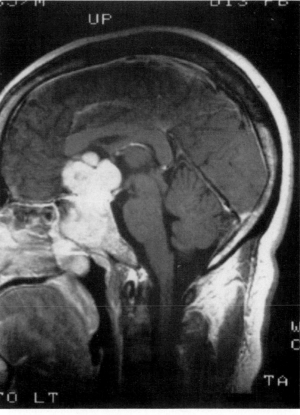

Medical Treatment of Giant Pituitary Prolactinomas

Mark E. Molitch, M.D.

The appellation *giant* has been reserved for pituitary tumors greater than 4 cm in diameter or those with more than 2 cm of suprasellar extension, or both.[12,34,40,47,58] Fortunately, such tumors are quite uncommon, representing only 9.6% of the 800 cases operated upon by Professor Jules Hardy.[12]

This patient has a giant prolactinoma with chiasmal compression causing bitemporal hemianopsia. We are not told the status of his pituitary gland, but it is likely that he has hypopituitarism and he may have diabetes insipidus. Before any treatment is undertaken, the patient should be evaluated for hypofunctioning of anterior pituitary hormones and diabetes insipidus, and any deficits found should be corrected.[35]

The basic controversy, in a patient such as this, is what type of therapy to try first. Before deciding upon the therapeutic modality, the goals of treatment need to be specified. Therapeutic goals may be divided into two categories: those relating to abnormal hormone production and those relating to tumor size. Prolactin (PRL) levels must be reduced to near normal to restore normal reproductive function. A reduction of 50% or even 90% may not mean much biologically, as the patient will still have sexual and reproductive dysfunction. With respect to tumor size, however, goals include preventing further tumor growth and reducing tumor size. For this tumor, which has likely been growing for many years, substantially reducing the size may not reverse the visual field defects or the hypopituitarism and a reasonable goal may be to prevent further growth. The benefits of therapy designed to achieve these goals must be balanced against the risks of such therapy.

The primary consideration in this patient is whether to use surgery or bromocriptine as initial treatment. To aid in this decision-making, I will review the literature with regard to the efficacy of surgery versus bromocriptine as initial treatment of prolactin-secreting macroadenomas in general and giant invasive prolactinomas in particular.

SURGERY

The transsphenoidal approach is usually used for microadenomas and most macroadenomas. Both the transsphenoidal and craniotomy approaches have been used for giant tumors, such as this.[9,21,34,47,58,68] Table 1 summarizes the surgical results from 27 published series for macroadenomas of all sizes, recording only the results from the latest series from a given neurosurgical/endocrinological team and not including data from earlier papers.[2,3,5,7-9,13,14,16,18,20-22,28,42,43,45,46,49,51-55,59,62,70] In these series, 400 (31.8%) of 1256 tumors were reported as being curatively resected; that is, having the patient's PRL levels normalized by 1 to 12 weeks after surgery. Within these series, the success rates were quite variable: for series with at least 10 patients, the surgical cure rate varied from 11 to 80%. From a mail survey of 80 neurosurgeons, Zervas reported a surgical cure rate of 30% for 1022 PRL-secreting macroadenomas.[71] Clearly, the success rate in large part depended upon the size of tumors in patients chosen for surgery. In many series, the object was, appropriately, debulking of a large tumor rather than cure and, in other series, patients with large tumors were not operated on.

Operative cure rates have been reported in a limited number of patients with giant pituitary tumors; these tumors have been operated on through the transsphenoidal, craniotomy, and combined transsphenoidal-craniotomy routes. Of tumors with a suprasellar extension greater than 20 mm operated upon through the transsphenoidal approach, Mohr and colleagues[34] reported no residual tumor on postoperative CT scans in 29 of 48 patients with normal PRL levels and in 8 of 14 patients with prolactinomas. Ciric and colleagues,[9] however, reported that, of 14 such patients undergoing the transsphenoidal approach, they found such a removal difficult or impossible, although they did not give specific figures. Guidetti and associates[21] noted that, of 21 patients with giant adenomas undergoing a fronto-temporal approach, gross total removal was obtained in 8 but normalization of PRL levels was not obtained in any of 6 patients with prolactinomas. Of 4 patients reported by Davis and co-workers[12] and 2 reported by Murphy and associates[40] with prolactinomas of sizes comparable to the patient in this case, none had a return of PRL to normal by surgery and all had significant residual tumor after surgery.

In 2 older surgical series of giant adenomas, the particular tumor types with respect to hormone secretion were not specified, nor were the cure rates given. They are included here, however, because of the discussions of the complication rates of surgery (see below). Symon and colleagues[58] found that, of 16 patients undergoing a craniotomy, in only 11 could a radical excision to remove all intradural tumor be done and all patients underwent postoperative irradiation. Pia and associates[47] operated on 77 such tumors, 23 through the transsphenoidal route and 54 through a craniotomy; of the 77, 22 tumors recurred.

In patients with normal PRL levels after surgery, the postoperative recurrence of hyperprolactinemia has also been a problem. Most recurrences of hyperprolactinemia occur within the first year after surgery, probably because of the regrowth of tumor remnants rather than the formation of a new tumor.[37] Recurrence rates vary from 0[53,59,70] to 91%[45] for patients with macroadenomas. From the series compiled in Table 1, the recurrence rate for macroadenomas is 48 (18.6%) of 235. In almost all of these cases, the recurrence is that of hyperprolactinemia and not documented radiological evidence of tumor regrowth. As yet, no long-term follow-up studies of these recurrences of hyperprolactinemia has been done to determine the rate of radiologically evident tumor regrowth. Nonetheless, recurrence of hyperprolactinemia is usually accompanied by a recurrence of sexual and reproductive dysfunction, which is usually an indication for medical therapy to reduce the patient's PRL levels.

Complications of Surgery

In general, surgery for patients with macroadenomas has a relatively low complication rate. The mortality rate for transsphenoidal surgery for all types of secreting and nonsecreting macroadenomas is 0.9%; the major morbidity rate is 6.5% (visual loss 1.5%, stroke/vascular injury 0.6%, meningitis/abscess 0.5% and oculomotor palsy 0.6%), and the rate of cerebrospinal fluid rhinorrhea is 3.3%.[29,71] Transient diabetes insipidus is quite common (6%) and permanent diabetes insipidus occurs in about 1% of patients undergoing surgery for a macroadenoma.[71]

Table 1. Surgical Cure Rates for Macroprolactinomas

Series	Number of Tumors	Tumors Cured	Recurrence
Domingue et al.[13]	25	10	–
Randall et al.[49]	46	13	–
Hardy[22]	89	34	4/5
Rodman et al.[52]	23	9	1/5
Tucker et al.[62]	18	8	–
Arafah et al.[3]	46	29	10
Faria and Tindall[18]*	28	13	4/11
Parl et al.[45]	–	11	10
Charpentier et al.[8]	289	134	10
Nelson et al.[42]	11	4	1
Ciric et al.[9]	41	11	–
Guidetti et al.[21]	120	11	4
Pelkonen et al.[46]	53	6	–
Antunes et al.[2]	8	3	–
Bevan et al.[5]	28	8	1
Rawe et al.[51]	9	3	–
Schlechte et al.[54]	24	11	4
Smallridge and Martins[55]	5	0	–
Grisoli et al.[20]	20	6	–
Nicola et al.[43]	40	16	–
Landolt[28]	37	10	–
Woosley et al.[70]	14	5	0
Dupuy et al.[14]	78	7	–
Thomson et al.[59]	8	4	0
Fahlbusch and Buchfelder[16]	139	15	1/15
Brabant et al.[7]	37	14	–
Scanlon et al.[53]	20	16	0
TOTAL	**1256**	**411 (32.7%)**	**50/235 (21.3%)**

*Classified on the basis of prolactinoma level ≤200 ng/ml (81% microadenoma) or >200 ng/ml (86% macroadenoma), rather than tumor size.

Patients may have hypopituitarism before surgery and, because of the extent of surgery sometimes performed, may have significant changes in pituitary function postoperatively. In an analysis of 84 patients with macroadenomas (36 of which were prolactinomas), Nelson and colleagues[41] found that, of those with normal preoperative pituitary function, only 78% retained normal function postoperatively. One third of patients with some pituitary deficits before surgery improved and one third with such deficits had worsened pituitary function after surgery. None of the patients with panhypopituitarism improved after surgery.[41]

For patients with giant tumors, the morbidity and mortality rates are considerably higher that those for patients with macroadenomas, although this seems to be improving in more recent series. Of the 16 patients undergoing a craniotomy by Symon and colleagues,[58] 3 died in the immediate postoperative period and 2 others died within 6 months of surgery. In the series of 77 patients operated upon by Pia and associates,[47] 8 patients died during surgery and considerable morbidity occurred, consisting of increased visual loss in 4, oculomotor disturbances in 8, diabetes insipidus in 15, mental deterioration in 14, and cerebrospinal fluid fistulas in 5 (3 requiring surgical repair). In their series of 21 patients, Guidetti and colleagues[21] also noted high complication rates, with 2 perioperative deaths, 4 patients with permanent diabetes insipidus, 1 with postoperative hemiparesis and 1 with hypothalamic failure. Furthermore, of 16 patients able

to be evaluated, they found the quality of life to be good in 4, fair in 9, and poor in 69. In the most recent series of Mohr and colleagues,[34] all patients being operated on through the transsphenoidal approach, operative mortality stemmed primarily from the development of postoperative hematomas. In addition, the risk of significant organic brain syndrome was 3% and that of permanent diabetes insipidus was 6.5%.[34]

Thus, surgery for giant prolactinomas is often successful in debulking tumors but actual cure is uncommon in almost all series, although Mohr and colleagues reported the exceptional hormonal cure rate of 57%.[34] The complication rates are high, however; the mortality rate ranges from 5.2[34] to 31.2%[58] and the major morbidity rate ranges from 10[34] to 62%.[58]

BROMOCRIPTINE

Dopamine is the primary inhibitory factor for PRL, and dopamine receptors are present on normal lactotrophs and prolactinoma cells. Bromocriptine is a long-acting dopamine receptor agonist that decreases the synthesis and secretion of PRL.[23,63] In several large early studies in the literature, including more than 1000 patients with hyperprolactinemia treated with bromocriptine, normoprolactinemia or return of ovulatory menses occurred in 80 to 90% of patients.[39,63]

In vitro studies have shown that bromocriptine not only decreases PRL synthesis but also DNA synthesis, cell multiplication, and tumor growth.[11,31,32] Clinical studies have shown that bromocriptine can often decrease the size of a prolactinoma. Table 2 lists the response of tumor size to bromocriptine from 19 different series of patients, totaling 236 patients with macroadenomas.[4,5,10,17,19,24,26,30,31,33,38,44,48,54,56,57,64–67,69] Each series was examined carefully to exclude duplication, patients with coexistent acromegaly, and patients who had received prior radiotherapy. Of these 236 patients analyzed, 77% had some decrease in tumor size in response to bromocriptine, with periods of observation ranging from 6 weeks to over 10 years.

In eight series, the degree of tumor reduction was quantitated.[4,5,17,38,44,48,64,67,69] Quantitation gave a total of 106 patients; in 45 (42.5%) tumors were reduced by more than 50%, in 30 (28.3%) tumors were reduced from 25 to 50%, in 12 (11.3%) tumors were reduced by less than 25%, and in 19 (17.9%) there was no evidence of any reduction in tumor size.

The time course of tumor reduction is variable. The tumors in some patients may decrease rapidly, with significant changes in visual fields noted within 24 to 72 hours and significant changes noted on a CT scan within 2 weeks.[61] In others, little change may be noted at 6 weeks but scanning again at 6 months may show significant changes.[38] In about two thirds of patients, a tumor reduction is noted by 6 weeks but, in others, improvement was not noted until later scans.[38] In many patients, continuing decreases were noted progressively after 1 year for up to several years.[6]

In a multicenter study,[3] visual field improvement occurred in 9 of 10 patients with significant visual field abnormalities; 80 to 90% of patients in other studies have had substantial improvement as well.[5,6,17,30,33,44,48,57,65,67] Visual field improvement generally parallels and often precedes the changes seen on scans.[38,48] Determining before treatment whether visual defects are temporary or permanent is difficult, and only the patient's response to therapy (medical or surgical) provides an answer. These studies with medical therapy are reassuring, in that a relatively slow chiasmal decompression over several weeks provides excellent restoration of visual fields and immediate surgical decompression is not absolutely necessary in this regard. Usually, when there is no significant change in visual fields despite significant evidence of tumor reduction on a scan, subsequent surgery does not improve these fields.[17]

In general, the extent of tumor reduction does not correlate with basal PRL levels, nadir PRL levels achieved, the percentage of decrease in PRL, or whether PRL levels reached normal.[10,38] Some patients have excellent reduction in PRL levels into the normal range but only modest changes in tumor size, and others have persistent hyperprolactinemia (although greater than an 88% suppression from basal values) with almost complete disappearance of the tumor. A reduction in PRL levels always precedes any detectable change in tumor size and patients whose PRL levels do not respond also do not have a reduction in tumor size. Once maximum size reduction is achieved, the dose of bromocriptine can often be gradually reduced.[6,12,30]

A permanent reduction in tumor size is likely related to the extent of scarring and fibrosis that occurs.[6] A striking, time-dependent increase in tumor fibrosis occurs with bromocriptine.[15] With short-term use, when bromocriptine is discontinued in a patient with a macroadenoma that has decreased, the tumor can re-expand within 2 weeks.[60] However, this re-expansion is not common with long-term use. When bromocriptine has been used for more than 3 years and then discontinued, 80 to 90% of tumors do not re-expand, although PRL levels remain normal in only 10 to 20% of patients.[26,50,64,65]

In many of the reported series, giant prolactinomas were included but specific details regarding their results were not given. Of the 9 patients with giant prolactinomas treated with bromocriptine reported by Davis and colleagues,[12] 1 had no response, one had minimal tumor reduction, 5 had modest decreases in tumor size, and 2 had marked reductions in tumor size. In 4 of these patients, PRL levels returned to normal but,

Table 2. Size Responses of Macroadenomas to Bromocriptine Treatment

| Series | Total | Tumor size reduction | | | | | Length of treatment (months) |
		>50%	25–50%	0–25%	Not quant.	No change	
Molitch et al.[38]	27	13	5	9	–	0	12
Bevan et al.[5]	7	5	2	0	–	0	1.5
Wang et al.[64]	3	3	0	0	–	0	24–144
McGregor et al.[33]	5	–	–	–	5	0	3
Sobrinho et al.[56]	12	–	–	–	9	3	6
Spark et al.[57]	10	–	–	–	8	2	8–27
Nissim et al.[44]	7	4	–	–	–	3	1.5
Wass et al.[66]	14	–	–	–	9	5	3–22
Wollesen et al.[69]	4	4	–	–	–	0	15–45
Horowitz et al.[24]	6	–	–	–	3	3	6
Corenblum and Taylor[10]	16	–	–	–	11	5	60–108
Weiss et al.[67]	19	–	10	0	–	9	1.5
Johnston et al.[26]	14	–	–	–	10	4	18–84
Warfield et al.[65]	6	–	–	–	4	2	6
Barrow et al.[4]	11	3	2	0	–	6	1.6
Liuzzi et al.[30]	38	–	–	–	29	9	30–88
Pullan et al.[48]	5	4	0	1	–	0	6–24
Gasser et al.[19]	9	–	–	–	6	3	
Fahlbusch et al.[17]	23	9	11	2	–	1	0.5–1.5
TOTAL	**236**	**45**	**30**	**12**	**94**	**55**	

in the other 5, PRL levels remained significantly elevated. Of the 2 similar patients reported treated with bromocriptine by Murphy and colleagues,[40] 1 had reduction of the tumor to 80% of its original size with a lowering of PRL from greater than 5000 to 193 ng/ml, and another had complete disappearance of the tumor associated with a lowering of PRL from 5600 to l0 ng/ml.

Adverse Effects of Bromocriptine Treatment

Bromocriptine is certainly not without side effects but, in general, patients tolerate it well. The most common adverse effects are nausea and sometimes vomiting; these are usually transient but may recur with each increase in dosage. Orthostatic hypotension usually is a problem only when initiating therapy and rarely recurs with increased dosages. Limited nausea and vomiting occurs in 3 to 5% of patients and digital vasospasm, nasal congestion, and depression occur rarely when doses less than 7.5 mg/day are used.[23,63] Side effects can be minimized by starting with 1.25 mg daily, with the dose being gradually increased. Rarely, the prolactinoma serves as a "cork" and tumor reduction with bromocriptine may cause cerebrospinal fluid rhinorrhea.[1,27] In patients intolerant of bromocriptine, other dopamine agonists, such as pergolide, can be tried. Bromocriptine may be given to women intravaginally to avoid adverse gastrointestinal effects.[36]

SUMMARY

Because of the excellent results with bromocriptine and the rather poor results of surgery in most patients, I recommend dopamine agonists as the initial therapy for patients with PRL-secreting macroadenomas, especially giant prolactinomas. Surgery can always be carried out later in patients with tumors that do not respond adequately to such medications. Even if subsequent surgery is necessary for tumor debulking, it rarely is curative and bromocriptine or some other dopamine agonist is usually necessary to treat the hyperprolactinemia. The goals of therapy must be kept in mind; complete tumor removal may not be achievable by any means and control of further growth may be sufficient. It is important to balance the benefits of therapy with the complications of therapy. Radiation therapy has a very limited role here, being used for those who have absolutely no response to dopamine agonists or with a tumor that was documented to actually grow while on dopamine agonists, and after incomplete surgical removal. Whether surgery should be considered for removing a shrunken tumor during dopamine-agonist treatment is not established. Some tumors show increased fibrosis after bromocriptine treatment and tumor removal has been impaired in some series,[5] but not others.[25] However, as complete surgical removal is rarely achieved and dopamine agonists are still necessary for controlling hyperprolactinemia, there seems to be little reason for surgical intervention if the tumor has satisfactorily decreased in size.

When dopamine-agonist therapy is stopped, the prolactinoma may return to its original size, often within days or weeks. With prolonged therapy, however, the tumor does not re-expand in most patients. This potential return to pretherapy size dictates extreme caution when withdrawing a patient from dopamine-agonist therapy, however, as rapid tumor expansion may produce far more clinical symptoms than slow tumor enlargement. This is particularly important in patients with giant prolactinomas. Often, however, the dose can be gradually tapered once maximum size reduction has occurred and, in suitable patients, stopped entirely if no re-expansion occurs.

Surgical Treatment of Giant Pituitary Prolactinomas

Ivan Ciric, M.D.

This patient has a giant and invasive macroprolactinoma. The tumor has eroded the sphenoid bone and the clivus and presents itself in the epipharynx. Superiorly, the tumor extends through a relatively constricted diaphragma sellae into the suprasellar space, where it compresses the anterior third ventricle. The dome of the tumor is close to the foramen of Monro, but does not obstruct it. The anterior cerebral arteries are elevated and straddled by the tumor, and are partially encased. The chiasm cannot be identified but, based on the patient's clinical presentation, it is evident that the chiasm is compressed. The cavernous sinuses are involved on both sides, more so on the left.

The fundamental goals of any neurosurgical intervention should be cure and, thus, prevention of recurrence, palliation if cure is not possible, and in some instances diagnosis. The same principles also apply to the surgical treatment of pituitary tumors. The patient's safety (no mortality and morbidity) must be the overriding prerequisite before surgery is considered. In addition, the treatment should be relatively painless. The recovery period before the patient returns to his premorbid lifestyle, work, and activities should be as short as possible and the treatment should be cost-effective.

The definition of cure implies complete resolution of the morbid state with no need for further therapy and with no prospects for recurrence. I do not believe this is attainable in this patient, regardless of the therapy or combination of treatments used. In this patient, the anatomic relationship of the tumor to the skull base, to the cavernous sinuses and their contents, and to the surrounding neurovascular structures is intimate and is likely an inseparable one. To be sure, complete removal of this tumor could be carried out as an unsavory surgical exercise with unacceptable morbidity, possibly even mortality. Thus, it would be highly unrealistic, naive and, yes, inconsistent with professional honesty to suggest that this tumor can be cured surgically, be it through a craniotomy, the transsphenoidal approach, or even a more extensive combined approach, regardless of the surgeon's aggressiveness and experience.

If we accept the premise that this patient is not curable with surgery alone, could he be cured or should his symptoms at least be palliated with a sequence of treatments, starting with surgical decompression and followed with medical therapy with bromocriptine or radiation therapy? For several reasons, I do not think so. First, giant and invasive macroprolactinomas are frequently tough and stringy in consistency, secondary to a pronounced desmoplastic reaction of the tissues invaded by the tumor. Thus, decompression is often very difficult to achieve. Second, the relatively constricted diaphragma sellae probably precludes safe and effective transsphenoidal decompression of the supradiaphragmatic tumor segment. In fact, such an attempt would likely be associated with hemorrhage and swelling into the residual tumor tissue, with the possibility of postoperative visual impairment and hydrocephalus. True, a craniotomy would be safer in this regard, but it could prove to be an exercise in futility as far as a meaningful decompression is concerned and would certainly be associated with considerable risk factors. In short, I do not recommend any operative procedure for this patient, especially not as the initial treatment.

Our experience with giant and invasive macroprolactinomas, some much worse than the tumor in this patient, shows that these tumors respond promptly and effectively to medical treatment with dopamine agonists regardless of their size, extent, and clinical presentation (Figs. 1, 2). Symptoms in patients with these tumors can be palliated rapidly with bromocriptine as a result of a decrease in the tumor size, improvement in the visual and other compressive symptoms and a decrease in the prolactin level. Six of 7 such patients with truly giant and invasive macroprolactinomas, who had either visual or oculomotor nerve impairment, 2 with hydrocephalus and 1 who was lethargic at the time of admission, improved rapidly with bromocriptine and had eventual complete resolution of all symptoms. In 3 of these patients, bromocriptine therapy was initially combined with dexamethasone. The bromocriptine was maintained on an indefinite basis in all 6 patients with the longest follow-up of 7 years. Symptoms have not recurred and the demonstrable residual tumor tissue has not increased in size. In 1 patient, cerebrospinal

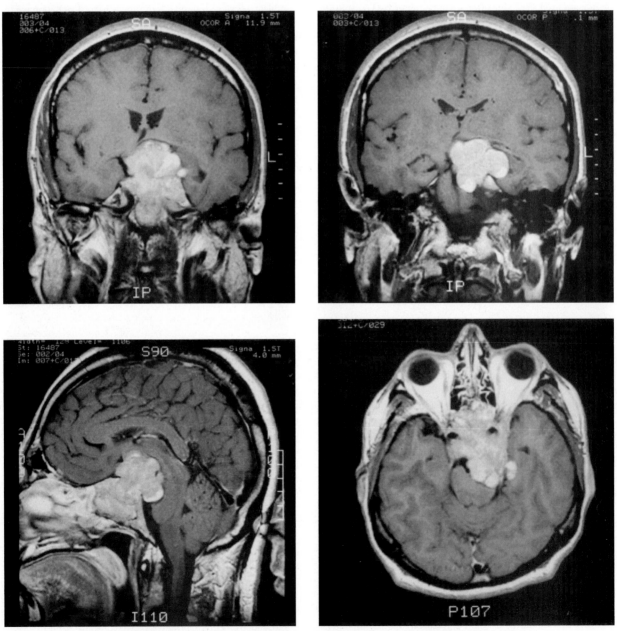

Fig. 1 Preoperative magnetic resonance images from a 42-year-old physicist with a giant macroprolactinoma who presented with confusion, lethargy, and severe visual impairment (light perception only on the left, finger counting at 1 foot on the right).

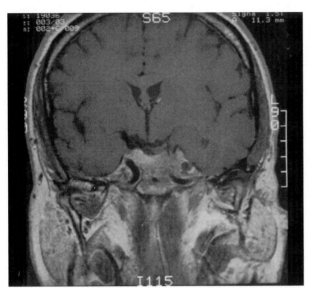
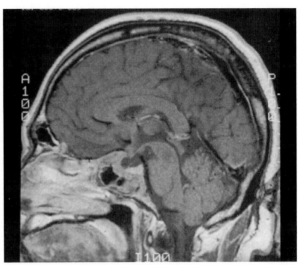

Fig. 2 Magnetic resonance images in the same patient 3 months after treatment with bromocriptine; the patient fully recovered all neurological function.

fluid rhinorrhea occurred 3 months after bromocriptine therapy was initiated, but spontaneously resolved. Only 1 patient with ophthalmoplegia resulting from cavernous sinus involvement failed to improve with bromocriptine and underwent a craniotomy and transcavernous tumor decompression followed by radiation therapy.

My recommendation, therefore, is to treat this patient with bromocriptine, starting with 2.5 mg twice a day and gradually increase the dosage to as much as 20 to 25 mg a day. The patient's visual symptoms should improve within a matter of days and the tumor should show demonstrable reduction within 3 to 6 weeks. The bromocriptine dosage should be titered in accordance with the patient's clinical course, the evidence of a reduction in the tumor size, the serum prolactin level, and the patient's tolerance of bromocriptine. This patient will require bromocriptine therapy on an indefinite basis, and it is imperative to involve the services of a competent pituitary endocrinologist in the patient's treatment. I would not accept a cursory trial with bromocriptine administered by a neurological surgeon as failure of medical therapy. I believe this patient has an excellent prognosis for a very effective and sustained palliation of symptoms as well as for long-term containment of his tumor with no need for further therapy. In the unlikely instance that this patient does

not respond to or is intolerant of bromocriptine therapy, surgical decompression through a craniotomy followed by radiation therapy should be considered.

The treatment issues are completely different in patients harboring contained macroprolactinomas. Our preference is to treat patients with large, but contained, macroprolactinomas with bromocriptine for a period of 3 months, titering the bromocriptine dosage so as to achieve the maximum reduction in tumor size and decrease the serum prolactin level. With these goals achieved, consideration should be given to either continuing bromocriptine on an indefinite basis or to removing the residual tumor. The latter option is exercised if the overall perception is that the patient can be cured or, at a minimum, that the tumor can be decreased and the serum prolactin level reduced further and in a way that would allow for a much smaller bromocriptine dosage postoperatively. Patients with smaller contained macroprolactinomas can be occasionally operated upon with cure as a goal without prior bromocriptine therapy.

Radiation therapy should not be used as an initial treatment in any patient with a macroprolactinoma. Even as adjuvant therapy, radiation should be used reluctantly and sparingly because it is rarely curative, and its effectiveness in reducing the serum prolactin level is still controversial, at best.

Medical vs. Surgical Treatment of Giant Pituitary Prolactinomas

Rudolf Fahlbusch, M.D.

Controversy about medical versus surgical treatment for patients with macroprolactinomas is a fact. The controversy began in the mid-1970s, when dopamine agonists became available and it became clear that results concerning normalizing prolactin levels were less favorable in patients with these tumors than those with other kinds of hormone-secreting pituitary adenomas. Today, the neurosurgical position is clear, and was recently defined at the conference of the Research Committee on Medical versus Surgical Treatment of Pituitary Adenomas of the

European Association of Neurological Surgeons (January, 1993, Nuremburg, Germany). On one hand, the current position is weak because of a continuous loss of original surgical cases. On the other hand, the position is strong, because the neurosurgeon maintains a place. With the increasing number of patients who do not respond to dopamine agonists, surgical treatment has become technically more difficult.

Both authors discuss and document that there is no doubt about the outcome of treating this patient with a giant prolactinoma if surgery alone is available. The outcome of such an operation would be a higher morbidity rate, the lack of total removal, and little chance for normalizing the elevated prolactin level. Therefore, the initial treatment for patients with macroprolactinomas should always be medical, with dopamine agonists such as bromocriptine. It is unclear why the second author recommends dexamethasone in addition to bromocriptine; the neuroimaging studies do not show edema around the tumor. Treatment of a macroprolactinoma should initially include replacing pituitary deficits to optimize the patient's general health even before surgery, as the first author emphasizes. Surgical treatment is clearly indicated if the patient has not responded to dopamine agonists, and has no tumor shrinkage; tumor shrinkage can be expected within the first weeks in up to 80% of patients. Many cystic tumors do not shrink. Among those that do not respond, I also include tumors with shrinkage insufficient to completely restore visual function and optomotoric deficits.

A patient's affinity to dopamine agonists can be predicted through dopamine-2-receptor scanning in a nuclear medicine laboratory. Only a few centers offer monitoring of dopamine-2-receptors with positron-emission tomography.

The patient discussed here would show good results with respect to tumor shrinkage, and could tolerate oral bromocriptine. For some years, I have used the injectable form of bromocriptine, which some patients tolerate better and presents adverse events—albeit transient—within 24 hours in two thirds of patients. Furthermore, prolactin levels would decrease in this patient. These levels must be normal or nearly normal to reach the goal of normoprolactinemia. Residual hyperprolactinemia still may cause problems; for example, with osteoporosis and, of course, residual hypogonadism including infertility. We must consider that further growth of a prolactinoma can occur in rare cases despite normal prolactin levels.

The only controversy in this patient and, also, in general is that, if surgery still has its place even when such a tumor has shrunk, the second author would have removed as much tumor tissue as possible to nearly normalize the prolactin level and then used long-term bromocriptine with a lower dosage. The first author argues that surgery to remove the tumor subtotally after shrinkage is not generally accepted. This attitude reflects a non-neurosurgical one.

My personal series includes a special group of about 100 patients with macroprolactinomas now undergoing long-term follow-up. These patients reflect the concept of short-term shrinkage of a tumor within 3 to an utmost of 12 weeks, followed by transsphenoidal resection. Currently, we have results for 35 patients observed for more than 5 years. These patients are taking a low dose of bromocriptine and have no documented residual tumor. Only one third of these patients, however, have threefold elevated prolactin levels after withdrawal of the drug. Not a single patient has a normal prolactin value after withdrawal. In light of poor long-term medical treatment in which, in general, the tumor does not totally disappear, we are waiting for a 10-year follow-up period to present our final results.

The role of radiotherapy is still open. Some agree that it has its place for invasive tumors, especially if we are to expect noncompliance in difficult patients, particularly among those in the nonregenerative age. In these patients, subjective cessation of medication may be accompanied by acute and spontaneous reexpansion of the tumor, which then can present in a very aggressive way and complicate subsequent treatment.

REFERENCES AND SUGGESTED READINGS

Mark E. Molitch, M.D.

1. Afshar F, Thomas A: Bromocriptine-induced cerebrospinal fluid rhinorrhea. *Surg Neurol* 1982; 18:61–63.
2. Antunes JL, Housepian EM, Frantz AG, et al.: Prolactin-secreting pituitary tumors. *Ann Neurol* 1977; 2:148–153.
3. Arafah BM, Brodkey JS, Pearson OH: Gradual recovery of lactotroph responsiveness to dynamic stimulation following surgical removal of prolactinomas: long-term follow-up studies. *Metabolism* 1986; 35:905–912.
4. Barrow DL, Tindall GT, Kovacs K, et al.: Clinical and pathological effects of bromocriptine on prolactin-secreting and other pituitary tumors. *J Neurosurg* 1984; 60:1–7.
5. Bevan JS, Adams CBT, Burke CW, et al.: Factors in the outcome of transsphenoidal surgery for prolactinoma and non-functioning pituitary tumour, including pre-operative bromocriptine therapy. *Clin Endocrinol* 1987; 26:541–556.
6. Bevan JS, Webster J, Burke CW, et al.: Dopamine agonists and pituitary tumor shrinkage. *Endocrine Revs* 1992; 13:220–240.
7. Brabant G, Brennecke I, Herrmann H, et al.: Hyperprolactinamie und Prolactinome. *Dtsch Med Wschr* 1985; 110:1564–1567.
8. Charpentier G, de Plunkett T, Jedynak P, et al.: Surgical treatment of prolactinomas. Short- and long-term results, prognostic factors. *Hormone Res* 1985; 22:222–227.
9. Ciric I, Mikhael M, Stafford T, et al.: Transsphenoidal microsurgery of pituitary macroadenomas with long-term follow-up results. *J Neurosurg* 1983; 59:395–401.
10. Corenblum B, Taylor PJ: Long-term follow-up of hyperprolac-tinemic women treated with bromocriptine. *Fertil Steril* 1983; 40:596–599.
11. Davies C, Jacobi J, Lloyd HM, et al.: DNA synthesis and the secretion of prolactin and growth hormone by the pituitary gland of the male rat: Effects of diethylstilboestrol and 2-bromo-alpha-ergocriptine methanesulphonate. *J Endocrinol* 1974; 61:411–417.
12. Davis JR, Sheppard MC, Heath DA: Giant invasive prolactinoma: A case report and review of nine further cases. *Q J Med* 1990; 74:227–238.
13. Domingue JN, Richmond IL, Wilson CB: Results of surgery in 114 patients with prolactin-secreting pituitary adenomas. *Am J Obstet Gynecol* 1980; 137:102–108.
14. Dupuy M, Derome PJ, Peillon F, et al.: Prolactinoma in man. Pre- and post-operative study in 80 cases. *Sem Hop Paris* 1984; 60:2943–2954.
15. Esiri MM, Bevan JS, Burke CW, et al.: Effect of bromocriptine treatment on the fibrous tissue content of prolactin-secreting and nonfunctioning macroadenomas of the pituitary gland. *J Clin Endocrinol Metab* 1986; 63:383–388.
16. Fahlbusch R, Buchfelder M: Present status of neurosurgery in the treatment of prolactinomas. *Neurosurg Rev* 1985; 8:195–205.
17. Fahlbusch R, Buchfelder M, Schrell U: Short-term preoperative treatment of macroprolactinomas by dopamine agonists. *J Neurosurg* 1987; 67:807–815.
18. Faria MA Jr, Tindall GT: Transsphenoidal microsurgery for prolactin-secreting pituitary adenomas. *J Neurosurg* 1982; 56:33–43.

19. Gasser RW, Mueller-Holzner E, Skrabal F, et al.: Macroprolactinomas and functionless pituitary tumours. Immunostaining and effect of dopamine agonist therapy. *Acta Endocrinol* 1987; 116: 253–259.

20. Grisoli F, Vincentelli F, Jaquet P, et al.: Prolactin secreting adenoma in 22 men. *Surg Neurol* 1980; 13:241–247.

21. Guidetti B, Fraioli B, Cantore GP: Results of surgical management of 319 pituitary adenomas. *Acta Neurochir* 1987; 85:117–124.

22. Hardy J: Transsphenoidal microsurgery of prolactinomas, in Black PM, Zervas NT, Ridgway EC, et al. (eds): *Secretory Tumors of the Pituitary Gland*. New York, Raven Press, 1984, pp 73–81.

23. Herman TN, Molitch ME: Bromocriptine: Indications and use in patients with endocrine disease. *Hosp Formulary* 1984; 19:784–791.

24. Horowitz BL, Hamilton DJ, Sommers, et al.: Effect of bromocriptine and pergolide on pituitary tumor size and serum prolactin. *AJNR* 1983; 4:415–417.

25. Hubbard JL, Scheithauer BW, Abboud CF, et al.: Prolactin-secreting adenomas: The preoperative response to bromocriptine treatment and surgical outcome. *J Neurosurg* 1987; 67:816–821.

26. Johnston DG, Hall K, Kendall-Taylor P, et al.: Effect of dopamine agonist withdrawal after long-term therapy in prolactinomas: Studies with high-definition computerised tomography. *Lancet* 1984; 2:187–192.

27. Kok JG, Bartelink AK, Schulte BP, et al.: Cerebrospinal fluid rhinorrhea during treatment with bromocriptine for prolactinoma. *Neurology* 1985; 35:1193–1195.

28. Landolt AM: Surgical treatment of pituitary prolactinomas: Postoperative prolactin and fertility in seventy patients. *Fertil Steril* 1981; 35:620–625.

29. Laws ET: Pituitary surgery. *Endocrinol Metab Clin North Am* 1987; 16:647–665.

30. Liuzzi A, Dallabonzana D, Oppizzi G, et al.: Low doses of dopamine agonists in the long-term treatment of macroprolactinomas. *N Engl J Med* 1985; 313:656–659.

31. Lloyd HM, Meares JD, Jacobi J: Effects of oestrogen and bromocryptine on in vivo secretion and mitosis in prolactin cells. *Nature* 1975; 255:497–498.

32. MacLeod RM, Lehmeyer JE: Suppression of pituitary tumor growth and function by ergot alkaloids. *Cancer Res* 1973; 33: 849–855.

33. McGregor AM, Scanlon MF, Hall R, et al.: Effects of bromocriptine on pituitary tumour size. *Br Med J* 1979; 2:700–703.

34. Mohr G, Hardy J, Comtois R, et al.: Surgical management of giant pituitary adenomas. *Can J Neurol Sci* 1990; 17:62–66.

35. Molitch ME: Hypopituitarism, in Rakel RE (ed.): *Conn's Current Therapy*. Philadelphia, WB Saunders Co., 1993, pp. 623–626.

36. Molitch ME: Pathological hyperprolactinemia. *Endocrinol Metab Clin North Am* 1992; 21:877–901.

37. Molitch ME: Pathogenesis of pituitary tumors. *Endocrinol Metab Clin North Am* 1987; 16:503–527.

38. Molitch ME, Elton RL, Blackwell RE, et al.: Bromocriptine as primary therapy for prolactin-secreting macroadenomas: Results of a prospective multicenter study. *J Clin Endocrinol Metab* 1985; 60:698–705.

39. Molitch ME, Reichlin S: The amenorrhea, galactorrhea and hyperprolactinemia syndromes. *Adv Intern Med* 1980; 26:37–65.

40. Murphy FY, Vesely DL, Jordan RM, et al.: Giant invasive prolactinomas. *Am J Med* 1987; 83:995–1002.

41. Nelson AT Jr, Tucker HSG Jr, Becker DP: Residual anterior pituitary function following transsphenoidal resection of pituitary macroadenomas. *J Neurosurg* 1984; 61:577–580.

42. Nelson PB, Goodman M, Maroon JC, et al.: Factors in predicting outcome from operation in patients with prolactin-secreting pituitary adenomas. *Neurosurgery* 1983; 13:634–641.

43. Nicola GC, Tonnarelli GP, Griner A: One hundred and ten prolactin secreting adenomas: Results of surgical treatment, in Faglia G, Giovanelli MA, MacLeod RM (eds): *Pituitary Microadenomas*. New York, Academic Press, 1980, pp 483–486.

44. Nissim M, Ambrosi B, Bernasconi V, et al.: Bromocriptine treatment of macroprolactinomas: Studies on the time course of tumor shrinkage and morphology. *J Endocrinol* 1982; 5:409–415.

45. Parl FF, Cruz VE, Cobb CA, et al: Late recurrence of surgically removed prolactinomas. *Cancer* 1986; 57:2422–2426.

46. Pelkonen R, Grahne B, Hirvonen E, et al.: Pituitary function in prolactinoma: Effect of surgery and postoperative bromocriptine therapy. *Clin Endocrinol* 1981; 14:335–348.

47. Pia HW, Grote E, Hildebrandt G: Giant pituitary adenomas. *Neurosurg Rev* 1985; 8:207–220.

48. Pullan PT, Carroll WM, Chakera TMH, et al.: Management of extra-sellar pituitary tumours with bromocriptine: Comparison of prolactin secreting and non-functioning tumours using half-field visual evoked potentials and computerized tomography. *Aust NZ J Med* 1985; 15:203–208.

49. Randall RV, Laws ER, Abboud CF, et al.: Transsphenoidal microsurgical treatment of prolactin-producing pituitary adenomas. *Mayo Clin Proc* 1983; 58:108–121.

50. Rasmussen C, Bergh T, Wide L: Prolactin secretion and menstrual function after long-term bromocriptine treatment. *Fertil Steril* 1987; 48:550–554.

51. Rawe SE, Williamson HO, Levine JH, et al.: Prolactinomas: Surgical therapy, indications and results. *Surg Neurol* 1980; 14: 161–167.

52. Rodman EF, Molitch ME, Post KD, et al.: Long-term follow-up of trans-sphenoidal selective adenomectomy for prolactinoma. *JAMA* 1984; 252:921–924.

53. Scanlon MF, Peters JR, Thomas JP, et al.: Management of selected patients with hyperprolactinemia by partial hypophysectomy. *Br Med J* 1985; 291:1547–1550.

54. Schlechte J, Sherman B, Halmi N, et al.: Prolactin-secreting pituitary tumors in amenorrheic women: A comprehensive study. *Endocrine Rev* 1980; 1:295–308.

55. Smallridge RC, Martins AN: Transsphenoidal surgery for prolactin-secreting pituitary tumors. *So Med J* 1982; 75:963–968.

56. Sobrinho LG, Nunes MC, Jorge-Calhaz C, et al.: Effect of treatment with bromocriptine on the size and activity of prolactin producing pituitary tumours. *Acta Endocrinol* 1981; 96:24–29.

57. Spark RF, Baker R, Bienfang DC, et al.: Bromocriptine reduces pituitary tumor size and hypersecretion: Requiem for pituitary surgery? *JAMA* 1982; 247:311–316.

58. Symon L, Jakubowski J, Kendall B: Surgical treatment of giant pituitary adenomas. *J Neurol Neurosurg Psychiatry* 1979; 42: 973–982.

59. Thomson JA, Teasdale GM, Gordon D, et al.: Treatment of presumed prolactinoma by transsphenoidal operation: Early and late results. *Br Med J* 1985; 291:1550–1553.

60. Thorner MO, Martin WH, Rogol AD, et al.: Rapid regression of pituitary prolactinomas during bromocriptine treatment. *J Clin Endocrinol Metab* 1980; 51:438–445.

61. Thorner MO, Perryman RL, Rogol AD, et al.: Rapid changes of prolactinoma volume after withdrawal and reinstitution of bromocriptine. *J Clin Endocrinol Metab* 1981; 53:480–483.

62. Tucker HSG, Grubb SR, Wigand JP, et al.: Galactorrhea-amenorrhea syndrome: follow-up of forty-five patients after pituitary tumor removal. *Ann Intern Med* 1981; 94:302–307.

63. Vance ML, Evans WS, Thorner MO: Bromocriptine. *Ann Intern Med* 1984; 100:78–91.

64. Wang C, Lam KSL, Ma JTC, et al.: Long-term treatment of hyperprolactinaemia with bromocriptine: Effect of drug withdrawal. *Clin Endocrinol* 1987; 27:363–371.

65. Warfield A, Finkel DM, Schatz NJ, et al.: Bromocriptine treatment of prolactin-secreting pituitary adenomas may restore pituitary function. *Ann Intern Med* 1984; 101:783–785.

66. Wass JAH, Williams J, Charlesworth M, et al.: Bromocriptine in management of large pituitary tumours. *Br Med J* 1982; 284:1908–1911.

67. Weiss MH, Wycoff RR, Yadley R, et al.: Bromocriptine treatment

of prolactin-secreting tumors: Surgical implications. *Neurosurgery* 1983; 12:640–642.

68. Wilson CB: Neurosurgical management of large and invasive pituitary tumors, in Tindall GT, Collins WF (eds): *Clinical Management of Pituitary Disorders*. New York, Raven Press, 1979, pp 335–342.

69. Wollesen F, Andersen T, Karle A: Size reduction of extrasellar pituitary tumours during bromocriptine treatment. *Ann Intern Med* 1982; 96:281–286.

70. Woosley RE, King JS, Talbert L: Prolactin-secreting pituitary adenomas: Neurosurgical management of 37 patients. *Fertil Steril* 1982; 37:54–60.

71. Zervas NT: Surgical results for pituitary adenomas: Results of an international survey, in Black PMcL, Zervas NT, Ridgway EC, et al. (eds): *Secretory Tumors of the Pituitary Gland*. New York, Raven Press, 1984, pp 377–385.

Ivan Ciric, M.D.

1. Al-Mefty O, Woodhouse N: Microprolactinoma and large prolactinoma: Are they two different diseases (letter). *Neurosurgery* 1985: 17:379.

2. Aubourg PR, Derome PJ, Peillon F, et al.: Endocrine outcome after transsphenoidal adenomectomy for prolactinoma: prolactin levels and tumor size as predicting factors. *Surg Neurol* 1980; 14:141–143.

3. Barrow DL, Mizuno J, Tindall GT: Management of prolactinomas associated with very high serum prolactin levels. *J Neurosurg* 1988; 68:554–558.

4. Bevan JS, Adams CBT, Burke CW, et al.: Factors in the outcome of transsphenoidal surgery for prolactinoma and non-functioning pituitary tumor, including preoperative bromocriptine therapy. *Clin Endocrinol* 1987; 26:541–556.

5. Black PM, Zervas NT, Candia G: Management of large pituitary adenomas by transsphenoidal surgery. *Surg Neurol* 1988; 29:443–447.

6. Bronsteim MD, Cardin CS, Marino R: Short-term management of macroprolactinomas with a new injectable form of bromocriptine. *Surg Neurol* 1977; 28:31–37.

7. Candrina R, Galli G, Bollati A, et al.: Results of combined surgical and medical therapy in patients with prolactin-secreting pituitary adenomas. *Neurosurgery* 1987; 21:894–896.

8. Ciric I, Mikhael M, Stafford T, et al.: Transsphenoidal microsurgery of pituitary macroadenomas with long-term follow-up results. *J Neurosurg* 1983; 59:395–401.

9. Domingue JN, Richmond IL, Wilson CB: Results of surgery in 114 patients with prolactin-secreting pituitary adenomas. *Am J Obstet Gynecol* 1980; 137:102–108.

10. Faglia G, Conti A, Muratori M, et al.: Dihydroergocriptine in management of microprolactinomas. *J Clin Endocrinol Metab* 1987; 65:779–784.

11. Fahlbusch R, Buchfelder M, Schrell U: Short-term preoperative treatment of macroprolactinomas by dopamine agonists. *J Neurosurg* 1987; 67:807–815.

12. Godo G, Koloszar S, Szilagyi I, et al.: Experience relating to pregnancy, lactation, and the after-weaning condition of hyperprolactinemic patients treated with bromocriptine. *Fertil Steril* 1989; 51:529–531.

13. Hardy J: Transsphenoidal microsurgery of prolactinomas: Report on 355 cases, in *Prolactin and Prolactinomas*. New York, Raven Press, 1983, pp 431–440.

14. Hashimoto N, Handa H, Yamashita J, et al.: Long-term follow-up of large or invasive pituitary adenomas. *Surg Neurol* 1986; 25:49–54.

15. Heidvall K, Hulting AL: Rapid progression of a growth hormone producing tumor during dopamine agonist treatment. *Br Med J* 1987; 294:546–547.

16. Hildebrandt G, Zierski J, Christophis P, et al.: Rhinorrhea following dopamine agonist therapy of invasive macroprolactinoma. *Acta Neurochir* 1989; 96:107–113.

17. Hubbard JL, Scheithauer BW, Aboud CF, et al.: Prolactin-secreting adenomas: the preoperative response to bromocriptine treatment and surgical outcome. *J Neurosurg* 1987; 67:816–821.

18. Jefferson G: Extrasellar extension of pituitary adenomas. *Proc R Soc Med* 1940; 33:433–458.

19. King LW, Molitch ME, Gittinger JW, et al.: Cavernous sinus syndrome due to prolactinoma: resolution with bromocriptine. *Surg Neurol* 1983; 19:280–284.

20. Laws ER Jr, Trautmann JC, Hollenhorst RW Jr: Transsphenoidal decompression of the optic nerve and chiasm. *J Neurosurg* 1977; 46:717–722.

21. Lawton NF: Prolactinomas: Medical or surgical treatment? *Q J Med* 1987; 64:557–564.

22. Loyo M, Kleriga E, Mateos H, et al.: Combined suprainfrasellar approach for large pituitary tumors. *Neurosurgery* 1984; 14: 485–488.

23. Maira G, Anile C, De Marinis L, et al.: Prolactin-secreting adenomas: Surgical results and long-term follow-up. *Neurosurgery* 1989; 24:736–743.

24. Marcovitz S, Hardy J: Combined medical and surgical treatment of prolactin-producing pituitary tumors. *Sem Reprod Endocrinol* 1984; 2:73–81.

25. Mohr G, Hardy J: Hemorrhage, necrosis, and apoplexy in pituitary adenomas. *Surg Neurol* 1982; 18:181–189.

26. Nelson PB, Goodman ML, Flickenger JC, et al.: Endocrine function in patients with large pituitary tumors treated with operative decompression and radiation therapy. *Neurosurgery* 1989; 24:398–400.

27. Pellegrini R, Rasolonjanahary G, Gunz G, et al.: Resistance to bromocriptine in prolactinomas. *J Clin Endocrinol Metab* 1989; 69: 500–509.

28. Shirataki K, Chihara K, Shibata Y, et al.: Pituitary apoplexy manifested during a bromocnptine test in a patient with a growth hormone and prolactin-producing pituitary adenoma. *Neurosurgery* 1988; 23:395–397.

29. Shucart WA: Implications of very high serum prolactin levels associated with pituitary tumors. *J Neurosurg* 1980; 52:226–228.

30. Snow RB, Lavyne MH, Lee BC, et al.: Craniotomy versus transsphenoidal excision of large pituitary tumors: The usefulness of magnetic resonance imaging in guiding the operative approach. *Neurosurgery* 1986; 19:59–64.

31. Srivastava VK, Narayanawamy KS, Vasudevrao T: Giant pituitary adenomas. *Surg Neurol* 1983; 20:379–382.

32. Symon L, Jakubowski J, Kendall B: Surgical treatment of giant pituitary adenomas. *J Neurol Neurosurg Psychiatry* 1979; 42: 973–982.

33. Van't Verlaat JW, Lancranjan I, Hendricks MJ, et al.: Primary treatment of macroprolactinomas with Parlodel LAR, in Van't Verlaat JW (ed): *Secreting Pituitary Adenomas* (Thesis, University of Utrecht, The Netherlands). Rotterdam, Tripiti, 1988, pp 45–55.

34. Wang C, Lam KS, Ma JT, et al.: Long-term treatment of hyperprolactinemia with bromocriptine: effect of drug withdrawal. *Clin Endocrinol* 1987; 27:363–371.

35. Wilson CB: Neurosurgical management of large and invasive pituitary tumors in Tindall GT, Collins WF (eds): *Clinical Management of Pituitary Disorders*. New York, Raven Press, 1979, pp 335–342.

36. Wilson CB, March CM: Prolactinoma. *Neurosurgery* 1982; 10: 283–284.

2

Surgical Approaches to Pituitary Macroadenomas with Cavernous Sinus Extensions: The Transcranial vs. the Transsphenoidal Approach

CASE

A 50-year-old, right-handed man came to medical attention with decreased vision in his right eye and headache. On examination, he had a partial third nerve palsy. Vision in his right eye was 20/200. Neuroendocrinological tests showed a prolactin level of about 40 IU and the patient had panhypopituitarism.

PARTICIPANTS

The Transcranial Approach to Pituitary Macroadenomas with Cavernous Sinus Extensions– Kenji Ohata, M.D., Akira Hakuba, M.D.

The Transsphenoidal Approach to Pituitary Macroadnomas with Cavernous Sinus Extensions– Wesley A. King, M.D., Donald P. Becker, M.D.

*Moderator–*George T. Tindall, M.D.

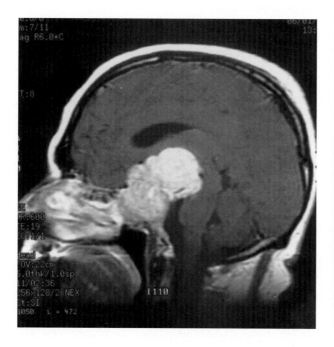
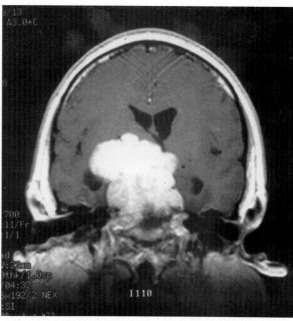

The Transcranial Approach to Pituitary Macroadenomas with Cavernous Sinus Extensions

Kenji Ohata, M.D., Akira Hakuba, M.D.

To demonstrate our practice and experience treating patients with nonsecreting pituitary macroadenomas with cavernous sinus extensions, we describe the following case.

CASE MATERIAL

A 55-year-old woman came to medical attention with visual loss in the right eye. At the time of admission, her visual acuity was 20/40 on the right side and 20/200 on the left side. A nonfunctioning pituitary adenoma with a moderate suprasellar extension was removed through the transcranial approach. After surgery, her left visual acuity improved to 20/64, although her visual field defect remained. The patient did not return to the clinic for follow-up for 9 years, apparently because her vision was stable.

Twelve years after her first treatment, the patient, now 68 years old, came to our attention with bilateral visual deterioration. Her neurological examination showed visual acuity in the right eye of 20/200 and in the left eye of 20/800 with temporal hemianopsia of the left eye and temporal quadranopsia of the right eye. Magnetic resonance images showed a huge recurrent mass involving both cavernous sinuses and extending to the temporal base bilaterally (Fig. 1). Both internal carotid arteries were engulfed by the tumor between C5 and C2 bilaterally. During a balloon occlusion test of the right internal carotid artery, disturbance of consciousness and left hemiparesis developed with 15 mm Hg of stump pressure after 80 seconds of balloon inflation.

SURGICAL APPROACH

The patient underwent a right orbitozygomatic infratemporal approach for radical removal of the tumor.[4] She was placed in a semisitting position with her head turned to the left side. The coronal incision used for her initial surgery was reopened and extended down to the level of the inferior end of the ear lobe, running along the anterior margin of the ear cartilage. An additional incision was made backward transversely about 4 cm above the upper margin of the ear lobe. Subgaleal dissection of the superficial temporal artery and vein was accomplished and a pericranial and galeal flap with intact blood flow was made to later reconstruct the skull base. In addition to the frontotemporal craniotomy, an orbitozygomatic osteotomy was made, hinging on the masseter muscle. The remaining major sphenoid wing was divided lateral to the superior orbital fissure and the foramen ovale.

The middle meningeal artery was coagulated and divided after plugging the foramen spinosum with dacron balls. The major petrosal nerve was exposed and divided. Through a subtemporal epidural approach, the petrosal tip was drilled out and the inner layer of the lateral wall of the cavernous sinus, consisting of the V1 through V3 nerve roots and the oculomotor and trochlear nerves, were carefully exposed while the temporal dura propria was elevated medially. The remaining minor sphenoid wing was removed up to the anterior clinoid process. The anterior clinoid process and its pedicles forming the optic

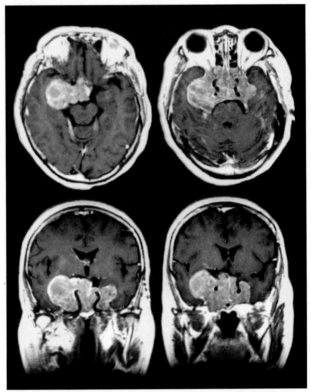

Fig. 1 Gd-DTPA enhanced, T1-weighted preoperative magnetic resonance image showing a huge mass, involving both cavernous sinuses and extending to the temporal base bilaterally. The internal carotid arteries were engulfed by the tumor between the C5 and C2 portions bilaterally.

canal were drilled, and the optic nerve sheath and both proximal and distal carotid rings were fully exposed. The dura mater was opened along the optic nerve, and the lateral leaf of the optic nerve sheath was retracted laterally and divided along the lateral margin of the optic nerve and the carotid ring. The carotid ring was also opened medially to expose the C3 portion of the left carotid artery.

The medial side of the medial triangle was opened with its posterior side. The dura propria of the lateral wall of the right cavernous sinus was further separated from the deep layer and was retracted backward together with the lateral fringe of the dura mater of the medial triangle in the superior wall of the right cavernous sinus. The third, fourth, and sixth cranial nerves were fully exposed to their dural entrances. Radical removal of the tumor took place through Parkinson's, Mullan's, and the medial triangles, from the right cavernous and sphenoid sinuses. The tumor was relatively soft and suckable, although highly vascular.

The tuberculum sellae was drilled out and the left optic nerve sheath was exposed. A transverse incision of the dura mater of the tuberculum sellae was made close to the left optic nerve. The

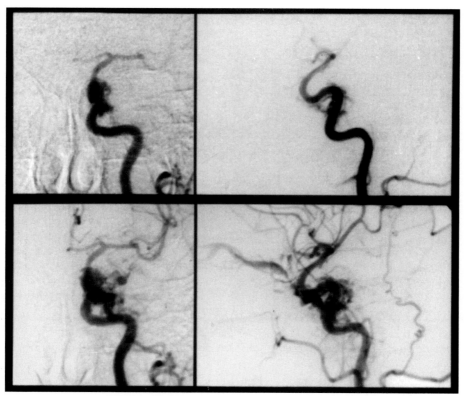

Fig. 2   Left carotid angiogram 6 days after the first operation showing a carotid-cavernous fistula at the C5 portion: left, anteroposterior view; right, lateral view.

tumor under the tuberculum sellae and the left optic nerve was removed with good decompression of the left optic nerve. The tumor partially extending into the left medial cavity of the left cavernous sinus was removed. We could see the medial wall of the C4 portion of the left internal carotid artery.

While packing the left cavernous sinus and the left portion of the sphenoid sinus through Mullan's triangle after the tumor was removed, a forceps accidentally penetrated and lacerated the left internal carotid artery. The laceration was located on the ventral wall of the C5 portion of the left internal carotid artery. The massive bleeding was controlled by sealing off the laceration with a fibrin-soaked collagen sponge and further packing with abdominal fat.

After surgery, the patient recovered well, although angiography revealed a traumatic carotid-cavernous fistula on the left side (Fig. 2). On the eighth day after surgery, she experienced sudden blindness in her left eye, and an emergency craniotomy was performed to repair the fistula. Because collateral circulation through the circle of Willis was poor, an extracranial-intracranial bypass graft was placed between the external carotid artery and the proximal M2 portion of the left middle cerebral artery to trap the cavernous portion of the internal carotid during the repair of the laceration at the C5 portion. The residual tumor in the left cavernous sinus was removed and the laceration repaired. The lacerated portion of the internal carotid artery was first repaired with 10-0 and 8-0 monofilament nylon, resulting in incomplete closure. The lacerated portion was then wrapped with a collagen sponge and the wrapping was tightened by clipping the free edges of the sponge.

A postoperative angiogram showed complete obliteration of the carotid-cavernous fistula (Fig. 3) and the patient recovered

her visual acuity. One year after the operation, the patient's visual acuity was 20/64 on the right and 20/40 on the left, although partial bitemporal hemianopsia remained. Her eye movement was normal on the left, but limited upwards and downwards on the right. A computed tomogram did not show any residual tumor (Fig. 4).

OTHER EXPERIENCE

Our strategy for treating patients with nonfunctioning pituitary adenomas is radical extirpation, even for recurrence, through the transcranial or transsphenoidal approach. Conventional radiotherapy is considered for rare cases of recurrence deemed unresectable.

During a period of 10 years (1981 to 1991), we operated on 33 patients with nonfunctioning pituitary adenomas. The average follow-up period was 6.7 years. The operative approach was selected depending upon extensions into the cavernous sinus and the suprasellar area. If the cavernous sinus was involved medially, we chose the transsphenoidal or bifrontobasal approach.[5] For more extensive involvement, we used the orbitozygomatic infratemporal approach.[4] For the first operation in these patients, we used the transsphenoidal approach 16 times, the bifrontobasal 11 times, and the orbitozygomatic approach 6 times. After the first operation, no residual mass was seen radiologically in 21 patients. In 6 of these 21 patients, the tumor extended into the cavernous sinus, which was totally resected.

In 10 of 12 patients who had residual mass radiologically after the first operation, the second operation was carried out because the mass regrew. In the remaining 2 patients, residual tumors were locally controlled without regrowth; 1 with stereotactic radiosurgery and the other without any adjuvant therapy. At the

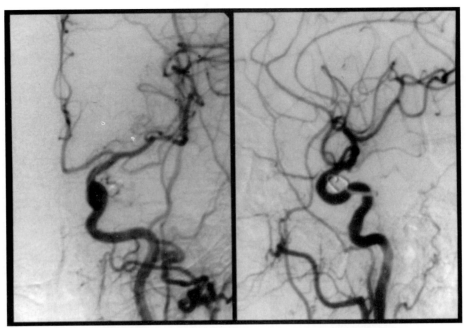

Fig. 3 Left carotid angiogram 40 days after the second operation documenting obliteration of the carotid-cavernous fistula: left: anteroposterior view; right: lateral view.

second operation in these 10 patients, we used 5 transsphenoidal approaches, 1 bifrontobasal and 4 orbitozygomatic infratemporal approaches. Postoperatively, 5 patients were free from a residual mass radiologically. The cavernous sinus was involved by the tumor in 7 of these 10 patients, and 2 of 7 were free from a residual mass postoperatively. In the other 5 patients, the tumors were subtotally removed because of invasive growth or a hard consistency in the cavernous sinus. The epidural spaces were the main sites of recurrence. Two of the 5 patients underwent conventional radiotherapy and stereotactic radiosurgery, respectively. One of these 5 patients underwent 2 more operations. In the remaining 2 of these 5 patients, the residual mass did not regrow for 3 and 5 years, respectively. Conclusively, 26 (79%) of the total 33 patients were free from residual tumor radiologically after 1 or 2 surgical resections without adjuvant therapy. In 3 of the remaining 7 patients with residual mass, regrowth was not apparent for 5, 3, and 2 years, respectively.

No operative mortality occurred in our series. The outcome in all patients was classified as excellent or good, as they all returned to their previous jobs or were able to work. Although paralysis of the oculomotor and abducens nerves occurred after radical manipulation of the cavernous sinus in patients undergoing the orbitozygomatic infratemporal approach, most of these resolved within 6 months.

DISCUSSION

We believe that nonfunctioning pituitary adenomas, even recurrence, should be treated only through radical extirpation, and that conventional radiotherapy should be avoided.

In general, a nonfunctioning pituitary adenoma is a slow-growing benign tumor. In contrast to craniopharyngioma and meningioma, this tumor is less adherent to the central nervous system, including the hypothalamus, and has a relatively soft consistency. Extirpation of the suprasellar compartment is much easier in pituitary adenoma than in craniopharyngioma and meningioma. What makes the total removal difficult, in some patients, is its tendency to invade the skull base including the cavernous sinus. Skull base surgery has advanced over the past decade, and the cavernous sinus is no longer considered a "no man's land."[2,4] Conceivably, it is possible not only to decrease the recurrence rate of tumors invading the cavernous sinus but also to resect the recurrent masses in the skull base. In our series, 80% (26 of 33) of patients were free from residual mass radiologically. It is now time to reconsider the surgical strategy for nonfunctioning pituitary adenomas.

We question the safety of postoperative radiation therapy. Al-Mefty and colleagues[1] reported the long-term adverse effects of radiation therapy for benign brain tumors in adults, such as visual disturbance, radiation necrosis, and pituitary dysfunction. Of 58 patients analyzed in their report, 46 had pituitary adenomas, and delayed side effects of radiotherapy were observed in 22 (38%). Postoperative radiotherapy should not be routinely carried out for a residual mass. With respect to efficacy, however, a decrease in recurrence rate after postoperative radiotherapy has been described by many authors.[3,6,7,11,12] A study by Valtonen and Myllymaki[10] suggests that postoperative radiation does not prevent recurrence, but may allow long-term tumor control. Although the efficacy is acceptable, postoperative radiotherapy is not necessarily a safe treatment for patients with benign brain tumors. We do not advocate the use of postoperative radiotherapy after biopsy or partial resection of a tumor.[8,9]

The development of microsurgical techniques and the improved skill of skull base surgeons will lead to better outcomes in the surgical extirpation of nonfunctioning pituitary adenomas. Postoperative radiation should be restricted to recurrences for which surgical resection is contraindicated.

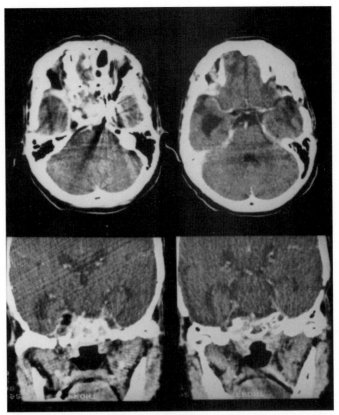

Fig. 4 Enhanced computed tomograms (upper, axial; lower, coronal) 1 year after surgery showing no apparent residual mass.

The Transsphenoidal Approach to Pituitary Macroadenomas with Cavernous Sinus Extensions

Wesley A. King, M.D., Donald P. Becker, M.D.

Judging by the marked enlargement and destruction of the sella turcica, the tumor in this patient is likely a nonsecreting or hormonally inactive pituitary adenoma. The presenting signs and symptoms in the patient include the classic triad seen in those with hormonally inactive tumors; namely, marked visual disturbance, headache, and hypopituitarism. The patient's hormonal abnormalities are limited to a modest elevation in prolactin of 40 ng/ml, which is entirely consistent with compression of the pituitary stalk caused by this large tumor. The neurological finding of an oculomotor nerve palsy is unusual in patients with pituitary tumors, but is occasionally seen with very large neoplasms or with tumors that have enlarged rapidly because of an apoplectic event. This finding can be related to perineural invasion within the cavernous sinus but, more frequently, cranial neuropathies with pituitary adenomas result from subarachnoid stretching or compression of the nerve rather than from violation of the cavernous sinus.

Several technical points of concern are raised by the magnetic resonance image (MRI) and must be considered when planning surgery. First, this is not merely a macroadenoma, but rather a giant pituitary adenoma; its suprasellar extension reaches the level of the foramen of Monro. Second, the tumor may involve the right cavernous sinus, although this cannot be determined

with any certainty until the time of surgery. Third, as can be seen on the sagittal MRI, the tumor compresses the brain stem at the level of the midbrain, although this compression has produced no symptoms. Finally, the tumor is broad and without a "waist" caused by the diaphragma sella, and has grown in a postero-superior direction. The tumor has neither grown anteriorly under the frontal lobe nor has it a significant lateral eccentric extension. These latter points are important and provide an optimal situation in this case when considering a transsphenoidal approach.

The goal of surgery in this patient is primarily to decompress the neural structures, especially the optic apparatus, because the tumor is hormonally inactive. Correcting the panhypopituitarism is unusual after pituitary surgery and should not be considered a surgical indication or expected goal.[10] We strongly believe that, as an initial procedure, the transsphenoidal avenue should be used to approach this tumor. A craniotomy or, alternatively, radiotherapy can be undertaken as a second stage if the initial operation is incomplete. The transsphenoidal approach allows complete removal of all of the tumor within the sphenoid sinus and immediate decompression of the optic nerves and brain stem, with low associated morbidity. In our experience, large tumors and tumors invading the cavernous sinus can be

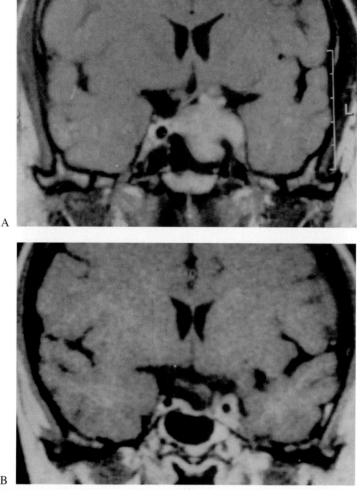

Fig. 1 (*A*) **Preoperative MRI of a 27-year-old woman with an invasive pituitary tumor involving the left cavernous sinus (arrows).** (*B*) **Postoperative MRI after a transsphenoidal procedure showing near-complete removal of the tumor.**

removed completely through this route (Fig. 1). Pituitary tumors are typically soft and gelatinous and have a propensity to descend into the sphenoid sinus, thus, making transsphenoidal resection feasible. The adenoma can be further encouraged to collapse into the sinus through elevation of the subarachnoid fluid pressure with intermittent Valsalva maneuvers carried out by the anesthesiologist or, alternatively, by injecting intrathecal saline through a lumbar subarachnoid catheter.

Although most pituitary tumors are avascular, larger adenomas such as that seen in this patient can develop a blood supply and can be quite hemorrhagic at the time of surgery. Histologically, one does not always see the sheets of monotonous cells typical of pituitary adenomas, but rather one may see nests of cells separated by a fibrovascular stroma (Fig. 2). This may, indeed, be the case in the present patient, as shown by the contrast enhancement on the MRI. One does not see this enhancement with smaller tumors. Concomitant with the increased vascularity is a tendency of the tumor to become fibrotic, firm, and multiseptated. The result is that tumor extirpation will be more difficult and may require sharp dissection to divide fibrous septations and to open tumor loculations. Further, the risk of cerebrospinal fluid leakage in this setting is significantly higher than during surgery on more routine macroadenomas.

CAVERNOUS SINUS INVOLVEMENT OF PITUITARY TUMORS

Growth Characteristics of Pituitary Adenomas

A relationship exists between the invasiveness of a pituitary tumor and its hormone-secretory status.[13] Specifically, hormonally active tumors tend to behave in more of an invasive fashion than the hormonally silent adenomas. In general, previous studies have looked at histological evidence of dural invasion by the tumor or the surgeon's observations at the time of surgery. MRI allows preoperative assessment of the relationship of the tumor to cranial base structures and a determination of the degree of invasiveness.[8] In regard to the cavernous sinus, we have found 2 distinct patterns of tumor involvement. First, adenomas can truly invade the sinus, such that the venous spaces are obliterated and the internal carotid artery is partially or completely surrounded by the tumor. This behavior is frequent with and is typical of prolactin-secreting micro- or macroadenomas and is occasionally seen in growth hormone-secreting macroadenomas. Second, a tumor can compress the cavernous sinus without invading it. On MRI, the internal carotid artery may appear to have tumor partially surrounding it but, in no case, is the artery completely encased. A fibrous or dural layer is main-

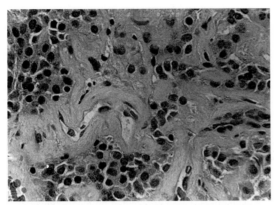

Fig. 2 Histological specimen from a giant pituitary adenoma showing nests of cells separated by a fibrovascular stroma; one does not see the sheets of monotonous adenoma cells characteristic of typical pituitary tumors.

tained between the tumor and the cavernous sinus. This situation is most typical of the nonsecreting or hormonally inactive tumors. Frank invasion of the cavernous sinus is rare, even when these tumors have reached a very large or giant size. At the time of surgery, one will find an intact capsule adjacent to the cavernous sinus and internal carotid artery, allowing easy tumor removal without bothersome venous bleeding.

The reason for the difference in growth characteristic is unclear. It may partially be explained by the fact that most prolactin- and growth hormone-secreting cells in the normal pituitary gland are located laterally within the anterior lobe of the gland;

consequently, tumors arising from them are more likely to spread into the cavernous sinus. This does not explain why some large tumors, that have completely destroyed the gland, fail to invade the vascular compartment. Most likely there are, in addition, biochemical factors inherent to the invasive (hormonally active) tumors that facilitate invasion of the cavernous sinus.

Surgical Anatomy

A complete familiarity with and understanding of the inferomedial anatomy of the cavernous sinus is essential before undertaking surgery through the transsphenoidal approach. As with lateral and superomedial approaches to the cavernous sinus, familiarity with the anatomy is best achieved through meticulous cadaveric dissections.[4,6,12,14,15] The dura of the medial wall of the cavernous sinus is thick, like that of the outer layer of the lateral wall. But, unlike the lateral wall, an inner layer is absent. The dura of the pituitary fossa, which does have two layers, is contiguous with that of the medial cavernous sinus. Interdural venous channels, in continuity with the cavernous sinus, can frequently be seen passing beneath the pituitary gland and can be the source of bleeding at the time of surgery. Dura separating the gland from the internal carotid artery is drawn in many diagrammatic representations of the parasellar area, but is not always present.

The internal carotid artery lies close to the medial wall of the cavernous sinus, and is usually separated from it by a thin medial venous space. Along the vertical segment of the internal carotid artery, there are usually no venous channels medial to the artery. All segments of the intracavernous portion of the internal carotid artery can be visualized through the transsphenoidal approach (Fig. 3). The posterior vertical segment is found after it appears,

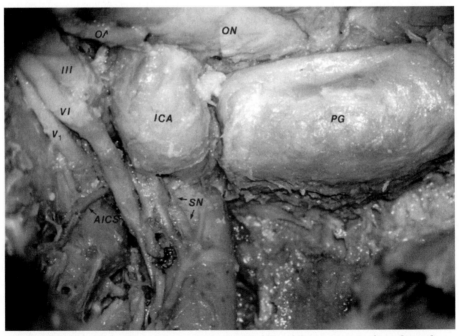

Fig. 3 Cadaveric dissection of the medial aspect of the right cavernous sinus through the transsphenoidal approach. The horizontal segment of the internal carotid artery (ICA) lies immediately adjacent to the pituitary gland (PG). Cranial nerves lll, V, and Vl can be seen lateral to the ICA as they enter the superior orbital fissure. The artery of the inferior cavernous sinus (AICS) passes over the abducens nerve. The optic nerve (ON) and ophthalmic artery (OA) pass superolateral to the pituitary fossa into the optic canal.

distal to the foramen lacerum. After the posterior bend, the artery runs anterior as the horizontal segment that ends at the anterior bend before leaving the cavernous sinus. To enter the subdural space, the artery must pierce the dural ring, which is tenaciously attached to the internal carotid artery. This dural ring actually consists of two fibrous rings that fuse medially where they are continuous with the dura of the diaphragma sellae. Laterally, the dural ring continues as the dura overlying the anterior clinoid. Several branches of the internal carotid artery can be visualized through the sphenoid sinus. The meningo-hypophyseal trunk and its branches can be seen arising from the convex portion of the posterior bend, and the artery of the inferior cavernous sinus is seen lateral to the internal carotid artery as it passes above the abducens nerve. Less frequently visualized arteries include the inferior hypophyseal and McConnell's capsular artery.

The neural relationships of the medial parasellar area are extraordinarily intricate, perhaps more than any other part of the central nervous system. The optic nerve exits through the optic canal superomedial to the cavernous sinus, with the ophthalmic artery applied to its inferior surface. The ophthalmic artery can occasionally arise from the horizontal segment of the internal carotid artery, in which case it enters the orbit through the superior orbital fissure. Cranial nerves lll, IV, and Vl can be seen lateral to the internal carotid artery. The ophthalmic and maxillary branches of the trigeminal nerve can be exposed transsphenoidally and are rarely injured during surgery of the medial cavernous sinus. Sympathetic nerve fibers run along the internal carotid artery before joining the abducens nerve and ultimately supplying the intraorbital structures.

Preoperative Considerations and Patient Selection

A careful and complete physical and neurological examination of the patient is required before undertaking surgery on the cavernous sinus, regardless of the approach. Because of the risk of vascular and neural injury, patient selection is very important. In all cases, an MRI is performed to delineate the extent of the lesion and assess any vascular involvement or abnormality. The MRI can suggest a sellar, clival, or cavernous sinus origin of the lesion, which is a critical distinction when making a differential diagnosis and planning surgery. Computed tomography supplements MRI by better defining bony destruction in selected cases. Usually, MRI will adequately demonstrate the relationship of the neoplasm to the internal carotid artery and document patency of the artery and cavernous sinus, making preoperative angiograms unnecessary. With pituitary adenomas, the caliber of the internal carotid artery is invariably normal, even when the artery is completely encased by the tumor. This is because of the soft consistency of the tumor and the fact that, unlike meningiomas, pituitary adenomas tend not to invade the arterial adventitia.

When an invasive pituitary tumor is suspected, preoperative blood studies, including hormonal levels, are essential. These studies may determine the use of a less-aggressive surgical approach supplemented postoperatively by medical treatment (e.g., bromocriptine) or radiation therapy. The role of surgery in the treatment of prolactinomas remains controversial. When surgery is undertaken on prolactinomas, we prefer to proceed with the operation before beginning bromocriptine or beginning shortly thereafter because this medication may promote fibrosis of the tumor and make surgical resection difficult. The chance of a hormonal cure in a patient with a prolactinoma invading the cavernous sinus is small with surgery alone and bromocriptine

will usually be required postoperatively. Overly-aggressive surgery with undue risk of cranial nerve injury is not indicated in this group of pituitary tumors.

Surgery remains the first-line treatment modality in patients with acromegaly, Cushing's disease, and hormonally inactive pituitary tumors. In these patients, the surgeon must take a particularly aggressive stance, even if this means entering the cavernous sinus transsphenoidally. This is especially true with the ACTH- and growth hormone-secreting tumors; these have a significant associated morbidity, including malignancy in the case of acromegaly, when left untreated. An analog of somatostatin, octreotide, has recently been introduced as a medical treatment modality for acromegaly.[1] Although it does not have the dramatic effect on tumor size that bromocriptine does with prolactinomas, octreotide has a high efficacy rate at lowering growth hormone levels and will likely serve as a pre- and postoperative adjunct to surgery in patients with acromegaly.

We do not believe that cavernous sinus involvement should be a criteria for deciding whether to operate on a pituitary tumor transsphenoidally or transcranially. This decision should be based on the patient's age and health, preoperative symptoms, and the direction of growth of the tumor. The surgeon's experience is also an important consideration. In our opinion, a craniotomy should be reserved for the patient who is otherwise in good health, whose tumor has grown either eccentrically under the temporal lobe or anteriorly under the frontal lobe. Posterosuperior growth, as in the patient described here, can usually be dealt with satisfactorily through the transsphenoidal route. A craniotomy can also be considered when a transsphenoidal procedure has been unsuccessful at complete tumor removal.

Giant pituitary adenomas are worrisome tumors. Symon and colleagues[17] reported a 19% operative mortality in 16 patients with giant pituitary adenomas operated on transcranially. This is in contrast to his group of patients with suprasellar extension that were not believed to be giant[16] who had an operative mortality of only 1%. We have also seen a significantly higher morbidity rate with these larger tumors. In these patients, a staged resection beginning with the transsphenoidal approach, should be considered. In older or debilitated patients, transsphenoidal biopsy and limited resection followed by irradiation, rather than a craniotomy, would be the preferred treatment.

Surgical Procedure

Entry into the sphenoid sinus is usually achieved through a standard transnasal transsphenoidal approach. When the tumor involvement is limited to the medial side of the internal carotid artery, this exposure is sufficient. If the lesion extends further laterally or involves the clivus and infratemporal structures, as is frequently the situation with clival chordomas and schwannomas, better exposure can be gained by performing a medial maxillotomy contralateral to the involved cavernous sinus. This allows placement of the nasal speculum at an angle to improve the view of the lateral wall of the sphenoid sinus (Fig. 4). The maxillary wall is removed to the inferior turbinate, which is fractured as the speculum is opened.

A wide bony opening into the sphenoid sinus is made to enhance the lateral exposure. After removing all of the mucosa within the sinus, several bony prominences are immediately visualized and should be noted before any bone within the sinus is removed. The carotid prominence, a bulge of the lateral wall of the sphenoid sinus, overlies the vertical and horizontal segment as well as the anterior bend of the internal carotid artery.

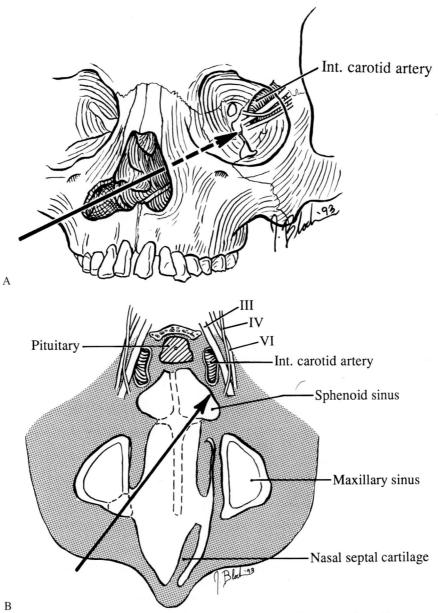

Fig. 4 (*A*) and (*B*) **Artist's conception of the transsphenoidal approach to the cavernous sinus; removing the anterior and medial maxillary walls facilitates better access into the medial cavernous sinus.**

Frequently, a bony prominence from the maxillary nerve will also be identified. The location of the optic nerves can usually be identified along the superolateral aspect of the sellar portion of the sinus and, at times, has no overlying bone. In the case of neoplasms, the sella, lateral walls, or clivus can appear attenuated or distorted. Not infrequently, tumors will extend into the sphenoid sinus.

The bone overlying the sella and medial cavernous sinus can be removed to expose the dura of the pituitary fossa and the internal carotid artery. In many cases, intercavernous sinuses involving the pituitary fossa will be encountered. Consequently, incising the dura will often result in vigorous venous bleeding that is easily controlled with oxidized cellulose. Bleeding can also be controlled, in some instances, by grasping both dural

leaves with the bipolar cautery and coagulating them closed. Tumors involving the medial cavernous sinus will, typically, obliterate the vascular space and can be removed in a piecemeal fashion using ring curettes and microdissectors. These instruments can be passed gently around the internal carotid artery to remove tumor that has extended lateral to it. Significant venous bleeding is not usually a problem until the final stages of tumor removal as the patent part of the sinus is exposed. Again, as with other approaches to the cavernous sinus, tumor should be removed in a systematic manner, controlling bleeding with carefully placed cellulose and pressure.

Intraoperative complications of the transsphenoidal approach include cerebrospinal fluid leakage, rare laceration of the internal carotid artery, and cranial nerve palsies. Most cerebrospinal fluid leaks, which have been no more frequent than with standard transsphenoidal procedures, can be repaired using autologous fascia lata and fibrin glue at the time of surgery. Postoperative diversion of cerebrospinal fluid with a lumbar subarachnoid catheter, left in place for 3 to 5 days after surgery, helps to ensure good healing of the leak. We have had only one laceration of the internal carotid artery, in a patient with an invasive pituitary adenoma. Likely, an intracavernous branch of the internal carotid artery was avulsed during tumor removal. Because of the narrow operative field, temporary carotid occlusion and suture placement is impossible in this situation. In most patients, this type of injury can be treated by holding pressure on the laceration with oxidized cellulose and cotton patties. An intraoperative angiogram, if feasible, should be done immediately to document patency of the internal carotid artery and rule out contrast extravasation. A cerebral angiogram must be repeated before the patient is discharged from the hospital and repeated again 3 months after surgery to confirm that a traumatic aneurysm has not developed. Our patient had no detrimental sequelae from this injury.

SUMMARY

Advances in microsurgical technique have allowed lesions of the cavernous sinus to be approached surgically.[2,7,11] One of the more challenging problems, that has received considerable attention recently, is encountered when a pituitary tumor invades the medial cavernous sinus.[3,5,9] We have successfully treated lesions involving the medial cavernous sinus using the transsphenoidal approach. As with other approaches to the cavernous sinus, injury of the internal carotid artery and cranial nerve palsies are potential surgical risks. In carefully selected patients, aggressive surgery should be undertaken. This approach allows exposure of the anterior and medial surfaces of the anterior bend of the internal carotid artery and the medial surface of the horizontal and vertical segments. The disadvantages of this approach include the narrow viewing angle, limited exposure of the medial wall of the cavernous sinus, and the inability to adequately occlude the internal carotid artery. When tumor involvement is extraordinarily extensive, the transsphenoidal approach should be combined with other approaches to the cavernous sinus.

Surgical Approaches to Pituitary Macroadenomas with Cavernous Sinus Extensions: The Transcranial vs. the Transsphenoidal Approach

George T. Tindall, M.D.

ILLUSTRATIVE CASE

The patient is a 68-year-old woman with bilateral visual deterioration caused by a large, recurrent, invasive pituitary tumor involving both cavernous sinuses. The patient's vision at the time of treatment of the recurrence was 20/200 O.D., 20/800 O.S. The patient had undergone a transcranial operation 12 years previously for a nonfunctional pituitary tumor.

The current magnetic resonance image (MRI) demonstrates an extensive recurrent mass involving both cavernous sinuses and extending to the temporal bases bilaterally. Both carotid arteries are encircled by the tumor. The authors elected to use a transcranial approach to the tumor. A right frontotemporal craniotomy was performed, and an orbitozygomatic osteotomy was done to increase the exposure. The tumor was first approached in the right cavernous sinus and, after opening the sinus, the third, fourth, and sixth cranial nerves were fully exposed. A radical removal of the tumor was accomplished from the right cavernous and sphenoid sinuses. During this operation, tumor was removed from beneath the left optic nerve, and the medial portion of the left cavernous sinus was removed. The left internal carotid artery was injured, however, and massive bleeding resulted. Postoperatively, the patient developed a traumatic carotid-cavernous fistula on the left side and, 8 days after the operation, sudden blindness in the left eye, after which an emergency craniotomy was performed. An extracranial-intracranial bypass graft was done on the left side in advance of trapping the cavernous portion of the internal carotid while the laceration was repaired. At the time of the second operation, a radical removal of residual pituitary tumor in the left cavernous sinus was accomplished.

Postoperative angiograms showed complete obliteration of the carotid-cavernous fistula. At 1 year follow-up, her visual acuity was 20/64 O.D. and 20/40 O.S. A bitemporal hemianopsia remained and extraocular movement was limited on the right side. A computed tomogram did not show any apparent residual tumor mass.

Comment

Judging by the postoperative computed tomogram, the authors are to be congratulated on their surgical accomplishment. However, I would not have advised such a radical procedure for this recurrent tumor. True, the patient was experiencing visual loss from the tumor mass, but the MRI reveals extensive involvement of both cavernous sinuses and, in my opinion, this would preclude a gross total removal of the tumor by any method of surgery. The fact that the patient developed a carotid-cavernous fistula from an arterial injury during surgery illustrates the complications that can occur whenever radical cavernous sinus surgery is undertaken for a pituitary tumor, or any tumor for that matter.

I would consider two options in the treatment of this patient. One option would be to simply perform a transsphenoidal operation and carry out a partial removal of the tumor, possibly enough to decompress the optic chiasm and nerves and, thus, alleviate the visual loss. With the knowledge that this operation would not remove the large amount of tumor in the cavernous sinuses, I would follow this procedure with conventional radiation therapy using 4500 cGy. If there was no immediate improvement in vision, I would consider using the second option; that is, to combine a frontal (pterional) craniotomy with a simultaneous transsphenoidal operation, choosing the side of the largest tumor mass for the craniotomy. I have used this combined approach now in more than 10 patients, and it has been effective in removing tumor that extends in other than a purely suprasellar direction. By combining the craniotomy and transsphenoidal approaches simultaneously, the surgeon performing the crani-

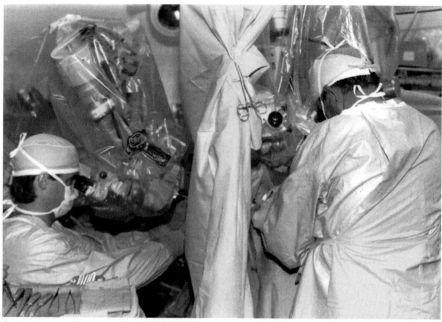

Fig. 1 Operative setup with transcranial surgeon seated on the left and transsphenoidal surgeon standing on the right, each with a separate microscope. (Reprinted with permission from Barrow DL, Tindall GT, Tindall SC: Combined simultaneous transsphenoidal transcranial operative approach to selected sellar tumors, in *Perspectives in Neurological Surgery*. vol 3, no. 2. St. Louis, Quality Medical Publishing, 1992, pp 49–58.)

otomy can carefully and gently push the tumor down into the sella so that the transsphenoidal surgeon can recover it (Fig. 1). In this way, a more effective removal of the intracranial portion of the tumor can be accomplished. Even if I chose the second option of combining a craniotomy with a transsphenoidal operation, I would still not attempt to remove the tumor in the cavernous sinus, particularly in a patient of this age. Pituitary tumors are radiosensitive and, if the tumor can be adequately decompressed, radiation therapy can effectively treat the residual portion.

I have not been impressed with the use of focused radiation in patients with pituitary tumors because I am concerned about the contiguous structures, particularly the optic apparatus. Even though this is an effective form of therapy for certain lesions, I believe there is some danger to vision unless there is a sizable margin between the optic nerve chiasm and the pituitary tumor.

PRESENTED CASE

This patient is a 50-year-old man who presented with headaches and decreased vision in the right eye (acuity 20/200). The patient also had a partial third nerve paresis and a prolactin of approximately 40 ng/ml. The latter finding tells us that we do not have an effective medical option (e.g., bromocriptine) in treating the tumor. While the authors strongly advocate an initial transsphenoidal exposure to this tumor, they further state that a craniotomy, or alternatively radiotherapy, can be undertaken as a second stage if the initial operation is incomplete. They note that, in their experience, very large tumors and tumors invading

the cavernous sinus can be removed completely through a transsphenoidal route.

Comment

I agree with the authors that the transsphenoidal procedure is an appropriate method for treating many of these tumors with an extensive suprasellar extension. However, this tumor is massive and, in addition to projecting directly suprasellar, it also shows lateral extension of the uppermost part of the tumor on the coronal view and a posterior extent of the tumor on the sagittal view. Thus, it is unlikely that a transsphenoidal procedure alone would accomplish removal of most of this tumor.

In this case, I would advise a combined approach using a simultaneous right frontal craniotomy (pterional) and a transsphenoidal approach as described above. The first step is the transsphenoidal approach with exposure of the tumor. The transsphenoidal surgeon then waits while the transcranial surgeon exposes the tumor through a right frontal pterional craniotomy. After the transcranial surgeon has exposed the tumor, he can use blunt dissectors to gently push the tumor down into the sella so that the transsphenoidal surgeon can recover it. With gentle and patient technique, most tumors can be delivered in this fashion, often without tearing the diaphragma sellae. Once most of the tumor is safely pushed down into the sella, the transsphenoidal surgeon then performs as complete a removal as possible.

The two operative fields must be kept separate to avoid any contamination of the craniotomy by the transsphenoidal procedure. With proper draping and care, this can be accomplished.

Once the patient has recovered, a MRI is obtained in 3 months to determine whether any residual tumor remains; if significant residual appears. Then conventional radiation therapy can be used.

I agree with the authors that transsphenoidal removal of large tumors (certainly tumors smaller than the one presented in this case) by intrathecal infusion of sterile Ringer's solution is a valuable adjunct. I routinely use spinal drains on all macroadenomas during surgery and have found this to be a very effective adjunct to surgery.

REFERENCES

Kenji Ohata, M.D., Akira Hakuba, M.D.

1. Al-Mefty O, Kersh JE, Routh A, et al.: The long-term side effects of radiation therapy for benign brain tumors in adults. *J Neurosurg* 1990; 73:502–512.
2. El-Kalliny M, Van Loveren H, Keller JT, et al.: Tumors of the lateral wall of the cavernous sinus. *J Neurosurg* 1992; 77:508–514.
3. Guidetti B, Fraioli B, Cantore GP: Results of surgical management of 319 pituitary adenomas. *Acta Neurochir (Wien)* 1987; 85: 117–124.
4. Hakuba A, Tanaka K, Suzuki T, et al.: A combined orbitozygomatic infratemporal epidural and subdural approach for lesions involving the entire cavernous sinus. *J Neurosurg* 1989; 71:699–704.
5. Iwai Y, Hakuba A, Khosla VK, et al.: Giant basal prolactinoma extending into the nasal cavity. *Surg Neurol* 1992; 37:280–283.
6. MacCarty CS, Hanson EJ, Randall RV, et al.: Indications for and results of surgical treatment of pituitary tumours by transfrontal approach, in Kohler PO, Ross GT (eds): *Diagnosis and Treatment of Pituitary Tumours*. International Congress Series, No. 303. Amsterdam, Excerpta Medica, 1973, pp 136–145.
7. Ray BS, Patterson RH: Surgical experience with chromophobe adenomas of the pituitary gland. *J Neurosurg* 1971; 34:726–729.
8. Srivastava VK, Narayanaswamy KS, Rao TV: Giant pituitary adenoma. *Surg Neurol* 1983; 20:379–382.
9. Symon L, Jakubowski J, Rendall B: Surgical treatment of giant pituitary adenomas. *J Neurol Neurosurg Psychiatry* 1979; 42:973–982.
10. Valtonen S, Myllymaki K: Outcome of patients after transcranial operation for pituitary adenoma. *Ann Clin Res* 1986; 47:43–45.
11. Van Alphen HAM: Microsurgical fronto-temporal approach to pituitary adenomas with extrasellar extension. *Clin Neurol Neurosurg* 1975; 78:246–256.
12. Van Lindert EJ, Grotenhuis JA, Meijer E: Results of follow-up after removal of non-functioning pituitary adenomas by transcranial surgery. *Br J Neurosurg* 1991; 5:129–133.

Wesley A. King, M.D., Donald P. Becker, M.D.

1. Barkan AL, Kelch RP, Hopwood NJ, et al.: Treatment of acromegaly with the long-acting somatostatin analog SMS 201-995. *J Clin Endocrinol Metab* 1966; 66:16–23.
2. Dolenc V: Direct microsurgical repair of intracavernous vascular lesions. *J Neurosurg* 1983; 58:824–831.
3. Fahlbusch R, Buchfelder M: Transsphenoidal surgery of parasellar pituitary adenomas. *Acta Neurochir (Wien)* 1988; 92:92–99.
4. Fujii K, Chambers SM, Rhoton AL: Neurovascular relationships of the sphenoid sinus. *J Neurosurg* 1979; 50:31–39.
5. Hashimoto N, Kikuchi H: Transsphenoidal approach to infrasellar tumors involving the cavernous sinus. *J Neurosurg* 1990; 73: 513–517.
6. Inoue T, Rhoton AL, Theele D, et al.: Surgical approaches to the cavernous sinus: A microsurgical study. *Neurosurgery* 1990; 26: 903–932.
7. Laws ER, Onofrio BM, Pearson BW, et al.: Successful management of bilateral carotidcavernous fistulae with a transsphenoidal approach. *Neurosurgery* 1979; 4:162–167.
8. Lundin P, Nyman R, Burman P, et al.: MRI of pituitary macroadenomas with reference to hormonal activity. *Neuroradiology* 1992; 34:43–51.
9. Mackay A, Hosobuchi Y: Treatment of intracavernous extensions of pituitary adenomas. *Surg Neurol* 1978; 10:377–383.
10. Nelson AT, Tucker HSG, Becker DP: Residual anterior pituitary function following transsphenoidal resection of pituitary macroadenomas. *J Neurosurg* 1984; 61:577–580.
11. Parkinson D: A surgical approach to the cavernous portion of the carotid artery: Anatomical studies and case report. *J Neurosurg* 1969; 23:474–483.
12. Rhoton AL, Hardy DG, Chambers SM: Microsurgical anatomy and dissection of the sphenoid bone, cavernous sinus and sellar region. *Surg Neurol* 1979; 12:63–104.
13. Scheithauer BW, Kovacs KT, Laws ER, et al.: Pathology of invasive pituitary tumors with special reference to functional classification. *J Neurosurg* 1986; 65:733–744.
14. Sekhar LN, Burgess J, Akin O: Anatomical study of the cavernous sinus emphasizing operative approaches and related vascular and neural reconstruction. *Neurosurgery* 1987; 21:806–816.
15. Sekhar LN, Sen CH, Jho HD, et al.: Surgical treatment of intracavernous neoplasms: A four year experience. *Neurosurgery* 1989; 24:18–30.
16. Symon L, Jakubowski J: Transcranial management of pituitary tumors with suprasellar extension. *J Neurol Neurosurg Psychiatry* 1979; 42:123–133.
17. Symon L, Jakubowski J, Kendall B: Surgical treatment of giant pituitary adenomas. *J Neurol Neurosurg Psychiatry* 1979; 42:973–982.

3

Conservative vs. Aggressive
Treatment of Craniopharyngiomas

CASE

A 14-year-old girl came to medical attention for growth retardation and frequent urination. On examination, she was noted to have a bitemporal hemianopsia. Laboratory findings were consistent with diabetes insipidus.

PARTICIPANTS

Conservative Treatment of Craniopharyngiomas–Robert A. Sanford, M.D.

Aggressive Treatment of Craniopharyngiomas–Harold J. Hoffman, M.D.

Moderator–Frederick A. Boop, M.D.

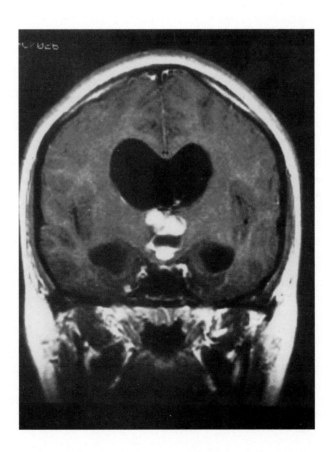

Conservative Treatment of Craniopharyngiomas

Robert A. Sanford, M.D.

This 14-year-old girl has a bitemporal hemianopsia, growth retardation, and frequent urination. The bitemporal hemianopsia is secondary to pressure on the optic chiasm by the tumor mass and obstructive hydrocephalus. The coronal section of the magnetic resonance image shows that the cystic component of the tumor has extended upward, filling the third ventricle, producing hydrocephalus and increasing the compressive effects of the tumor. The growth retardation indicates that this long-standing tumor is already producing hypofunction of the pituitary gland. I suspect that the frequent urination is early diabetes insipidus.

The multiple views provided by the magnetic resonance images show the precise anatomic relationship between the hypothalamus, chiasm, and the solid portion of the tumor. The computed tomogram shows the amount and type of calcification. With this information, the preoperative diagnosis of craniopharyngioma is relatively secure, but must be confirmed through a biopsy.

DISCUSSION

For most children with a craniopharyngioma, the surgeon is faced with two options: radical surgery or limited surgery supplemented with radiotherapy. I always discuss the advantages and disadvantages of each treatment regimen with the patient and the family, but my recommendation for this child is conservative surgery and radiotherapy. After carefully considering the anatomic relationship of the tumor and chiasm, if I believed the patient's vision could be improved through stereotactic drainage of the cyst, I would carry out a stereotactic biopsy, drain the cyst, and place a reservoir before the patient underwent radiotherapy. If the solid component of the tumor seemed to compress the posterior chiasm, I would undertake a limited craniotomy using a right pterional approach to carefully drain the cyst and remove enough tumor to decompress the chiasm. I would not attempt to dissect the cyst capsule from the hypothalamus, thereby preserving the infundibulum. Of the children undergoing this treatment at our institution, all have had their vision preserved or improved and none has developed permanent diabetes insipidus.

After surgery, the patient and her family are given the option of standard radiotherapy or stereotactic radiotherapy. A 14-year-old can be placed in the stereotactic frame and given a fraction of 160 cGy each day. Although the hypothalamus and pituitary gland are included in the radiation field, the frontal and temporal lobes are completely spared, negating concern about the harmful effects of radiation on intelligence.

Standard radiotherapy has an 85% chance of controlling the tumor and, in children older than 10 years, has little morbidity, with a 3 to 7% complication rate. Stereotactic radiotherapy is a new modality offered only in an experimental protocol, but there is every reason to believe it will be equally effective because the radiation to the tumor is exactly the same as it is in conventional treatment. Sparing the temporal and frontal lobes reduces the problems of cerebral radiation effect or damage to intelligence. Stereotactic radiotherapy is extremely appealing for patients between 3 and 10 years of age, in which significant loss of intelligence has been documented.

RATIONALE FOR LIMITED SURGERY WITH RADIOTHERAPY

A survey of the literature[2] reveals that the rate of recurrence after complete tumor removal is 25%. After partial removal supplemented with radiotherapy, the recurrence rate is 21%. Because tumor control is about equal with both modes of therapy, the most important consideration is the patient's quality of life. My recent survey of institutions belonging to the American Society of Pediatric Neurosurgery (ASPN) details the quality of life in 144 patients treated at 8 pediatric hospitals.[3] A good outcome was achieved in 83% of the children who underwent limited surgery or biopsy and radiation. The good outcome varied significantly in the 7 centers whose primary goal was total removal. The surgeons who operated on 1 or fewer children per year achieved a good outcome in 52.2% of patients; surgeons at 2 institutions who had operated on 1.5 to 2.5 patients per year had a good outcome in 86% of the patients. Unfortunately, in only 75% were they able to achieve a gross total resection. The remainder of the children underwent radical surgery, with its complications, and then required irradiation to achieve a good outcome in 50%. This series confirms the superiority of limited surgery and irradiation in all but the most expert hands.

Endocrine complications are high after both types of therapy and major hormone replacement is required in 95% of patients. In the radical surgical group, these complications occur immediately after surgery. In children undergoing limited surgery followed by irradiation, endocrinopathy is delayed, but occurs within 2 years. After radical surgery, however, diabetes insipidus occurred in 79% of the patients in the ASPN series and 90% of those reported in the literature.[1,5,6] Diabetes insipidus occurs in only 6% of children undergoing limited surgery and irradiation.[3] Not only does diabetes insipidus present significant long-term hazards to children and limit their outside activities during the summer, but the additional expense of desmopressin acetate of (DDAVP) at this time is about $75 to $300 per month.

OTHER COMPLICATIONS

Death is not an infrequent complication in those undergoing attempted total removal; it is reported in 2 to 4% even in the most expert hands[1,4,6] and 4 to 9% in the ASPN survey.[3] No deaths were reported in those undergoing limited surgery; the expected death rate for this treatment should be less than 1%.

Serious complications occurred in 3 to 7% of patients undergoing standard irradiation. Radiation vasculitis, radiation-induced malignant gliomas, radiation necrosis, and visual loss were reported. With stereotactic radiotherapy, radiation vasculitis and damage to the optic chiasm are still possible, but secondary malignant tumors should be rare because the radiation field is limited.

The last factor that must be considered is the overall expense of treatment. If stereotactic biopsy and shunting is used, the total time the patient spends in the hospital should be less than 48 hours, which greatly reduces the medical expense.

Based on these factors, I conclude that limited surgery and

stereotactic radiotherapy in this child offers the best chance for improving vision and preventing permanent diabetes insipidus.

Furthermore, it has minimal complications and the best chance for an excellent quality of life.

Aggressive Treatment of Craniopharyngiomas

Harold J. Hoffman, M.D.

This 14-year-old child has a retrochiasmic craniopharyngioma, which is both cystic and solid. The tumor fills the third ventricle and has occluded the foramina of Monro and produced hydrocephalus. The child already has evidence of endocrine problems, including growth retardation and diabetes insipidus. Furthermore, this retrochiasmic tumor is compressing the chiasm and producing a bitemporal hemianopsia.

HISTORICAL PERSPECTIVE

In the era before the development of steroid therapy, the morbidity and mortality rates of surgical treatment of craniopharyngioma were prohibitive. With the advent of steroid therapy in the early 1950s, Matson and Crigler[14] were able to remove craniopharyngiomas safely and totally. Despite this, many believed that there was no line of cleavage between a craniopharyngioma and adjacent brain, and that forcible removal of the tumor could severely damage the hypothalamus and optic apparatus.[15] Radiotherapy was and still is widely advocated for the treatment of craniopharyngiomas.[8,11,13] An increasing number of reports, however, have identified various complications of radiotherapy for this tumor. These include the development of a second tumor, moyamoya disease, the failure of the radiotherapy to control the tumor's growth, and adverse intellectual and endocrine sequelae of the radiotherapy, particularly in young children.[5,16,18–20,22,23]

During the past 15 years, the techniques for investigating and treating a patient with a craniopharyngioma have changed radically. Neuroimaging allows earlier diagnosis of these lesions and better assessment of what surgery has accomplished. When tumor has been left behind, it is now possible to reoperate and remove the remnant. The operating microscope has allowed visualization of important structures and performance of the maneuvers necessary to separate the craniopharyngioma from the surrounding structures. Surgical tools such as the ultrasonic aspirator, which can decompress solid craniopharyngiomas, and the laser beam, which can vaporize foci of tumor and even fragment pieces of calcium, have facilitated safe excision. These have rendered tumors formerly considered inoperable both safely accessible and totally removable.

Craniopharyngiomas are primarily tumors of childhood and are the most common intracranial tumors of nonglial origin in children. Their treatment has always presented a challenge to the neurosurgeon. Despite the benign histological appearance of these tumors, many patients progressively deteriorate regardless of therapy and die of their disease. The method of treating this tumor remains controversial, with proponents of radical removal, radiation therapy, or a combination of these modalities vigorously espousing their points of view.[8,9,11,13,15,25]

One choice for therapy in this child consists of diverting cerebrospinal fluid through a shunt, aspirating the small cyst and using some form of radiotherapy to deal with the tumor. In contrast to that approach, one can attempt to remove the tumor.

With such removal, the cerebrospinal fluid pathways would open up, obviating the need for a diversionary shunt. If the tumor is totally removed, radiotherapy, with its possible deleterious effects on the brain, is not necessary.

PATHOLOGY

Craniopharyngiomas arise from embryonic cell rests in the pituitary stalk.[7] As a result, the tumor closely adheres to the area of the tuber cinereum, where it insinuates itself into the brain parenchyma. Elsewhere, the tumor is covered with meninges and, thus, is distinct from brain tissue. It is in the tuber cinereum that tumor "nests" surrounded by glial tissue are found. Concern has been expressed that surgical removal always leaves nests of tumor cells in this region.[1] These so-called "nests," however, are always continuous with the main tumor capsule, which sends fingers of tumor into the adjacent tuber cinereum. When pathologists section the hypothalamus post mortem, they cut these fingers transversely. Thus, the resulting specimen appears to contain isolated tumor cells. Sweet[21] has pointed out that these nests of tumor cells cause an intense glial reaction which, in itself, helps to effect total removal of the tumor. As the surgeon pulls on the tumor capsule, the glial tissue containing the tumor nests aids in dissecting the tumor free of the hypothalamus.

INVESTIGATION

This child requires a complete neuroendocrinological investigation to confirm the presence of diabetes insipidus and to ascertain whether the functions of the pituitary-adrenal axis and the pituitary-thyroid axis are impaired. Neuropsychological evaluation should be carried out to rule out memory disorder and any other intellectual malfunction produced by the tumor. This is particularly true in the case of a craniopharyngioma, which can distort the columns of the fornices and, thus, affect memory function.[4,24] Vasopressin, which can be deficient, as in this patient, has been noted to have an effect on memory.[6]

SURGICAL TREATMENT

A commonly accepted view of these tumors is that no line of cleavage exists between the tumor and adjacent brain, so that removal of the tumor is accompanied by severe damage to the important adjacent structures, including the hypothalamus and optic apparatus.[15] These beliefs restrain many surgeons and encourage palliative treatment for what is essentially a benign tumor. These beliefs are reinforced by numerous reviews of the treatment of these tumors that go back over many years and include cases done without the benefit of modern technology.[8,17,19] Modern neuroimaging has allowed for earlier diagnosis. Furthermore, accurate imaging has allowed the surgeon to plot an appropriate surgical approach. The operating microscope has allowed surgeons to see important structures and carry out the delicate maneuvers necessary to free the craniopharyngioma from the vital structures on which it impinges. Surgical tools, such as the ultrasonic aspirator and the laser beam, allow one to deal with calcified and solid craniopharyngiomas in a fashion undreamed of by surgeons in the past. Although they did not have these magnificent tools, they were still able to operate on craniopharyngiomas.[14]

In 1950, Donald Matson began to attempt complete removal of every craniopharyngioma.[14] He had no operative mortality, and a review of his cases in 1975[10] showed that the tumor had not recurred in 53% of patients he had operated on. Surely, if Matson could accomplish such results without the advantages that we now have available, we should be able to cure most of these tumors through surgical excision. Furthermore, the more conservative techniques, including external beam irradiation, Gamma knife radiation, and implantation of ^{90}Y seeds and ^{32}P, carry with them morbidity and a significant risk of failure.[2,3,18,19] In addition, the patient in whom surgery has failed can still be treated through one of these more conservative approaches; however, the tumor in a patient in whom a conservative approach has failed usually becomes inoperable because of the dense adhesions between radiated tumor and the adjacent brain.

SURGICAL APPROACH

Craniopharyngiomas require meticulous dissection from the adjacent optic apparatus, the internal carotid, and anterior cerebral arteries, and the overlying floor of the third ventricle. To carry out this dissection safely, these structures must be in view. A transcranial approach, which allows these structures to be safely seen and separated from the tumor, is necessary, except for the rare sellar craniopharyngiomas in which a transsphenoidal approach frequently meets with success.

Because the surgeon must be aware of all the structures in the region of the tumor, the patient's head is positioned with the nose pointing directly up. The patient's neck must be extended so that the frontal lobes can literally fall away from the floor of the anterior fossa. This position removes the risk of traction injury to the frontal lobes. A pin-fixation head rest is mandatory to immobilize the patient's head and allow for securing of self-retaining retractors.

In preparation for surgery, the patient is medicated with dexamethasone and given mannitol in a dose of 2 g/kg just as the skin is incised. The scalp incision extends from temple to temple, and a right frontal bone flap is turned to the midline and the pterion is removed. Once the dura is exposed, a brain needle is inserted into the right frontal horn and cerebrospinal fluid siphoned out of the ventricle, thus decompressing the brain. The dura is opened just above the supraorbital ridge, and the dural incision is extended across the region of the sylvian fissure to the anterior temporal lobe. Once the dura is opened, the frontal and temporal lobes are retracted away from the sphenoid wing, exposing the bifurcation of the internal carotid artery and the right optic nerve. In addition, the frontal lobe is elevated from the floor of the anterior fossa. To elevate the lobe, the polar veins are coagulated and divided and the olfactory tract is coagulated and divided just behind the olfactory bulb. This prevents avulsion of the olfactory bulb from the cribriform plate.

With elevation of the frontal lobe, the chiasmatic cistern is exposed and opened. In this patient with a retrochiasmic tumor, the chiasm is pushed forward to the tuberculum and the chiasm forms a sheet over the dome of the tumor. With the temporal lobe and frontal lobe elevated from the sphenoid wing, the termina-

tion of the internal carotid artery and its apposition to the optic nerve are well exposed. One then has the choice of separating the internal carotid artery from the optic nerve and visualizing the tumor as it pushes upon the third ventricle. This particular tumor is large, filling the entire third ventricle, and I would choose to open the lamina terminalis just in front of the A1 segment of the anterior cerebral artery. The lamina terminalis has a grayish hue and is distinct from optic fibers. On opening of the lamina terminalis, the floor of the third ventricle is seen. This is stretched and thinned out, so that frequently one can see tumor within the third ventricle upon opening the lamina terminalis. The cyst within the tumor is emptied and, with the aid of the ultrasonic aspirator, the tumor is decompressed within the third ventricle. As this is done, the chiasm moves back from the tuberculum, allowing access to the tumor between the optic nerves. The route between the internal carotid artery and the optic nerve is also available. It may be necessary to use all 3 of these routes to effect total removal of the tumor.

It is helpful to place a cotton patty into the third ventricle through the lamina terminalis.[12] As one pushes down on the patty, the tumor comes into view between the optic nerves.

In attempting to remove a craniopharyngioma, it is helpful to keep the capsule in continuity, which allows one to apply traction to the remaining tumor and thus help secure total removal. The use of a dental mirror helps detect remnants of craniopharyngioma that may have been left behind as one pulls on the tumor.

With the tumor decompressed, it must be separated from the internal carotid artery and its branches on both sides, and from the optic nerve and chiasm. If calcified components are too large to remove through these various access routes, one could drill away the tuberculum, thus creating a large opening between the 2 optic nerves. This opening allows one to remove large fragments of tumor between the optic nerves.[17]

The membrane of Liliequist is always intact at the time of initial removal of a craniopharyngioma; this membrane provides a useful barrier between the tumor, the basilar artery, and the brain stem.

Postoperative Care

This retrochiasmic tumor has distorted the hypothalamus and produced endocrine problems preoperatively. These endocrine problems can be aggravated postoperatively and children with these problems must be monitored by a skilled pediatric endocrinologist. The preoperative doses of dexamethasone are continued for 48 to 72 hours, at which time maintenance doses of cortisone are substituted. Because this patient already has diabetes insipidus, treatment with desmopressin acetate will bring this condition under control. Thyroid function, sexual function, and growth must be carefully watched after a craniopharyngioma is removed to document those patients who need replacement therapy.

Prophylactic doses of phenytoin are administered for a period of 5 to 10 days. A computed tomogram should be done within the first 12 to 24 hours to ensure that no areas of calcification or enhancing tumor are left behind. With the tumor removed, cerebrospinal fluid pathways should open and the ventricles should return to their normal size.

Surgical Morbidity

This patient has a bitemporal hemianopsia. One hopes that removing the tumor and decompressing the chiasm will improve her visual field. There is a possibility, however, that this child's visual acuity may deteriorate because of injury to the chiasm or optic nerve.

Craniopharyngiomas distort the columns of the fornix.[24] In sophisticated testing, patients with craniopharyngiomas can be found to have a memory deficit,[9] which becomes clinically relevant if the patient has a significant drop in intelligence. This is rarely a problem in a patient who has undergone surgical removal of a tumor, but it can become a problem in patients with recurrent tumors, particularly those who have received radiotherapy.

Excessive weight gain can be a problem in 10 to 15% of patients who have had a craniopharyngioma removed. Pathologic overeating is extremely rare, however, and occurs in less than 1% of patients. Cortisone and thyroid replacement therapy are necessary in 75% of patients undergoing surgery for a craniopharyngioma. Growth hormone is necessary in 25% of children after the removal of a craniopharyngioma, and replacement of sex hormones is necessary in 30% of young adults and adults after the removal of a craniopharyngioma.

DISCUSSION

Total excision of a craniopharyngioma is possible and, with the modern technological aids available, can be carried out without significant morbidity or mortality.[9] Although radiotherapy decreases the amount of cyst fluid, it probably does not completely destroy craniopharyngioma epithelia. A computed tomogram rarely shows complete disappearance of the tumor mass. Amacher[1] has shown that the mass remaining after radiotherapy can be largely necrotic, with some viable tumor cells that can lead to recurrence. Radiotherapy does, however, cause degenerative changes in brain parenchyma and vasculature.[5] The changes

induced progress slowly over a period measured in decades, resulting in an increased rate of vascular catastrophes in later years and enhancing the possibility of tumors within the irradiated volume.[16,19,20,22,23] The risk of tumor induction by irradiation in a young child with a benign lesion can be significant. Several reports attest to this possibility. I believe, therefore, that the first approach to a child with a craniopharyngioma is to attempt total removal. If this approach fails, then more conservative approaches with radiotherapy can be used. Attempting to remove a craniopharyngioma that has been treated with radiotherapy presents a serious problem; the irradiation can cause numerous adhesions that often make total removal impossible.

Perhaps the most important factor governing operative treatment of a craniopharyngioma is the surgeon's attitude towards the tumor. If the surgeon regards the tumor as nonresectable, it will be treated as such and no attempt will be made to remove it. If, on the other hand, the surgeon believes that craniopharyngiomas can be totally removed, the surgical approach is likely to be successful.

CONCLUSION

My experience indicates that more than 60% of craniopharyngiomas in children can be totally resected with minimal significant morbidity and mortality. The morbidity and mortality rates in patients who undergo an attempt at total resection of a craniopharyngioma are reasonable. Increasing experience with resection of these tumors and the advanced technology available should reduce these rates further, so that children with craniopharyngiomas can look forward to functioning in a more normal fashion. Their chances of leading a fully normal life are greatest when their tumors are diagnosed and treated early.

Conservative vs. Aggressive Treatment of Craniopharyngiomas

Frederick A. Boop, M.D.

As stated by both authors, craniopharyngioma is the most common nonglial tumor of childhood. Even so, Dr. Sanford's study shows that, at the largest of pediatric referral centers, a given surgeon's experience is not likely to exceed 2 or 3 cases per year. It is also clear that centers treating patients with craniopharyngiomas frequently have much more acceptable morbidity and mortality than those treating this tumor only occasionally. Therefore, in interpreting the available literature, one cannot assume that the surgical morbidity and mortality reported by Hoffman or Yasargil will apply to one's own practice. The most important message to be learned regarding this tumor is that the practicing neurosurgeon who encounters a patient with a craniopharyngioma only once every 2 or 3 years should send the child to a major referral center where pediatric neurosurgery, pediatric endocrinology, and pediatric neuroradiology are established.

SURGERY

Microsurgical resection continues to be the mainstay of treatment for craniopharyngiomas and clearly offers the best opportunity for a cure. Whereas surgical mortality and morbidity continue to improve, one must not forget that three quarters of patients undergoing radical surgery have deficiencies of 4 or

more hormones. Although better neuroendocrine replacement therapies have made long-term survival possible, the psychosocial and financial burden placed upon the family trying to care for the child with hypocortisolemia or diabetes insipidus is tremendous.[1] Add to this the facts that half of these children develop obesity, most will have learning disabilities, and, despite what was believed to be a curative resection, 20 to 25% experience recurrence of their tumor, there remains much room for improvement in the surgical treatment of this disease.

The application of radiotherapy to craniopharyngiomas must likewise be interpreted with caution. True, the neuroendocrine sequelae are significantly less with this form of therapy than with surgery, but one can anticipate a 20 to 25% rate of recurrence with either microsurgery or radiation. Seventy percent of recurrences appear within 3 years of initial treatment. Many of the reports in the older literature involved the use of conventional external beam radiation for these tumors, and outcome after this treatment modality does not necessarily apply to treatment with stereotactic radiosurgical modalities or intracavitary irradiation. We must recognize, however, that conventional radiotherapy increases the long-term risk of secondary neoplasia more than fivefold. The literature documents at least 2 children who developed highly malignant gliomas within their radiation ports after treatment for a craniopharyngioma. The development of radiation-induced vasculitis, moyamoya disease, or radiation injury to optic nerves, cranial nerves, or hypothalamic structures can be anticipated if significant radiation (greater than 8 to 10 cGy) is delivered to these structures. Given that their recurrence rates are similar, surgery carries a one-time risk for most patients. The long-term risks associated with either stereotactic radiosurgery or intracystic radioisotope treatment have yet to be determined.

CONCLUSIONS

For a current comprehensive review of this topic, the reader is referred to the monograph published after a consensus conference held in New York in December of 1993.[2] This publication reviews all major issues associated with the treatment of craniopharyngiomas, and it is from this meeting that the following conclusions are drawn:

1. The goal of treating craniopharyngiomas should be to control tumor growth while preserving the patient's cognitive, visual, and endocrine function.
2. Microsurgical resection should be the initial treatment in any patient with rapid visual or neurological decline or obstructive hydrocephalus. Tumors having a small or moderate noncystic mass are most amenable to resection.
3. Microsurgical resection should be the initial treatment in children younger than 5 years of age in an effort to avoid the deleterious effects of radiation on the developing brain.
4. Microsurgical resection should be the initial treatment in patients with a large solid component to their tumor.
5. Transsphenoidal resection should be considered the initial treatment of tumors located primarily within the sella turcica.

6. Surgical removal should be considered only for patients for whom there is ready access to appropriate endocrinological follow-up and replacement hormones, and for whom the family is capable of reliably providing for postoperative endocrinological needs. Patients returning to underdeveloped countries or rural areas are at increased risk of death if these needs are not considered preoperatively. As Dr. Sanford has shown, compared to surgery, radiation therapy clearly reduces the likelihood of diabetes insipidus and the need for multiple hormone placement.
7. For patients with primarily cystic tumors, intracystic radiotherapy with ^{32}P or ^{90}Y appears to be efficacious, is less expensive, and carries minimal morbidity compared to surgery. If this modality fails, it does not appear to increase the difficulty of subsequent resection.
8. Patients in whom a complete resection has been attempted by a skilled surgeon and has failed because of tumor adhering to vital structures should be followed closely with postoperative computed tomograms. Two thirds of these patients will have a recurrence within 3 years of the initial operation. Focused radiotherapy should be given at the time of radiographic progression. It should not be given for a fleck of residual calcification seen on a postoperative computed tomogram.
9. Patients presenting with solid or mixed tumor recurrence after what was initially believed to be a complete resection should undergo surgical re-exploration. More than half of these can be "cured" through a second resection.
10. Stereotactic radiosurgery is best reserved for solid components of craniopharyngiomas that are small (less than 20 mm in diameter) and are separated from the optic apparatus by 5 mm or more.

REFERENCES

Robert A. Sanford, M.D.

1. Hoffman HJ, De Silva M, Humphreys RP, et al.: Aggressive surgical management of craniopharyngiomas in children. *J Neurosurg* 1992; 76:47–52.
2. Sanford RA, Donahue DJ: Intraventricular Tumors, in Cheek WR, Marlin AE, McLone DG, et al. (eds): *Pediatric Neurosurgery*. Philadelphia, WB Saunders, 1994, pp 403–408.
3. Sanford RA, Muhlbauer MS: Craniopharyngioma in children. *Neurol Clin* 1991; 9:453–465.
4. Symon L, Pell MF, Hibib HA: Radical excision of craniopharyngioma by the temporal route: A review of 50 patients. *Br J Neurosurg* 1991; 5:539–549.
5. Tomita T, McLone DG: Radical resection of childhood craniopharyngiomas. *Pediatr Neurosurg* 1993; 19:6–14.
6. Yasargil MG, Curcic M, Kis M, et al.: Total removal of craniopharyngiomas: Approaches and long-term results in 144 patients. *J Neurosurg* 1990; 73:3–11.

Harold J. Hoffman, M.D.

1. Amacher AL: Craniopharyngioma: The controversy regarding radiotherapy. *Child Brain* 1980; 6:57–64.
2. Backlund EO: Studies on craniopharyngiomas: III. Stereotaxic treatment with intracystic yttrium-90. *Acta Chir Scan* 1973; 139: 237–247.
3. Backlund EO: Studies on craniopharyngiomas: IV. Stereotaxic treatment with radiosurgery. *Acta Chir Scan* 1973; 139:344–351.
4. Barbizet J: Defect of memorizing of hippocampal-mam-millary origin: A review. *J Neurol Neurosurg Psychiatry* 1963; 26:127–135.
5. Bleyer WA, Griffin TW: White matter necrosis, mineralizing microangeopathy, and intellectual abilities in survivors of childhood leukemia, in Gilbert HA, Kogan AR (eds.): *Radiation Damage to the Nervous System*. New York, Raven Press, 1980, pp 155–174.
6. De Wied D, Van Greidanus W, Bohus B, et al.: Vasopressin and memory consolidation. *Prog Brain Res* 1976; 45:181–194.
7. Erdheim J: Uber hypophysengangsyeschwulse und Hurnocholesteatome. *Sitzargsb Akad Wissensch* 1904; 113:537–726.
8. Fischer EG, Welch K, Shillito J Jr, et al.: Craniopharyngiomas in children. Long-term effects of conservative surgical procedures combined with radiation therapy. *J Neurosurg* 1990; 73:534–540.
9. Hoffman HJ, Da Silva M, Humphreys RP, et al.: Aggressive surgical management of craniopharyngiomas in children. *J Neurosurg* 1992; 76:47–52.
10. Katz EL: Late results of radical excision of craniopharyngiomas in children. *J Neurosurg* 1975; 42:86–90.
11. Kramer S, Southard M, Mansfield CM: Radiotherapy in the man-

agement of craniopharyngiomas. Further experiences and late results. *Am J Roentgenol Radium Ther Nucl Med* 1968; 103:44–52.

12. Lapras C, Patet JD, Mottolese C, et al.: Craniopharyngiomas in childhood: Analysis of 42 cases. *Prog Exp Tumor Res* 1987; 30:350–358.

13. Manaka S, Teramoto A, Takakura K: The efficacy of radiotherapy for craniopharyngioma. *J Neurosurg* 1985; 62:648–656.

14. Matson DD, Crigler JF Jr: Management of craniopharyngiomas in childhood. *J Neurosurg* 1969; 30:377–390.

15. Mori K, Handa H, Murata T, et al.: Results of treatment for craniopharyngioma. *Child Brain* 1980; 6:303–312.

16. Olds MV, Griebel RN, Hoffman HJ, et al.: Surgical treatment of Moya moya disease. *J Neurosurg* 1987; 66:675–680.

17. Patterson RH Jr, Danylevich A: Surgical removal of craniopharyngiomas by a transcranial approach through the lamina terminalis and sphenoid sinus. *Neurosurgery* 1980; 7:111–117.

18. Richards GE: Effects of irradiation on the hypothalamic pituitary regions, in Gilbert HA, Kagan AR (eds): *Radiation Damage to the Nervous System*. New York, Raven Press, 1980, pp 175–180.

19. Shillito J Jr: Treatment of craniopharyngioma. *Clin Neurosurg* 1985; 33:533–546.

20. Sogg RL, Donaldson SS, Yorke CH: Malignant astrocytoma following radiotherapy of a craniopharyngioma. Case Report. *J Neurosurg* 1987; 48:622–627.

21. Sweet WH: Radical surgical treatment of craniopharyngioma. *Clin Neurosurg* 1976; 23:52–79.

22. Ushio Y, Arita N, Yoshimine T, et al.: Glioblastoma after radiotherapy for craniopharyngioma: Case report. *Neurosurgery* 1987; 21:33–38.

23. Waga S, Handa H: Radiation-induced meningioma: With review of literature. *Surg Neurol* 1976; 5:215–219.

24. Williams M, Pennybacker J: Memory disturbances in third ventricle tumours. *J Neurol Neurosurg Psychiatry* 1954; 17:115–123.

25. Yasargil MG, Curcic M, Kis M, et al.: Total removal of craniopharyngiomas: Approaches and long-term results in 144 patients. *J Neurosurg* 1990; 73:3–11.

Frederick A. Boop, M.D.

1. Cavazzuti V, Fischer EG, Welch K, et al.: Neurological and psychophysiological sequelae following different treatments of craniopharyngioma in children. *J Neurosurg* 1983; 59:409–417.

2. Epstein FJ, Handler MH (eds): Craniopharyngioma: the answer. *Pediatric Neurosurgery*, vol. 21 (S1). Philadelphia, WB Saunders, 1994.

4

Approaches to Colloid Cysts:
Transcranial vs. Stereotactic

CASE

A 35-year-old, right-handed man came to medical attention with a new onset of headaches. His fundoscopic exam showed bilateral papilledema; the rest of his neurological exam was normal.

PARTICIPANTS

Colloid Cysts: The Case for Craniotomy–Michael L.J. Apuzzo, M.D.

The Stereotactic Approach to Colloid Cysts–Christoph B. Ostertag, M.D., Friedrich W. Kreth, M.D.

Moderator–Isao Yamamoto, M.D.

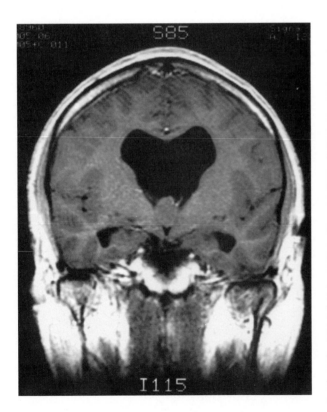
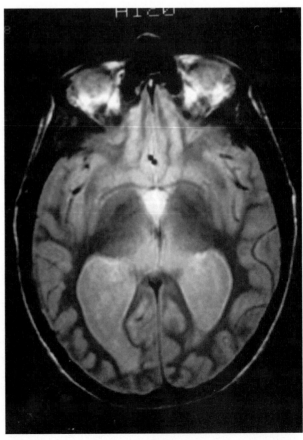

Colloid Cysts: The Case for Craniotomy

Michael L.J. Apuzzo, M.D.

The colloid cyst represents a seemingly simple, but frequently complex, strategic and technical problem for the neurosurgeon. With the advent of sophisticated imaging modes, more frequently the lesion is found incidentally, commonly in young individuals with complaints of headache. In these patients, no ventriculomegaly is present and lesions usually measure a centimeter or less in size. The cysts are quite characteristic, particularly on magnetic resonance images. In a second major group, the lesions are found in symptomatic patients who manifest, not only the presence of the cyst, but attendant ventriculomegaly with associated appropriate clinical symptoms and signs.

In each one of these major groups, from a technical standpoint, modern neurosurgery offers the capability to treat as follows: craniotomy including cyst aspiration and wall excision, procedures to divert cerebrospinal fluid, and stereotactic aspiration.

For patients with an incidental lesion, a fourth option may be considered—simply following the patient with serial clinical (history, neurological examination, psychometrics) and imaging studies.

This discussion approaches both the incidental and symptomatic presentation of colloid cysts, arguing for the use of a craniotomy and against the options of clinical observation, cerebrospinal fluid diversion, and stereotactic aspiration.

SYMPTOMATIC COLLOID CYSTS

Clinical Observation

The case against clinical observation is clear for the established symptomatic colloid cyst because the symptoms in attendant, progressive ventriculomegaly are striking and these are time-honored indications for surgical intervention of some type.

Diversion of Cerebrospinal Fluid

Diversion of cerebrospinal fluid is a suboptimal treatment mode because it does not treat the cause of the obstruction and does not offer definitive treatment of the disorder. Shunt function is inconsistent and failures may sometimes occur that are inopportune for rapid resolution, thus, establishing a substrate for continued risk for the patient.

In addition, obstruction of the foramen of Monro requires bilateral catheter placement, which increases the risk of the intracranial procedure. Reason would dictate that bilateral shunt procedures are more at risk for segmental failure than the placement of a single catheter.

Stereotactic Aspiration

Although potentially an attractive procedure, stereotactic aspiration has a number of risks and shortcomings. Colloid cysts vary in wall thickness and consistency. An inability to puncture and aspirate is a frequently encountered phenomenon. The global experience with stereotactic aspiration of these lesions is meager and hardly justifies a universal statement regarding the advisability of such an approach. Even in the most experienced of hands, aspiration of the cyst contents is the ultimate endpoint with no safe capability available for excising all, or components,

of the cyst wall. Finally, aspirations of colloid cysts are complicated stereotactic techniques that should be undertaken only by experienced stereotactic neurosurgeons who regularly perform stereotactic neurosurgery, and who are experienced with endoscopic methods. Both from the standpoint of difficulty and current available experience, stereotactic methods are not in the general scope of expertise of most neurosurgeons or the "occasional" stereotactic surgeon.

Craniotomy

In experienced and competent hands, microsurgical aspiration and excision of the wall of the colloid cyst offers the patient absolute definitive treatment of this disorder. It relieves the risk of future obstruction of cerebrospinal fluid pathways. For experienced microsurgeons, particularly in patients with attendant ventriculomegaly, the procedure is relatively simple and offers the opportunity to aspirate and maximize excision of the cyst wall while maximizing a diversity of egress pathways for cerebrospinal fluid. This includes the potential for a callosotomy, fenestration of the septum pellucidum, third ventriculostomy, and absolute assurance of patency at the foramen of Monro and anterior third ventricular space.

Any risks incurred during a craniotomy are compacted within the time of the surgical event and the immediate postoperative period. With a properly executed procedure, patients are free of risk for the rest of their lives.

INCIDENTAL COLLOID CYSTS

As has been noted, the incidental colloid cyst is often found in young people who complain of headache. Occasionally, it is seen in older individuals, at times with attendant *ex vacuo* hydrocephalus. My approach is to carefully assess the images in 3 planes with our neuroradiologist to ascertain the potential for cerebrospinal fluid flow in the situation. Frequently, even in cysts 1.5 cm or larger, in *ex vacuo* situations there is evidence of flow, with patent spinal fluid pathways apparent at the region of the foramen of Monro that decrease the concern about obstruction. In addition, it is not uncommon for us to obtain psychometric examinations as part of the baseline of appraisal. Being clinically assured that the patient truly has an incidental cyst, the issue of treatment or nontreatment may be approached as follows.

Clinical Appraisal and Follow-up Without Surgery

The argument against clinical appraisal and follow-up without surgery is that the patient is frequently stressed by the clinical truism that the potential for obstruction and rapid demise exists in each one of these cases. Patients can rarely tolerate the "sword" over their head. Surgical treatment terminates this risk and the patient can resume a normal life without concern.

Diversion of Cerebrospinal Fluid

Diversion of cerebrospinal fluid in these patients is illogical, as no ventriculomegaly exists. Even through stereotactic methods, placement of bilateral ventricular catheters potentially carries a high risk in patients without ventriculomegaly. Valve-related problems may evolve, associated with iatrogenic headache and added risk for intracranial hematoma. Shunt failure may go unrecognized and, therefore, the diversionary system may offer no protection at the time it is needed.

Stereotactic Aspiration

Particularly for cysts noted incidentally, the lesion is less than 1 cm; even in the most experienced hands, stereotactic puncture and aspiration is difficult. The use of endoscopic methods in patients with normal ventricles carries more difficulty and potential risks than when ventriculomegaly is present. Visualiza-

tion and the capability for manipulating the cyst and its wall are cumbersome technical problems.

Craniotomy

With the symptomatic colloid cyst, craniotomy offers the greatest and safest opportunity to correct a problem associated with potential obstruction of cerebrospinal fluid pathways. Although the cerebrospinal fluid pathways and corridors are reduced in size in patients with colloid cysts, experienced surgeons using microsurgical methods offer the opportunity for cure and relieve the risk of future obstruction. Additionally, the opportunity to create alternate pathways for the egress of cerebrospinal fluid is presented.

The Stereotactic Approach to Colloid Cysts

Cristoph B. Ostertag, M.D., Friedrich W. Kreth, M.D.

The T2-weighted axial magnetic resonance image of this patient reveals high signal intensity within the cyst in the floor of the third ventricle. The coronal T1-weighted image shows the isointense round mass in the third ventricle with resulting hydrocephalus. The quality of the image is not good enough to decide whether there is also a cavum septi pellucidi. The lesion is considered compatible with a colloid cyst of the anterior third ventricle, although other isointense lesions, such as gliomas, ependymomas, and plexus papillomas, are not positively excluded.

SURGICAL TECHNIQUE

A computed tomography (CT)-based stereotactic approach is used in all patients, including stereotactic angiography and endoscopy. With the patient under general anesthesia, the stereotactic head ring, part of a modified Riechert stereotactic system, is secured on the patient's head with four plastic posts, each holding a Mayfield pin.[25] Target localization is carried out in a standard CT scanner (Somatom High Q) with the head ring fixed. At a workstation, coordinates of the frame are then directly derived from the CT image without further calculation, once the image cross-hair and the axes of the head ring are made to coincide. The accuracy of the stereotactic procedure is guaranteed when the coordinate system of the imaging and the localization procedure and that of the intervention are in a fixed relationship.

After CT scanning, the patient is transferred to the stereotactic operating room. After the target is localized and the site of the burr hole is determined, the stereotactic system is attached to the head ring. A 2-cm skin incision and a paramedian precoronal 5-mm burr hole in the line of the probe are made. After incision of the dura and point-like coagulation of the pia mater, a guide cannula is introduced until it reaches the frontal horn. The guide cannula is replaced by a guide cannula with a trocar. This trocar is then removed and an endoscope (Stortz, Tuttlingen type Hopkins forward-viewing endoscope with a 2-mm diameter) is introduced down the guide cannula. The right frontal horn and the foramen of Monro are then inspected and the colloid cyst identified, including the position of the thalamostriate vein and the choroid plexus. The colloid cyst usually is seen as a green or grayish mass filling the foramen of Monro.

After a portion of the cyst that is free of vessels is identified, the 2-mm guide cannula with a smaller inner cannula is introduced with a small sharp trocar and the cannula placed in the center of the cyst. A drop of contrast medium mixed with saline solution helps delineate the size of the cyst and define evacuation. The completeness of evacuation depends on the consistency of the contents. The cannulas are not withdrawn without a final endoscopic inspection to exclude any bleeding into the ventricles. The skin incision is closed.

Under local anesthesia and mild sedation, the stereotactic procedure usually takes 1 to 1.5 hours, including CT-scanning, calculating the setting parameters and aspiration, and closing the wound.

AUTHORS' EXPERIENCE

Over the course of 12 years (1980 to 1992), we treated 39 patients with the expected diagnosis of a colloid cyst using a stereotactic procedure. In 2 patients, however, this diagnosis could not be confirmed. One had an astrocytoma (WHO II) and the other had a plexus papilloma. Thus, our treatment results consist of 37 patients (20 men, 17 women) with biopsy-verified colloid cysts analyzed retrospectively. Follow-up examinations, both clinical and using X-ray computed tomography, took place 6 weeks, 6 months and, then, annually after the procedure. The findings on CT were classified as significant reduction when the volume of the cyst had decreased at least 50% compared to the preoperative volume.

Table 1 shows the distribution of important clinical and radiological findings. In 18 patients, the colloid cyst was completely evacuated by means of a stereotactic aspiration; in 12 patients, a considerable reduction (>50%) was obtained (Table 2). In 7 patients, findings were similar or unchanged in comparison to preoperative ones. Two patients of this group were operated on through the transcallosal approach at a later time. Ten patients came to the stereotactic procedure with a biventricular shunt already implanted. In 2 patients, we used no further measures because of minimal clinical symptoms and a cyst volume of less than 0.5 ml. Of the 25 patients with preoperative hydrocephalus, 11 had normal ventricles after the stereotactic aspiration of the colloid cyst. This was accomplished in 4 patients after complete aspiration and in 7 patients after considerable reduction of the

Table 1. Important Clinical and Radiographic Findings in a Series of 37 Patients with Colloid Cysts Treated with Stereotactic Surgery

Feature	Measurement
Age, mean (median) ± SD*	41 (41) ± 13.4 years
Duration of disease, mean ± SD*	27 ± 45 months
Leading symptom	
Headache, vomiting	15 patients
Nausea	20 patients
Mental clouding	2 patients
Preoperative cyst volume, mean ± SD	2 ± 2.3 ml
Cyst volume on last follow-up	0.6 ± 1.2 ml
CT* appearance, hyperdense/isodense	29/8 patients
Recurrent cyst	2 patients
Follow-up time, mean (range)	5.2 (1–14) years

*SD, standard deviation; CT, computed tomogram.

cyst. In 2 patients, recurrent cysts were observed 4 and 5 years after the stereotactic aspiration, which had been incomplete.

Prognostic Factors

Of the 8 patients harboring iso- or hypodense cysts, 6 showed complete evacuation of the cyst and 2 a significant reduction of the volume. These results were in contrast to patients with primarily hyperdense cysts (29 patients, 7 of which remained unchanged). The difference between both groups, however, was not significant (p>0.05). Patients with smaller treatment volumes (< 1 ml) more often had unchanged postoperative CT findings than patients with larger treatment volumes (X2 = 5.122, p<0.05). Treatment volumes in patients with hypo- or isodense cysts were larger than those with hyperdense cysts (Table 2). The combination of a hyperdense cyst with a treatment volume of less than 1 ml was prognostically unfavorable (Fisher's Exact Test: p<0.05). CT scans taken immediately after the procedure were important for predicting later results. All patients with a significant reduction of the cyst after surgery and with complete filling of the cavity with contrast medium had complete disappearance or a significant reduction of the cyst (p<0.01) on further CT follow-up.

Complications

In 1 patient, bleeding was seen on postoperative CT, in the area of the head of the caudate nucleus, that was asymptomatic and needed no further treatment. One patient suffered mild meningitis after the procedure. There was no mortality.

EXPERIENCE REPORTED IN THE LITERATURE

Colloid cysts are benign lesions of maldevelopmental origin that can cause considerable morbidity because of intermittent or permanent occlusion of the foramen of Monro.[6,22] It appears that, with improved digital computed imaging techniques, colloid cysts of the third ventricle are becoming easier to diagnose and, therefore, are apparently more commonly encountered. Most are well-delineated on CT, are hyperdense and exceptionally isodense masses in patients presenting with a history of episodic headache, or with fluctuating dementia in patients with or without headaches or paroxysmal attacks (the history and symptoms of which make the diagnosis of a colloid cyst highly likely).

Although the CT findings of a round, hyperdense, well-delineated mass strongly suggest the likelihood of a colloid cyst, CT and magnetic resonance do not allow a definitive pathologic diagnosis.[4,5,10,13,28,29,31] The differential diagnosis includes gliomas, meningiomas, ependymomas, and papillomas, as well as arachnoid cysts, all of which must be verified histologically through biopsy or extirpation.[14]

Because colloid cysts are benign curable lesions, they have always attracted the interest of neurosurgeons. Various surgical techniques have been used since Dandy's first description of the successful removal of a colloid cyst.[8] A variety of open surgical approaches has been described, mainly frontal transcortical, transventricular, or anterior transcallosal approaches, which have caused considerable mortality and morbidity in the past.[11,12,18,19,31] Microsurgical expertise has decreased operative mortality and morbidity considerably.[1,2,7,16,24] The standard approaches now are the transcortical transventricular approach or an anterior transcallosal approach which, in the hands of an experienced neurosurgeon, is associated with low morbidity and mortality.[30] With this approach and the operating microscope, excellent visibility is achieved.

Some, therefore, argue that a transcallosal approach affords reasonably good exposure and a chance for operative cure in general circumstances. The transcallosal approach, however, is not without functional consequences if the patient undergoes a careful neuropsychometrical examination.[15,22] However, the mucous fluid of the colloid cyst can be aspirated simply through a stereotactically guided cannula.[3,9,20,23,27] The method of stereotactic aspiration has continuously been improved. Ventriculoscopy and angiography under stereotactic conditions have been incorporated, which makes the procedure effective, harmless and, above all, avoids major operative trauma.[21,26] Our results show the effectiveness of the stereotactic procedure in the treatment of colloid cysts. The significance of the stereotactic intervention, first of all, lies in affirming the diagnosis, and second in local decompression and relief of the hydrocephalus

Table 2. CT Findings and Treatment Results in a Series of 37 Patients with Colloid Cysts Treated with Sterotactic Surgery

Feature	Hyperdense colloid cysts (n = 29)	Isodense/hypodense colloid cysts (n = 8)
Cyst volume, mean (median) ± SD	1.6 (0.9) ± 1.6 ml	3.3 (2.2) ± 3.6
Total aspiration	12 patients	6 patients
Partial aspiration (≥50%)	10 patients	2 patients
Unchanged	7 patients	–

*SD, standard deviation.

or temporary block of the foramen of Monro. Experience suggests that preoperative CT findings, such as density and volume, are indicators predicting the feasibility of aspiration.[17] Recurrence is rare, even after incomplete stereotactic aspiration. Despite a long follow-up (even up to 12 years), only 2 patients had recurrence. Successful aspiration in the 4 patients with subsequent relief without any morbidity or mortality proves the simplicity and easy repeatability of the procedure. Because colloid cysts seem to grow slowly, a single procedure seems to provide definitive cure for patients with follow-up as long as 12 years. Theoretical objections have been made to CT-guided stereotactic aspiration on the grounds of risks of hemorrhage, seizures, reaccumulation, and spilled contents provoking chemical ventriculitis and secondary aqueductal stenosis. The present series refutes these claims. The patients in our series experienced no mortality or significant morbidity. Even those with partially evacuated cysts did not have chemical ventriculitis or secondary aqueductal stenosis.

Therefore, we conclude that stereotactic aspiration is effective and can be the primary and definitive curative procedure for most patients with colloid cysts. This suggestion is also valid when considering the cost-effectiveness of treatment. Stereotactic aspiration is carried out under local anesthesia, and requires a minimum of manpower and resources compared to that needed for open surgery. The open microsurgical approach is recommended only for those patients in whom aspiration is not feasible or is likely to be grossly incomplete. Many neurosurgeons still consider the stereotactic technique "nonsurgical." The belief of most neurosurgeons who are not yet ready to give up the exquisite surgical delight of exposing and removing a colloid cyst of the third ventricle is not in the best interest of the patient and is ethically unacceptable.[26] A controlled trial proving the efficacy of both methods should be carried out before sides are drawn between those who are sure a procedure offers exquisite surgical delight and those who are offering an atraumatic and cost-effective alternative.

Approaches to Colloid Cysts: Transcranial vs. Stereotactic

Isao Yamamoto, M.D.

Colloid cysts of the third ventricle represent between 0.3% and 2.7% of all intracranial tumors.[13] With the advances in modern imaging techniques, however, this benign lesion is now diagnosed with increasing frequency. These lesions appear in patients of any age group, but mostly in those between the ages of 30 and 50 years.[27] Although Nitta and Symon[22] reported a male-to-female ratio of 2.5:1, these tumors usually have no sexual predominance. Ibrahim and colleagues[15] described the case of an exceptional occurrence in identical twins.

Since Dandy[9] first successfully removed a colloid cyst in 1921, various surgical approaches have been used for these lesions. However, the ideal surgical treatment of colloid cysts remains controversial.

The illustrative case is a 35-year-old, right-handed man presenting with a headache resulting from increased intracranial pressure. In this symptomatic patient with a colloid cyst of the third ventricle, 3 treatments may be considered: the placement of a ventricular shunt, excision through a transcallosal or transcortical approach, and removal through a stereotactic approach.

VENTRICULAR SHUNT

The clinical course of a colloid cyst is rather variable; some patients experience symptoms for more than 20 years, whereas others may suddenly deteriorate and die. Camacho and associates[7] described the nonsurgical treatment of 24 symptomatic patients with colloid cysts at a mean follow-up period of 19.3 months. Of these patients, 71% had a normal ventricular size. However, Little and MacCarty[20] reported that sudden death in patients with colloid cysts was thought to occur in up to 10% of cases. Ryder and associates[28] speculated that ventricular enlargement might disturb the hypothalamus-mediated cardiovascular control to cause sudden deterioration and death in patients with colloid cysts of the third ventricle. Therefore, the use of a palliative method of placing a shunt in the lateral ventricles is justified and the surgical results of this conservative approach are relatively good. Nonetheless, patients were left at risk of progressive effects of local tumor pressure, and the risks

associated with the placement of a ventricular shunt include shunt dependency, malfunction, and infection. Northfield[23] argued against shunting procedures on the grounds of a significant mortality rate because unsupported pressure within the cyst caused a relative increase in its size and subsequent acute damage to the diencephalon. For these reasons, a direct surgical approach has been generally preferred.

CYST EXCISION

Dandy[9] first successfully removed a colloid cyst using a frontal transcortical approach in 1921. If the ventricles are enlarged, a wide operative field is obtainable with a transcortical transventricular approach (Table 1). As the coronal magnetic resonance image in this case revealed an isodense round mass at the foramen of Monro with resulting hydrocephalus, the transcortical route through the right middle frontal gyrus is an easier approach. The main complication associated with the cortical incision is the development of seizures, the incidence of which varies from 0 to 10%.[1,13,20] Once the anterior horn is opened,

Table 1. The Transcortical Approach to Colloid Cysts

Advantages	Disadvantages
A wide operative field	Requires hydrocephalus
Ease of landmark identification	Poor visualization of ipsilateral third ventricular wall
Good visualization of ipsilateral foramen of Monro	Divides the cortex in the frontal region
Good visualization of contralateral third ventricular wall	
No need to sacrifice parasagittal cortical bridging veins	
Less chance of injuring the pericallosal artery	

anatomic landmarks such as thalamostriate, septal and caudate veins, the choroid plexus, and the foramen of Monro are better identified with this approach than the transcallosal one because of the enlarged ventricular cavity. The cyst wall is usually firm, smooth and greenish-blue or gray in color. Therefore, the cyst in this patient can probably be dissected from the adjacent neural structures without sacrificing any foraminal structures.

When a cyst itself is large or attached to the column of the fornix, thalamus, or choroid plexus, the contents of the cyst, which are usually jelly-like in consistency, are removed after the capsule is opened and then delivered through the foramen of Monro. During this procedure, care is taken to avoid traction or manipulation of the cyst's attachment at the tela choroidea adjacent to the foramen to avoid arterial or venous injury. The fact that the genu of the internal capsule touches the wall of the ventricle in the area lateral to the foramen of Monro near the anterior pole of the thalamus should be kept in mind. Little and MacCarty,[20] however, found that, in 6 of 21 patients in their series, the foramen of Monro needed to be enlarged to remove the cyst wall in the third ventricle. For this purpose, a number of surgical alternatives to enter the third ventricle are required.

Transforniceal Approach

When the exposure through the foramen of Monro is not adequate to visualize deeper portions of the anterior third ventricle, it is safe to incise the ipsilateral column of the fornix at the anterosuperior edge of the foramen. However, dividing the fornix on both sides should be avoided to prevent postoperative impairment of memory. Ehni[11] has noted that it is safer to enlarge the foramen of Monro to see within the third ventricle by removing a little of the anterior tuberculum of the thalamus than to divide a column of the fornix.

Subchoroidal Approach

The subchoroidal transvelum interpositum approach also gives access to the central portion of the third ventricle through an opening in the choroidal fissure by incising the tenia choroidea.[8,19] This approach, however, risks damage to the thalamus and vessels that pass through the thalamic side of the fissure by penetrating the tenia choroidea.[26]

Resecting the Thalamostriate Vein

To prevent the complications associated with sectioning the fornix, several authors[10,14,19] have reported cases in which the thalamostriate vein was interrupted at the posterior margin of the foramen of Monro to enlarge the opening into the third ventricle. The interruption of this vein was usually harmless because of the presence of connections between deep medullary and superficial subependymal venous systems, permitting transcerebral and subependymal anastomosis. However, some patients developed drowsiness, hemiplegia, and mutism. Hemorrhagic infarction of the basal ganglia has been reported after the ligation of the thalamostriate vein in treating a colloid cyst of the third ventricle.[22] Stein[30] noted that cautery of the choroid plexus and manipulation of the medial posterior choroidal arteries, in addition to the section of the thalamostriate vein, provide excellent exposure of the entire third ventricle.[8] The advantages of the transcortical approach are good visualization of the ipsilateral lateral ventricle and the contralateral third ventricular wall, compared with the view provided by the transcallosal route. On the contrary, the ipsilateral third ventricular wall offers a less satisfactory visual alignment.

Transcallosal Approach

The major advantage of the transcallosal approach[6,21] is that the foramen of Monro can be easily explored regardless of the ventricular size, and the distance to the foramen is shorter than that obtained transcortically without disruption of hemispheric tissue.[26,29] One of the disadvantages of this approach, however, is a risk of damage to the parasagittal cortical draining veins (Table 2). These draining veins anterior to the coronal suture can usually be sacrificed with impunity, but a large draining vein should be preserved whenever possible.[3] When both pericallosal arteries are identified, the callosal section, no more than 2 or 3 cm in length, is usually performed between these two arteries to avoid dividing penetrating branches going to either hemisphere. This short anterior callosal incision usually produces no long-term neurological or behavioral sequelae.[2] With a normal-sized ventricle, the corpus callosum is considerably thicker and the line of both bodies of fornices is often identified. In the presence of hydrocephalus, as in the patient described here, the corpus callosum is quite thin and the precise midline landmarks can seldom be defined. Therefore, the callosotomy should be done a little ipsilateral to the midline to avoid damage to both fornices. Once either the right or left lateral ventricle is entered, the operative principles are the same as described for the transcortical approach. With the transcallosal approach, other surgical alternatives to enter the third ventricle are required, such as the interforniceal, transchoroidal, or transseptal approach.

Interforniceal Approach

With normal ventricles, especially in the presence of a cavum septi pellucidum or septal leaves, the midline forniceal raphe is easily identified. At this time, the third ventricle can be entered directly by way of the midline exposure of the corpus callosum. Although this technique affords excellent visualization primarily of the anterior and mid-third ventricular cavity,[3] it is at times difficult to identify the forniceal raphe. Therefore, in many cases, the left rather than the right lateral ventricle may be entered on an approach from the right side. During the midline raphe incision, an attempt should be made not to incise beyond the region of the column-anterior commissure interface.[4]

Transchoroidal Approach

In the transchoroidal approach, the midportion of the third ventricle is exposed by dividing the tenia fornices from the choroid plexus and displacing the body of the fornix to the opposite side without damaging important vascular structures.[25]

Table 2. The Transcallosal Approach to Colloid Cysts

Advantages	Disadvantages
Ventricular size is irrelevant	Section of the anterior corpus callosum
Shorter transit to the diencephalic roof	Risks of bilateral forniceal damage
Largely extra-axial on the medial hemispheric surface	Difficulty in landmark identification
No disruption of hemispheric tissue	Risk of sacrifice of major parasagittal cortical bridging veins
Good visualization of both lateral walls of the third ventricle	

Transseptal Approach

When one can enter either the right or the left lateral ventricle through a midline callosal approach, the thalamostriate, septal and caudate veins, and the choroid plexus are seen to converge on the foramen of Monro. The septum pellucidum is then incised to expose the openings of the foramen of Monro into both lateral ventricles. At this stage, the interforaminal, transforniceal, transforaminal, or transchoroidal approach is selected to expose an appropriate part of the third ventricle.

In this illustrative case, either the transcortical or transcallosal approach could be expected to provide a satisfactory outcome. Although I personally prefer the transcallosal approach to deal with such a small colloid cyst, the selection of the appropriate direct approach should depend upon the surgeon's experience.

STEREOTACTIC APPROACH

Aspiration of the cyst contents has been done by free hand,[12] ventriculoscopy,[24] and the stereotactic technique.[5] Free-hand needle aspiration is more dangerous than the use of a precise stereotactic technique. The problems with ventriculoscopy are similar to those encountered in the transcortical approach, the necessity for cortical incision: limitation of exposure and applicability only in patients with hydrocephalus.[26] Since Bosch and colleagues[5] first performed a stereotactic aspiration of a cyst, CT-guided stereotactic techniques have become accurate and relatively safe. The advantage of this approach is that it can be employed even when the ventricles are small[7] (Table 3). Successful stereotactic aspiration, however, depends upon the viscosity of the cyst contents, the size of the cyst, and the penetration of the cyst wall.[18] If the cyst contents are thick and highly viscous, aspiration is unsuccessful or excessive suction may be required. Technical difficulties with cyst puncture are noted in lesions less than 1.0 ml in volume, not only because of the high

Table 3. Stereotactic Aspiration of Colloid Cysts

Advantages	*Disadvantages*
Less strain on the patient	Limited indication
Ventricular size is irrelevant	Danger of bleeding from
Avoidance of the callosal or	ventricular vessels
forniceal injury	Risk of recurrence
Minimal injury to the cerebral	
matter	

intracystic viscosity, but also because of the technical difficulties of proper cyst wall penetration in small cysts. If the cyst wall is not punctured by the cannula, this may distort the anatomy defined by stereotactic imaging techniques, then creating a possibility for injury to the surrounding important neurovascular structures of the foramen of Monro.[16] Although I have no experience with stereotactic puncture, based on the imaging findings of this patient, CT-guided cyst aspiration may be feasible as an initial procedure of choice.

Kelly and colleagues[17] recently described a stereotactic microsurgical laser craniotomy for the removal of a colloid cyst through the middle frontal gyrus or the superior frontal sulcal route with a 1.5-inch cranial trephine. Several rewards have been realized by coupling the benefits of stereotactic precision and localization to the microsurgical treatment of colloid cysts: (1) only a limited cortical incision is needed; (2) the hazards of callosal or forniceal injury can be avoided; (3) the lesion is easily localized regardless of ventricular size; (4) hemostasis can be readily achieved with bipolar cautery or defocused laser power; and (5) a total resection is possible with little risk to the patient.[1]

SUGGESTED READING AND REFERENCES

Michael L.J. Apuzzo, M.D.

1. Apuzzo MLJ: *Surgery of the Third Ventricle.* Baltimore, Williams and Wilkins, 1987.
2. Apuzzo MLJ, Litofsky NS: Surgery in and around the anterior third ventricle, in Apuzzo MLJ (ed): *Brain Surgery: Complication Avoidance and Management.* New York, Churchill Livingstone, 1993, pp 541–579.

Christoph B. Ostertag, M.D., and Friedrich W. Kreth, M.D.

1. Abernathey CD, Davis DH, Kelly PJ: Treatment of colloid cysts of the third ventricle by stereotaxic microsurgical laser craniotomy. *J Neurosurg* 1989; 70:525–529.
2. Antunes JL, Louis KM, Ganti SR: Colloid cysts of the third ventricle. *Neurosurgery* 1980; 7:450–455.
3. Bosch DA, Rahn T, Backlund EO: Treatment of colloid cysts of the third ventricle by stereotactic aspiration. *Surg Neurol* 1978; 9: 15–18.
4. Bullard DE, Osborne E, Cook WA: Colloid cysts of the third ventricle presenting as a ring-enhancing lesion on computed tomography. *Neurosurgery* 1982; 11:790–791.
5. Camacho A, Abernathey CD, Kelly PJ, et al.: Colloid cysts: Experience with the management of 84 cases since the introduction of computed tomography. *Neurosurgery* 1989; 24:693–700.
6. Chan RC, Thompson GB: Third ventricular colloid cysts presenting with acute neurological deterioration. *Surg Neurol* 1983; 19:358–362.
7. Ciric I, Zivin I: Neuroepithelial (colloid) cysts of the septum pellucidum. *J Neurosurg* 1975; 43:69–73.
8. Dandy WE: *Benign Tumors of the Third Ventricle: Diagnosis and Treatment.* Springfield, Charles C. Thomas, 1933.
9. Donauer E, Moringlane JR, Ostertag CB: Colloid cysts of the third ventricle: Open operative approach or stereotactic aspiration? *Acta Neurochir (Wien)* 1986; 83:24–30.
10. Ganti SR, Antunes JL, Louis KM, et al.: Computed tomography in the diagnosis of colloid cysts of the third ventricle. *Radiology* 1981; 138:385–391.
11. Gardner WJ, Turner M: Neuroepithelial cysts of the third ventricle. *Arch Neurol Psychol* 1937; 38:1055–1061.
12. Greenwood J: Paraphyseal cysts of the third ventricle. *J Neurosurg* 1949; 6:153–159.
13. Guner M, Shaw MDM, Tuner JW, et al.: Computed tomography in the diagnosis of colloid cysts. *Surg Neurol* 1976; 6:345–348.

14. Gutierrez-Lara F, Patino R, Hakim S: Treatment of tumors of the third ventricle: A new and simple technique. *Surg Neurol* 1975; 3: 323–325.

15. Jeeves MA, Simpson DA, Geffen G: Functional consequences of the transcallosal removal of intraventricular tumors. *J Neurol Psychiatry* 1979; 42:134–142.

16. Kelly R: Colloid cysts of the third ventricle. *Brain* 1951; 74:23–65.

17. Kondziolka D, Lunsford LD: Stereotactic management of colloid cysts: Factors predicting success. *J Neurosurg* 1991; 75:45–51.

18. Little JR, MacCarty SC: Colloid cysts of the third ventricle. *J Neurosurg* 1974; 39:230–235.

19. McKissock W: The surgical treatment of colloid cysts of the third ventricle. *Brain* 1951; 74:18.

20. Mohadjer M, Teshmar E, Mundinger F: CT-sterotaxic drainage of colloid cysts in the foramen of Monro and the third ventricle. *J Neurosurg* 1987; 67:220–223.

21. Moringlane JR, Lippitz B, Ostertag CB: Cerebral angiography under stereotaxic conditions. *Acta Neurochir (Wien)* 1988; 91: 147–150.

22. Mosberg WH, Blackwood W: Mucus secreting cells in colloid cysts of the third ventricle. *J Neuropathol Exp Neurol* 1954; 13:417–422.

23. Musolino A, Fosse S, Munari C, et al.: Diagnosis and treatment of colloid cysts of the third ventricle by stereotactic drainage: Report on 11 cases. *Surg Neurol* 1989; 32:294–299.

24. Nitta M, Symon L: Colloid cysts of the third ventricle: A review of 36 cases. *Acta Neurochir (Wien)* 1985; 76:99–104.

25. Ostertag CB: New head fixation for the Riechert stereotaxic system: Technical note. *Acta Neurochir (Wien)* 1985; 94:99–105.

26. Powell MP, Torrens MJ, Thomson JL, et al.: Isodense colloid cysts of the third ventricle: A diagnostic and therapeutic problem resolved by ventriculoscopy. *Neurosurgery* 1983; 13:234–237.

27. Rivas JJ, Lobato RD: CT assisted stereotaxic aspiration of colloid cysts of the third ventricle. *J Neurosurg* 1985; 62:238–242.

28. Roosen N, Gahlen D, Stork W, et al.: Magnetic resonance imaging of colloid cysts of the third ventricle. *Neuroradiology* 1987; 29: 10–14.

29. Sackett JF, Messina AV, Petito CK: Computed tomography and magnification vertebral angiotomography in the diagnosis of colloid cysts of the third ventricle. *Radiology* 1975; 116:95–100.

30. Shucart WA, Stein BM: Transcallosal approach to the anterior ventricular system. *Neurosurgery* 1978; 3:339–343.

31. Yenermen MH, Bowerman CI, Haymaker W: Colloid cyst of the third ventricle: A clinical study of 54 cases in the light of previous publications. *Acta Neurosurg (Wien)* 1958; 17:211–277.

Isao Yamamoto, M.D.

1. Abernathey CD, Davis DH, Kelley PJ: Treatment of colloid cysts of the third ventricle by stereotaxic microsurgical laser craniotomy. *J Neurosurg* 1989; 70:525–552.

2. Antunes JL, Louis KM, Ganti SR: Colloid cysts of the third ventricle. *Neurosurgery* 1980; 7:450–455.

3. Apuzzo MLJ, Chikovani OK, Gott PS, et al.: Transcallosal interforniceal approaches for lesions affecting the third ventricle: Surgical considerations and consequences. *Neurosurgery* 1982; 10:547–554.

4. Apuzzo MLJ, Giannotta SL: Transcallosal interforniceal approach, in Apuzzo MLJ (ed): *Surgery of the Third Ventricle*. Baltimore, Williams & Wilkins, 1987, pp 354–380.

5. Bosch DA, Rahn T, Backlund EO: Treatment of colloid cysts of the third ventricle by streotactic aspiration. *Surg Neurol* 1978; 9:15–18.

6. Busch E: A new approach for the removal of tumors of the third ventricle. *Acta Psychiatr Scand* 1944; 19:57–60.

7. Camacho A, Abernathey CD, Kelly PJ: Colloid cysts: Experience with the management of 84 cases since the introduction of computed tomography. *Neurosurgery* 1989; 24:693–700.

8. Cossu M, Lubinu F, Orunesu G, et al.: Subchoroidal approach to the third ventricle: Microsurgical anatomy. *Surg Neurol* 1984; 21:325–331.

9. Dandy WE: *Benign Tumors of the Third Ventricle. Diagnosis and Treatment*. Springfield, Charles C. Thomas, 1933.

10. Deladsheer J, Guyot J, Jomin M, et al.: Acces au troisieme ventricule par voie inter-thalamo-trigonale. *Neurochirurgie* 1978; 24: 419–422.

11. Ehni G: Interhemispheric and pericallosal (transcallosal) approach to the cingulate gyri, intraventricular shunt tubes, and certain deep placed brain lesions. *Neurosurgery* 1984; 14:99–110.

12. Gutierrez-Lara F, Patino R, Hakim S: Treatment of tumors of the third ventricle: A new and simple technique. *Surg Neurol* 1975; 3: 323–325.

13. Hall WA, Lunsford LD: Changing concepts in the treatment of colloid cyst. An 11-year experience in the CT era. *J Neurosurg* 1987; 66:186–191.

14. Hirsch J, Zouaoui A, Reiner D, et al.: A new surgical approach to the third ventricle with interruption of the striothalamic vein. *Acta Neurochir (Wien)* 1979; 47:135–147.

15. Ibrahim AWM, Farag H, Naguib M, et al.: Neuroepithelial (colloid) cyst of the third ventricle in identical twins. *J Neurosurg* 1986; 65:401–403.

16. Kelly PJ: Nonglial mass lesions, in Kelly PJ (ed): *Tumor Stereotaxis*. Philadelphia, WB Saunders, 1991, pp 358–386.

17. Kelly PJ, Alker GJ, Goerss S: Computer-assisted sterotactic laser microsurgery for the treatment for the intracranial neoplasms. *Neurosurgery* 1982; 10:324–331.

18. Kondziolka D, Lundsford LD: Stereotactic management of colloid cysts: Factors predicting success. *J Neurosurg* 1991; 75:45–51.

19. Lavyne MH, Patterson RH: Subchoroidal trans-velum interpositum approach to mid-third ventricular tumors. *Neurosurgery* 1983; 12: 86–94.

20. Little JR, MacCarty CS: Colloid cysts of the third ventricle. *J Neurosurg* 1974; 39:230–235.

21. Milhorat TH, Baldwin M: A technique for surgical exposure of the cerebral midline: Experimental transcallosal microdissection. *J Neurosurg* 1966; 24:687–691.

22. Nitta M, Symon L: Colloid cysts of the third ventricle: A review of 36 cases. *Acta Neurochir (Wien)* 1985; 76:99–104.

23. Northfield DWC: *The Surgery of the Central Nervous System*. London, Blackwell Scientific Publication, 1973, pp 206–210.

24. Powell MP, Torrens MJ, Thomson JL, et al.: Isodense colloid cysts of the third ventricle: A diagnostic and therapeutic problem resolved by ventriculoscopy. *Neurosurgery* 1983; 13:234–237.

25. Rhoton AL, Yamamoto I, Peace DA: Microsurgery of the third ventricle: Part 2. Operative approaches. *Neurosurgery* 1981; 8: 357–373.

26. Rhoton AL: Microsurgical anatomy of the lateral ventricle, in Wilkins RH, Rengachary SS (eds): *Neurosurgery Update I. Diagnosis, Operative Technique and Neuro-oncology*. New York, McGraw-Hill, 1990, pp 354–368.

27. Russel DS, Rubinstein LJ (eds): *Pathology of Tumours of the Nervous System*, ed. 5. London, Edward Arnold, 1989.

28. Ryder JW, Kleinschmidt-DeMasters BK, Keller T: Sudden deterioration and death in patients with benign tumors of the third ventricle area. *J Neurosurg* 1986; 64:216–223.

29. Shucart WA, Stein BM: Transcallosal approach to the anterior ventricular system. *Neurosurgery* 1978; 3:339–343.

30. Stein BM: Transcallosal approach to tumors of the third ventricle, in Schmidek HH, Sweet WH (eds): *Operative Neurosurgical Techniques: Indication, Methods and Results*, vol 1. New York, Grune & Stratton, 1988, pp 381–387.

5

Surgical Approaches to Pineal Tumors

CASE

A 20-year-old girl came to medical attention with headaches. A physical examination revealed Parinaud's syndrome.

PARTICIPANTS

The Infratentorial Supracerebellar Approach to Pineal Tumors–Jeffrey Bruce, M.D.

The Supratentorial Three-Quarters Prone Approach to Pineal Tumors–Jacques Brotchi, M.D.

Moderator–Kintomo Takakura, M.D.

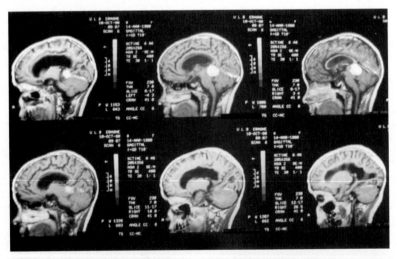

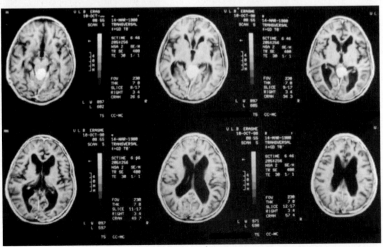

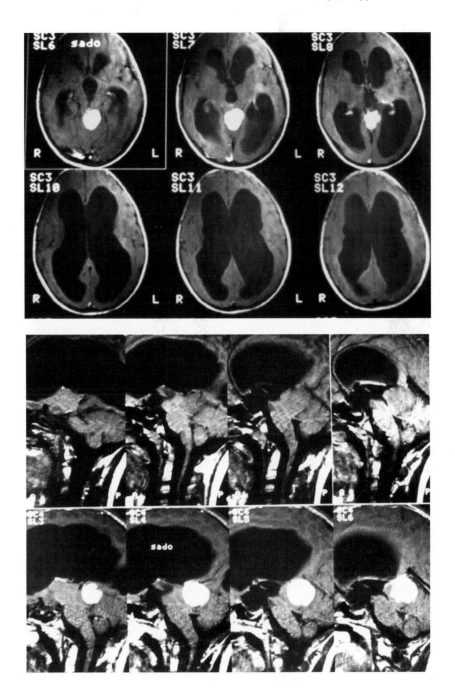

The Infratentorial Supracerebellar Approach to Pineal Tumors

Jeffrey Bruce, M.D.

The central principles governing the treatment of patients with pineal region tumors are derived from the histological diversity of these neoplasms and the prominent role of surgery in their diagnosis and treatment. A wide spectrum of pathologic entities can be found in the pineal region, ranging along a continuum of benign to highly malignant tumors, in addition to numerous cysts and non-neoplastic vascular lesions.[3] This spectrum is further complicated by the high incidence of tumors that are of a mixed-cell variety. Because of this diversity, an accurate determination of a tumor's histopathology is essential for guiding patient treatment. Open surgery, as opposed to stereotactic biopsy, provides the best method for obtaining a tumor specimen of sufficient quantity to maximize the diagnostic accuracy.[7,19] Furthermore, nearly one third of all pineal lesions are benign and curable with surgery alone, and a significant percentage of malignant tumors can be completely resected or significantly debulked to improve their response to adjuvant therapy.[3,12,19]

The patient in this case study has advanced hydrocephalus secondary to obstruction of third ventricle outflow resulting from a pineal region mass. The mass enhances homogeneously with gadolinium and, rather than extending anteriorly into the third ventricle like most tumors in the pineal region, it extends posteriorly into the posterior fossa, compressing the quadrigeminal plate and anterior vermis of the cerebellum. The veins of the deep venous system, seen best on the sagittal view, lie dorsal to the mass. A small portion of the anterior tumor border on the right is indistinct, suggesting the possibility that it is an exophytic tumor from the brain stem or that it may be locally invasive. As explained later, these radiographic features have important implications for differential diagnosis as well as for choosing the best operative approach to the tumor.

TREATING THE HYDROCEPHALUS

Before any consideration is given to surgically approaching this lesion, the hydrocephalus must be addressed. Because of the acute symptomatic presentation of hydrocephalus, the patient should undergo placement of a right ventriculoperitoneal shunt immediately. Once the shunt has been placed, definitive surgery for the tumor can be delayed for a few days, or even weeks, to allow gradual decompression of the ventricles. Although shunt placement is associated with some risk of abdominal seeding in the setting of a malignant pineal tumor, in my experience this happens rarely.[9] I would, therefore, not use a shunt filter because it would increase the risk of shunt malfunction.[7] On the rare occasions when a patient presents with insidious symptoms from a small pineal tumor and long-standing or minimally symptomatic hydrocephalus, a decision can be made to place a ventricular drain at the time of surgery.[2] If the tumor is completely removed at surgery, thereby relieving the hydrocephalus, then the ventricular drain can be removed after 2 or 3 days, avoiding the problems of a permanent shunt.

During shunt placement, cerebrospinal fluid should be obtained for cytological examination and analysis of the alpha fetoprotein and beta-HCG tumor markers.[1,17] Beta-HCG and alpha fetoprotein levels may also be measured in the serum, but cerebrospinal fluid measurements are more sensitive. Elevation of either of these markers occurs in the presence of malignant germ cell tumors.

DIFFERENTIAL DIAGNOSIS

Most tumors in the pineal region fall within 3 categories: germ-cell tumors, pineal-cell tumors, and glial-cell tumors. Because germ-cell tumors of the pineal region rarely occur in female patients, the most likely differential diagnosis in this patient includes a pineal-cell tumor, such as a pineocytoma or pineoblastoma, or a glial-cell tumor, such as an astrocytoma, glioblastoma, or ganglioglioma. The fact that this tumor appears to be either arising in the vermis of the cerebellum or exophytic from the quadrigeminal plate supports the glial-cell diagnosis. The radiographic suggestion of infiltration is indicative of both pineal and glial-cell tumors. Other types of enhancing masses to be considered include hemangioblastoma, choroid plexus papilloma, and meningioma, although these are encapsulated and are less common, particularly in this age group. Despite increased experience and advances in radiographic imaging, one cannot accurately predict the histology of a pineal-region tumor preoperatively.[1,8,21] A tissue specimen is essential to guide subsequent therapy.[3,6,7,10,19]

CHOOSING SURGERY

Although computed tomography (CT)-guided stereotactic biopsy has been advocated by some as an alternative for obtaining tumor tissue, I nearly always prefer an open resection for several reasons:

1. One third of pineal tumors, including nearly all benign tumors, can be totally resected and cured with surgery alone. In patients with malignant tumors, aggressive surgical resection can often result in a gross total removal or significant debulking to improve the response to adjuvant therapy.[3,12,16,19]

2. The wide variety of tumor types that occur in the pineal region makes histological analysis by even an experienced pathologist very difficult.[3,4,7] Many tumors are heterogeneous and contain mixed cell types so that the small specimens provided by stereotactic biopsy run a high risk of sampling error.[5,11]

3. There are risks due to hemorrhage within the tumor, as well as potential damage to the confluence of the deep venous system adjacent to the tumor. These risks are best controlled with open surgery.[14,15]

CHOOSING THE APPROACH

The pineal region can be approached either supratentorially or infratentorially.[1] The supratentorial approach has 2 major variations, the transcallosal interhemispheric approach and the occipital transtentorial approach. I generally prefer the infratentorial supracerebellar approach in the sitting-slouch position and would recommend it specifically for this patient.[18] The location of this tumor gives the infratentorial supracerebellar approach several natural advantages.[20] The tumor is in the midline and lies mostly in the infratentorial space, having extended into the posterior fossa rather than into the third ventricle. The supracerebellar infratentorial approach provides a more direct central trajectory to the mass and specifically avoids the inconvenience of working around the deep venous system that usually (as in this case) lies dorsally. The sitting-slouch position allows gravity to assist in the dissection. Furthermore, minimal brain retraction is needed, unlike the supratentorial approaches in which significant parietal or occipital retraction is required.[4] The supratentorial approaches also require the division of bridging veins between the medial hemisphere and the sagittal sinus. This combination of brain retraction and venous interruption can cause neurological deficits. I generally reserve the supratentorial approaches for several situations:

1. Tumors that are large and extend laterally to the trigone of the lateral ventricle,
2. tumors that have a significant extension supratentorially,
3. tumors that are located dorsal to the deep venous system, such as meningiomas.

I generally reserve stereotactic biopsies for patients with an unstable medical condition or who have evidence of metastatic disease at the time of diagnosis.

SURGICAL PROCEDURE

The infratentorial supracerebellar approach can be performed with the patient in the sitting-slouch position, prone in the Concorde position, or in the lateral position.[1] I generally prefer the sitting-slouch position because it enables gravity to work in the surgeon's favor. Blood pooling in the operative field is minimized and gravity aids in dissecting the tumor from the roof of the third ventricle. Although the sitting position carries a risk of air embolus, subdural hematoma, or air from cortical collapse, this is rarely a source of significant morbidity.[4]

For the infratentorial supracerebellar approach in the sitting-slouch position, the patient's head is flexed and the body should assume a C-shaped configuration to place the tentorium as closely horizontal as possible.[2,4] A suboccipital craniectomy or craniotomy is done through a midline incision extending just above the transverse sinus and torcula without opening the foramen magnum. The dura is opened in a semicircular fashion, extending from the most lateral portion of the craniectomy at the lateral sinus. The bridging veins between the cerebellum

and the tentorium are cauterized and divided, allowing the cerebellum to drop downward with gravity. A retractor is placed on the cerebellum, retracting it inferiorly and posteriorly. Opening the arachnoid overlying the tumor exposes the precentral cerebellar vein, which is cauterized and divided. The dorsal surface of the tumor can then be visualized. A variety of techniques can be used for tumor removal, depending on the consistency of the tumor, including large-bore variable suctions, laser, ultrasonic aspirators, or sharp dissection and pituitary forceps. Following internal decompression, the tumor is gradually dissected from the surrounding structures. The entrance into the third ventricle serves as a convenient anatomic landmark. For additional insurance against blockage of cerebrospinal fluid pathways, the infratentorial supracerebellar approach allows the surgeon to leave a ventricular catheter in the third ventricle anchored in the cisterna magna to act as an internal shunt. After this, the dura is closed as completely as possible. Recently, I have observed fewer postoperative inflammatory complications when a craniotomy with replacement of the bone flap has been done rather than a craniectomy.

Further treatment depends upon the histological diagnosis of the tumor. Patients with malignant tumors require radiation therapy.[1,17] Chemotherapy is reserved for nongerminomatous malignant germ-cell tumors.[1] If the tumor is an ependymoma, pineal-cell tumor, or malignant germ-cell tumor, a complete spinal magnetic resonance image with contrast is done to detect metastasis. Spinal radiation is given only when metastases are present radiographically, and is not given prophylactically.[3,7,13]

RESULTS

Based on my experience with 150 patients undergoing surgery of the pineal region, an excellent outcome can be expected in more than 90% of patients.[19] Most operative morbidity is transient, and related to minor dysfunction of extraocular movement.[4] Operative mortality is about 4%, with permanent major morbidity about 3%. A complete resection can be expected in 40 to 50% of cases. When a benign tumor is present, surgical resection results in a nearly 100% cure rate. With malignant tumors, I believe some correlation exists with improved prognosis when a gross total removal is accomplished.

The Supratentorial Three-Quarters Prone Approach to Pineal Tumors

Jacques Brotchi, M.D.

In this 20-year-old girl with acute hydrocephalus secondary to a pineal tumor, I would first treat the hydrocephalus with a ventriculoperitoneal shunt. The shunt allows us several days to get the serum and cerebrospinal fluid markers to approach the diagnosis. If there is any doubt about the diagnosis, I recommend a biopsy, even if a magnetic resonance image with strong gadolinium enhancement in a 20-year-old girl favors the diagnosis of a dysgerminoma. One must remember that the markers are not specific for dysgerminomas and, in my experience, determining the tumor's histological process is mandatory. I am not in favor of radiotherapy first, without diagnostic certainty, particularly in a child. The final diagnosis may be an uncommon tumor in that area, for example, a ganglioglioma, which is nonresponsive to radiotherapy; this illustrates the need to deter-

mine the tumor's histological process. A biopsy may be done through a stereotactic procedure or a direct approach, which is the best decision whenever one thinks that the tumor can be extirpated. In this patient, the magnetic resonance image shows a well-defined lesion located in the pineal area and quadrigeminal plate, with no infiltration of the walls of the third ventricle. I would take a direct approach in such a patient.

SURGICAL ROUTES

Many surgical routes have been proposed for tumors in the pineal region, the transcallosal,[5] occipital-transtentorial,[1,4,6,9,10,11] and infratentorial supracerebellar.[7,8,14] Several positions have been recommended, the sitting,[6,8,9,11,14] prone,[13] Concorde,[7] and three-quarters prone.[1,4,10,15] This variety of recommendations probably stems from the difficult surgical access. Some authors[12] already have compared infratentorial to supratentorial approaches. After having used all of these approaches and positions, I recommend the three-quarters prone position with the operative side down. In contrast with the first descriptions of this approach,[1,4,10] we have simplified the technique.[2,3]

Operative Details

The patient is placed in the three-quarters prone position, lying on the side on which surgery is done. The patient's head is tilted up at a 30-degree angle to the upper shoulder, moderately flexed, and turned to a 30-degree angle with the horizontal plane. The operating table is kept horizontal and may be rotated during surgery if one desires more or less head rotation. A parieto-occipital bone opening is made, 8 to 10 cm long (6 to 8 cm in children) and 4 cm wide, along the midline, which is not crossed, stopping 1 to 2 cm over the lateral sinus.

The dura is opened in a conventional horseshoe fashion, with the base on the superior sagittal sinus and preservation of the parieto-occipital parasagittal draining veins, which are not numerous in that area. Mannitol and furosemide are given at the beginning of the operation. When the hydrocephalus is not obstructive, a spinal drain should be placed. In this patient, I prefer a ventricular tap.

With the operative side down, the brain falls by gravity and may be slightly retracted without injury. The tentorium is then divided parallel to the straight sinus, 2 or 3 mm from it, giving an excellent view of the splenium, Galenic venous complex, quad-

rigeminal plate, and superior vermis after the arachnoid is removed. The tumor is now ready to be attacked. A smear biopsy is done first. If the tumor does not prove to be a dysgerminoma, we debulk the lesion with the ultrasonic aspirator and, under the microscope, we gently dissect it from all the vital structures met in that area. In the case of a ganglioglioma, we should be able to do a total resection. At the end of the procedure, the dura is closed in a watertight manner, the bone flap is replaced and wired in position, and the scalp is closed in two layers. In this patient, radiotherapy should not be necessary.

COMMENTS ON THE SURGICAL PROCEDURE USED

With the surgical table kept in a horizontal plane, the risk of air embolism encountered in the sitting position is avoided. The supracerebellar approach has been developed to avoid postoperative visual deficits resulting from the brain retraction in the supratentorial approach. In our experience, these deficits no longer occur because the operative side is kept down, taking advantage of gravity, which offers a wide operative corridor and eliminates the need for the sitting position.

In conclusion, the three-quarters prone position allows the surgeon comfort and good access to the posterior third ventricle, the superior vermis, and the brain stem. The venous complex may be easily protected, and there is no risk of air embolism or visual deficit. In this way, it is possible to have an overview on both sides, with the help of a retractor on the falx after the tentorium is divided. A right approach is generally recommended but, if necessary, an opening may be made on the left.

Surgical Approaches to Pineal Tumors:
The Infratentorial Supracerebellar vs. the Supratentorial Three-Quarters Prone Approach

Kintomo Takakura, M.D.

A variety of histologically different tumors develop in the pineal region. It is quite curious but evident that there is an epidemiological difference regarding the incidence of pineal-region tumors in different parts of the world. The incidence of pineal-region tumors verified by surgery in Japan[3] is shown in Table 1. The statistical data are quite accurate but different statistics come from North America or Europe.

TYPES OF PINEAL TUMORS

In male patients, 60.3% of all pineal tumors were germinomas. Benign teratomas constituted 9.7% and malignant germ-cell tumors (teratocarcinoma, choriocarcinoma, etc.) constituted 6.4%. On the other hand, gliomas and pineal parenchymal tumors (pineocytoma and pineoblastoma) composed only 5.2 and

Table 1. Incidence of Tumors in the Pineal Region in Patients in Japan

Diagnosis	Males	Females	Total
Germinoma	430 (60.3%)	43 (33.3%)	473 (56.2%)
Teratoma	69 (9.7%)	4 (3.1%)	73 (8.7%)
Malignant teratoma	36 (5.0%	3 (2.3%)	39 (4.6%)
Choriocarcinoma	10 (1.4%)	1 (8.8%)	11 (1.3%)
Dermoid	5 (0.7%)	0 (0.0%)	5 (0.6%)
Epidermoid	10 (1.4%)	3 (2.3%)	13 (1.5%)
Pineocytoma	20 (2.8%)	11 (8.5%)	31 (3.7%)
Pineoblastoma	21 (2.9%)	10 (7.8%)	31 (3.7%)
Glioma	37 (5.2%)	32 (24.8%)	69 (8.2%)
Others	75 (10.5%)	20 (15.5%)	95 (11.3%)
Total	713 (100.0%)	127 (100.0%)	840 (100.0%)

5.7%, respectively. In female patients, the incidence of germinoma was only one tenth of that in males and it constituted one third of all pineal tumors. Teratomas and malignant germ-cell tumors in the pineal region were quite rare, while gliomas and pineal parenchymal tumors were more common in females, constituting 24.8 and 8.5% of female tumors, respectively.

Intracranial germ-cell tumors are classified into 3 major histological categories: germinoma, teratoma, and malignant or anaplastic germ-cell tumors. However, mixed tumor types of those cellular components are quite commonly found in the pineal region. A pure germinoma has histological characteristics of the so-called two-cell pattern, which is composed of large round tumor cells and lymphocytes. A germinoma never secretes human beta-chorionic gonadotropin (beta-HCG). A pure teratoma is a benign tumor. On the contrary, malignant germ-cell tumors, such as choriocarcinoma, endodermal sinus tumor (yolk sac tumor), teratocarcinoma, and embryonal carcinoma, show several histologically different cellular components. Only trophoblastic cells of choriocarcinoma produce beta-HCG, and endodermal sinus tumors produce alpha fetoprotein. Some carcinomatous cells produce tumor marker proteins, such as carcinoembryonic antigen, CA-199, CA-125, and so on. In my opinion, the term *non-germinomatous germ-cell tumor* should not be used because such a tumor can be classified as a teratoma, a malignant germ-cell tumor or a mixed tumor.

A germinoma is quite sensitive to radiation and it is fully controlled by radiotherapy. Only disseminated cases require treatment with chemotherapy.[11] A pure germinoma can now be cured with radiotherapy. The historical improvement of long-term survival rates in Japan has clearly proved the efficacy of radiation[3] (Fig. 1). The 5-year survival rates with germinoma after surgical verification were 59% for patients treated during the years 1969 to 1973, 70.6% for those treated from 1974 to 1978, 85.2% for those treated from 1979 to 1983 and 100% for those treated from 1984 to 1987. Surgical mortalities (the death rate 1 month after surgery) were 10.5% (73 in 1989), 5.2% (78 in 1974), 3.1% (83 in 1979) and 3.2% (87 in 1984), respectively. These data suggest that all patients who survived longer than 1 month after surgical intervention have been cured by radiotherapy. All patients treated during the years 1984 to 1987 have survived well. These data also suggested that, if we can diagnose a pineal germinoma without surgical intervention, all patients can be cured with radiotherapy.

On the other hand, a teratoma can be treated only through surgical removal and malignant germ-cell tumors must be reduced in volume through surgery followed by radiation and chemotherapy.[4,11,14,15] The current, most effective chemotherapy might be cisplatin or carboplatin combined with etoposide, vinblastine, and bleomycin.[6,8,9,15]

Benign tumors, such as meningioma, dermoid, epidermoid, and pineocytoma, can be successfully treated through surgery. Falcotentorial meningiomas can be diagnosed through computed tomography (CT), magnetic resonance imaging (MRI) and, especially, through angiography. The surgical indication for an arachnoid cyst is determined by the patient's clinical signs and symptoms. Arachnoid cysts in some of my patients have shown no enlargement for many years, even with careful follow-up using MRI.

Gliomas in the pineal region infiltrate into parenchymal tissue. The tumor generally shows some heterogeneity of density on CT and intensity on MRI. The tumor border is not sharply demarcated and has an irregular shape. However, the type of glioma cannot be diagnosed without histological examination. Gliomas and pineal parenchymal tumors are treated through

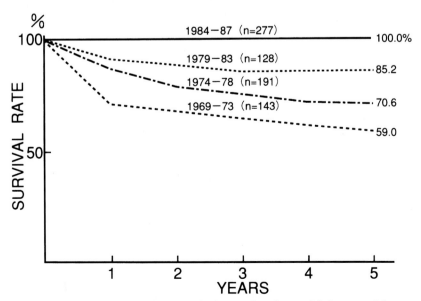

Fig. 1 Historical improvement of the survival rate of patients with intracranial germinoma; all tumors were verified by surgery and all patients underwent postoperative radiosurgery (data from the Brain Tumor Registry of Japan, 1993[3]).

surgery and chemo- or radiotherapy[13] in the same way as gliomas in other parts of the brain.

METHODS OF DIAGNOSIS

Recent imaging diagnosis by CT and MRI is quite accurate and provides much information not only about the morphological structure, but also about the tumor's size, shape, homogeneity, infiltration to adjacent brain tissue, and even some histological characteristics of the tissues. Although a variety of histologically different tumors develop in the pineal region, the histological diagnosis can be established fairly well by the images, as well as the age and sex of the patient and tumor-marker studies of the serum or cerebrospinal fluid. Non-neoplastic lesions, such as arachnoid cysts, can also be differentiated almost definitively with MRI. A pure germinoma is round or oval, with a clearly demarcated smooth border and homogeneous density on CT scans or intensity on MRI, extending into the third ventricle, and never infiltrating the adjacent brain parenchymal tissue or demonstrating cystic imaging. Almost all pineal germinomas develop in boys or young men. If the morphological figure of the tumor on CT or MRI does not show a typical germinoma pattern, the accurate diagnosis requires histological verification. In such cases, I always do open surgery because it is performed quite safely today under the microscope. Enough tumor tissue can be obtained for histological diagnosis and the tumor can be removed radically. The reduction of the tumor mass can provide better response to radio- and chemotherapy, if it is required, bringing a better prognosis. On the other hand, stereotactic biopsy in this region still involves considerable risk of hemorrhage and not enough tissue can be obtained for histological examination because some pineal-region tumors have a heterogeneic nature.

DISCUSSION

This particular patient complained of headaches, and the physical examination revealed Parinaud's syndrome. CT scans and MRI show advanced hydrocephalus. Both experts recommend placement of a ventriculoperitoneal shunt for the initial stage of treatment. I agree with this procedure; the hydrocephalus appears to be advancing quite rapidly because of the obstruction of the aqueduct by the tumor. The seeding of tumor cells in the peritoneal cavity rarely occurs, except in patients with malignant germ-cell tumors. I agree with the author regarding this and would not use a shunt filter in this case.

On the CT scan and MRI, the tumor is round but the border is irregular and not clearly demarcated. The tumor extends mostly into the posterior fossa and not into the third ventricle. It compresses the cerebellar vermis and quadrigeminal plate. Although the tumor enhances homogeneously with gadolinium DTPA, the anterior border of the tumor is indistinct and invasive, as one of the authors realized. The tumor is possibly an exophytic tumor from the brain stem. Based on the findings on CT and MRI, as well as the age and sex of the patient, the diagnosis of glioma is most likely. I have an almost similar case of pineoblastoma in an infant, which showed the same pattern on CT and MRI.[13] No possibility of a germ-cell tumor is suspected, and the surgical verification of the histological diagnosis is required.

Both authors favor open surgery over stereotactic biopsy.[2,4,5,10] A major part of this tumor can be removed. They have, however, different opinions about the approach and the patient's position. One selected the occipital transtentorial approach[1] in the three-quarters prone position with the operative side down. The other selected the supracerebellar infratentorial approach[2,7,12] in the sitting-slouch position. Because of the location of the tumor, the supracerebellar infratentorial approach might be the most logical and recommendable for this patient. The merits of this approach are well described by the author. The sitting-slouch position might be recommendable for removing the tumor easily. I prefer the prone Concorde position, however, or a semilateral position to avoid any risk of air embolism. On the other hand, the tumor can also be removed through the occipital transtentorial approach, if the surgeon is accustomed to this avenue; there is no complication caused by air embolism in this approach.

When the histological diagnosis of this tumor is malignant glioma, such as a glioblastoma, anaplastic astrocytoma, or pineoblastoma, postoperative radiotherapy and chemotherapy are generally required. A ganglioglioma, which is described by one of the authors, is quite rare in the pineal region. Ganglioglioma is a well-differentiated tumor and the prognosis is fairly good when the tumor is radically removed. The efficacy of conventional radiotherapy and chemotherapy for this tumor has not been analyzed in detail. In this case, the portion of the tumor infiltrating the quadrigeminal plate might not be removable. Chemo- or radiotherapy for a general malignant glioma is indicated.

In conclusion, based on my experience, this pineal region tumor cannot be diagnosed as a germ-cell tumor based on the findings on CT and MRI and the age and sex of the patient. The most likely diagnosis is a malignant glioma. Histological examination and radical removal of the tumor through open surgery are recommended. A good outcome can be expected with radical surgical removal followed by radiotherapy and chemotherapy.

REFERENCES

Jeffrey Bruce, M.D.

1. Bruce JN: Management of pineal region tumors. *Neurosurg Q,* (in press).
2. Bruce JN, Stein BM: Infratentorial approach to pineal tumors, in Wilson CB (ed): *Neurosurgical Procedures: Personal Approaches to Classic Operations.* Baltimore, Williams and Wilkins, 1992, pp 63–76.
3. Bruce JN, Stein BM: Pineal tumors. *Neurosurg Clin North Am* 1990; 1:123–138.
4. Bruce JN, Stein BM: Supracerebellar approaches in the pineal region, in Apuzzo MLJ (ed): *Brain Surgery: Complication Avoidance and Management.* New York, Churchill Livingstone, 1993, pp 511–535.
5. Chandrasoma PT, Smith MM, Apuzzo MLJ: Stereotactic biopsy in the diagnosis of brain masses: Comparison of results of biopsy and resected surgical specimen. *Neurosurgery* 1989; 24:160–165.
6. Dempsey PK, Kondziolka D, Lunsford LD: Stereotactic diagnosis

and treatment of pineal region tumours and vascular malformations. *Acta Neurochir (Wien)* 1992; 116:14–22.

7. Edwards MSB, Hudgins RJ, Wilson CB, et al.: Pineal region tumors in children. *J Neurosurg* 1988; 68:689–697.

8. Ganti SR, Hilal SK, Stein BM, et al.: CT of pineal region tumors. *AJNR* 1986; 7:97–104.

9. Hoffman HJ, Yoshida M, Becker LE, et al.: Pineal region tumors in childhood: Experience at the Hospital for Sick Children, in Humphreys RP (ed): *Concepts in Pediatric Neurosurgery*, vol. 4. Basel, S Karger, 1983, pp 360–386.

10. Jooma R, Kendall BE: Diagnosis and management of pineal tumors. *J Neurosurg* 1983; 58:654–665.

11. Kraichoke S, Cosgrove M, Chandrasoma PT: Granulomatous inflammation in pineal germinoma. *Am J Surg Pathol* 1988; 12: 655–660.

12. Lapras C, Patet JD: Controversies, techniques, and strategies for pineal tumor surgery, in Apuzzo MLJ (ed): *Surgery of the Third Ventricle*. Baltimore, Williams and Wilkins, 1987, pp 649–662.

13. Linstadt D, Wara WM, Edwards MS, et al.: Radiotherapy of primary intracranial germinomas: The case against routine craniospinal irradiation. *Int J Radiat Oncol Biol Phys* 1988; 15:291–297.

14. Pecker J, Scarabin JM, Vallee B, et al.: Treatment in tumours of the pineal region: Value of stereotaxic biopsy. *Surg Neurol* 1979; 12: 341–348.

15. Peragut JC, Dupard T, Graciani N, et al.: De la prevention des risques de la biopsie stereotaxique de certaines tumeurs de la region pineale. *Neurochir (Paris)* 1987; 33:23–27.

16. Sano K: Diagnosis and treatment of tumors in the pineal region. *Acta Neurochir (Wien)* 1976; 34:153–157.

17. Sawaya R, Hawley KD, Tobler WD, et al.: Pineal and third ventricle tumors, in Youmans JR (ed): *Neurological Surgery*. Philadelphia, WB Saunders, 1990, pp 3171–3203.

18. Stein BM: The infratentorial supracerebellar approach to pineal lesions. *J Neurosurg* 1971; 35:197–202.

19. Stein BM, Bruce JN: Surgical treatment of pineal region tumors. *Clin Neurosurg* 1992; 39:509–532.

20. Stein BM, Bruce JN, Fetell MR: Surgical approaches to pineal tumors, in RH Wilkins, Rengachary SS (eds): *Neurosurgery Update 1: Diagnosis, Operative Technique, and Neuro-oncology*. New York, McGraw-Hill, 1990, pp 389–390.

21. Tien RD, Barkovich AJ, Edwards MS: MR imaging of pineal tumors. *Am J Roentgenol* 1990; 155:143–151.

Jacques Brotchi, M.D.

1. Ausman JI, Malik GM, Dujovny M, et al.: Three-quarter prone approach to the pineal-tentorial region. *Surg Neurol* 1988; 29: 298–306.

2. Brotchi J, Levivier M, Raftopoulos C, et al.: Three-quarter prone approach to the pineal-tentorial region: Experience with seven cases. *Acta Neurochir* (Suppl) 1991; 53:144–147.

3. Brotchi J, Raftopoulos C, Levivier M, et al.: Lésions de la région pinéale et falco-tentorielle. *Neurochirurgie* 1991; 37:410–415.

4. Clark WK: Occipital transtentorial approach, in Apuzzo MLJ (ed): *Surgery of the Third Ventricle*. Baltimore, Williams and Wilkins, 1987, pp 591–610.

5. Dandy W: An operation for the removal of pineal tumors. *Surg Gynecol Obstet* 1921; 33:113–119.

6. Jamieson KG: Excision of pineal tumors. *J Neurosurg* 1971; 35:550–553.

7. Kobayashi S, Sugita K, Tanaka Y, et al.: Infratentorial approach to the pineal region in the prone position: Concorde position. *J Neurosurg* 1983; 58:141–143.

8. Krause F: Operative freilegug der vierhugel nebst beobachtunger über hirnbrisk und dekonpression. *Zentralbl Chir* 1926; 53:2812–2819.

9. Lapras C, Patet JD: Controversies, techniques, and strategies for pineal tumor surgery, in Apuzzo MLJ (ed): *Surgery of the Third Ventricle*. Baltimore, Williams and Wilkins, 1987, pp 649–662.

10. McComb JG, Apuzzo MLJ: Posterior intrahemispheric retrocallosal and transcallosal approaches, in Apuzzo MLJ (ed): *Surgery of the Third Ventricle*. Baltimore, Williams and Wilkins, 1987, pp 611–648.

11. Poppen JL: The right occipital approach to a pinealoma. *J Neurosurg* 1966; 25:706–710.

12. Reid NS, Clark WK: Comparison of the infratentorial and transtentorial approaches to the pineal region. *Neurosurgery* 1978; 3:1–8.

13. Sano K: Pineal region tumors: Problems in pathology treatment. *Clin Neurosurg* 1983; 30:59–91.

14. Stein BM: The infratentorial supracerebellar approach to pineal lesions. *J Neurosurg* 1971; 35:197–202.

15. Stone JL, Cybulski GR, Crowell RM, et al.: The lateral position-dependent occipital approach-to pineal and medial occipitoparietal lesions. *Acta Neurochir* 1990; 102:133–136.

Kintomo Takakura, M.D.

1. Apuzzo MLJ, Tung H: Supratentorial approaches to the pineal region, in Apuzzo MLJ (ed): *Brain Surgery: Complication Avoidance and Management*. New York, Churchill Livingstone, 1993, pp 451–486.

2. Bruce JN, Stein BM: Supracerebellar approaches in the pineal region, in Apuzzo MLJ (ed): *Brain Surgery: Complication Avoidance and Management*. New York, Churchill Livingstone, 1993, pp 511–535.

3. Committee of the Brain Tumor Registry of Japan: *Brain Tumor Registry of Japan*, Tokyo, National Cancer Center, 1993.

4. Edwards MSB, Hudgins RJ, Wilson CB, et al.: Pineal region tumors in children. *J Neurosurg* 1988; 68:689–697.

5. Hoffman HJ, Yoshida M, Becker LE, et al.: Pineal region tumors in childhood: Experience at the Hospital for Sick Children, in Humphreys RP (ed): *Concepts in Pediatric Neurosurgery*, vol. 4. Basel, S Karger, 1983, pp 360–386.

6. Kobayashi T, Yoshida J, Ishiyama J, et al.: Cisplatin and etoposide for malignant intracranial germ cell tumors. *J Neurosurg* 1989; 70: 676–681.

7. Lapras C, Patel JD: Controversies, techniques, and strategies for pineal tumor surgery, in Apuzzo MLJ (ed): *Surgery of the Third Ventricle*. Baltimore, Williams and Wilkins, 1987, pp 649–662.

8. Matsukado Y, Abe H, Tanaka R, et al.: Cisplatin, vinblastin, and belomycin (PVD) combination chemotherapy in the treatment of intracranial malignant germ cell tumors—a preliminary report of a phase II study—The Japanese Intracranial Germ Cell Tumor Study Group. *Gan No Rinsho (Jpn)* 1986; 32:1387–1393.

9. Neuwelt EA, Frenke EP: Germinomas and other pineal tumors: Chemotherapeutic responses, in Neuwelt EA (ed): *The Diagnosis and Treatment of Pineal Region Tumors*. Baltimore, Williams and Wilkins, 1984, pp 332–343.

10. Sano K: General considerations: 17 pineal region masses, in Apuzzo MLJ (ed): *Brain Surgery, Complication Avoidance and Management*. New York, Churchill Livingstone, 1993, pp 473–485.

11. Sawaya R, Hawley KD, Tobler WD, et al.: Pineal and third ventricle tumors, in Youmans JR (ed): *Neurological Surgery*. Philadelphia, WB Saunders, 1990, pp 3171–3203.

12. Stein BM: The infratentorial supracereberallar approach to pineal regions. *J Neurosurg* 1971; 35:197–202.

13. Takakura K, Matsutani M: Selection of an operative approach, in

Apuzzo MLJ (ed): *Brain Surgery: Complication Avoidance and Management*, New York, Churchill Livingstone, 1993, pp 473–485.

14. Takakura K, Matsutani M: Therapeutic modality selection in management of germ cell tumors, in Apuzzo MLJ (ed): *Surgery of the Third Ventricle*, Baltimore, Williams and Wilkins, 1987, pp 844–846.

15. Takakura K, Matsutani M, Shitara N: Diganosis and treatment of pineal region tumors, in Paoletti P, Takakura K, Walker M, et al. (eds): *Neuro-oncology*. Dordrecht, Kluwer Academic Publishers, 1991, pp 283–289.

6

Treatment of Intracranial Metastases:
Surgery vs. Radiosurgery

CASE

A 60-year-old man was diagnosed with adenocarcinoma of the lung 2 years ago. At that time, he had a lung lobectomy and radiation therapy. His systemic disease is stable. Recently, he developed headaches and mild paresis of the left arm. An MRI showed multiple lesions.

PARTICIPANTS

Surgical Treatment of Intracranial Metastases–Rajesh K. Bindal, M.D., Raymond Sawaya, M.D.

Radiosurgical Treatment of Intracranial Metastases–Eben Alexander III, M.D., Jay S. Loeffler, M.D.

Moderator–Dennis E. Bullard, M.D.

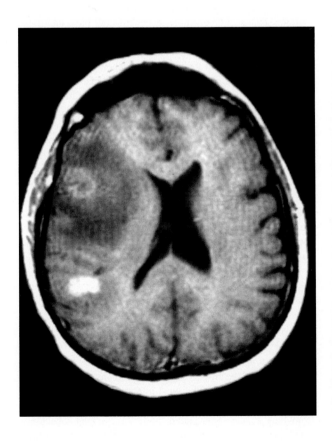 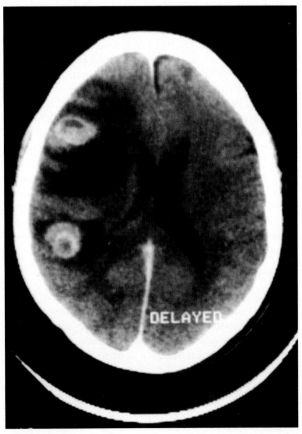

Surgical Treatment of Intracranial Metastases

Rajesh K. Bindal, M.D., Raymond Sawaya, M.D.

Metastatic brain tumors are the most common type of intracranial tumor, with an estimated incidence of 82,000 per year.[7] More than 50% of these tumors have a primary lesion in the lung. Furthermore, 72% of all patients who develop brain metastasis from adenocarcinoma of the lung have multiple lesions.[13] Thus, in many ways, this case is typical of a patient developing brain metastasis. However, the median interval for developing brain metastasis from lung cancer is 6 to 9 months.[11] This patient had an interval of 2 years.

HISTORICAL PERSPECTIVE

Surgery for the treatment of a single brain metastasis has been practiced for many years. Overall, early results of surgery were not very encouraging. Few investigators reported median survivals of more than 6 months.[5] These results were not significantly superior to the results of treatment with whole brain radiation therapy alone, which increased survival of 3 to 6 months, given the more selected nature of surgically treated patients.[4] Operative mortality was 10 to 40% and morbidity rates were also high.[9]

Since then, however, the results of surgery have improved dramatically. With the introduction of advances, such as the use of corticosteroids, the advent of computed tomography (CT) and magnetic resonance imaging (MRI), the operative microscope and ultrasound, stereotactic localization, and cortical mapping, operative mortality and morbidity rates have declined dramatically. This, coupled with the improved treatment of systemic cancer, has resulted in significantly improved survival for surgically treated patients. The first study of patients who all had a preoperative CT scan reported a median survival of 9 months.[8] Since then, reported survivals have generally ranged from 10 to 15 months.[3,6,10,12] Additionally, operative mortality and morbidity rates have both fallen to 3 to 5%.

In 1990, Patchell and colleagues[10] reported the results of a randomized trial comparing the use of surgery followed by whole-brain radiation therapy to the use of whole-brain radiation alone for treating patients with a single brain metastasis, limited systemic disease, and good neurological status. The results clearly support the use of surgery for these patients as the surgically treated patients survived 40 weeks, vs. 15 weeks for patients receiving radiation therapy alone (p <0.001). Surgery has been proven beyond doubt to be effective therapy for patients with a single accessible brain metastasis, limited systemic disease, and good neurological status.

MULTIPLE METASTASES

Many authors have indicated that the presence of multiple brain metastases is a strong contraindication to surgery. This is despite the fact that no study has ever specifically analyzed the role of surgery in the treatment of these patients. We recently evaluated the results of surgery for patients with multiple metastases at our institution.[3] This review indicated that surgery can play a very important role in treating these patients. Over a period of 8 years (1984 to 1992), 56 patients underwent surgery for multiple brain metastases. Thirty of these patients had one or more lesions remaining after surgery (Group A) and 26 had all lesions re-

moved (Group B). Those patients having all multiple lesions removed were matched with 26 patients undergoing surgery for a single lesion (Group C). Patients were matched by type of primary tumor, presence or absence of systemic disease, Karnofsky performance status, and time from first diagnosis of cancer to diagnosis of brain metastases. Median survival for patients in Group A was 6 months, for Group B was 14 months, and for Group C was 14 months. There was a significant difference in survival between both Groups A and B (p = 0.003) and Groups A and C (p = 0.012), but not between Groups B and C (p >0.5). Additionally, recurrence, morbidity, mortality, and neurological improvement rates were similar between Groups B and C. Furthermore, multiple craniotomies in a single operation were not associated with a higher per-craniotomy complication or 30-day mortality rates than a single craniotomy. This is important because the lesions in many patients with multiple lesions are located too far apart to be resected in a single craniotomy. This study indicated that surgery for patients with multiple metastatic lesions is just as effective as surgery for a single lesion if all metastases can be removed.

SELECTING PATIENTS

The selection of appropriate patients for surgical treatment depends on a number of factors. The status of the systemic disease is crucial in determining appropriate therapy. Most patients with brain metastasis have advanced, widespread, and uncontrolled systemic cancer. For example, a patient may have additional lung, liver, and bone metastases that are growing and spreading. These patients have a limited life expectancy and the goal of treatment is short-term palliation. They should be treated with whole-brain radiation therapy and corticosteroids, which usually provide adequate relief from symptoms for the duration of their expected survival. Patients with absent, controlled, or limited systemic cancer, such as the patient in this case, are considered for more aggressive therapy. In this category, those patients with especially radio- or chemosensitive tumors are generally treated with whole-brain radiation therapy or chemotherapy as appropriate. Metastases from small-cell lung cancer, lymphoma, and germ-cell tumors generally fall into this category. Unfortunately, adenocarcinoma of the lung is not a radio- or chemosensitive tumor. Patients with this lesion are carefully evaluated specifically with the goal of surgical excision in mind. The exact number and location of brain lesions is the most important factor in making this determination. This patient has 2 lesions, both easily accessible in a single craniotomy. The use of intraoperative ultrasound is appropriate to help localize the more deep-seated posterior lesion.

CASE DISCUSSION

This patient is without a doubt an excellent surgical candidate. He meets all of the criteria for classification as such. Treatment of the primary tumor is the most important factor determining survival of patients undergoing resection of brain metastasis from lung cancer. This patient underwent a lung lobectomy, which portends a good prognosis. The lack of other metastases and the patient's good neurological performance status are other favorable indicators. Surgical excision can be performed with operative morbidity rates of less than 5% and equivalent 30-day mortality rates. The median hospital stay after a craniotomy is 3 days. More than 80% of patients have improved Karnofsky scores after surgery. Local recurrence occurs in 15 to 20% of tumor beds.[3,10,11] This is in contrast to the 85 to 96% local control provided by radiosurgery.[2] The physician must remember, however, that local control in radiosurgery includes lesions that have merely stabilized in size, whereas local control in surgery requires no evidence of tumor in a treated bed at any time in a patient's life. Also, in many radiosurgery studies, the follow-up time is too limited to allow accurate determination of what fraction of treated lesions eventually fail.

Surgery provides a number of benefits over radiosurgery. First, very few patients remain steroid-dependent, whereas in radiosurgery, up to 27% of patients must be retained or restarted on steroids to control edema.[1] Second, relief of symptoms is often achieved quite rapidly after surgery but, in one radiosurgery study, only 42% of patients improved neurologically within the first 3 months.[2] Third, with surgery, tissue is available to confirm the diagnosis. In one study, 11% of patients with a previous cancer history and a brain lesion radiologically consistent with metastasis proved to have nonmetastatic diseases upon biopsy or resection; including those with gliomas and abscesses.[10] These lesions may require alternative treatment and would not be recognized without a biopsy.

We use radiosurgery to treat patients with brain metastasis at our institution; however, our use is largely limited to patients with surgically inaccessible lesions and those who refuse or cannot physically tolerate surgery. Although we find the results of radiosurgery encouraging, the fact that most reports contain small numbers of patients and relatively limited follow-up times deters us from using it as primary therapy for brain metastasis except in select instances.

Radiosurgical Treatment of Intracranial Metastases

Eben Alexander III, M.D., Jay S. Loeffler, M.D.

Metastases are the most common malignant tumors of the brain. More than 150,000 people in the United States (50% of all patients with cancer) develop metastatic disease to the brain from systemic cancer each year. Autopsy series have shown that up to 50% of patients dying of cancer will have intracerebral metastases, of which 40% are single lesions.[21] Untreated patients have a median survival of about a month, while patients treated with whole-brain radiotherapy have a median survival of 3 to 6 months, with most patients ultimately dying of systemic disease.[4,5,27] However, there exists a subset of patients who develop solitary brain metastasis as the only site of metastatic disease. The role of surgery in the treatment of these patients has been controversial, with uncontrolled retrospective studies showing conflicting results.[3,9,19,24] A recent study was completed in which patients with single metastatic lesions were randomized to surgery and postoperative whole-brain radiotherapy versus whole-brain radiotherapy alone.[20] The results of this study showed that recurrence at the site of the original metastasis was less frequent in the surgical group than in the radiation group (20% vs. 52%, p <0.02). The overall length of survival was significantly longer in the surgical group (median 40 weeks vs. 15 weeks in the radiation group, p <0.01), with a better quality of life than similar patients treated with radiotherapy alone. There is still a high recurrence rate for patients treated with either whole-brain radiotherapy alone and those treated with surgery and whole-brain radiotherapy, resulting in a difficult therapeutic dilemma. The use of systemic chemotherapy has added little to the treatment of these patients with recurrent disease of the central nervous system. Attempts have been made using conventional radiotherapy techniques to retreat selected patients with recurrent metastatic disease. In one recent study, 42% of patients responded to the second course of radiotherapy with neurological improvement of at least one functional level.[6]

FAVORABLE FEATURES OF METASTASES

The patient described here exemplifies the standard indications for radiosurgical treatment of metastatic lesions in the brain. The following features illustrate the main reasons that metastases are particularly well-suited to radiosurgical treatment:

1. Discrete, quasi-spherical lesions,
2. rarely infiltrating beyond radiographically-defined margins,[22,25]
3. preferably a size under 3 cm in maximum diameter,[23]
4. steep dose gradient allows dose escalation, enabling treatment of even the most radioresistant lesions,[16]
5. optimal margin coverage in spite of deep or critical location (surgical margins adequate only in noneloquent locations),
6. geometry of treatment is closely linked with radiographic images of three-dimensional lesion configuration,
7. no risk of hemorrhage, infection, or mechanical spread of tumor cells,
8. even high-dose single-fraction irradiation allows a differential biological effect against tumor cells adjacent to eloquent neural structures,
9. local control rate of 88% in our series (other centers range from 73 to 98%). See Tables 1 and 2.

The Harvard-Brigham & Women's Experience

Patient characteristics, histology, treated and radiosurgical treatment details for the first 330 metastatic lesions in 217 patients treated at the Brigham & Women's Hospital and the Joint Center for Radiation Therapy of Harvard Medical School are shown in Tables 3, 4, and 5. A description of the preparation of the linear accelerator, patient alignment and immobilization, target localization, and treatment planning have been previously published.[1,10,17,26] Following is a discussion of the arguments for radiosurgery in the treatment of intracranial metastases based on this experience.

DISCUSSION

Most metastatic tumors within the brain parenchyma are roughly spherical in shape because of their natural growth pattern.[25] In most patients, they tend to displace the surrounding brain parenchyma circumferentially without actually infiltrating. En-

Table 1. Patterns of Failure Within the Central Nervous System After Radiosurgery for 282 Brain Metastases at the Brigham & Women's Hospital

Local (within radiosurgery volume)	27/330 (8%)
Interval (months from radiosurgery to local failure)	
median	10
range	2–28
Marginal—at margin of prescribed dose	9/300 (3%)
Interval (months) from radiosurgery to marginal failure	
median	5
range	3–9
Distant sites in central nervous system	69/217 (32%)
Interval (months) from radiosurgery to distant failure	
median	6
range	1–27

Table 4. Histologies of the 300 Metastatic Lesions Treated with Radiosurgery Between May 1986 and August 1992 at the Brigham & Women's Hospital

Primary site	Number
Lung nonsmall-cell carcinoma	134
Lung small-cell carcinoma	22
Melanoma	60
Breast	44
Soft tissue sarcoma	18
Renal	25
Colon	10
Germ cell	7
Others	10

hanced imaging of these lesions, whether obtained using computed tomography (CT) or magnetic resonance imaging (MRI), represents the absolute target volume in most cases. This is in contradistinction to gliomas, which are infiltrative and often have changes in enhancement on CT or MRI only in the region of high tumor-cell density, with infiltrated regions less well defined.

Most metastatic lesions present before they are greater than 3 cm in maximum diameter.[23] One of the greatest limitations in the use of high-dose single-fraction radiation (stereotactic radiosurgery) involves the inability to safely treat lesions greater than a certain volume. This inverse relationship between dose and volume is one of the major biological premises of radiosurgery.[13] Important variables in this consideration also include location, histology, and anticipated dose for tumor control. As an example of the effect of location, the incidence and severity of nausea and vomiting were directly correlated to the dose delivered to the area postrema. In our series of radiosurgery patients with metastases, as well as other diagnoses, all patients who received more than 275 cGy (range 275 to 1340 cGy) to the area postrema developed these symptoms, compared to only one of 174 patients who received less than 256 cGy (p <0.001).[2] In terms of the effect of histology, we have found that the neurological complication rate associated with the treatment of metastatic lesions is often lower than one would have for similar-sized lesions in similar locations where the histology is that of a glioma, benign tumor (acoustic neurinoma or meningioma), or vascular malformation. Metastatic lesions, in general, demon-

Table 2. Summary of Radiosurgery Results for Brain Metastases

Institution	RS*	Lesions treated	Dose* (cGy)	% Local control	FU* (months)
Harvard (current series)	LA*	330	1675	92	9
Heidelberg**	LA	124	1700	94	7
Stanford[8]	LA	47	2460	85	5
Wisconsin[18]	LA	45	1800	73	8.5
Pittsburgh[7]	GU*	53	1600	85	10
Karolinska*	GU	59	3000	98	NS*

*RS, radiation source; LA, linear accelerator; GU, gamma unit; Dose, median peripheral dose; FU, median follow-up in months; NS, not stated.
**Data presented at the International Stereotactic Radiosurgery Symposium, June 19–21, 1991, Pittsburgh, PA.

Table 3. Characteristics of 217 Patients Treated with Radiosurgery for Brain Metastases at the Brigham & Women's Hospital

Age (years)	median	46
	range	14–81
Karnofsky performance status	median	80
	range	50–100
Time (months) from initial treatment to radiosurgery	median	8
	range	0–183
Dose of prior radiotherapy (cGy)	median	3600
	range	3000–9000
Follow-up (months) from radiosurgery	median	9
	range	2–77

Table 5. Radiosurgery Details of 330 Metastatic Lesions Treated at the Brigham & Women's Hospital

Volume (cc) of lesions treated	median	32
	range	0.1–53
Collimator size (mm) used	median	27.5
	range	12.5–40
Dose to periphery (cGy)	median	1650
	range	900–2500
Dose to the isocenter (cGy)	median	2031
	range	1400–3125

strate significant radiographic response in a period as short as a few months after treatment with radiosurgery, when compared with other histological groups. Within the rubric of all metastatic lesions, the radiographic response to radiosurgery is dependent on the histology of the primary disease and volume of the metastasis.[11,12,14–16] In general, responses have been rapid and dramatic in adenocarcinomas, squamous-cell carcinomas, small-cell carcinomas, and germ-cell tumors. Melanomas, sarcomas, and renal-cell carcinomas have, alternatively, either radiographically decreased slightly over time or have stabilized with the development of a new central region of hypodensity.

Because of this relatively rapid radiographic response and, to a lesser degree, the release of toxic cytokines and substances that induce vasogenic edema, neurological complications after radiosurgery for metastatic tumors are lower than one would anticipate in comparison with other histological subgroups. Neurological complications cannot be predicted solely on the basis of the dose and volume distribution of radiation in regions of the brain adjacent to the lesion. Histology is a critical factor.

Although we have found that the traditionally "radiosensitive" lesions, such as squamous-cell carcinoma and adenocarcinoma, have a slightly higher local failure rate than the more "radioresistant" lesions (melanoma, sarcoma, and renal cell tumor), based on CT and MRI scans, the former are more likely to respond quickly than the latter. In addition, we have found that the edema often associated with metastatic lesions is frequently reduced in weeks to months after radiosurgery, and that this has serious implications in considering whether surgery or radiosurgery should be done. One common argument is that mass effect and edema resolve much more rapidly after surgery, but we have found that radiosurgery often leads to a fairly rapid reduction in edema. This is not as true with the treatment of gliomas and benign tumors (meningiomas and acoustic neurinomas) in which posttreatment edema, especially several months afterwards, can present a formidable problem.

Because of the very steep dose gradients (commonly going from 80 to 10% of the maximum dose over a distance of 5 to 7 mm), the dose may be escalated into a therapeutically effective range, even with the most radioresistant lesions. The failure of standard fractionated radiation therapy with relatively large treatment fields to treat more radioresistant tumors stems largely from the inability to obtain significant tumor kill without excessive neurological complications. However, the enhancement of dose delivery to the tumor using radiosurgery, in which the advantage is more a geometric than a biologic one, enables successful treatment of even the most radioresistant tissue types known. This specific geometric advantage is reduced with the treatment of larger lesions. In general, lesions greater than 35 to 40 mm in maximum diameter are frequently associated with

such excessive complications that treatment with radiosurgery can become unsafe. The advantage of radiosurgery is, in a sense, providing safe radiation "dose escalation."

A deep location does not in and of itself significantly interfere with successful radiosurgical treatment of a metastasis. We have treated a number of lesions (40, or 12% of 330 total metastases) in deep gray structures, as well as in and adjacent to the brain stem, with good results and few complications. In fact, metastases are probably more readily treated in these critical locations because of their propensity to resolve rapidly after radiosurgery, compared to other histologies. We, therefore, obtain optimal coverage of the tumor margin in spite of a deep or critical location. Surgical margins are frequently adequate only in noneloquent locations.

An additional advantage of radiosurgery over current techniques of surgical extirpation with metastatic lesions has to do with the benefits offered by modern three-dimensional treatment-planning software, because the full anatomic extent of the lesion corresponds with its three-dimensional imaging characteristics. Because there is no alteration of this three-dimensional geometry during treatment (as opposed to the anatomic alterations that occur during surgical resection), radiosurgery is especially well-suited to treating the entire image-visualized target. This is a particularly compelling argument for those metastases that do not have obvious visual or tactile cues as to their margins during surgical resection. In the future, more technologically advanced links between three-dimensional imaging and surgical removal may become possible to enhance the efficiency and success of the latter technique.

Although radiosurgery has been referred to as a technique for defining a "kill zone," wherein every living cell within the target zone is eradicated, this is actually untrue when considering dosages currently used to treat metastatic tumors (1000 to 2500 cGy). There is often a significant differential biologic effect against tumor cells adjacent to neural structures with high-dose single fractionated irradiation, such that necrosis is much more likely to occur within the tumor than within the adjacent brain. Radionecrosis is a complex event having to do with the effect of radiation on normal tissue and tumor tissue, as well as normal and tumor blood vessels. There is a complex statistical relationship between the distribution of abnormal and normal cells within a certain treatment volume and the subsequent distribution of necrosis. We have frequently used postoperative stereotactic radiosurgery to obtain a differential tumor effect at the edge of the surgical margin when it is immediately adjacent to eloquent cortex or critical white-matter tracts.

Finally, there are the obvious advantages of radiosurgery over surgery in that there is no risk of hemorrhage, postoperative infection, or the mechanical spread of tumor cells that is inherent with surgical removal of a tumor.

Multiple metastases are easily treated at a single session without excessive additional planning time, discomfort to the patient or cost. In our institution, multiple lesions are only treated if: (a) the patient's systemic disease is well-controlled with surgery, radiation, or chemotherapy; (b) the overall dose-volume considerations are acceptable with minimal risk of neurological complications; and (c) we expect overall improvement in quality and time of survival for the patient to warrant the cost and discomfort involved. As a general rule, we would only rarely consider treating a patient with more than 4 intracranial lesions, and we would require an overall scenario in which the benefits would be obvious (i.e., that control of the intracranial lesions would offer a reasonable chance of long-term quality survival). The long-accepted conservative neurosurgical thinking about the treatment of multiple metastases requires revision in the presence of a modality with higher control rates and lower morbidity and risk, even for deep lesions.

CONCLUSION

Overall, metastases are almost an ideal indication for radiosurgery. In addition to the reasons given above, radiosurgery is generally much less expensive than a craniotomy, can be performed as a single-day outpatient procedure, and is much less traumatic to the patient overall. There are probably about 150,000 patients with intracranial metastases annually in the United States, many of which would be suited to radiosurgery. Over the next decade, radiosurgery may be much more frequently used for metastatic tumors than for vascular lesions, gliomas, and residual or recurrent benign tumors that are not believed to be candidates for reoperation. There are currently several major centers investigating the potential benefits of high single-dose convergent-beam radiation to treat lesions throughout the body. It is very likely that the most significant beneficial impact of radiosurgery on patients' lives and overall health care may be in the treatment of metastases.

Treatment of Intracranial Metastases: Surgery vs. Radiosurgery

Dennis E. Bullard, M.D.

In the sections above, two very differing opinions are given concerning the spectrum of treatment for intracranial metastases. Both groups of authors provide clear and logical arguments for their respective approaches to controversial issues using state-of-the-art technology. The data from each suggest that these are clinically appropriate ways to treat a variety of problems. However, the value of any treatment modality is only equal to how well it can be applied by the individual practitioner. Not everyone who reads these arguments has access to intraoperative cortical stimulation, stereotactic facilities, or radiosurgery. After reading and absorbing these articles, the question posed to readers is, which of these treatment modalities is appropriate for their use? It remains to be seen whether both of these potentially promising approaches will provide consistent benefit compared to current treatment modalities.

Neurosurgery very much remains an art based upon science. For most problems, there is no standard form of treatment. However, most neurosurgeons probably agree that single, surgically accessible metastases from tumors that are moderately radiosensitive or radioresistant in patients without diffuse disease should be treated through surgery. Most clinicians recommend radiation therapy if a patient has multiple intracranial lesions, but not systemic involvement. They also generally agree that patients with multiple intracranial lesions and diffuse systemic disease are best treated through palliation, which may or may not include radiation therapy. The authors challenge these general policies.

Many clinicians still assume a natural disease history based upon outdated treatment regimens. It is unfair to judge current treatment modalities based upon results generated before their full development. This point is well addressed by the authors advocating a more aggressive surgical approach for multiple metastases. The advent of MRI, the widespread use of the operating microscope, better intraoperative localization techniques with ultrasound, stereotactic technology, and the use of cortical mapping have significantly reduced operative mortality and morbidity. This has been clearly shown in the multiple studies cited. The operative mortality and morbidity for an individual surgeon treating intracranial metastases should be less than 10% and, in most cases, should fall within the reported range of 3 to 5%. This certainly makes surgery a viable option for patients with a single lesion. In their hands, multiple craniotomies at a single operative time were not associated with a higher per craniotomy complication or 30-day mortality rates than a single craniotomy. This begs the question, however, because relatively few surgeons currently perform multiple craniotomies on the same patient. The overall morbidity and mortality, however, do appear to be excellent for multiple lesions. The advantage of this approach is in the relief of mass affect, the ability to reduce steroid dependence, and in the confirmation that all intracranial lesions were, in fact, metastatic disease. These are all valid considerations.

The authors recommending the use of radiosurgery argue that their data show that radiosurgery, in contrast to standard surgical techniques, is the treatment of choice in those patients with single or multiple well-defined lesions without systemic involvement. Their argument that the well-defined nature of metastatic disease makes it more amenable to radiation than primary brain tumors is well taken. Their conjecture that radiosurgery is effective appears to be supported with excellent responses in their hands. The issues of whether the morbidity or effectiveness associated with multiple craniotomies is less than that associated with radiosurgery is not directly answered. One obvious question raised is how important clinically is the immediate relief of mass effect. The authors advocating radiation therapy suggest that this is not a major issue in most patients. In those patients with melanomas, sarcomas, and renal-cell carcinomas, the answer is still not available. This question must be better defined and quantitated. The extensive patient population to which these authors have access should allow this information to be generated by retrospective historical comparisons of complication rates, neurological performance, and duration of life at Karnofsky levels above 70 after either surgery or radiation therapy.

Patchell and colleagues' eloquent work has answered the first in a series of important questions concerning metastatic cancer; surgery combined with whole-brain irradiation is superior to whole-brain radiation alone for the treatment of single, surgically accessible lesions. The next point to be answered is whether radiosurgery is the equivalent to surgery and to define the optimal use for it on a comparative basis. Both groups of authors have suggested that a more aggressive approach should be taken to the treatment of multiple lesions in an otherwise stable patient. The data from the first authors indicates that surgery combined with whole-brain radiation therapy is superior to radiation therapy alone if all lesions can be removed. The next logical question is that, assuming radiosurgery is equal to surgery for single lesions, is it equal for multiple lesions and, if so, what is the maximum number of lesions that can be treated?

Treatment must be individualized to consider the general medical condition of the patient, the extent of the cancer, the tempo of disease progression, and the resources available. Both groups of authors are to be congratulated on their excellent presentation and on their willingness to be aggressive in the treatment of this disease. Only by pursuing such an aggressive approach can we define optimal treatment regimens. Patients with more than one intracranial lesion but without systemic involvement should be approached aggressively through either surgery or radiosurgery, with increasing numbers of patients evolving from more aggressive and effective treatment of primary cancers as the questions are being answered.

REFERENCES

Rajesh K. Bindal, M.D., and Raymond Sawaya, M.D.

1. Adler J, Cox R, Kaplan I, et al.: Stereotactic radiosurgical treatment of brain metastases. *J Neurosurg* 1992; 76:444–449.
2. Alexander E III, Loeffler J: Radiosurgery using a modified linear accelerator. *Neurosurg Clin North Am* 1992; 3:167–190.
3. Bindal R, Sawaya R, Leavens M, et al.: Surgical treatment of multiple brain metastases. *J Neurosurg* 1993; 79:210–216.
4. Borgelt B, Gelber R, Kramer S, et al.: The palliation of brain metastases: Final results of the first two studies by the Radiation Therapy Oncology Group. *Int J Radiat Oncol Biol Phys* 1980; 6:1–9.
5. Cairncross G, Posner J: The management of brain metastases, in Walker M (ed): *Oncology of the Nervous System*. Boston, Martinus Nejhoff Publishers, 1983, pp 341–377.
6. Ferrara M, Bizzozzero F, Talamonti G, et al.: Surgical treatment of 100 single brain metastases. *J Neurosurg Sci* 1990; 34:303–308.
7. Galicich J, Arbit E: Metastatic brain tumors, in Youmans JR (ed): *Neurological Surgery*. Philadelphia, WB Saunders, 1990, pp 3204–3222.
8. Galicich J, Sundaresan N, Thaler H: Surgical treatment of single brain metastasis: Evaluation of results by computerized tomography scanning. *J Neurosurg* 1980; 53:63–67.
9. Horwitz N, Rizzoli H: *Postoperative Complications of Intracranial Neurological Surgery*. Baltimore, Williams and Wilkins, 1982.
10. Patchell R, Tibbs P, Walsh J, et al.: A randomized trial of surgery in the treatment of single metastases. *N Engl J Med* 1990; 322: 494–545.
11. Sorensen J, Hansen H, Hansen M, et al.: Brain metastases in adenocarcinoma of the lung: Frequency, risk groups, and prognosis. *J Clin Oncol* 1988; 9:1474–1480.
12. Sundaresan N, Galicich J: Surgical treatment of brain metastases: Clinical and computerized tomography evaluation of the results of treatment. *Cancer* 1985; 55:1382–1388.
13. Takakura K, Sano K, Hojo S, et al.: *Metastatic Tumors of the Nervous System*. New York, Igaku-Shoin, 1982.

Eben Alexander III, M.D., and Jay S. Loeffler, M.D.

1. Alexander E III, Loeffler JS: Stereotactic radiosurgery using a modified linear accelerator, in Lundsford LD (ed): *Neurosurgery Clinics of North America*, Philadelphia, WB Saunders, 1991, pp 167–191.
2. Alexander E III, Siddon RL, Loeffler JS: The acute onset of nausea and vomiting following stereotactic radiosurgery: Correlation with total dose to area postrema. *Surg Neurol* 1989; 32:40–44.
3. Burt M, Wronski M, Arbit E, et al.: Resection of brain metastases from nonsmall-cell lung carcinoma: Results of therapy. *J Thorac Cardiovasc Surg* 1992; 103:399–410.
4. Cairncross JG, Kim JH, Posner JB: Radiation therapy for brain metastases. *Ann Neurol* 1980; 7:529–541.
5. Coia LR, Aaronson N, Linggood R, et al.: A report on the consensus workshop panel on the treatment of brain metastases. *Int J Radiat Oncol Biol Phys* 1992; 23:223–227.
6. Cooper J, Steinfeld A, Lerch I: Cerebral metastases: Value of re-irradiation in selected patients. *Radiology* 1990; 174:883–885.
7. Flickinger JL, Lunsford LD, Kondziolka D, et al.: Improved local control of brain metastases with radiotherapy and whole brain radiotherapy. *Cancer* (in press).
8. Fuller BG, Kaplan ID, Adler J, et al.: Stereotaxic radiosurgery for brain metastases: The importance of adjuvant whole brain irradiation. *Int J Radiat Oncol Biol Phys* 1992; 23:413–418.
9. Hendrickson FR, Lee MS, Larson M, et al.: The influence of surgery and radiation therapy on patients with brain metastases. *Int J Radiat Oncol Biol Phys* 1983; 9:623–627.
10. Kooy HM, Nedzi L, Loeffler JS, et al.: Treatment planning for stereotactic radiosurgery of intracranial lesions. *Int J Radiat Oncol Biol Phys* 1991; 21:683–693.
11. Loeffler JS, Alexander E III: Radiosurgery for the treatment of intracranial metastases, in Alexander E III, Loeffler JS, Lunsford LD (eds): *Stereotactic Radiosurgery*. New York, McGraw-Hill, 1993.
12. Loeffler JS, Alexander E III: The role of stereotactic radiosurgery in the management of intracranial tumors. *Oncology* 1990; 4:21–31.
13. Loeffler JS, Larson DA: Radiosurgery in the management of intracranial lesions: A radiation oncology prospective, in Dewey WC, Edington M, Frye RJM, et al. (eds): *Radiation Research: A Twentieth-Century Perspective*. San Diego, Harcourt Brace Jovanovich, 1992, pp 535–540.
14. Loeffler JS, Alexander E III, Kooy HM, et al.: Radiosurgery for brain metastases, in DeVita VT, Hellman S, Rosenberg SA (eds): *Cancer: Principles and Practice of Oncology, Update*, vol. 5. Philadelphia, JB Lippincott, 1991, pp 1–13.
15. Loeffler JS, Alexander E III, Wen PY, et al.: Radiosurgery for brain metastases: Five year experience at the Brigham and Women's Hospital, in Lunsford LD (ed): *Stereotactic Radiosurgery Update*. New York, Elsevier, 1992, pp 383–392.
16. Loeffler JS, Kooy HM, Wen PY, et al: The treatment of recurrent brain metastases with stereotactic radiosurgery. *J Clin Oncol* 1990; 8:576–582.
17. Lutz W, Winston KR, Maleki N: A system for stereotactic radiosurgery using a standard linear accelerator. *Int J Radiat Oncol Biol Phys* 1988; 14:373–381.
18. Mehta MP, Rozental JM, Levin AB, et al.: Defining the role of radiosurgery in the management of brain metastases. *Int J Radiat Oncol Biol Phys* 1992; 24:619–625.
19. Patchell RA, Cirrincione C, Thaler HT, et al.: Single brain metastases: Surgery plus radiation or radiation alone. *Neurology* 1986; 36:447–453.
20. Patchell RA, Tibbs PA, Walsh JW, et al.: A randomized trial of surgery in the treatment of single metastases to the brain. *N Engl J Med* 1990; 322:494–500.
21. Posner J: Management of central nervous system metastases. *Semin Oncol* 1977; 4:81–91.

22. Russell DS, Rubinstein JL: *Pathology of Tumors of the Nervous System*. Baltimore, Williams and Wilkins, 1971.

23. Smalley S, Schray M, Lans E, et al.: Adjuvant radiation therapy after surgical resection of solitary brain metastasis: Association with pattern of failure and survival. *Int J Radiat Oncol Biol Phys* 1987; 13:1611–1616.

24. Sundaresan N, Galicich JH, Beattie EJ Jr.: Surgical treatment of brain metastases from lung cancer. *J Neurosurg* 1983; 58:666–671.

25. White KT, Fleming TR, Laws ER: Single metastasis to the brain: Surgical treatment in 122 consecutive patients. *Mayo Clin Proc* 1981; 56:426–428.

26. Winston KR, Lutz W: Linear accelerator as a neurosurgical tool for stereotactic radiosurgery. *Neurosurgery* 1988; 22:454–464.

27. Zimm S, Wampler GL, Stablein D, et al.: Intracranial metastases in solid-tumor patients: Natural history and results of treatment. *Cancer* 1981; 48:384–394.

7

Treatment of Supratentorial Low-Grade Gliomas: Surgical vs. Conservative

CASE

A 43-year-old, right-handed woman came to medical attention with focal motor seizures that subsequently became generalized. The patient's neurological exam was normal. Magnetic resonance images show the lesion.

PARTICIPANTS

Surgical Treatment of Supratentorial Low-Grade Gliomas–Mitchel S. Berger, M.D., Evren Keles, M.D.

Conservative Treatment of Supratentorial Low-Grade Gliomas–Joanne N. Bacchus, M.D., J. Gregory Cairncross, M.D.

Moderator–Robert A. Morantz, M.D.

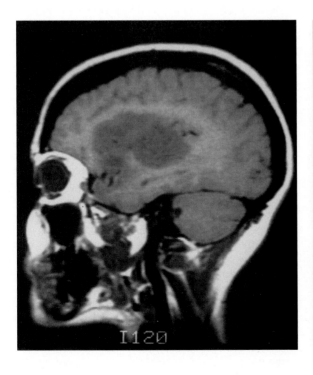 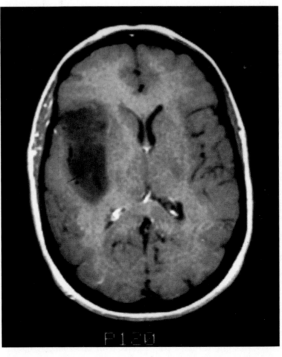

Surgical Treatment of Supratentorial Low-Grade Gliomas

Mitchel S. Berger, M.D., Evren Keles, M.D.

Currently, the treatment of patients with low-grade gliomas is controversial, especially as it pertains to the timing of surgical intervention, the extent of tumor resection, and adjuvant radiotherapy. In the literature, the timing of surgical intervention varies from surgery immediately after the initial diagnostic imaging study to conservative treatment, although few studies address the issue of nonsurgical treatment when the patient initially comes to medical attention. Furthermore, no prospective randomized clinical study analyzes the impact of the extent of tumor resection on recurrence patterns and survival rates. Although several retrospective studies compare the effect of gross total, near-total, and subtotal resections and biopsy alone,[27,33,37,41,47,49] these results are difficult to interpret because of the considerable variability in patient characteristics and therapeutic modalities. In these studies, assessment of the extent of resection is usually based on the neurosurgeon's description in the operative report, which is not quantitative and often not correlated with postoperative imaging studies.

Another important factor to be taken into account is the potential of low-grade gliomas to recur at a higher histological grade; that is, dedifferentiation or upgrading.[2,27,28,36,37,41,47] This well-documented phenomenon may result in part from histological heterogeneity or errors in tissue sampling at the time of the initial diagnosis.[27,50,51]

CASE EVALUATION

The patient's history is that of a previously healthy individual who experienced simple partial, that is, focal motor seizures that subsequently spread and became generalized. Although it is not disclosed, we assume that the patient was treated with antiepileptic drugs and the seizures were easily controlled. The neurological exam was within normal limits and, when the patient's condition was stable, a magnetic resonance imaging (MRI) study was done.

The axial and parasagittal T1-weighted MRIs showed a hypointense signal originating in an expanded area throughout the right insula. The lesion does not involve the temporal lobe and is located within the insular cortex and subcortical white matter. Neither the internal capsule nor the basal ganglia are involved. Because the patient is right-handed and has no language deficit associated with the seizure, the tumor is almost certainly located within the nondominant cerebral hemisphere. Injection of an intravenous contrast agent showed no evidence of enhancement within the mass. Although about 10% of noncontrast-enhancing lesions can be histologically malignant,[14] the most likely diagnosis is a low-grade glial tumor.

TREATMENT STRATEGIES

Surgical Approach

The insula is a cortical region located within the depths of the Sylvian fissure. Anatomically, the dominant hemisphere insula is covered with lateral language cortex and the inferior aspect of the Rolandic cortex, which is intimately associated with Broca's area. Mesially, descending motor fibers within the internal capsule may become directly contiguous with an enlarged insula

infiltrated by a tumor. Various somatosensory and special sensory functions (olfactory, gustatory, autonomic, somatic) are localized to the insular cortex, although it is not clear which deficits stem from the removal of this area.[11,26,34,40,53] The most common presenting sign or symptom secondary to neoplastic involvement of the insula is seizure activity with the associated sensory phenomena.

Technically, the nondominant insula is safe to completely resect because language function does not have to be tested or localized in this or the overlying cortical area. The motor pathways are an important consideration, however, and must be localized before the tumor is removed and during the resection. In this case, after exposure of the temporal, posterior frontal, and anterior parietal cortices, ultrasound is used to define the limits of the lesion.[30–32] Typically, low-grade, noncontrast-enhancing lesions are homogeneously hyperechoic with regard to the surrounding hypoechoic brain. Small letter tags are placed on the cortical surface to define the underlying tumor before functional localization.

The motor cortex is then identified by stimulation mapping with a bipolar electrode (5-mm spacing) and a current between 6 and 16 mA (in the sleeping patient). Further details regarding the stimulation parameters and the method necessary to map motor cortex and subcortical motor pathways can be found in previous publications.[3–7] After the face motor cortex is identified and marked with numbered tickets, the overlying superior temporal gyrus and frontal operculum are resected to expose the tumor-infiltrated insula. The arterial loops covering the insular surface are usually stretched and elongated from the underlying tumor and run parallel to each other. A cortical incision is made between the arteries and the tumor is removed with the ultrasonic aspirator. At a depth of 1.0 to 1.5 cm, the bipolar electrode is used to stimulate subcortical white matter to identify mesial descending motor pathways. Previous testing for current spread using this stimulation method revealed little dispersion of current from the electrode contact points.[23,24]

The cortical sites previously localized and marked should be retested to confirm that the functional connections between the cortex and subcortical white matter are still intact. The resection should then proceed in millimeter increments, and the surgeon should alternate the ultrasonic aspirator with the bipolar electrode until the depth is reached according to the ultrasound dimensions, or when motor responses are identified. In general, the resection cannot extend past an imaginary line drawn perpendicular to any cortical site representing stimulation-induced motor movements. If necessary, the face motor cortex may be completely removed without permanent sequelae[31] if this improves exposure of the underlying middle to posterior section of the insular surface. As long as no subcortical stimulation responses are identified and, if the cortical sites remain functional in assessing the viability of the descending motor loops, the tumor resection can be as radical and extensive as the surgeon desires without any permanent complications. It would not be unexpected for this patient to have transient weakness on the left side if the resection came within 5 to 10 mm of the motor pathways.

Control of Seizure Activity

Assuming this patient had well-controlled seizures while taking antiepileptic drugs, a radical tumor resection would have a high likelihood of further preventing or controlling the seizure activity with or without medication.[12,13,19,25] The etiology of epilepsy associated with low-grade glial tumors is linked to the chronic nature of an indolent, slow-growing tumor mass affecting the surrounding cortex.[18,39,42] We have recently reported the molecular alterations within cortical neurons that are responsible for this phenomenon in a series of patients with low-grade gliomas and intractable epilepsy. In this retrospective analysis of epileptic cortex compared with electrically silent tissue, as documented with electrocorticography, there was a statistically significant decrease in both somatostatin and gamma-aminobutyric acid immunoreactive neurons in the hyperexcitable cortex taken from the same patient.[22]

In our experience with patients who have low-grade gliomas associated with intractable epilepsy, seizure control was maximized without antiepileptic drugs if electrocorticography was used to map seizure foci during tumor removal.[8,9] Other investigators disagree with this approach, citing evidence that a radical tumor resection encompassing adjacent cortex or mesial structures typically associated with epileptic spike activity, for example, the amygdala, parahippocampal gyrus, and hippocampus, often reduces seizure activity without requiring extraoperative mapping or electrocorticography at the time of surgery.[16,20,48] In the treatment of the patient presented for evaluation in this case, however, no perioperative monitoring (including electrocorticography) is necessary as an adjunct to surgery because of the presumed controlled nature of the seizure activity.

EXPERIENCE WITH RADICAL TUMOR REMOVAL

We have previously described a quantitative volumetric assessment method[15] that has allowed us to retrospectively analyze our patients with low-grade gliomas and determine from their preoperative and postoperative imaging studies: (1) the degree of tumor resection, and (2) the volume of residual disease. Both of these factors were then related to the time until tumor progression was documented, the likelihood of recurrence, and the histological subtype at recurrence. The tumor volume measured and quantitated was based on the T2-weighted hyperintense signal abnormalities seen on magnetic resonance images and the hypodense areas seen on axial computed tomograms. In only a few of our cases (4 of 53 patients), slight contrast enhancement was identified. About 20% of our patients with low-grade glial tumors developed a recurrence. This was defined by comparing the preoperative imaging study to the first scan done after surgery. Although this latter time interval has varied over the years, it has been our policy to obtain images with and without contrast enhancement within 48 to 72 hours after the operation using computed tomography. This study is then followed by a magnetic resonance imaging evaluation within the next 4 to 8 weeks. Most recurrent tumors were found to show a higher histological grade. However, the time it took to develop a recurrence and the histology at that time were critically dependent on the amount of tumor present before and after surgery, indicating that the extent of tumor resection was a significantly important variable in this patient population.

For example, patients in whom the tumor (preoperatively) was quantitatively determined to be less than 10 cm³ never developed a recurrence when followed to the end of the current analysis, about 50 months. However, the time to tumor progression decreased with an increasing preoperative tumor volume, so that most patients with initial tumor volumes of 30 cm³ and greater had a recurrence within 30 months of surgery and all of these tumors were of a malignant histological type.

When the volume of residual tumor was evaluated, the same trends were documented. If a patient had no evidence of tumor remaining on the postoperative imaging studies, no recurrence was identified at a follow-up of over 50 months. Yet, when the remaining postoperative disease measured over 10 cm³, the likelihood of developing a recurrence was nearly 50% at 30 months versus less than half that percentage at a longer time interval for those patients with a tumor volume of less than 10 cm³. As expected, the degree of tumor resection was indirectly proportional to the volume of residual disease, indicating that a radical resection of tumor decreased the incidence of recurrence and the chances of having a more malignant phenotype at that time.

REVIEW OF THE LITERATURE

Resection and Its Influence on Recurrence Patterns

The influence of the extent of resection on a patient's outcome has been addressed in several retrospective studies. Despite the lack of prospective randomized studies to evaluate the effect of the extent of resection on outcome for patients with low-grade gliomas, recent retrospective studies suggest that survival may be improved when extensive surgical resection is carried out.[21,27,37,47] In all studies that address this issue, the extent of resection is determined either according to the surgeon's intraoperative estimation or based on postoperative computed tomograms. To eliminate the surgeon's bias on the evaluation of the extent of resection, we quantified tumor volumes on preoperative and postoperative scans using volumetric image analysis.

Although immediate surgical intervention, after a tumor is documented on diagnostic imaging studies, is recommended in several recent reviews,[28,35,51] other studies advocate a less urgent approach or even question the necessity of surgical treatment for patients with low-grade gliomas.[10,43] Preoperative tumor volume has not been evaluated as an independent variable, except for a few studies in which preoperative tumor diameter, involvement of multiple lobes, or the diameter of the surgical specimen was analyzed in terms of affecting survival.[27,37,45] Contrary to some opinions that patients with low-grade gliomas can be conservatively followed with serial imaging studies,[10,43] our retrospective analysis showed evidence that delayed surgical intervention may increase the risk of recurrence and malignant transformation in a shorter time period, in comparison to patients operated on when the tumor is smaller. This increased risk caused by deferring surgical therapy is also exacerbated by the fact that tumors less than 10 cm³ did not recur in any of our patients.

It has been reported that 13 to 85% of glial tumors initially diagnosed as low-grade recur at a higher histological grade.[1,2,27,36,37,41,47,50,51] However, the factors resulting in the change to a malignant phenotype remain unclear. In our series, no high-grade recurrence was documented in patients who underwent total resection and had no evidence of residual tumor radiographically. Our data suggest that the risk of recurrence, either as low-grade or at a higher histological grade, is minimized when less residual tumor volume is present after surgery.

In addition, residual tumor volume is found to be more important than the degree of resection in predicting the histological phenotype of recurrence. Similarly, time to tumor progression is longer with more extensive resections associated with a smaller residual tumor volume. In a recent study, 58% of patients who did not initially undergo biopsy and treatment of a suspected low-grade glioma after diagnostic imaging studies eventually required surgery at a median interval of 29 months, and 50% of the tumors then showed anaplastic features.[43] The authors of this study stated that no difference was observed in terms of survival, despite a higher incidence of malignant transformation at the time of operation and shorter time to tumor progression compared with that in patients who initially were operated upon. However, factors analyzed in our study, including pre- and postoperative tumor volumes and degree of resection, were not included in that report.

Adjuvant Radiotherapy

For our patients, postoperative radiotherapy did not influence the outcome with regard to recurrence and time to tumor progression. In the literature, the effect of this treatment modality is not well established, partly because of various dose regimens administered, improved technical properties of the radiotherapy equipment used, and a common tendency to forego radiation therapy for patients with gross total resection. In addition to reports that favor the use of postoperative radiotherapy for patients with low-grade glial tumors,[44–46,52] several studies failed to show any significant affect on survival.[27,38,41,47,50] The use of postoperative radiotherapy only for incompletely resected low-grade gliomas is advocated in some reviews.[17,29,35,51] Although the patient population in our series was not randomized to assess the effectiveness of postoperative radiotherapy, our results did not show any evidence to support the use of postoperative radiotherapy. This was especially true in patients with a preoperative tumor volume of less than 10 cm^3 or in those patients who had a complete resection with no residual tumor. However, the follow-up period in our series was not long enough to make a final assessment regarding the effectiveness of radiotherapy, especially as it influences survival.

CONCLUSION

In our opinion, patients with low-grade glial tumors should have an attempt at a radical resection of as much of the lesion as possible. This may be achieved in the dominant hemisphere with the patient awake and language mapping of the cortex. Identifying the motor pathways from the surface to the internal capsule is possible with stimulation-induced responses, using the bipolar electrode to elicit individual movements of the face and extremities. A thorough review of our patient population indicated that smaller tumors, documented on preoperative imaging studies, were less likely to recur or have a malignant histological grade. Yet, even with larger tumors, if the resection achieved a greater extent of resection with less residual tumor, there was also a significant difference in the recurrence patterns of tumors in patients with low-grade gliomas. Whether radiotherapy is useful after a radical tumor resection with minimal residual disease is, as of yet, to be determined. We would, however, advocate its use when a less aggressive resection must be done, leaving a large amount of tumor within or adjacent to critical functional areas.[10]

Acknowledgment. This work was supported by NIH Grant KO8 NS01253-01, The American Cancer Society Professor of Clinical Oncology (M.S. Berger), and NIH Grant T32NS07144-13.

Conservative Treatment of Supratentorial Low-Grade Gliomas

Joanne N. Bacchus, M.D., J. Gregory Cairncross, M.D.

A 43-year-old, right-handed woman came to medical attention with recent-onset, left-sided focal motor seizures with secondary generalization. Headaches, drowsiness, nausea and vomiting, and visual obscurations, symptoms often indicative of raised intracranial pressure, were absent. She had no interictal, left-sided motor or sensory complaints. The neurological examination was normal with no evidence of papilledema. Magnetic resonance images done with and without gadolinium disclosed a nonenhancing right insular abnormality with slight mass effect. The radiological appearance was typical of a low-grade glioma. Moreover, the clinical and radiological features, considered together, effectively excluded other diagnostic considerations such as infarct, hemorrhage, abscess, encephalitis, and demyelinating disease.

RECOMMENDATION

Given that the diagnosis is reasonably secure, how should this patient be treated? We advocate a noninterventionist, wait-and-see approach; that is, clinical and magnetic resonance imaging follow-up at 3-month intervals for the first year and every 6 months thereafter.[6] Is it not reasonable in this case to defer surgery and, of course, radiotherapy until such time as clinical deterioration or radiological progression occurs? Progressive focal neurological dysfunction with or without raised intracranial pressure, intractable seizures, unequivocal tumor growth, or the emergence of enhancing regions within the tumor would lead us to abandon conservative treatment in favor of surgery and, in all likelihood, radiotherapy. Others have also suggested that conservative treatment may be appropriate for some patients with low-grade gliomas.[24,25]

DISCUSSION

For low-grade glioma of the cerebral hemispheres, many specialists recommend the maximum feasible surgical resection, or stereotactic biopsy if the risks of resection are judged too great, followed by limited-field radiotherapy. Most studies of the treatment of low-grade glioma, all of which are retrospective, have concluded that time to tumor progression and survival are prolonged by gross total resection and, in the case of incomplete resection, by postoperative irradiation.[3,11,12,16,17,19–23,27–30] Based on an analysis of "levels of evidence,"[10] one is almost certainly on thin ice concluding that early aggressive treatment is undoubtedly superior to other treatment strategies for low-grade hemispheric gliomas. True, retrospective studies generate useful hypotheses, but their conclusions do not have the scientific validity of those gleaned from randomized trials, or even case-control studies.[7,10] The indolent nature of these tumors makes it difficult, in the absence of a properly controlled trial, to evaluate the effectiveness of any intervention and raises the possibility that the alleged benefits of aggressive treatment will, sooner or later, be offset by treatment-related toxic effects. Maximum feasible surgical resection followed by limited-field radiotherapy may, indeed, be good treatment for patients with low-grade gliomas, but the evidence supporting this approach is not strong, scientifically speaking, and, in our opinion, should not dictate treatment policy worldwide.

Surgery has an important role in the treatment of some low-grade gliomas. For example, surgery may save the lives of patients with threatened herniation from large hemispheric tumors, tumor-associated cysts, or hydrocephalus. Surgery may help those patients with low-grade glioma who have seizures refractory to anticonvulsants. Most importantly, small polar tumors may be curable through surgery and serious consideration should be given to early aggressive resection. However, surgery is not curative treatment for most patients with low-grade hemispheric gliomas. Surely even the most enthusiastic surgical oncologist would agree that this woman's tumor cannot be completely resected without unacceptable morbidity. Surgery can establish the diagnosis with reasonable certainty, but with no chance for surgical cure and, in the absence of unequivocally effective follow-up therapy for a disease with a relatively long natural history, it is open to question whether all patients should be exposed early on to the risks of surgery simply to obtain a diagnosis. Admittedly, surgical misadventure is unusual these days, less than 5% for computed tomographic or magnetic resonance-directed stereotactic biopsy.[2,4,5,15] Morbidity and mortality rates are somewhat higher for patients undergoing aggressive surgical resection, but these more extensive procedures do not have the 5 to 20% misdiagnosis rate associated with stereotactic biopsy.[4,9] It can be argued that routine biopsy is justified on the grounds that it permits the identification of nonenhancing anaplastic tumors thought to be low-grade according to radiological criteria.[8] We acknowledge that neither computed tomography nor magnetic resonance imaging reliably predict tumor grade, but believe that careful clinical and radiological follow-up of patients with suspected low-grade gliomas identifies those with an accelerated course (that is, anaplastic glioma) requiring more aggressive treatment. We think frequent reassessment is a satisfactory alternative to immediate surgery for many patients with lesions seen on computed tomograms or magnetic resonance images compatible with low-grade glial tumors of the cerebral hemispheres.

Of course, the major controversy in the treatment of low-grade glioma centers not on surgery, but on the use of radiation therapy. Anecdotal evidence shows that radiotherapy benefits individual patients and, as discussed, most retrospective studies have concluded that postoperative radiotherapy prolongs tumor control after partial removal. Even if true, the decision to radiate the human brain must never be taken lightly; other issues besides tumor control must be considered. The potential benefits of radiation must be weighed against its risks. Gains in tumor control may be offset by treatment-related cognitive impairment

or other difficulties.[1,13,18] Low-grade gliomas grow slowly, leaving ample time for the toxic effects of treatment to become manifest. We know, for example, that radiotherapy to large volumes of brain in doses sufficient to control a malignant glioma leads to dementia in a substantial proportion of long-term survivors, and to cerebral necrosis in a few.[14,26] Will high-dose, limited-field radiotherapy (5000 to 6000 cGy spanning 5 to 6 weeks), as currently prescribed for low-grade gliomas, be so much less toxic that the overall risk-benefit ratio clearly favors early treatment? If not, then delaying radiation as long as possible may be the prudent course of action for many patients with low-grade glioma. One could make a stronger case for early radiation if it prevented or delayed malignant degeneration in patients with low-grade gliomas, but there is no evidence that this is so.[25] Until these issues are clarified by new data, we will continue to make treatment decisions on a case-by-case basis and delay radiation whenever possible. For the patient under discussion, we would postpone radiation and, of course, would not treat her in the absence of a tissue diagnosis.

Nor would we recommend systemic therapy for this patient. Chemotherapy has no established role in the treatment of low-grade glioma. The acute toxic effects and the potential long-range complications of cytotoxic drugs, including neurotoxic effects and second malignancies, weigh heavily against their use. Likewise, there is no established role for the long-term administration of differentiation-inducing agents or other biological response modifiers. In our view, systemic therapies for low-grade glioma should only be administered within the context of a well-designed, carefully monitored, phase II or phase III clinical trial.

Lest we be misunderstood, early surgery and radiation are undoubtedly appropriate for some patients with low-grade glioma of the cerebral hemispheres, but we are most reluctant to endorse early aggressive treatment for all patients. Neither surgery nor radiotherapy is without risk. We hesitate to recommend surgery for patients with small tumors in eloquent areas of the brain, especially when they have few symptoms and, reassurances not withstanding, focal radiotherapy for big central tumors inevitably means treatment of large volumes of the brain and will impair intellect in some patients. Lastly, we question whether the "published" natural history of low-grade glioma is based on a representative cross-section of patients with these tumors. We suspect those with indolent gliomas seen by neurologists for seizure control are not always referred to a neurosurgeon or a brain-tumor center. These patients with a better prognosis are hidden from neuro-oncologists and undoubtedly under-represented in descriptions of the natural history of these tumors by clinical investigators at special referral centers.

All things considered, we favor a wait-and-see approach for many patients with suspected low-grade gliomas, including the 43-year-old woman whose case is presented here. The prevailing view in neuro-oncology runs contrary to our own,[3,6,7,10–12,16,17,19–25,27–30] and so we were pleased to see that the data from Recht and colleagues from the University of Massachusetts[25] support our contention that the noninterventionist treatment plan is both safe and effective.

Treatment of Supratentorial Low-Grade Gliomas: Surgical vs. Conservative

Robert A. Morantz, M.D.

In a perfect world, all neurosurgical patients with a specific disease would be referred to a regional tertiary-care center, which could then rapidly accrue a sufficiently large number of patients to carry out prospective randomized studies evaluating alternative treatment regimens for each particular disease. In those circumstances, it would soon become apparent which treatment option was best in each case. Obviously, such a scenario will never be realized in the United States. The difficult task facing the clinician, then, is to decide on the most appropriate course of therapy in situations in which definitive scientifically valid data are simply not available. In making such therapeutic decisions, one should be guided by the dictum, "First, do not harm." In addition to its literal meaning, one must also interpret this dictum to require that the risks or probability of producing a complication or untoward event from the therapy advocated be outweighed by the advantages that accrue to the patient from the proposed treatment.

When the problem is formulated in this manner, we realize that few universal rules of patient care can be promulgated because, at the very least, the risks associated with a particular procedure vary with the individual patient and the physicians, and depend on such factors as the patient's age, medical condition, and neurological status, as well as the skill and experience of the surgeon. The case history presented here is a perfect reflection of the above dilemma as it relates to the neurosurgeon. In this scenario, we are presented with a young woman whose only neurological complaint was the presence of focal motor seizures that became generalized. She suffered from no neurological deficit, and I believe that we may assume that her seizures could be controlled with medication. Magnetic resonance images show a low-density, rather large insular lesion that did not enhance after the administration of a contrast agent. What then should we recommend as treatment to this patient and her family? Before evaluating the pros and cons of each position, let us first briefly summarize the arguments of each author.

SURGICAL THERAPY

The first group of authors agree that this woman most likely has a low-grade glial tumor located within the nondominant insular cortex and subcortical white matter. They advocate a radical surgical approach in which an ultrasound device is used to define the limits of the lesion, and intraoperative neurophysiological monitoring techniques are used to allow such a resection to be carried out with only a small risk of producing a permanent motor deficit. These authors do, however, indicate that it would not be surprising for this patient to have transient left-sided weakness if the resection came within 5 to 10 mm of the motor pathways.

In defending their recommendation for radical surgery in this patient, the authors rely upon several lines of evidence. First and foremost, they rely on their own data, in which they used a computer-based system to quantitate volumetrically the extent of tumor present both before and after surgery. Using this method, they found a correlation between preoperative tumor size and recurrence or time to tumor progression. Most relevant to this case, the authors appear to have also found a similar trend

in which a correlation exists between the volume of postoperative residual tumor and evidence of tumor recurrence. Thus, in their hands, a radical resection of a low-grade tumor decreased the incidence of recurrence and the chances of finding a more malignant phenotype when the tumor did recur. In addition to this data, the writers indicate that several recent retrospective studies have also suggested that there is an improvement in the length of survival when an extensive surgical resection is performed.

With respect to adjuvant therapy, the authors indicate that their nonrandomized study did not support the use of postoperative radiation therapy in patients with low-grade gliomas. They conclude, however, that the literature is unclear on this point, and they ultimately advocate the use of radiotherapy when a large amount of tumor is left within or adjacent to critical functional areas of the brain.

CONSERVATIVE THERAPY

The second group of authors believe that the findings on the magnetic resonance images are typical of a low-grade glioma and, when taken in conjunction with the clinical findings, effectively rule out other non-neoplastic diagnoses such as infarct, abscess, and demyelinating disease. In these circumstances, they advocate a noninterventionist approach, in which the patient will be closely followed clinically and have imaging studies ordered initially at 3-month intervals and then every 6 months thereafter. Surgery and possibly radiation therapy will be withheld until such time as there is documented clinical deterioration or radiographic progression. Such a change will be manifested either by the onset of focal neurological dysfunction, intractable seizures, enlargement of the tumor on successive images, or the emergence of areas of enhancement within the currently nonenhancing lesion.

In support of this position, these authors maintain that the several retrospective studies advocating maximal surgical resection followed by radiation therapy are not scientifically valid because they were not prospective randomized trials, and thus should not cause us to advocate an aggressive treatment policy. They admit that surgery would have an excellent chance of establishing the diagnosis with certainty, but believe that it is almost certain that this woman's tumor could not be completely resected without an unacceptable risk of morbidity.

With respect to adjuvant therapy, these authors agree that most retrospective studies have concluded that postoperative radiotherapy prolongs tumor control, but stress that there are significant long-term risks of radiation toxicity in this group of patients. Most importantly, these writers maintain that there is no definitive evidence that the use of early radiation prevents the occurrence of malignant degeneration. Thus, for this specific patient, they would advocate delaying radiation therapy for as long as possible—probably until she showed definite evidence of tumor progression or malignant degeneration.

Consensus

Before reviewing the important areas that are currently unsettled with respect to low-grade gliomas, perhaps it would be beneficial to discuss briefly what I believe are the few areas in which a consensus exists, although we must be aware that what is said here is based on information that could change in the future. In the current era, by far the most common patient presenting with this tumor is a relatively young man or woman (median age about 35 years), who presents with epileptic seizures. Today, magnetic resonance imaging is the diagnostic procedure of choice, and such a study allows the diagnosis to be made with a high degree of probability. In a fairly large number of patients who harbor anaplastic astrocytomas or even glioblastoma multiforme, however, the imaging studies do not show enhancement.[1] With respect to pathology, almost all would agree that patients with the gemistocytic variant of low-grade astrocytoma have a worse prognosis and, conversely, that patients with related tumor types such as the pilocytic astrocytoma, ganglioglioma, and pleomorphic xanthoastroma have a better prognosis. All would agree that dedifferentiation, or change to a more malignant form, does occur in a varying number of these patients, and that such evidence of malignancy is *not* solely a reflection of initial sampling error.

With respect to treatment, almost all would agree that surgery is warranted in patients with large tumors or cystic lesions who are at risk of impending herniation, because of either the tumor itself or its obstruction of the cerebrospinal fluid pathways. Finally, no current place appears for postoperative adjuvant chemotherapy or immunotherapy in the treatment of these patients.

POINTS OF DIFFERENCE

Unfortunately for the clinician, far more areas remain unsettled with respect to low-grade gliomas than those on which a consensus has been reached. I will list here only the most important ones:

1. There is conflicting evidence as to whether enhancement on the computed tomogram in a patient with a low-grade glioma is a poor prognostic indicator. Similarly, it is not certain whether the presence of a cyst confers a better prognosis.
2. Although all agree that dedifferentiation does occur, the percentage of patients in which it occurs varies from 15 to 80% in the literature.
3. Almost all authors agree that a young age at the time of diagnosis is the most important positive prognostic indicator for a patient. There is no agreement, however, as to the potential beneficial effect conferred by other factors such as a pre- or postoperative neurological deficit or the duration of symptoms before diagnosis.
4. Most relevant to this discussion, there is no consensus as to when surgery should be undertaken.
5. It has never been proven that there is a difference in outcome depending on whether the patient undergoes a gross total removal compared to either a biopsy or a subtotal resection.
6. It is unclear whether postoperative radiation therapy should be used.
7. The optimal type of radiation therapy (traditional external beam radiation therapy versus newer modalities, such as interstitial radiation therapy or radiosurgery) is not certain. If external beam radiation therapy is used, the optimal portals as well as the most effective dose rate and total dose have not been determined.
8. The true incidence of long-term adverse effects of radiation therapy in these patients, such as intellectual decline, has not been determined.
9. What we should tell our patients and their families with respect to both the quality and length of expected survival is still controversial.

In spite of the many unsettled areas listed above, neurosurgeons are forced to make treatment decisions for patients such as the one presented here. Both groups of authors are to be commended for cogently presenting their point of view. To the authors advocating radical resection for this patient, I would point out that, because recent studies have confirmed the presence of tumor cells at a distance from the lesion as seen on radiological imaging,[3] in this particular patient, the achievement of anything approaching a total resection is unlikely. Furthermore, in spite of the elegant neurophysiological mapping techniques this group has pioneered, radical surgery on a lesion such as this one would have a substantial risk of leaving the patient in worse condition postoperatively. Even the most conservative surgeons would advocate an attempt at radical removal if a small lesion is located in a silent area of the brain, such as the frontal or temporal poles. In the patient presented here, however, most conservative surgeons and even some with a more radical inclination would be reluctant to recommend such an attempt in a young patient who is neurologically intact. The risk of performing a stereotactic biopsy to confirm the nature of the lesion would probably be lower than an attempt at radical resection, and so our options should not be limited to either an open procedure attempting to achieve gross total removal or no surgery at all.

On the other hand, to the group that recommends a "noninterventionist wait-and-see approach," I would indicate that, in a small percentage of patients, *not* knowing the precise histological diagnosis (that is, whether the patient harbors a variant with a better prognosis, such as pilocytic astrocytoma or an anaplastic astrocytoma, which does not enhance) *will* make a difference as to what treatment options are chosen and what the patient is told with respect to the prognosis. Furthermore, the thrust of recent molecular genetic research on low-grade gliomas indicates that a reasonable hypothesis of the events underlying dedifferentiation is that a glial cell experiences a small number of "genetic hits" to change it into a low-grade astrocytoma. If these cells or their daughter cells then experience further alteration in their genetic make-up (for example, by mutation of a tumor suppressor gene such as p53), they will undergo dedifferentiation to a more malignant phenotype.[2] The implication of this data would seem to be that we should remove as much of the low-grade astrocytoma cells as feasible to decrease the probability of dedifferentiation. Certainly one could not fault the clinician who would recommend careful follow-up and "watchful waiting" in this particular patient. However, in the situation of a more favorably located, smaller lesion, in which the chance of complete removal is greater and the chance of complications less, I would maintain that the patient's best interests are served by an attempt at gross total removal.

CONCLUSION

Ultimately, then, in a particular situation such as that which we are faced with here, the role of the neurosurgeon is to honestly present to the patient and the family the data as they are presently known. Specifically, one must honestly evaluate in a particular patient what one believes to be one's *own* chances of carrying out a successful biopsy or gross total resection (whichever is the goal) and, in addition, what one believes to be the honest risks of producing (neurological or nonneurological) morbidity from the operation. Finally, we must retrospectively be totally honest in evaluating our *own* patients' outcomes with respect to the degree of tumor removal that we have achieved and the postoperative morbidity that we have produced. This is certainly an imperfect solution to a most difficult problem, but until more valid scientific data (derived from ongoing prospective randomized studies) become available, it would appear to be the only available choice.

REFERENCES

Mitchel S. Berger, M.D., Evren Keles, M.D.

1. Afra D, Muller W, Benoist G, et al.: Supratentorial recurrences of gliomas, results of reoperations on astrocytomas, and oligodendrogliomas. *Acta Neurochir (Wien)* 1978; 43:217–227.
2. Afra D, Muller W, Slowik F, et al.: Supratentorial lobar pilocyticastrocytomas: Report of 45 operated cases, including 9 recurrences. *Acta Neurochir (Wien)* 1986; 81:90–93.
3. Berger MS, Ojemann GA: Techniques of functional localization during removal of tumors involving the cerebral hemisphere, in Traynelis VC, Loftus CM (eds): *Intraoperative Monitoring Techniques in Neurosurgery.* New York, McGraw-Hill, 1994, pp 113–127.
4. Berger MS, Ojemann GA: Intraoperative brain mapping techniques in neuro-oncology. *Stereotac Funct Neurosurg* 1992; 58:153–161.
5. Berger MS, Ojemann GA: Stimulation mapping and recording techniques used during pediatric brain tumor surgery, in Bleyer WA, Pochedly C (eds): *Pediatric Neuro-Oncology: New Trends in Clinical Research.* New York, Harwood Academic Publishers, 1992, pp 136–160.
6. Berger MS, Ojemann GA, Lettich E: Neurophysiological monitoring to facilitate resection during astrocytoma surgery. *Neurosurg Clin North Am* 1990; 1:65–80.
7. Berger MS, Kincaid J, Ojemann GA, et al.: Brain mapping techniques to maximize resection, safety, and seizure control in children with brain tumors. *Neurosurgery* 1989; 25:786–792.
8. Berger MS, Ghatan S, Geyer JR, et al.: Seizure outcome in children with hemispheric tumors and associated intractable epilepsy: The role of tumor removal combined with seizure foci resection. *Pediatr Neurosurg* 1991–92; 17:185–191.
9. Berger MS, Ghatan S, Haglund MM, et al.: Low-grade gliomas associated with intractable epilepsy: Seizure outcome utilizing electrocorticography during tumor resection. *J Neurosurg* 1993; 79:62–69.
10. Cairncross JG, Laperrier NJ: Low-grade glioma. To treat or not to treat? *Arch Neurol* 1989; 46:1238–1239.
11. Cancelliere AEB, Kertesz A: Lesion localization in acquired deficits of emotional expression and comprehension. *Brain Cognit* 1990; 13:133–147.
12. Cascino GD: Epilepsy and brain tumors: Implications for treatment. *Epilepsia* 1990; 31 (Suppl 3):S37–S44.
13. Cascino GD, Kelly PJ, Hirschhorn KA, et al.: Stereotactic resection of intra-axial cerebral lesions in partial epilepsy. *Mayo Clin Proc* 1990; 65:1053–1060.
14. Chamberlain MC, Murovic J, Levin VA: Absence of contrast enhancement on CT brain scans of patients with supratentorial malignant gliomas. *Neurology* 1988; 38:1371–1373.
15. Duong DH, Rostomily RC, Haynor DR, et al.: Measurement of tumor resection volumes from computerized images: Technical note. *J Neurosurg* 1992; 77:151–154.
16. Falconer MA, Cavanagh JB: Clinico-pathological considerations of temporal lobe epilepsy due to small focal lesions: A study of cases submitted to operation. *Brain* 1959; 82:483–504.
17. Fazekas JT: Treatment of grades I and II brain astrocytomas: The role of radiotherapy. *Int J Radiat Oncol Biol Phys* 1977; 2:661–666.
18. Franceschetti S, Binelli S, Casazza M, et al.: Influence of surgery and antiepileptic drugs on seizures symptomatic of cerebral tumors. *Acta Neurochir (Wien)* 1990; 103:47–51.
19. Goldring S, Rich KM, Picker S: Experience with gliomas in patients presenting with a chronic seizure disorder, in Little JR (ed): *Clinical Neurosurgery,* vol. 33. New York, Raven Press, 1986, pp 15–42.
20. Goldring S: Pediatric epilepsy surgery. *Epilepsia* 1987; 28:S82–S102.
21. Guthrie BL, Laws ER: Supratentorial low-grade gliomas. *Neurosurg Clin North Am* 1990; 1:37–48.
22. Haglund MM, Berger MS, Kunkel DD, et al.: Changes in GABA and somatostatin in epileptic cortex associated with low-grade gliomas. *J Neurosurg* 1992; 77:209–216.
23. Haglund MM, Ojemann GA, Blasdel GG: Video imaging of bipolar cortical stimulation. *Epilepsia* 1991; 32(Suppl 3):22.
24. Haglund MM, Ojemann GA, Hochmann D: Optical imaging of epileptiform and functional activity in human cerebral cortex. *Nature* 1992; 358:668–671.
25. Hirsch JR, Rose CS, Pierre-Khan A, et al.: Benign astrocytic and oligodendrocytic tumors of the cerebral hemispheres in children. *J Neurosurg* 1989; 70:568–572.
26. Kaada BR, Pribram KH, Epstein JA: Respiratory and vascular responses in monkeys from temporal pole, insula, orbital surface, and cingulate gyrus. *J Neurophysiol* 1949; 12:347–356.
27. Laws ER, Taylor WF, Clifton MB, et al.: Neurosurgical management of low-grade astrocytoma of the cerebral hemispheres. *J Neurosurg* 1984; 61:665–673.
28. Laws ER, Taylor WF, Bergstralh EJ, et al.: The neurosurgical management of low-grade astrocytoma. *Clin Neurosurg* 1985; 33: 575–588.
29. Leibel SA, Sheline GE, Wara WM, et al.: The role of radiation therapy in the treatment of astrocytomas. *Cancer* 1975; 35:1551–1557.
30. LeRoux PD, Berger MS, Ojemann GA, et al.: Correlation of intraoperative ultrasound tumor volumes and margins with preoperative computerized tomography scans: An intraoperative method to enhance tumor resection. *J Neurosurg* 1989; 71:691–698.
31. LeRoux PD, Berger MS, Haglund MM, et al.: Resection of intrinsic tumors from nondominant face motor cortex using stimulation mapping: Report of two cases. *Surg Neurol* 1991; 36:44–48.
32. LeRoux PD, Berger MS, Wang K, et al.: Low grade gliomas: Comparison of intraoperative ultrasound characteristics with preoperative imaging studies. *J Neuro-Oncol* 1992; 13:189–198.
33. Medbery CA, Straus KL, Steinberg SM, et al.: Low-grade astrocytomas: Treatment results and prognostic variables. *Int J Radiat Oncol Biol Phys* 1988; 15:837–841.
34. Mesulam MM, Mufson EJ: Insula in the old monkey. III: Efferent cortical output and comments on function. *J Comp Neurol* 1982; 212:38–52.
35. Morantz RA: Radiation therapy in the treatment of cerebral astrocytoma. *Neurosurgery* 1987; 20:975–982.
36. Muller W, Afra D, Schroder R: Supratentorial recurrences of gliomas: Morphological studies in relation to time intervals with astrocytomas. *Acta Neurochir (Wien)* 1977; 37:75–91.
37. North CA, North RB, Epstein JA, et al.: Low-grade cerebral astrocytomas: Survival and quality of life after radiation therapy. *Cancer* 1990; 66:6–14.
38. Palma L, Guidetti B: Cystic pilocytic astrocytomas of the cerebral hemispheres. *J Neurosurg* 1985; 62:811–815.
39. Penfield W, Erickson TC, Tarlov IM: Relation of intracranial tumors and symptomatic epilepsy. *Arch Neurol Psychiatry* 1940; 44: 300–315.

40. Penfield W, Faulk ME: The insula: Further observations on its function. *Brain* 1955; 78:445–470.

41. Piepmeier JM: Observations on the current treatment of low-grade astrocytic tumors of the cerebral hemispheres. *J Neurosurg* 1987; 67:177–181.

42. Rasmussen TB: Surgery of epilepsy associated with brain tumors. *Adv Neurol* 1975; 8:227–239.

43. Recht LD, Lew R, Smith TW: Suspected low-grade glioma: Is deferring treatment safe? *Ann Neurol* 1992; 31:431–436.

44. Scanlon PW, Taylor WF: Radiotherapy of intracranial astrocytomas: Analysis of 417 cases treated from 1960 through 1969. *Neurosurgery* 1979; 5:301–308.

45. Shaw EG, Daumas-Duport C, Scheithauer BW, et al.: Radiation therapy in the management of low-grade supratentorial astrocytomas. *J Neurosurg* 1989; 70:853–861.

46. Sheline GE: Radiation therapy of brain tumors. *Cancer* 1977; 39: 873–881.

47. Soffietti R, Chio A, Giordana MT, et al.: Prognostic factors in well-differentiated cerebral astrocytomas in the adult. *Neurosurgery* 1989; 24:686–692.

48. Spencer DD, Spencer SS, Mattson RH, et al.: Intracerebral masses in patients with intractable partial epilepsy. *Neurology* 1984; 34:432–436.

49. Steiger HJ, Markwalder RV, Seiler RW, et al.: Early prognosis of supratentorial grade 2 astrocytomas in adult patients after resection or stereotactic biopsy. *Acta Neurochir (Wien)* 1990; 106:99–105.

50. Vertosick FT, Selker RG, Arena VC: Survival of patients with well differentiated astrocytomas diagnosed in the era of computed tomography. *Neurosurgery* 1991; 28:496–501.

51. Weingart J, Olivi A, Brem H: Supratentorial low-grade astrocytomas in adults. *Neurosurg Q* 1991; 1:141–159.

52. Weir B, Grace M: The relative significance of factors affecting postoperative survival in astrocytomas, grades one and two. *Can J Neurol Sci* 1976; 3:47–50.

53. Yaxley S, Rolls ET, Sienkiewcz ZJ: Gustatory responses of single neurons in the insula of the Macaque monkey. *J Neurophysiol* 1990; 63:689–700.

Joanne N. Bacchus, M.D., J. Gregory Cairncross, M.D.

1. Al-Mefty O, Kersh JE, Routh A, et al.: The long-term side effects of radiation therapy for benign brain tumors in adults. *J Neurosurg* 1990; 73:502–512.

2. Apuzzo MLJ, Chandrasoma PT, Cohen D, et al.: Computed imaging stereotaxy: Experience and perspective related to 500 procedures applied to brain masses. *Neurosurgery* 1987; 20:930–937.

3. Bloom HJG: Intracranial tumors: Response and resistance to therapeutic endeavours, 1970–1980. *Int J Radiat Oncol Biol Phys* 1982; 8:1083–1113.

4. Bullard DE: Role of stereotaxic biopsy in the management of patients with intracranial lesions. *Neurol Clin* 1985; 3:817–830.

5. Bullard DE, Osborne D, Burger PC, et al.: Further experience utilizing the Gildenberg technique for computed tomography-guided stereotactic biopsies. *Neurosurgery* 1986; 19:386–391.

6. Cairncross JG, Laperriere NJ: Low-grade glioma: To treat or not to treat? *Arch Neurol* 1989; 46:1238–1239.

7. Cairncross JG, Laperriere NJ: Low-grade gliomas: To treat or not to treat? (A reply). *Arch Neurol* 1990; 47:1139–1140.

8. Chamberlain MC, Murovic J, Levin VA: Absence of contrast enhancement on CT brain scans of patients with supratentorial malignant gliomas. *Neurology* 1988; 38:1371–1373.

9. Chandrasoma PT, Smith MM, Apuzzo MLJ: Stereotactic biopsy in the diagnosis of brain masses: Comparison of results of biopsy and resected surgical specimens. *Neurosurgery* 1989; 24:160–165.

10. Cook DJ, Guyatt GH, Laupacis A, et al.: Rules of evidence and clinical recommendations on the use of antithrombotic agents. *Chest* 1992; 102 (Suppl):305–311.

11. Fazekas JT: Treatment of grades I and II brain astrocytomas: The role of radiotherapy. *Int J Radiat Oncol Biol Phys* 1977; 2:661–666.

12. Gol A: The relatively benign astrocytomas of the cerebrum. *J Neurosurg* 1961; 18:501–506.

13. Hochberg FH, Slotnick B: Neuropsychologic impairment in astrocytoma survivors. *Neurology* 1980; 30:172–177.

14. Hohwieler ML, Lo T, Silverman ML, et al.: Brain necrosis after radiotherapy for primary intracerebral tumor. *Neurosurgery* 1986; 18:67–74.

15. Kelly P: Stereotactic technology in tumor surgery. *Clin Neurosurg* 1987; 35:215–253.

16. Laws ER, Taylor WF, Clifton MB, et al.: Neurosurgical management of low-grade astrocytoma of the cerebral hemispheres. *J Neurosurg* 1984; 61:665–673.

17. Leibel SA, Sheline GE, Wara WM, et al.: The role of radiation therapy in the treatment of astrocytomas. *Cancer* 1975; 35:1551–1557.

18. Maire JPH, Coudin B, Guerin J, et al.: Neuropsychologic impairment in adults with brain tumors. *Am J Clin Oncol* 1987; 10:156–162.

19. Marsa GW, Goffinet DR, Rubinstein LJ, et al.: Megavoltage irradiation in the treatment of gliomas of the brain and spinal cord. *Cancer* 1975; 36:1681–1689.

20. McCormack BM, Miller DC, Budzilovich GN, et al.: Treatment and survival of low-grade astrocytoma in adults—1977–1988. *Neurosurgery* 1992; 31:636–642.

21. Medbery CA, Straus KL, Steinberg SM, et al.: Low-grade astrocytomas: Treatment results and prognostic variables. *Int J Radiat Oncol Biol Phys* 1988; 15:837–841.

22. Morantz RA: Radiation therapy in the treatment of cerebral astrocytoma. *Neurosurgery* 1987; 20:975–982.

23. North CA, North RB, Epstein JA, et al.: Low-grade cerebral astrocytomas: Survival and quality of life after radiation therapy. *Cancer* 1990; 66:6–14.

24. Piepmeier JM: Observations on the current treatment of low-grade astrocytic tumors of the cerebral hemispheres. *J Neurosurg* 1987; 67:177–181.

25. Recht LD, Lew R, Smith TW: Suspected low-grade glioma: Is deferring treatment safe? *Ann Neurol* 1992; 31:431–436.

26. Shapiro WR: Treatment of neuroectodermal brain tumors. *Ann Neurol* 1982; 12:231–237.

27. Shaw EG, Daumas-Duport C, Scheithauer BW, et al.: Radiation therapy in the management of low-grade supratentorial astrocytomas. *J Neurosurg* 1989; 70:853–861.

28. Soffietti R, Chio A, Giordana MT, et al.: Prognostic factors in well-differentiated cerebral astrocytomas in the adult. *Neurosurgery* 1989; 24:686–692.

29. Wallner KE, Gonzales MF, Edwards MSB, et al.: Treatment results of juvenile pilocytic astrocytoma. *J Neurosurg* 1988; 69:171–176.

30. Weir B, Grace M: The relative significance of factors affecting postoperative survival in astrocytomas, grades one and two. *Can J Neurol Sci* 1976; 3:47–50.

Robert A. Morantz, M.D.

1. Chamberlain MC, Murovic JA, Levin VA: Absence of contrast enhancement on CT brain scans of patients with supratentorial malignant gliomas. *Neurology* 1988; 38:1371–1374.

2. Fults D, Brockmeyer D, Tullous MW, et al.: *p53* mutation and loss of heterozygosity on chromosomes 17 and 10 during human astro-cytoma progression. *Cancer Res* 1992; 52:674–679.

3. Kelly PJ, Daumos-Duport C, Scheithauer BW, et al.: Stereotactic histologic correlations of computed tomography- and magnetic imaging-defined abnormalties in patients with glial neoplasms. *Mayo Clin Proc* 1987; 62:450–459.

8

Treatment of de Novo Glioblastoma Multiforme: Radical Removal and Chemo- or Radiotherapy vs. Conservative Approaches

CASE

A 21-year-old man received a minor head injury in an altercation. His neurological exam was normal. Computed tomography demonstrated a lesion. The subsequent magnetic resonance image was consistent with a glioblastoma multiforme.

PARTICIPANTS

Radical Removal and Chemo- or Radiotherapy in the Treatment of de Novo Glioblastoma Multiforme–Michael Salcman, M.D.

Neurosurgical Treatment Considerations for Glioblastoma Multiforme– Jules M. Nazzaro, M.D., Edward A. Neuwelt, M.D.

Moderator–Walter A. Hall, M.D.

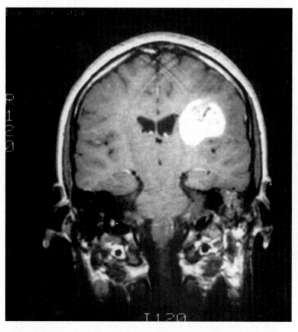 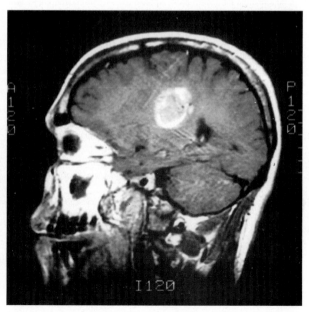

Radical Removal and Chemo- or Radiotherapy in the Treatment of *de Novo* Glioblastoma Multiforme

Michael Salcman, M.D.

Decision-making in the treatment of any patient with a brain tumor should be an individualized process, one that takes into account the specific biology and geography of the lesion, as well as the resources and aspirations of the patient.[32,34,38] The patient's emotional outlook, functional grade, age, and neurological status are usually just as important as the histologic grade or size and location of the tumor. In some patients, doing less than what is possible represents a type of therapeutic nihilism on the part of the physician and, in other patients, doing all that is possible is doing too much and exposes the patient to risks and discomforts out of proportion to the benefits to be derived from aggressive therapy.

In my personal experience with 400 consecutive and unselected patients with malignant astrocytoma, evaluated and treated by an interdisciplinary neuro-oncology team, 20% have survived 36 months or longer from the time of diagnosis and about 6% have lived at least 5 years. Before the current era of aggressive therapy, population surveys could identify only a handful of patients who did well on a long-term basis.[44] Faced with a definite increase in the number of such patients, it becomes even more critical to isolate the demographic and therapeutic features that contribute to the occasional successful outcome.[30,36] Within the context of the aggressive multimodality treatment plan carried out in our patients, all of the long-term survivors had extensive removal of their tumors, often on a repetitive basis, with a 30-day operative mortality of 3.5% and a neurological morbidity rate of 8%. In addition, they were exposed to more than 60 cGy of conventional radiation and underwent prolonged treatment with nitrosourea chemotherapy, as well as other more experimental agents. In our patients, these treatment variables were significantly associated with long-term survival independent of age and histological grade. Nevertheless, most long-term survivors were less than 40 years of age at the time of diagnosis, had tumors restricted to a single surgical field, and were highly functional when first seen. Of course, even patients selected for randomized clinical trials, as well as those who are offered interstitial brachytherapy or repeated surgery, often have favorable prognostic factors that complicate the analysis of treatment effect.[51]

PATIENT SELECTION

On the basis of prognostic and radiographic criteria, therefore, it is possible to define an ideal patient, one who is likely to respond to aggressive therapy with prolonged survival in a highly functional state; conversely, a "worst-case" scenario can also be defined, the patient in whom almost all therapeutic approaches are likely to fail. An ideal patient with a malignant glioma is in the third or fourth decade of life, has no neurological deficits, may have had a long history of seizures or other prodromal symptoms, and has a tumor of less than 5 cm in its greatest dimension that is localized to a noneloquent portion of one cerebral hemisphere. Note that these features are very similar to those used for the selection of patients for interstitial brachytherapy.[15,43] Patients with gliomas with the worst prognosis are in the seventh or eighth decade of life and present with the recent onset of mental change, incontinence, or hemiparesis; their tumors demonstrate bilateral spread through the corpus callosum or have invaded the thalamus and brain stem. Most patients with malignant gliomas can be placed somewhere along this clinical continuum, from those with the best prognosis to those with the worst, and their therapeutic options can be appropriately individualized.

RADICAL REMOVAL

As I have already indicated, even patients with good prognostic features do not achieve long-term survival in large numbers unless they are exposed to suitably aggressive therapy. Before 1980, more than 90% of patients with glioblastoma were dead 18 to 24 months after diagnosis and the 5-year survival rate was essentially zero.[39] Radical removal of the tumor should almost always be the first step in treatment (Table 1). The survival of patients with cancers outside the central nervous system is usually directly related to the surgical stage of the disease and the feasibility of wide excision.[14] The length of survival for patients suffering with a variety of benign and malignant brain tumors has been statistically associated with the extent of resection; this has been shown for medulloblastoma, meningioma, low-grade astrocytoma, and giant-cell astrocytoma.[1,18,21,23,26,46] Even patients with metastatic brain tumors benefit from surgical excision, as shown in a recent randomized trial.[27] It is logical to expect, therefore, that surgery should have a positive influence on the length of survival of patients with high-grade astrocytomas. Indeed, a number of prospective and retrospective clinical trials have isolated surgery as a significant prognostic variable, even when the effect was unexpected and initially unaccounted for.[12,25]

More to the point, several studies, some prospective and randomized in nature, have now shown that the amount of residual tumor on the postoperative images correlates with the length of survival in patients with malignant astrocytoma and glioblastoma multiforme.[3,4,9,17,52] The extent of resection also favorably influences the quality of survival and the amelioration

Table 1. Rate of Neurological Stability or Improvement by Type of Operation

Series	Number of patients	Incomplete	Complete
Ciric et al., 1987[9]	42	60%	96%
Fadul et al., 1988[13]	138	61–70%	80%
Hollerhage et al., 1991[17]	118	50–91%	74–77%

of neurological deficits.[3,17] Patients with complete removal have fewer early complications and a shorter stay in the intensive care unit.[13,17] Literature reviews denying the association between the extent of resection and the length of survival in patients with glioblastoma have generally failed to separate studies performed with and without postoperative scans for the amount of tumor removed. Patients with deeply placed tumors can sometimes achieve respectable survival times with just a stereotactic biopsy and external radiation.[11]

In some patients, of course, treatment with radiation and other therapeutic adjuvants is almost impossible without a preliminary surgical reduction in mass effect and intracranial pressure. The neurological and functional status of a patient with a malignant glioma is almost always improved or stabilized through surgery.[45] Some of this effect may result from beneficial changes in cerebral blood flow and metabolism.[5] There are also theoretical and experimental reasons for believing that surgical resection may potentiate the effectiveness of other treatments.[35] The removal of resistant cells, breakdown of the blood-brain barrier, a decrease in the tumor burden of the immunocompromised host, and a redistribution of noncycling cells into a more metabolically active state by reduction in population pressure are only some of the possible effects of surgery.[18,37,40] Laboratory studies have shown potentiation of chemotherapy and immunotherapy by surgical reduction of the tumor mass.[7,47] Similar mechanisms may serve to explain the effectiveness of reoperation in the context of multimodality therapy.[2,16,37,41,53] In the context of a multimodality treatment plan, reoperation provides a median additional survival of 37 weeks from the time of the second operation until another procedure or death.

RADIATION THERAPY

Radiation remains the single most useful therapeutic modality in the treatment of patients with malignant gliomas of all types.[49] No series has reported a measurable 2-year survival rate when patients with glioblastoma have not been given radiation.[39] In fact, the median length of survival of patients with malignant astrocytoma linearly increases with the total dose until a level of 60 to 70 cGy is reached, at which point the likelihood of neurotoxicity increases and any potential benefits are outweighed by the prospect of functional deterioration.[48] This limitation can be circumvented in a limited number of patients through the delivery of high doses of radiation to sharply restricted targets, with the use of such techniques as interstitial brachytherapy and fractionated stereotactic radiosurgery.[10,15,43] Unfortunately, the ultimate effectiveness of any purely local or regional therapy, including surgery, is limited by 3 factors based on the discrepancies between the target volume as defined by images and the actual geometry of the lesion in the brain (Table 2). Not only are astrocytomas locally invasive, but small columns or scattered "nests" of cells may extend for several centimeters into the

Table 2. Reasons for the Failure of Local Therapy

An inadequate dose is delivered to the target.
Nonvisualized tumor extends outside the target.
Too high a dose is delivered to surrounding brain tissue.

These three principles apply to any strictly local or image-based
therapeutic modality, including radiosurgery, brachytherapy,
hyperthermia, interstitial chemotherapy, and surgery.

surrounding neuropil.[8,19,33] Hence, it is necessary to deliver some type of therapy to a relatively large volume of the brain. For this reason, it is believed that conventional external radiation may confer some benefit when used "up front" to follow surgery. A similar rationale motivates the continued development of blood-borne agents, such as cytotoxic drugs or monoclonal antibodies linked to radiopharmaceuticals or toxins.

CHEMOTHERAPY

In general, the use of chemotherapy in the treatment of malignant brain tumors has been highly unsatisfactory.[49] It has not been possible to overcome the triad of problems associated with drug toxicity in the brain, selective access to the tumor, and inherent cell resistance.[40] In my experience, the brain tumors of elderly patients are resistant to almost all conventional chemotherapeutic agents. Furthermore, growth of the tumor during radiation, even in younger patients, usually predicts treatment failure with nitrosourea chemotherapy. However, those few young patients whose tumors respond to carmustine (those whose clinical exams and scans remain stable or improve over many cycles of chemotherapy, thereby requiring that the drug be discontinued only because of the risk of pulmonary or renal toxicity) are disproportionately represented among our long term (>36 months) survivors. In addition, no single agent or combination of agents has been shown to have a higher response rate (about 40%) than carmustine or procarbazine when used alone for patients with glioblastoma. Recently, a combination of agents known as PCV (procarbazine, CCNU, vincristine) has been shown to be superior to monotherapy in some patients with anaplastic astrocytoma.[22] Therefore, a trial of carmustine alone or in combination with procarbazine and vincristine is probably of benefit in young patients with malignant glioma.

CASE ANALYSIS

What to do, therefore, with the 21-year-old patient incidentally found to have the tumor illustrated? This tumor is almost certainly malignant and sits just anterior to the motor strip in the dominant hemisphere. It probably is less than 5 cm in diameter. Although the tumor's mesial margin sits perilously close to the wall of the lateral ventricle, the lesion appears to be sharply circumscribed. One should also note that a superficial sulcus enters the brain near the midportion of the tumor and that there is evidence for mass effect and left-to-right shift on the axial scan. The location of this tumor certainly is not the most desirable for a radical excision in a functionally intact patient, but the presence of the sulcus, the sharp margins of the lesion, and the vertical distance between the tumor and cortical language centers are relatively favorable features. The youth of the patient and his functional status are further arguments for taking an aggressive approach.

Surgical Technique

In this location and in this patient, the operation should be carried out with the aid of the microscope, a two-point suction cautery, and the carbon dioxide laser.[20,31,37,42] When a relatively large tumor must be removed through a restricted exposure in a critical area of the brain, the magnification and illumination of the operating microscope become essential. The transcortical approach required in this patient can be carried out by at least 2 different methods.[28,37] In the first technique, a 2-cm incision is made in the superior frontal gyrus, as perpendicular to the long axis of the motor strip as possible, and just in front of the most anterior edge of the enhancing margin of the tumor. The incision should be spread open superiorly and inferiorly by a self-retaining retractor without resection of a cortical plug. The tumor is gently vaporized or aspirated until glistening and edematous white matter is reached on every side and intraoperative measurements of the resection cavity in 3 dimensions match those of the preoperative scan.

Alternatively, this patient's tumor can be approached microsurgically through a sulcus or a fissure, as described by Pia and others.[28,31] This strategy shortens the working distance and reduces the possibility of inadvertently resecting the cortex. Of course, it also places a premium on fastidious handling of the superficial vasculature and arachnoidal spaces. To facilitate either approach, I would use an image-guided stereotactic craniotomy to bring the microscope to the specific gyrus or sulcus required for the procedure without risk of misidentification.[24,32,50] Some surgeons might prefer to use intraoperative corticography to further increase the safety of surgery in the vicinity of eloquent cortex and permit resection of the tumor to the very edge of a motor or language area.[6,29]

Radiotherapy Treatment

Postoperatively, the patient should receive at least 60 cGy of radiation, the first 45 cGy of which is delivered to a large region in the left hemisphere by conventional external means. In most cases, a boost of 18 cGy can then be delivered to the operative site through the same technique. As an alternative, a total dose higher than 60 cGy can be achieved by using interstitial brachytherapy to deliver a local boost of 50 to 60 cGy over a period of 3 to 5 days after external treatment to 45 cGy has been completed. Up front use of brachytherapy is more likely to be of benefit in patients with anaplastic astrocytoma than glioblastoma multiforme. I would also be less likely to recommend initial brachy-

therapy if the postoperative scan is essentially free of enhancement or if the ventricle was breached during surgery and there is risk of a cerebrospinal fluid leakage. The likelihood of subependymal spread occurring in this young patient is increased because of the proximity of the mesial edge of the tumor to the ventricle and would prompt me to start carmustine chemotherapy at the conclusion of radiation. The starting dose would be 80 to 100 mg/m^2 every 8 to 10 weeks given intravenously. I would be less likely to use up front chemotherapy if the tumor was not a glioblastoma, if there was no evidence of ventricular involvement and, especially, if the postoperative scan were free of enhancement. Chemotherapy would then be saved as a rescue modality for use alone or in combination with brachytherapy after repeated resection. In addition, I would not offer initial carmustine to a patient older than 40 years of age if alternative phase II or phase III agents were available for study. In older and sicker patients, when investigational agents are not available or appropriate, treatment with an oral agent such as lomustine (CCNU) or procarbazine may facilitate community-based care.

Post-Treatment Considerations

Unless the postoperative scan is negative for enhancement and the tumor fails to grow during radiation, I am not optimistic about long-term survival in this patient. Subependymal spread in the lateral ventricle is very likely and is an ominous sign of a rapidly downhill course in young patients with glioblastoma. Spread of the tumor to immediately contiguous functional regions would quickly impair the quality of survival and decrease the motivation of both patient and physician for further intensive therapy. On the other hand, the lack of ring-shaped enhancement and the young age of the patient may indicate that the tumor is really an anaplastic astrocytoma. This would obviously change both the prognosis and the therapeutic plan.

Neurosurgical Treatment Considerations for Glioblastoma Multiforme

Jules M. Nazzaro, M.D., Edward A. Neuwelt, M.D.

The present case is that of a neurologically intact 21-year-old man found to have a left-sided intracerebral lesion, and a subsequent needle biopsy showed glioblastoma multiforme. He is referred now for an opinion regarding further surgical treatment.

AIMS OF SURGERY

Surgery has 3 aims in adults with intermediate and high-grade astrocytomas. First is the need to establish a diagnosis, which may be done either through needle biopsy or at craniotomy. The accuracy and overall limited morbidity associated with needle biopsy techniques are now well established.[31] The second aim of surgery is to reduce mass effect, and the third aim is to significantly reduce the number of tumor cells. A consideration of the latter 2 aims as they pertain to the patient described above are discussed below.

Reduction of Mass Effect

This patient presents with a relatively large lesion, but he is asymptomatic and the lack of significant mass effect both clinically and radiographically is noted. The basal cisterns are well visualized and there appears to be minimal overall distortion of adjoining brain structures. Given these considerations, and the

fact that the lesion is deep and located within eloquent brain in the dominant hemisphere, we would not recommend surgery for mass effect at this juncture. In our opinion, a high risk of significant morbidity is associated with craniotomy and tumor resection in patients such as this. This consideration includes surgery which may be done with intraoperative brain mapping.[2] Further, although it may be proposed that computer-based stereotactic surgery be considered here, there is little, if any, data comparing morbidity after conventional surgery to the patient's function after stereotactic-directed surgery for glioblastoma.[30] This includes stereotactic methods in which catheters are placed to guide the resection,[13] as well as "volumetric" methods.[12,22] Regardless of the surgical method, few studies have examined either short- or long-term patient function and neurological status after supratentorial surgery for glioblastoma but, rather, have emphasized survival statistics.[30] In addition, computer-based stereotactic surgery requires an open route to the lesion and, thus, the attendant risks to associated eloquent structures. Other potential limitations of such methods are considered below. Finally, the lesion in this patient is too large to be considered for primary treatment with high-dose single- or limited-fraction stereotactic radiotherapy.[37]

This patient can be held in contrast to the patient who clearly has symptoms from a tumor and in whom surgery may provide decompression and relief of elevated intracranial pressure. However, the potential temporizing benefits of surgery in the latter situation must be weighed in regard to the patient's preoperative response to steroids, as well as to significant prognostic factors such as age, Karnofsky (functional) status, and the location of the lesion.

Cytoreductive Surgery

Frequently, neurosurgeons report that a gross total resection of visually apparent tumor was accomplished. The true oncologic meaning of gross total resection, however, or even some percentage thereof in patients with high-grade gliomas, is far from clear. Tumor cells invariably infiltrate adjoining brain tissue[5,35] and evidence suggests that a tumor may not only extend beyond areas of contrast enhancement on computed tomograms (CT) or magnetic resonance images (MRI),[24,25] but also beyond areas of increased signal on T2-weighted MRI.[26,29] Kelly[23] suggested that less than 50% of actual tumor volume may be delineated on contrast-enhanced CT, and enhanced MRI has yet to be shown to be more sensitive than contrast CT in defining the extent of the tumor.[3,26] Contrast enhancement only represents a breakdown of the blood-brain barrier and methods to detect infiltrative tumor beyond these areas remain investigational.[34] Considerable research is directed at finding methods of not only manipulating the blood-brain barrier to enhance the delivery of chemotherapy to a tumor, but also towards the biochemical and pharmacological alteration of agents to enhance delivery to areas protected by an intact barrier.[14,15,38] The gross infiltration of brain tissue by high-grade gliomas is further suggested by the fact that a lobectomy (that is, a wide and generous resection) has not been clearly shown to increase a patient's survival in comparison to more limited techniques.[30]

Investigators have compared pre- and postoperative contrast-enhanced studies as a measure of the degree of tumor removal. The broad estimation of tumor cell number and the overall inherent high degree of error of such methods are apparent. Further, the methods employed to compare pre- and postoperative areas of enhancement and, thus, measures of tumor volume vary widely among investigators. In this regard, there is no agreement concerning the timing of postoperative contrast studies and at what time such studies reflect gross tumor as opposed to operative changes.[30] Of note, authors[28] reported margin or ring enhancement on postoperative days 3 and 7, but not on day 30, in nontumor patients who had a lobectomy for epilepsy.

In accord with the broad and inherently optimistic estimation afforded by descriptions such as gross total resection, such estimates are most often translated to represent a 90 to 99% tumor resection. It must be recognized, however, that if a high-grade glioma represents 10^{11} or 10^{12} cells when it is detected,[20,29,36] a 90 or 99% resection (that is, 1- to 2-log cell kill) means that 10^9 to 10^{10} tumor cells remain after aggressive surgery, assuming 10^{11} as the original number.

Given these considerations, it is not surprising to find that there is no agreement in the literature as to whether cytoreductive surgery in adults with supratentorial glioblastoma increases survival.[6,7,9–11,19,21,27,30,33] This may also be due, in part, to the lack of or improper statistical handling of significant prognostic variables such as patient age, Karnofsky status, histopathological variables, tumor location, and adjuvant therapies in such

studies, all of which have been retrospective in design. Also considered are recent retrospective studies that have employed statistical methods, including multivariant analyses, recursive partitioning analyses, and further regression analyses although, again, there is little agreement or clear direction regarding patient survival and aggressive surgery for glioblastoma. In this regard, the only therapy that has been consistently associated with improved survival is conventional external radiation.[30] The need for a prospective randomized study to examine the relationship between cytoreductive surgery and patient survival is evident.

While considerable attention over recent years has been directed towards computer-based stereotactic methods, overall there is no clear data documenting significantly improved survival associated with such techniques in adults with supratentorial high-grade gliomas.[21,39] Such methods rely on available imaging techniques to detect infiltrative tumors. In addition, as the brain shifts during surgery and real-time intraoperative computer-assisted methods are not available, the ability of current computer-based stereotactic methods to truly direct glioblastoma surgery with regard to a significant and more meaningful oncologic reduction in tumor cell number, in comparison to more standard techniques, may be questioned. Recent investigators who have used volumetric stereotactic techniques have reported a high percentage of grossly incomplete (that is, 50 to 90%) resections of glioblastoma as measured through postoperative contrast-enhanced CT.[12] Thus, it is also not clear if there is any cost benefit associated with these more recent methods.

SUMMARY OF RECOMMENDED TREATMENT PLAN

The patient under discussion here is asymptomatic. After considering all factors, a surgical procedure for mass effect is not recommended. The tumor is left-sided, deeply situated and involves ganglionic structures. In our opinion and based on the available data, surgery would not *significantly* reduce the tumor cell number in this patient. We would refer the patient for radiation and chemotherapy. Should the patient become symptomatic during therapy, a course of steroids can be used, although the limitations and complications of the long-term use of steroids are readily recognized.[8] If the latter is exhausted, the overall temporizing nature of surgery with regard to mass effect must be weighed and based, in part, on the patient's expected function after surgery.

When this patient experiences the expected eventual disease progression after radiation and chemotherapy, further radiographs will be necessary to evaluate gross areas of brain involvement and the role of temporizing surgery. The role of surgery again must be weighed in view of the patient's clinical status, the attendant operative morbidity, and the lack of clear data indicating improved survival after aggressive surgery for glioblastoma. Surgery would also not be considered at that juncture unless the patient, as well as the consultant physicians, agreed preoperatively upon a plan of further adjuvant therapy after tumor surgery. However, adjuvant therapies such as brachytherapy or supplemental radiotherapy such as radiosurgery are not applicable here, given the size and location of the tumor and the overall rise of brain necrosis, swelling, and the need for further surgery associated with these therapies.[1,16,17] Other adjuvant therapies, such as immunotherapy, gene therapy, or polymer wafers impregnated with chemotherapy, have yet to be shown to significantly improve survival.[4,18,32] To date, all of these are limited by the blood-brain barrier and, thus, are local therapies for a nonlocalized disease. The role of cranial radiation in the treatment of brain tumor patients and its associated cognitive sequelae remain therapeutic dilemmas. In a soon to be initiated multi-institutional phase III randomized trial, we will evaluate the sequencing of enhanced combination chemotherapy delivery and cranial radiation with regard to both survival and cognitive outcome in patients with glioma.

Treatment of *de Novo* Glioblastoma Multiforme: Radical Removal and Chemo- or Radiotherapy vs. Conservative Approaches

Walter A. Hall, M.D.

The patient presented is a 21-year-old man with an asymptomatic brain tumor found incidentally after a minor head injury. Because the lesion is located in the deep posterior left frontal lobe, a stereotactic biopsy was initially performed to obtain a histological diagnosis. Although stereotactic biopsies can be associated with sampling error because of the limited amount of tissue obtained, the fact that glioblastoma multiforme was confirmed histologically argues against pathologic inaccuracy or misrepresentation. The presence of glioblastoma multiforme within the tissue sample dictates the biologic behavior of the lesion shown on magnetic resonance imaging (MRI).

There are 2 opposing viewpoints presented regarding the appropriate treatment of an individual with *de novo* glioblastoma multiforme. One approach favors an aggressive surgical resection after the results of the biopsy are known, and before initiating adjuvant external beam radiation therapy and systemic chemotherapy. The second opinion recommends conservative treatment and supports the use of immediate radiotherapy combined with chemotherapy.

This particular case has several prognostic factors that must be considered individually and in combination when recommending a rational treatment plan to the patient. These factors have been examined in numerous studies and include the histology of the tumor, the age of the patient, the patient's functional status or Karnofsky score, and the size and location of the tumor.[2–4,6,8,11,12,16,17,19] Each factor can influence both the current choice of therapy and the therapeutic options available in the future.

TUMOR HISTOLOGY

Two particular features intrinsic to the glioblastoma multiforme should be examined when choosing a route of treatment. These are the infiltrative nature of the tumor and the long-term survival of patients with this diagnosis. Infiltration of malignant cells into surrounding brain parenchyma for several centimeters, that is only detectable histologically, prevents complete resection of this neoplasm. This infiltration extends beyond the enhancing margin of the tumor that is apparent on radiologic images and well into surrounding edematous areas that are hypodense on the computed tomogram and have an increased signal on the T2-weighted MRI.[10] The dissemination of tumor cells into adjacent brain tissue provides the basis for adjuvant radiation therapy, which will deliver a defined amount to a region around the enhancing lesion combined with a boost to the mass, and systemic chemotherapy, that will permeate the whole brain.[5,16,20]

The long-term survival of patients with glioblastoma multiforme has been recently evaluated. Salcman and colleagues[17] reported a survival of more than 3 years for 20% of patients with malignant astrocytoma who were treated with an aggressive multi-disciplinary approach. The observed 5-year survival rate was 6%. A similar survival rate of 5% was seen in 22 of 449 patients with glioblastoma multiforme at 5 years who underwent aggressive tumor removal and multimodal therapy.[2] According to the Swedish Cancer Registry,[18] 6 (0.5%) of 1147 patients with grade III and IV astrocytomas lived for 12 to 28 years after surgery.

AGE AND KARNOFSKY SCORE

Probably the single most important variable that predicts a patient's response to therapy is the patient's age.[4,6,11,17,19] Salcman and colleagues[17] found that long-term survivors were more likely to be younger than 40 years of age. Franklin[6] found that patients with glioblastoma multiforme under the age of 30, as in the present case, survived longer. As the annual number of malignant brain tumors seen in the elderly increases, the appropriate treatment for these patients must be determined.[7,11,17] In patients with glioblastoma multiforme over the age of 65, Kelly and Hunt[11] reported a mean survival of 16.9 weeks for those who had biopsies and radiation compared to 30 weeks for those having resection before radiation therapy. A higher Karnofsky performance status has been associated with longer survival times.[4,19] The improved length of survival for younger patients with a good performance status is more likely related to their ability to tolerate more aggressive therapy, such as multiple resections, interstitial radiotherapy (brachytherapy), and changes in chemotherapeutic regimens before experiencing treatment-related toxicity, than a difference in the biologic behavior of their tumors.[17] Patients in poor neurological condition are less likely to tolerate repeated surgery and are prone to those systemic complications associated with malignant primary brain tumors.

TUMOR LOCATION AND SIZE

The location of the tumor often dictates the surgical approach most appropriate for the patient. Lesions located in eloquent brain are often not completely resectable without an increased risk of postoperative neurological morbidity. Lesions located deep, midline, and beneath the motor cortex are frequently treated through stereotactic biopsy in contrast to superficial, lobar lesions for which total resection is usually attempted.[4,6,12,16,17,19] Characteristically, most neurosurgeons overestimate the extent of their surgical resection for accessible tumors. The degree of residual disease can be ascertained by postoperative MRI obtained between 1 and 3 days after surgery to minimize surgically-induced contrast enhancement.[1] In these early postoperative studies, about 80% of tumor recurrences arise from enhancing remnants. In this same study, the neurosurgeon's estimation of the reduction of gross tumor burden was much less accurate, by a factor of 3, compared to imaging studies.[1] Patients with glioblastoma multiforme who were found to have postoperative enhancement had a 7 times higher risk of death than those without residual tumor.[1] Lesions that are large in diameter are difficult to resect completely and are more likely to show postoperative peripheral enhancement. Size is an important determinant for the applicability of other therapeutic modalities, such as brachytherapy and stereotactic radiosurgery. In addition to having a diameter of less than 6 cm, lesions considered for brachytherapy should not have an irregular shape.[8] Stereotactic radiosurgery has been considered useful in the initial treatment of malignant gliomas with a median tumor volume of about 5 cm^3.[15]

APPROACHES TO TREATMENT

Aggressive Approach

Factors that weigh heavily on the decision to recommend open surgical resection at this time are the patient's age and functional status. The diagnosis of glioblastoma multiforme in a 21-year-old is obviously more of a tragedy than for the elderly patient with a much shorter natural life expectancy. Even though some cerebral edema surrounds the lesion on MRI, the patient is asymptomatic with a Karnofsky performance status of 100 (normal, no evidence of disease). Clearly, with most neurosurgical procedures, patients in good condition do better than those who are impaired, and neurosurgeons are more able to preserve than restore neurological function with surgery.

Selected patients with glioblastoma multiforme treated with resection and radiation therapy have longer survival times than those who undergo biopsy and radiation therapy.[4] An open procedure would be best done with stereotactic guidance because of the deep, posterior location of this lesion in the dominant hemisphere. Cortical mapping or functional mapping with MRI may provide the neurosurgeon with useful information that will result in less neurological morbidity. The size of the lesion poses 2 problems with respect to radiation therapy. "Up front" brachytherapy without some degree of resection has a risk of neurological morbidity, and this modality may be best reserved for future recurrent disease. The potential for worsening cerebral edema during conventional radiotherapy that leads to emergent debulking cannot be ignored.

Cytoreductive surgery without additional adjuvant treatment is of limited benefit for patients. However, when an aggressive surgical approach is combined with radiation therapy, chemotherapy, brachytherapy, and repeated surgery, the 3-year survival for patients is 20% in some series.[17] For the young individual, 3 years is a considerable improvement over the average survival for glioblastoma multiforme of less than a year. In extending survival by 3 years, most neurosurgical oncologists hope that some of the more novel agents currently under development, such as immunotoxin therapy or gene therapy, will become available for clinical use.[9,14]

Conservative Approach

A conservative approach to this particular patient is related to the location of the lesion, the performance status of the patient and the tumor histology. Lesions located deep in the dominant hemisphere adjacent to the motor cortex have a higher surgical morbidity than those in superficial, lobar regions. This patient is neurologically normal with an excellent performance status and a good quality of life. If open surgical resection is attempted, potential postoperative deficits for this lesion include expressive aphasia and hemiparesis or hemiplegia. The effect of a major neurological deficit resulting from surgery on this patient's life must be considered. A young college athlete is unlikely to tolerate a hemiparesis or difficulty in communication. Profound motor weakness can lead to other problems associated with malignant brain tumors, such as deep venous thrombosis and pulmonary embolus. All of these issues must be clearly presented to the patient and the patient's family when therapeutic options are discussed.

The histology and biologic behavior of the glioblastoma multiforme must also be emphasized when counseling the patient. This is currently not a curable disease; the 5-year survival for patients who have received both aggressive and conservative treatment is about 5%.[2,17] Ten-year survivors are almost nonexistent.[18] Infiltration by a glioblastoma multiforme extends far beyond what can be resected using the microscope and laser, ensuring incomplete removal and future regrowth. The knowledge that the degree of surgical resection either initially or at recurrence has not influenced the overall survival rates for this disease process has strongly influenced the advocates of a conservative approach.[3,6,12,16,19] The likelihood of some postoperative residual enhancement along the posterior edge of the lesion anterior to the motor strip also supports conservative treatment.[1]

Two other features present on the MRI that may support a conservative approach are the presence of minimal mass effect and the proximity of the tumor to the lateral ventricle. In the absence of severe mass effect, the patient may tolerate radiation therapy without neurological decompensation. If the patient has evidence of subependymal spread of malignant disease, the prognosis is much worse, irrespective of the treatment plan proposed.

Agreement in Treatment

Both parties agree with respect to the utility of adjuvant therapies in treating a patient such as the one described here. The most effective treatment for malignant brain tumors, in this case the glioblastoma multiforme, is radiation therapy. Many reviews cite postoperative radiation therapy as a prognostic factor for extended survival in patients who complete this treatment.[1,4,12,13,16,17,20] Although patients in these series were treated with whole-brain radiation therapy, partial-brain radiotherapy delivered to the enhancing mass and a 3-cm peripheral margin is commonly administered today. A total dose of at least 60 Gy in conventional fraction sizes is usually administered for glioblastoma multiforme.[13,17] The effect of conventional radiotherapy and the inability to control local disease form the theoretical basis for treating malignant gliomas with brachytherapy and stereotactic radiosurgery, despite their infiltrative nature.[8,15,17] Controlling peripheral tumor extension is the intention behind instituting combined radiation therapy and chemotherapy after surgery. A recently published meta-analysis of 16 randomized clinical trials involving more than 3000 patients treated with combination radiation therapy and chemotherapy found an increase in survival of 10.1% at 1 year and 8.6% at 2 years.[5]

Personal Considerations

Taking into account the patient's individual situation cannot be overly emphasized. A young adult who is neurologically normal with glioblastoma multiforme is usually treated more aggressively than patients in their 40s or 50s who present with this tumor *de novo*. The treatment recommendations should represent a balance between an aggressive and conservative approach for a lesion in this location. The risk of neurological injury that can occur with an open surgical resection and the resultant alteration in quality of life must be clearly presented to and understood by the patient and his family. Similarly, the chances of neurological worsening during or after radiation therapy necessitating surgical intervention that may not restore lost function must be elucidated.

Personal Treatment

The best treatment strategy for this patient combines aspects of both therapeutic approaches. Initially, I would recommend conventional radiation therapy and chemotherapy. Stabilization of the tumor on radiographs can be managed with continued chemotherapy; progression dictates a change in the treatment regimen if the patient remains clinically stable. If this patient's neurological condition worsens during or after radiation therapy, I would carry out a limited resection using stereotactic guidance that is intended to restore neurological function and prevent further progression. Any postoperative enhancement detected on images done within 1 to 3 days after surgery may be considered for treatment with either brachytherapy or stereotactic radiosurgery. Prolonging survival to the longest possible extent may allow other potentially more effective therapies, such as gene therapy and immunotoxin therapy, to be further developed and investigated for future use. These newer, more potent agents might preclude many of our currently employed conventional therapeutic measures, such as surgical resection, radiation therapy, and chemotherapy.

REFERENCES

Michael Salcman, M.D.

1. Adegbite AB, Khan MI, Paine KWE, et al.: The recurrence of intracranial meningioma after surgical treatment. *J Neurosurg* 1983; 58:51–56.
2. Ammirati M, Galicich JH, Arbit E, et al.: Reoperation in the treatment of recurrent intracranial malignant gliomas. *Neurosurgery* 1987; 21:601–614.
3. Ammirati M, Vick N, Liao Y, et al.: Effect of the extent of surgical resection on survival and quality of life in patients with supratentorial glioblastomas and anaplastic astrocytomas. *Neurosurgery* 1987; 21:201–206.
4. Andreou J, George AE, Wise A, et al.: CT prognostic criteria of survival after malignant glioma surgery. *Am J Neuroradiol* 1983; 4:488–490.
5. Beaney RP, Brooks DJ, Leenders KL, et al.: Blood flow and oxygen utilization in the contralateral cerebral cortex of patients with untreated intracranial tumors as studied by positron emission tomography, with observations on the effect of decompressive surgery. *J Neurol Neurosurg Psychiatry* 1985; 48:310–319.
6. Berger MS, Cohen WA, Ojemman GA: Correlation of motor cortex brain mapping data with magnetic resonance imaging. *J Neurosurg* 1990; 72:383–387.
7. Brooks WH, Roszman TL: Cellular immune responsiveness of patients with primary intracranial tumors, in Thomas DGT, Graham DI (eds): *Brain Tumors: Scientific Basis, Clinical Investigation, and Current Therapy*. London, Butterworth, 1980, pp 121–132.
8. Burger PC: Pathologic anatomy and CT correlations in the glioblastoma multiforme. *Appl Neurophysiol* 1983; 46:180–187.
9. Ciric I, Ammirati M, Vick N, et al.: Supratentorial gliomas: Surgical considerations and immediate postoperative results. Gross total resection versus partial resection. *Neurosurgery* 1987; 21:21–26.
10. Coffey RJ, Lunsford LD, Flickinger JC: The role of radiosurgery in the treatment of malignant brain tumors. *Neurosurg Clin North Am* 1992; 3:231–244.
11. Coffey RJ, Lunsford LD, Taylor FH: Survival after stereotactic biopsy of malignant gliomas. *Neurosurgery* 1988; 22:465–473.
12. Cohadon F, Aouad N, Rougier A, et al.: Histologic and non-histologic factors correlated with survival time in supratentorial astrocytic tumors. *J Neuro-Oncol* 1985; 3:105–111.
13. Fadul C, Wood J, Thaler H, et al.: Morbidity and mortality of craniotomy for excision of supratentorial gliomas. *Neurology* 1988; 38:1374–1379.
14. National Gastrointestinal Tumor Study Group: Adjuvant therapy of colon cancer: Results of a prospectively randomized trial. *N Engl J Med* 1984; 310:737–743.
15. Gutin PH, Leibel SA, Wara WM, et al.: Recurrent malignant gliomas: Survival following interstitial brachytherapy with high-activity iodine-125 sources. *J Neurosurg* 1987; 67:864–873.
16. Harsh GR IV, Levin VA, Gutin PH, et al.: Reoperation for recurrent glioblastoma and anaplastic astrocytoma. *Neurosurgery* 1987; 21:615–621.
17. Hollerhage HG, Zumkeller M, Becker M, et al.: Influence of type and extent of surgery on early results and survival time in glioblastoma multiforme. *Acta Neurochir (Wien)* 1991; 113:31–37.
18. Hoshino T: A commentary on the biology and growth kinetics of low-grade and high-grade gliomas. *J Neurosurg* 1984; 61:895–900.
19. Kelly PJ, Daumas-Duport C, Kispert DB, et al.: Imaging-based stereotaxic serial biopsies in untreated intracranial glial neoplasms. *J Neurosurg* 1987; 66:865–874.
20. Kelly PJ, Kall BA, Goerss S, et al.: Computer-assisted stereotaxic laser resection of intra-axial brain neoplasms. *J Neurosurg* 1986; 64:427–439.
21. Laws ER, Taylor WF, Clifton MB, et al.: Neurosurgical management of low-grade astrocytoma of the cerebral hemispheres. *J Neurosurg* 1984; 61:665–673.
22. Levin VA, Silver P, Hannigan J, et al.: Superiority of postradiotherapy adjuvant chemotherapy with CCNU, procarbazine, and vincristine (PCV) over BCNU for anaplastic gliomas: NCOG 6G61 final report. *Int J Radiat Oncol Biol Phys* 1990; 18:321–324.
23. Mirimanoff RO, Dosoretz DE, Linggood RM, et al.: Meningioma: Analysis of recurrence and progression following neurosurgical resection. *J Neurosurg* 1985; 62:18–24.
24. Moore MR, Black PM, Ellenbogen R, et al.: Stereotactic craniotomy: Methods and results using the Brown-Roberts-Wells stereotactic frame. *Neurosurgery* 1989; 25:572–578.
25. Nelson DF, Nelson JS, Davis DR, et al.: Survival and prognosis of patients with astrocytoma with atypical or anaplastic features. *J Neuro-Oncol* 1985; 3:99–103.
26. Park TS, Hoffman HJ, Hendrick EB, et al.: Medulloblastoma: Clinical presentation and management: Experience at the Hospital for Sick Children, Toronto, 1950–1980. *J Neurosurg* 1983; 58:543–552.
27. Patchell RA, Tibbs PA, Walsh JW, et al.: A randomized trial of surgery in the treatment of single metastases to the brain. *N Engl J Med* 1990; 322:494–499.
28. Pia HW: Microsurgery of gliomas. *Acta Neurochir (Wien)* 1986; 80:1–11.
29. Rostomily RC, Berger MS, Ojemann GA, et al.: Postoperative deficits and functional recovery following removal of tumors involving the dominant hemisphere supplementary motor area. *J Neurosurg* 1991; 75:62–68.
30. Salcman M: Epidemiology and factors affecting survival, in Apuzzo

MLJ (ed): *Malignant Cerebral Glioma.* Park Ridge, American Association of Neurological Surgeons, 1990, pp 95–109.

31. Salcman M: Intrinsic cerebral glioma, in Apuzzo MLJ (ed): *Brain Surgery: Complication Avoidance and Management.* New York, Churchill Livingstone, 1993, pp 379–390.

32. Salcman M: Malignant glioma management. *Neurosurg Clin North Am* 1990; 1:49–63.

33. Salcman M (ed): *Neurobiology of Brain Tumors,* vol. 4. Baltimore, Williams and Wilkins, 1991.

34. Salcman M: Radical surgery for low-grade glioma. *Clin Neurosurg* 1990; 36:353–366.

35. Salcman M: Resection and reoperation in neuro-oncology: Rationale and approach. *Neurol Clin* 1985; 3:831–842.

36. Salcman M: The role of surgical resection in the treatment of malignant brain tumors: Who benefits? *Oncology* 1988; 2:47–59.

37. Salcman M: Supratentorial gliomas: Clinical features and surgical therapy, in Wilkins RH, Rengachary SS (eds): *Neurosurgery.* New York, McGraw-Hill, 1985, pp 550–579.

38. Salcman M: Surgical decision-making for malignant brain tumors. *Clin Neurosurg* 1989; 35:285–313.

39. Salcman M: Survival in glioblastoma: Historical perspective. *Neurosurgery* 1980; 7:435–439.

40. Salcman M, Broadwell RD: The blood-brain barrier, in Salcman M (ed): *Neurobiology of Brain Tumors,* vol. 4. Baltimore, Williams and Wilkins, 1991, pp 229–249.

41. Salcman M, Kaplan RS, Ducker TB, et al.: Effect of age and reoperation on survival in the combined modality treatment of malignant astrocytoma. *Neurosurgery* 1982; 10:454–463.

42. Salcman M, Robinson W, Montgomery E: Laser microsurgery: A review of 105 intracranial tumors. *J Neuro-Oncol* 1986; 3:363–371.

43. Salcman M, Sewchand W, Amin PP, et al.: Technique and prelimi-nary results of interstitial irradiation for primary brain tumors. *J Neuro-Oncol* 1986; 4:141–149.

44. Salford LG, Brun A, Nirfalk S: Ten-year survival among patients with supratentorial astrocytomas grade III and IV. *J Neurosurg* 1988; 69:506–509.

45. Shapiro WR: Treatment of neuroectodermal brain tumors. *Ann Neurol* 1982; 12:231–237.

46. Steiger HJ, Markwalder RV, Seiler RW, et al.: Early prognosis of supratentorial grade 2 astrocytomas in adult patients after resection or stereotactic biopsy: An analysis of 50 cases operated on between 1984 and 1988. *Acta Neurochir (Wien)* 1990; 106:99–105.

47. Tel E, Hoshino T, Barker M, et al.: Effect of surgery on BCNU chemotherapy in a rat brain tumor model. *J Neurosurg* 1980; 52:529–532.

48. Walker MD, Green SB, Byar DP, et al.: Randomized comparisons of radiotherapy and nitrosoureas for the treatment of malignant glioma after surgery. *N Engl J Med* 1980; 303:1323–1329.

49. Walker MD, Strike TA, Sheline GE: An analysis of dose effect relationship in the radiotherapy of malignant gliomas. *Int J Radiat Oncol Biol Phys* 1979; 5:1725–1731.

50. Watanabe E, Mayanagi Y, Kosugi Y, et al.: Open surgery assisted by the neuronavigator, a stereotactic, articulated, sensitive arm. *Neurosurgery* 1991; 28:792–800.

51. Winger MJ, Macdonald DR, Schold SC, et al.: Selection bias in clinical trials of anaplastic glioma. *Ann Neurol* 1989; 26:531–534.

52. Wood JR, Green SB, Shapiro WR: The prognostic importance of tumor size in malignant gliomas: A computed tomographic scan study by the Brain Tumor Cooperative Group. *J Clin Oncol* 1988; 6:338–343.

53. Young B, Oldfield EH, Markesbery WR, et al.: Reoperation for glioblastoma. *J Neurosurg* 1981; 55:917–921.

Jules M. Nazzaro, M.D., Edward A. Neuwelt, M.D.

1. Alexander E III, Loeffler J: Radiosurgery using a modified linear accelerator. *Neurosurg Clin North Am* 1992; 3:167–190.

2. Berger MS, Ojemann GA: Intraoperative brain mapping techniques in neuro-oncology. *Stereotact Funct Neurosurg* 1992; 58:153–161.

3. Brant-Zawadski M, Berry I, Osaki L, et al.: Gd-DTPA in clinical MR of the brain: 1. Intraaxial lesions. *AJR* 1986; 147:1223–1230.

4. Brem H, Walter KA, Langer R, et al.: Polymers as controlled drug delivery devices for the treatment of malignant brain tumors. *Eur J Pharm Biopharm* 1993; 39:2–7.

5. Burger PC, Heinz ER, Shibata T, et al.: Topographic anatomy and CT correlations in the untreated glioblastoma multiforme. *J Neurosurg* 1988; 68:698–704.

6. Chandler KL, Prados MD, Malec M, et al.: Long-term survival in patients with glioblastoma multiforme. *Neurosurgery* 1993; 31:716–720.

7. Curran WJ, Scott CB, Horton J, et al.: Recursive partitioning analysis of prognostic factors in three radiation therapy oncology group malignant glioma trials. *J Natl Cancer Inst* 1993; 85:704–710.

8. Delattre JY, Posner JB: Neurologic complications of chemotherapy and radiation therapy, in Aminoff MJ (ed): *Neurology and General Medicine.* New York, Churchill Livingstone, 1989, pp 365–388.

9. Devaux BC, O'Fallon JR, Kelly PJ: Resection, biopsy, and survival in malignant glial neoplasms. *J Neurosurg* 1993; 78:767–775.

10. Fischbach AJ, Martz KL, Nelson JS, et al.: Long-term survival in treated anaplastic astrocytomas: A report of combined RTOG/ECOG studies. *Am J Clin Oncol* 1991; 14:365–370.

11. Franklin CI: Does extent of surgery make a difference in high-grade malignant astrocytoma? *Australas Radiol* 1992; 36:44–47.

12. Giorgi C, Ongania E, Casolino SD, et al.: Deep seated cerebral lesion removal, guided by volumetric rendering of morphological data, stereotactically acquired clinical results, and technical considerations. *Acta Neurochir (Suppl)* 1991; 52:19–21.

13. Giunta F, Marini G: Open stereotactic neurosurgery: 57 cases. *Acta Neurochir (Suppl)* 1991; 52:13–14.

14. Greig NH: Drug delivery to the brain by blood-brain barrier circumvention and drug modification, in Neuwelt EA (ed): *Implications of the Blood-Brain Barrier and Its Manipulation,* vol. 1. New York, Plenum, 1989, pp 311–367.

15. Gumerlock MK, Drew Belshe B, Madsen R, et al.: Osmotic blood-brain barrier disruption and chemotherapy in the treatment of high grade malignant gliom: Patient series and literature review. *J Neuro-Oncol* 1992; 12:33–46.

16. Gutin PH, Leibel SA, Wara WM, et al.: Recurrent malignant gliomas: Survival following interstitial brachytherapy with high-activity iodine-125 sources. *J Neurosurg* 1987; 67:864–873.

17. Gutin PH, Prados MD, Phillips TL, et al.: External irradiation followed by an interstitial high activity iodine-125 implant 'boost' in the initial treatment of malignant gliomas: NCOG Study 6G82-2. *Int J Radiat Oncol Biol Phys* 1991; 21:601–606.

18. Hall WA, Fodstad Ø: Immunotoxins and central nervous system neoplasia. *J Neurosurg* 1992; 76:1–12.

19. Hollerhage HG, Zumkeller M, Becker M, et al.: Influence of type and extent of surgery on early results and survival time in glioblastoma multiforme. *Acta Neurochir (Wien)* 1991; 113:31–37.

20. Hoshino T, Wilson CB, Rosenblum ML, et al.: Chemotherapeutic implications of growth fraction and cycle time in glioblastomas. *J Neurosurg* 1975; 43:127–135.

21. Kelly PJ: Stereotactic biopsy and resection of thalamic astrocytomas. *Neurosurgery* 1989; 25:185–195.

22. Kelly PJ: Stereotactic craniotomy. *Neurosurg Clin North Am* 1990; 1:781–799.

23. Kelly PJ: Stereotactic technology in tumor surgery. *Clin Neurosurg* 1987; 35:215–253.

24. Kelly PJ, Daumas-Duport C, Kispert DB, et al.: Imaging-based stereotaxic serial biopsies in untreated intracranial glial neoplasms. *J Neurosurg* 1987; 66:865–874.

25. Kelly PJ, Daumas-Duport C, Scheithauer BW, et al.: Stereotactic

histologic correlations of computed tomography- and magnetic imaging-defined abnormalities in patients with glial neoplasms. *Mayo Clin Proc* 1987; 62:450–459.

26. Kent DL, Larson EB: Magnetic resonance imaging of the brain and spine: Is clinical efficacy established after the first decade? *Ann Intern Med* 1988;107:402–424.

27. Kreth FW, Wamke PC, Scheremet R, et al.: Surgical resection and radiation therapy versus biopsy and radiation therapy in the treatment of glioblastoma multiforme. *J Neurosurg* 1993; 78:762–766.

28. Laohaprasit V, Silbergeld DL, Ojeman GA, et al.: Postoperative CT contrast enhancement following lobectomy for epilepsy. *J Neurosurg* 1990; 73:392–395.

29. Lunsford LD, Martinez AJ, Latchaw RE: Magnetic resonance imaging does not define tumor boundaries. *Acta Radiol (Stockh)* (Suppl) 1986; 369:154–156.

30. Nazzaro JM, Neuwelt EA: The role of surgery in the management of supratentorial intermediate and high-grade astrocytomas in adults. *J Neurosurg* 1990; 73:331–344.

31. Neuwelt EA, Nazzaro JM, Gumerlock MK: Is there a role for biopsy in the treatment of supratentonal high-grade glioma? *Clin Neurosurg* 1990; 36:384–407.

32. Oldfield EH, Ram Z, Culver KW, et al.: Gene therapy for the treatment of brain tumors using intra-tumoral transduction with the thymidine kinase gene and intravenous ganciclovir. *Hum Gene Ther* 1993; 4:39–69.

33. Quigley MR, Maroon JC: The relationship between survival and the extent of the resection in patients with supratentorial malignant gliomas. *Neurosurgery* 1991; 29:385–389.

34. Sage MR, Turski PA, Levin A: CNS imaging and the brain barriers, in Neuwelt EA (ed): *Implications of the Blood-Brain Barrier and lts Manipulation*, vol. 2. New York, Plenum, 1989, pp 1–52.

35. Scherer HJ: The forms of growth in gliomas and their practical significance. *Brain* 1940; 63:1–35.

36. Shapiro WR: Treatment of neuroectodermal brain tumors. *Ann Neurol* 1982; 12:231–237.

37. Steiner L, Lindquist C, Steiner M: Radiosurgery. *Adv Tech Stand Neurosurg* 1992; 19:19–102.

38. Tamargo RJ, Brem H: Drug delivery to the central nervous system: A review. *Neurosurg Q* 1992; 2:259–272.

39. Walker RW, Posner JB: Central nervous system neoplasms. *Curr Neurol* 1984; 5:285–320.

Walter A. Hall, M.D.

1. Albert FK, Forsting M, Sartor K, et al.: Early postoperative magnetic resonance imaging after resection of malignant glioma: Objective evaluation of residual tumor and its influence on regrowth and prognosis. *Neurosurgery* 1994; 34:45–61.

2. Chandler KL, Prados MD, Malec M, et al.: Long-term survival with glioblastoma multiforme. *Neurosurgery* 1993; 32:716–720.

3. Coffey RJ, Lunsford LD, Taylor FH: Survival after stereotactic biopsy of malignant gliomas. *Neurosurgery* 1988; 22:465–473.

4. Devaux BC, O'Fallon JR, Kelly PJ: Resection, biopsy, and survival in malignant glial neoplasms. *J Neurosurg* 1993; 78:767–775.

5. Fine HA, Dear KBG, Loeffler JS, et al.: Meta-analysis of radiation therapy with and without adjuvant chemotherapy for malignant gliomas in adults. *Cancer* 1993; 71:2585–2597.

6. Franklin CIV: Does the extent make a difference in high-grade malignant astrocytoma? *Australas Radiol* 1992; 36:44–47.

7. Greig NH, Ries LG, Yancik R, et al.: Increasing annual incidence of primary brain tumors in the elderly. *J Natl Cancer Inst* 1990; 82:1621–1624.

8. Gutin PH, Leibel SA, Wara WM, et al.: Recurrent malignant gliomas: Survival following interstitial brachytherapy with high-activity iodine-125 sources. *J Neurosurg* 1987; 67:864–873.

9. Hall WA, Fodstad Ø: Immunotoxins and central nervous system neoplasia. *J Neurosurg* 1995; 76:1–12.

10. Kelly PJ, Daumas-Duport C, Kispert DB, et al.: Imaging-based stereotaxic serial biopsies in untreated intracranial glial neoplasms. *J Neurosurg* 1987; 66:865–874.

11. Kelly PJ, Hunt C: The limited value of cytoreductive surgery in elderly patients with malignant gliomas. *Neurosurgery* 1994; 34:62–67.

12. Kreth FW, Warnke PC, Scheremet R, et al.: Surgical resection and radiation therapy versus biopsy and radiation therapy in the treatment of glioblastoma multiforme. *J Neurosurg* 1993; 78:762–766.

13. Laperriere NJ, Bernstein M: Radiotherapy for brain tumors. *CA Cancer J Clin* 1994; 44:96–108.

14. Laske DW, Youle RJ, Ilercil O, et al.: Tumor regression with regional distribution of immunotoxin in patients with malignant brain tumors. *J Neurosurg* 1994; 80:412A.

15. Loeffler JS, Alexander E III, Shea WM, et al.: Radiosurgery as part of the initial management of patients with malignant gliomas. *J Clin Oncol* 1992; 10:1379–1385.

16. Nazzaro JM, Neuwelt EA: The role of surgery in the management of supratentorial intermediate and high-grade astrocytomas in adults. *J Neurosurg* 1990; 73:331–344.

17. Salcman M, Scholtz H, Kaplan RS, et al.: Long-term survival in patients with malignant astrocytoma. *Neurosurgery* 1994; 34:213–220.

18. Salford LG, Brun A, Nirfalk S: Ten-year survival among patients with supratentorial astrocytomas grade III and IV. *J Neurosurg* 1988; 69:506–509.

19. Stromblad LG, Anderson H, Malmstrom P, et al.: Reoperation for malignant astrocytomas: Personal experience and a review of the literature. *Br J Neurosurg* 1993; 7:623–633.

20. Walker MD, Green SB, Byar DP, et al.: Randomized comparisons of radiotherapy and nitrosoureas for the treatment of malignant glioma after surgery. *N Engl J Med* 1980; 303:1323–1329.

9

Conservative vs. Aggressive Treatment
of Recurrent Glioblastoma

CASE

A 35-year-old, right-handed man had a craniotomy 9 months ago for resection of a *de novo* glioblastoma. Surgery was followed by whole brain radiotherapy. He now has headaches and a mild left arm drift that appears only when he is fatigued. Magnetic resonance imaging revealed a recurrent lesion.

PARTICIPANTS

Aggressive Treatment of Recurrent Glioblastoma–Andrew H. Kaye, M.D.

Conservative Treatment of Recurrent Glioblastoma–David G.T. Thomas, M.D.

Moderator–Stephen K. Powers, M.D.

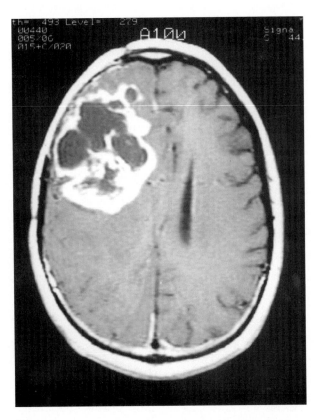
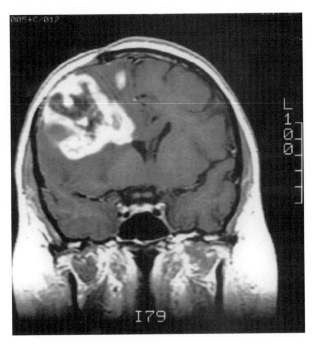

Aggressive Treatment of Recurrent Glioblastoma

Andrew H. Kaye, M.D.

For the recurrent glioblastoma in this patient, I would advise a radical resection of the tumor followed by adjuvant therapy. This treatment is most likely to provide symptomatic relief and a chance of continued good-quality life.

CRITERIA FOR REOPERATION

Glioblastoma multiforme inevitably recurs after treatment. Despite the best conventional treatment, the median survival is less than 1 year and only 5% of patients live longer than 2 years.[5,13,14] In general, the frequency of reoperation for recurrent glioblastoma multiforme has been low and undertaken only in a sporadic fashion.[1,4,8–12,15] The usual nihilistic approach to recurrent glioblastoma multiforme is believed to be justified because of the poor prognosis; however, this belief should be tempered by a realistic attitude that reoperation can be useful in some patients by both improving the patient's quality of life and lengthening the patient's survival.[6,7]

The patient described in this case satisfies many of the criteria used to identify patients most likely to benefit from reoperation.[1,4,6–8,12] The likelihood of improving the quality of and lengthening the patient's survival relates to the histologic grade of recurrent high-grade glioma, the length of time between recurrence and the initial operation, the intracerebral location of the recurrence, the morphological characteristics of the recurrent tumor, and the patient's age and clinical status.[6,7] The most important factors affecting the likelihood of improving survival through reoperation are the histologic characteristics of the recurrence and, as expected, patients with recurrent anaplastic astrocytoma have a significantly better prognosis than those with glioblastoma multiforme. Ammirati and colleagues[1] reported a median survival of 61 weeks for patients with anaplastic astrocytoma after reoperation compared to 29 weeks for those with glioblastoma multiforme.

Extending Survival

The patient's tumor-free interval is related to the prognostic factors at the time of initial treatment, most importantly the grade of the tumor, the patient's age, and the extent of initial resection. In general, the longer the tumor-free interval, the better the chance of lengthening the patient's survival with further treatment, but this is particularly influenced by changes in the biologic characteristics of the tumor. This patient has survived 9 months from the initial operation. For recurrent high-grade gliomas in general, the length of satisfactory high-quality life after reoperation is about half that of the initial tumor-free period. In only 2 of the past 50 patients with high-grade recurrent gliomas treated at the Royal Melbourne Hospital was the length of survival after resection greater than the initial tumor-free period if no adjuvant therapy was administered.

Although the malignant nature of the tumor in this patient and the relatively short period to tumor recurrence mitigate against lengthy survival after reoperation, younger patients retain greater benefits after further treatment. In the Royal Melbourne Hospital series, 14 of the 16 patients younger than 40 years survived more than half the initial tumor-free period compared with only 1 of the last 8 patients older than 70 years. In some series, the patient's performance status at the time of recurrence

indicates the likelihood of a satisfactory response after further treatment,[1,15] but many factors can cause a poor performance status and some of these may be reversible. If deteriorating consciousness stems from raised intracranial pressure, resecting the tumor mass may cause dramatic improvement. On the other hand, neurological deterioration stemming from invasion by the tumor into deep vital structures will not be improved with surgery.

Although this patient meets only some of the criteria that indicate a long survival after reoperation, the morphology of the tumor mass is such that a resection should rapidly palliate the debilitating symptoms of raised intracranial pressure. A vigorous radical resection of the tumor including excision of the margins extending out into the gliotic and edematous brain should be possible without significant morbidity. Although controversial, some evidence shows that vigorous tumor resection may sufficiently reduce the tumor burden to improve the effectiveness of subsequent adjuvant therapy.

SURGICAL TECHNIQUE AND RESULTS

Reoperation for recurrent glioblastoma multiforme requires careful planning and meticulous operative technique. The patients are often frail, having been debilitated by the neurological deficit, steroid medication, and sometimes chemotherapy. These factors also influence wound healing, blood coagulation, and the risk of infection. Surgery can be performed safely, however, and in the last 50 patients undergoing reoperation for glioblastoma multiforme at the Royal Melbourne Hospital no perioperative mortality has occurred. Six patients had initial worsening of their preoperative neurological deficit after reoperation and, in 2 of these, the neurological disability was significant and permanent. Sixteen patients had no substantial change in their preoperative neurological disability. Marked improvement was seen in the remainder with increases in the Karnofsky (functioning) score ranging from 10 to 45 points (median 25 points).

INVESTIGATIONAL TREATMENTS

The most common position of tumor recurrence after conventional therapy is locally in the tumor bed, indicating that the initial treatment has failed in local control.[2,3] In general, recurrence after reoperation is also locally in the tumor bed, but the edges of the tumor are often more widespread. This regional pattern of recurrence has encouraged the investigation of new adjuvant therapies for local disease. These include new radiotherapy techniques and photodynamic therapy. Forty-five patients with recurrent glioblastoma multiforme have been treated at the Royal Melbourne Hospital with photodynamic therapy as an adjuvant to reoperation. The median survival time was 8.7 months, with 3 patients still alive more than 18 months after treatment. These 3 patients were all younger than 40 years and a complete macroscopic excision had been attained at the time of reoperation.

CONCLUSION

Reoperation and adjuvant therapy will not cure this patient's malignant brain tumor, but surgery will almost certainly relieve his disabling symptoms, and there is a small but definite chance of providing a satisfactory period of high quality survival. In general, the decision to reoperate on patients with recurrent glioblastoma multiforme depends on careful evaluation of the patient and consideration of the criteria described. In the future, the main value of further surgery may lie in reducing the tumor burden so that adjuvant therapies or biologic response modifiers now being developed will have the greatest chance of controlling further growth.

Conservative Treatment of Recurrent Glioblastoma

David G.T. Thomas, M.D.

This relatively young patient has presented with clear clinical signs of tumor progression only 9 months after excisional surgery and postoperative radiotherapy for a brain tumor in the nondominant hemisphere. Although the histology from the original resection of a right frontal mass lesion yielded the diagnosis of glioblastoma, it is good practice to review this diagnosis at the time of recurrence and to confirm the histologic diagnosis. It is also important to confirm that the course of external beam radiotherapy has been completed to a satisfactory total dose in the range of 50 to 60 cGy, because this is the most effective treatment modality postoperatively in patients with glioblastoma.[2,8]

MEASURING THE VALUE OF TREATMENT

All further treatment is palliative in the context of current medical knowledge and must be tempered by the expectations of the patient and his relatives concerning the quality, as well as the extent, of survival. His medical advisors must, at least in their own minds, distinguish whether significant differences exist in the reported results of different types of treatment in this situation. This is judged by survival and clinical response, as well as by the burden likely to be imposed upon the patient by the adverse effects and complications that may be attached to further specific treatment. Thus, a scale has been proposed grading the value of treatment for patients with malignant gliomas.[4] According to this scale, treatment leading to increased survival of less than 6 months is hardly worthwhile, if it entails 3 months of treatment and includes a terminal period of 6 weeks. An increase in survival of 6 to 12 months is rated just worthwhile, 1 year definitely worthwhile, and 3 years or more very worthwhile.

SPECIFIC TREATMENT

This specific patient now has shown clinical and radiologic evidence of tumor progression, but remains at a relatively high performance level with only variable mild neurological deficits. One may assume that he is independent in his normal activities of daily living and self-care and it is specifically stated that his neurological deficit is apparent only when he is fatigued. It is, therefore, reasonable to advocate further specific treatment and logical that this treatment should initially be of the kind already shown scientifically to be effective in such a case. The patient has not already undergone chemotherapy; my recommendation is that he undergo this treatment at this stage because it can be effective either as an adjuvant[7] or at the time the glioblastoma recurs.

Chemotherapy with nitrosoureas, such as carmustine as a single agent,[9] or the triple-agent chemotherapy regime of lomustine, procarbazine, and vincristine,[1] might be expected within 2 cycles, given at 6-week intervals, to have about a 30% chance of inducing a remission in his symptoms. Such a remission might last 6 to 9 months. The treatment itself is generally associated with only small attendant adverse effects and an even smaller risk of major complications.

Clearly, it is possible to consider the alternative of more invasive measures. Reoperation might relieve this patient's symptoms temporarily, but probably not for a long period and certainly with a greater risk of morbidity and mortality related to the surgical treatment. Although he underwent a full course of whole brain radiotherapy 9 months previously, it is reasonable to consider further focused radiation treatment. The maximum diameter of the recurrent tumor is about 8 cm, which precludes the safe use of interstitial radiotherapy without prior surgery to debulk the tumor. However, some good short-term results have been reported in patients undergoing surgery.[6] The cumulative risks of further surgery with subsequent interstitial radiotherapy, however, are significantly greater than of those associated with chemotherapy. Alternatively, focused stereotactic external beam radiation treatment to the tumor volume, without the catheter implantation required for interstitial treatment, might be offered.[5] The chance of palliation with this type of focused radiation is probably in the region of 30 to 40%, with fewer risks of serious complications because no open neurosurgical intervention is required.

EXPERIMENTAL TREATMENT

This patient might also reasonably be offered treatment in an experimental protocol, for example, with antibody-targeted radiotherapy or with gene transfer therapy.[3] Such novel therapy might be justified on the basis that he is relatively young and is presently at a good level of performance, although he has a very dismal prognosis on the basis of the tumor histology and the recurrence.

Physicians as well as patients and their relatives must be aware that no progress will be made in treating this disease unless such attempts at experimental treatment are made. However, physicians, in particular, must be aware that such new methods seldom, or probably never, result in a change from a palliative to curative effect at the first attempt. Therefore, when persuading an individual patient to enter such an experimental protocol, one must temper one's enthusiasm for the experiment in light of the patient's individual circumstances and understanding of exactly what is being offered.

CONCLUSION

My own advice for this particular patient at this stage in the disease is to proceed to chemotherapy with the triple-agent regime of lomustine, procarbazine, and vincristine. If this were to fail to induce a tumor response, I would offer drug treatment with the experimental agent temozolamide (Cancer Research Campaign, London). If this also failed, I would propose focused fractionated stereotactic radiotherapy. As a last resort, I would enter the patient into the local research program employing antibody-targeted radiation with interstitial [125]I.

Conservative vs. Aggressive Treatment of Recurrent Glioblastoma

Stephen K. Powers, M.D.

Glioblastoma multiforme and anaplastic astrocytoma are highly complex and heterogeneous lesions that require a multimodality treatment approach to control growth and delay or prevent recurrence. The 5-year survival rate for patients with glioblastoma multiforme is only 6.6%.[13] Recurrence is seen in nearly every case of this tumor and occurs usually within 1 year of the original treatment, in spite of aggressive surgical decompression combined with radiation therapy with or without adjuvant chemotherapy. Most first-time recurrences (>80%) occur regionally at or adjacent to the primary tumor site.[9] Therefore, they can be considered for further treatment with various forms of regional therapies, which include surgical resection (reoperation), radiosurgery or stereotactic radiation therapy, regionally delivered chemotherapy (for example, intra-arterial or intratumoral infusion), brachytherapy, photodynamic therapy, and hyperthermia. Because the solid portion of the tumor that is defined by computed tomography and magnetic resonance imaging as the volume within the contrast-enhancing boundary has no viable neural parenchyma, it may be safely ablated by cytoreductive surgery or any of the regional therapies mentioned above. However, the infiltrative tumor that extends into the normal brain adjacent to the solid tumor mass is best treated through more cell-selective treatments, such as chemotherapy, conventional radiotherapy, immunotherapy, and possibly even photodynamic therapy and hyperthermia.

CONSIDERATIONS AND EXPERIMENTS

Any decision regarding treatment of a recurrence of a malignant brain tumor must take into consideration the patient's interests and expectations regarding outcome, the resources available to the neurosurgeon for use in treating the patient, and the inherent technical and practical limitations, including the risks of those treatments for the individual patient. Although numerous investigational studies are available for the treatment of patients with both *de novo* and recurrent primary malignant brain tumors, based on a practice survey of data from 1980 and 1985,[12,13] only 7.6% of the maximum number of eligible patients was placed into investigative protocols. According to this survey, the patients who enrolled in investigative studies had a threefold better 5-year survival rate than those who did not. Although the improved survival may simply reflect the fact that better-functioning patients who would be expected to have a better prognosis were placed into treatment protocols, it is also reasonable to conclude that the patients who were treated more aggressively by the very nature of entering a trial did better than patients who underwent a less aggressive approach.

In this case, both authors agree that the patient should receive treatment for his recurrent glioblastoma of the frontal lobe based upon radiologic evidence of local tumor recurrence and the patient's excellent clinical status. The authors disagree, however, about the choice of treatment for the recurrence.

When interpreting the results from recently reported series of patients who have undergone reoperation for the treatment of recurrent malignant gliomas,[1,2,8,14,16] it is important to note that the reported patient survival rates reflect overall aggressive treatment of the patients for recurrence. These patients often underwent additional therapy, including chemotherapy, which would be expected to contribute to a favorable outcome. It can be argued that reoperation rapidly lowers increased intracranial pressure and improves blood flow to the brain adjacent to the tumor, thus contributing to the recovery of neurological function that had been compromised by compression. Experimental studies indicate that cytoreductive surgery may potentiate both immunotherapy and chemotherapy.[3,15] Finally, although infrequently seen during the first year after treatment following conventional radiotherapy,[4] delayed radiation necrosis may occur and may present clinically and radiographically in a fashion similar to recurrent glioblastoma multiforme. Surgical biopsy to confirm tumor recurrence (required by some investigational studies) may be needed before the patient begins treatment.

SURGICAL TREATMENT

An aggressive treatment approach centered around surgical resection of recurrent tumor is favored in a young patient whose neurological function is compromised because of mass effect from a relatively large tumor, especially when the tumor is located near the hemispheric surface and in silent, noneloquent brain. It can be argued that recurrences with large necrotic centers in symptomatic patients should be debulked because, theoretically, these devascularized regions of tumor are not susceptible to systemically administered chemotherapy or immunotherapy, and viable tumor cells in these areas are resistant to radiation therapy because of the hypoxic environment.[7] Relative contraindications to reoperation include: advanced age (over 65), a small tumor, a patient who is neurologically intact, no or minimal mass effect from the tumor, a tumor that is located deep or in eloquent brain, and a tumor with poorly defined margins on imaging studies that is diffusely infiltrative into the brain (gliomatosis cerebri).

The patient's age, the length of time to recurrence or progression, the patient's functional status (Karnofsky functional scale), the tumor grade, and the extent of surgical resection have been identified in previous reports as prognostic factors influencing the length and the quality of survival after reoperation for patients with malignant gliomas.[2,5,6,8,14] Mean survival after reoperation for a Grade 3 astrocytoma is predictably longer than for a Grade 4 tumor, and patients under 40 years of age do better than those over 40 years of age after repeated resection.[8] Of course, the age relatedness of outcome may simply reflect the fact that higher grade gliomas are more prevalent in older patients.

CHOOSING CHEMOTHERAPY

When considering adjuvant chemotherapy, the physician must recognize that only about 1 in every 3 patients responds to treatment and that most drugs used have produced either no benefit or a short-term response.[11] Failures of drug treatment have been attributed to poor drug delivery, a low tumor growth fraction, low immunogenicity of the tumor cells, and cellular resistance and heterogeneity.[10] In general, drug delivery is poor in normal brain adjacent to tumor where microscopic infiltration occurs. Drug delivery is greatest at the periphery of the tumor bulk, where there is increased vascularity, and it is low in the central necrotic regions. Drug administration before resection may be more effective because of improved delivery to the tumor; residual tumor after surgical removal may lie in surgically devascularized regions of the brain.

CONCLUSION

For the patient described here, however, the proposal to reoperate should be followed by the caveat that reoperation alone can improve the quality of life and prolong survival only to the extent afforded by surgical debulking of the tumor mass, unless approached with the intent of radical surgical removal with at least a 2- to 3-cm margin of normal surrounding brain included in the excision. Radical surgery as such usually causes significant neurological deficits that are unacceptable to the patient. Cytoreductive surgery can relieve symptoms resulting from

mass effect but has only a minimal influence on prolonging the patient's survival. Chemotherapy, immunotherapy, and other novel treatments such as photodynamic therapy, which have the potential to kill tumor cells multiplying in the surrounding brain or arrest their growth, will, when effective, exert a greater influence on the patient's survival than can be expected with surgical excision of just the tumor bulk. On the other hand, antiproliferative therapies do not reduce mass effect initially and may, in some cases, aggravate it because of treatment-induced tumor necrosis, increased permeability of the blood-brain barrier, and a heightened host immune response to the tumor. Therefore, any treatment plan designed to maximize both the quality and length of survival in a patient with a recurrent malignant glioma must address the issues of relieving neurological symptoms resulting from mass effect and effectively inhibit the proliferation of tumor cells in the brain adjacent to the tumor.

REFERENCES

Andrew H. Kaye, M.D.

1. Ammati M, Galicich JH, Arbit E, et al.: Reoperation in the treatment of recurrent intracranial malignant gliomas. *Neurosurgery* 1987; 21:607.
2. Bashir R, Hochberg F, Oot R: Regrowth patterns of glioblastoma multiforme related to planning of interstitial brachytherapy radiation fields. *Neurosurgery* 1988; 23:27–30.
3. Choucair AK, Levin VA, Gutin PH, et al.: Development of multiple lesions during radiation therapy and chemotherapy in patients with gliomas. *J Neurosurg* 1986; 65:654–658.
4. Harsh GR, Levin VA, Gutin PH, et al.: Reoperation for recurrent glioblastoma and anaplastic astrocytoma. *Neurosurgery* 1987; 21:615–621.
5. Kaye AH: Adjuvant treatment of malignant brain tumors. *Aust NZ J Surg* 1989; 59:831–833.
6. Kaye AH: Reoperation for malignant brain tumours, in Little J, Awad I (eds): *Reoperative Neurosurgery*. Baltimore, Williams and Wilkins, 1992.
7. Kaye AH: Reoperation for malignant brain tumours—Is it worthwhile? *Aust NZ J Surg* 1992; 62:677–679.
8. Moser RP: Surgery for glioma relapse: Factors that influence a favourable outcome. *Cancer* 1988; 62:381–390.
9. Pool JL: The management of recurrent gliomas. *Clin Neurosurg* 1967; 15:265–287.
10. Ray BS: Surgery of recurrent intracranial tumors. *Clin Neurosurg* 1962; 10:1–30.
11. Roth JG, Elvidge AR: Glioblastoma multiforme: A clinical survey. *J Neurosurg* 1960; 17:736–750.
12. Salcman M, Kaplan RS, Ducker TB, et al.: Effect of age and reoperation on survival in the combined modality treatment of malignant astrocytoma. *Neurosurgery* 1982; 10:454–463.
13. Walker MD, Alexander E Jr, Hunt WE, et al.: Evaluation of BCNU and/or radiotherapy in the treatment of anaplastic gliomas: A cooperative clinical trial. *J Neurosurg* 1978; 49:333–343.
14. Walker MD, Green SB, Byar DP, et al.: Randomized comparisons of radiotherapy and nitrosoureas for the treatment of malignant glioma after surgery. *N Engl J Med* 1980; 303:1323–1329.
15. Young B, Oldfield EH, Markesbery WR, et al.: Reoperation for glioblastoma. *J Neurosurg* 1981; 55:917–921.

David G.T. Thomas, M.D.

1. Brufman G, Halpern J, Sulkes A, et al.: Procarbazine, CCNU, and vincristine (PCV) combination chemotherapy for brain tumours. *Oncology* 1984; 41:239–241.
2. Chang CH, Horton J, Schoenfeld D, et al.: Comparison of postoperative radiotherapy and chemotherapy in the multidisciplinary management of malignant gliomas: A joint Radiation Therapy Oncology and Eastern Cooperative Oncology Group Study. *Cancer* 1983; 52:997–1007.
3. Culver KW, Ram Z, Wallbridge S, et al.: In vivo gene transfer with retroviral vector-producer cells for treatment of experimental brain tumors. *Science* 1992; 256:1550–1553.
4. Gleave JRW: Surgery for primary brain tumours, in Bleehan NM (ed): *Tumours of the Brain*. Berlin, Springer-Verlag, 1986, pp 101–120.
5. Graham JD, Warrington AP, Gill SS, et al.: A non-invasive, relocatable stereotactic frame for fractionated radiotherapy and multiple imaging. *Radiother Oncol* 1991; 21:60–62.
6. Leibel SA, Gutin PH, Wara WM, et al.: Survival and quality of life after interstitial implantation of removable high-activity iodine-125 sources for the treatment of patients with recurrent malignant gliomas. *Int J Radiat Oncol Biol Phys* 1989; 17:1129–1139.
7. Levin VA, Silver P, Hannigan J, et al.: Superiority of post-radiotherapy adjuvant chemotherapy with CCNU, procarbazine, and vincristine (PVC) over BCNU for anaplastic gliomas: NCOG 6G61 Final Report. *Int J Radiat Oncol Biol Phys* 1990; 18:321–324.
8. Walker MD, Strike TA, Sheline GE: An analysis of dose-effect relationship in the radiotherapy of malignant gliomas. *Int J Radiat Oncol Biol Phys* 1979; 5:1725–1731.
9. Wilson CB, Boldrey EB, Enot KJ: 1,3-Bis (2-chloroethyl)-1-nitrosourea (NSC-409962) in the treatment of brain tumors. *Cancer Chemother Rep* 1970; 54:273–281.

Stephen K. Powers, M.D.

1. Ammirati M, Galicich JH: Reoperation in the treatment of recurrent intracranial malignant astrocytoma. *Dev Oncol* 1991; 66:171–173.
2. Ammirati M, Galicich JH, Arbit E, et al.: Reoperation in the treatment of recurrent intracranial malignant gliomas. *Neurosurgery* 1987; 21:607–614.
3. Brooks WH, Roszman TL: Cellular immune responsiveness of patients with primary intracranial tumors, in Thomas DGT, Graham Dl (eds): *Brain Tumors: Scientific Basis, Clinical Investigation, and Current Therapy.* London, Butterworth, 1980, pp 121–132.
4. Burger PC, Mahaley MS Jr, Dudka L, et al.: The morphologic effects of radiation administered therapeutically for intracranial gliomas. *Cancer* 1979; 44:1256–1272.
5. Davis LW: Presidential address: Malignant glioma—A nemesis which requires clinical and basic investigation in radiation oncology. *Int J Radiation Oncol Biol Phys* 1989; 16:1355–1365.
6. Franklin CI: Does the extent of surgery make a difference in high-grade malignant astrocytoma? *Australas Radiol* 1992; 36:44–47.
7. Gutin PH, Levin VA: Surgery, radiation, and chemotherapy in the treatment of malignant brain tumors, in Thompson RA, Green JR (eds): *Controversies in Neurology.* New York, Raven Press, 1983, pp 67–86.
8. Harsh GR, Levin VA, Gutin PH, et al.: Reoperation for recurrent glioblastoma and anaplastic astrocytoma. *Neurosurgery* 1987; 21: 615–621.
9. Hochberg FH, Pruitt A: Assumptions in the radiotherapy of glioblastoma. *Neurology* 1980; 30:907–911.
10. Janus TJ, Kyritsis AP, Forman AD, et al.: Biology and treatment of gliomas. *Ann Oncol* 1992; 3:423–433.
11. Kyritsis AP, Levin VA: Chemotherapeutic approaches to the treatment of malignant gliomas. *Adv Oncol* 1992; 8:9–13.
12. Mahaley MS Jr, Mettlin C, Nachimuthu N, et al.: Analysis of patterns of care of brain tumor patients in the United States: A study of the Brain Tumor Section of the MNS and the CNS and the Commission on Cancer of the ACS, in Black PM (ed): *Clinical Neurosurgery,* vol 19. Baltimore, Williams and Wilkins, 1990, pp. 347–362.
13. Mahaley MS Jr, Mettlin C, Nachimuthu N, et al.: National survey of patterns of care for brain-tumor patients. *J Neurosurg* 1989; 71: 826–836.
14. Salcman M, Kaplan RS, Ducker TB, et al.: Effect of age and reoperation on survival in the combined modality treatment of malignant astrocytoma. *Neurosurgery* 1982; 10:454–463.
15. Tel E, Hoshino T, Barker M, et al.: Effect of surgery on BCNU chemotherapy in a rat brain tumor model. *J Neurosurg* 1980; 52:529–532.
16. Young B, Oldfield EH, Markesbery WR, et al.: Reoperation for glioblastoma. *J Neurosurg* 1981; 55:917–921.

10

Aggressive vs. Conservative Treatment of Parasagittal Meningiomas Involving the Superior Sagittal Sinus

CASE

A 40-year-old, right-handed woman presented with headache and an onset of new, generalized seizures. A physical exam showed mild left hemiparesis.

PARTICIPANTS

Aggressive Treatment of Parasagittal Meningiomas Involving the Superior Sagittal Sinus–
   Marc Sindou, M.D., P. Hallacq, M.D.

Conservative Treatment of Parasagittal and Falx Meningiomas Involving the Superior Sagittal Sinus–Robert G. Ojemann, M.D.

Moderator–Edward R. Laws, Jr., M.D.

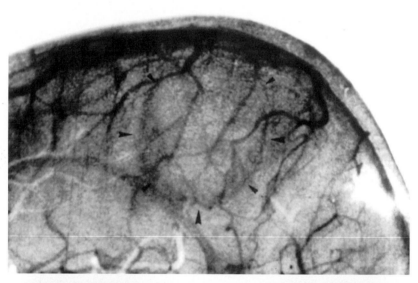

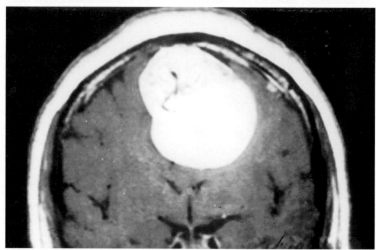

Aggressive Treatment of Parasagittal Meningiomas Involving the Superior Sagittal Sinus

Marc Sindou, M.D., P. Hallacq, M.D.

The case presented here is an excellent illustration of the difficulties of treatment decision-making. Although the T1-weighted magnetic resonance image (MRI) in the coronal plane shows that the tumor involves both lateral walls of the sinus and is believed to invade the lumen totally, on angiography this parasagittal meningioma actually appears to occlude the sinus only partially.

For this otherwise healthy young woman, two surgical attitudes are possible: gross tumor removal with coagulation of the sinus walls leaving an intrasinusal fragment in place, and radical removal with resection of the invaded sinus with or without restoring the venous circulation. In this particular patient, our preference is to plan a two-stage operation. The first stage consists of debulking the tumor with dissection of its so-called capsule from the brain cortex on both sides and removal of the extrasinusal meningioma. At the second stage (within 2 weeks), after having done an end-to-side bypass with an autologous internal saphenous vein, we would attempt a complete removal of the invaded portion of the sinus.

CASE DISCUSSION

To reduce the rate of recurrence of parasagittal meningiomas, our current attitude is to attempt, whenever possible, a total removal of the tumor, including the invaded portion of the sinus. Making the decision to systematically repair the sinus leads to a more aggressive surgical behavior, which favors total removal of the tumor.

In the dangerous case presented here, the decision to restore venous circulation is reinforced by this tumor's location within the province of Rolandic outflow. Impairment in this location would probably cause edema, hemorrhage, or infarction in sensorimotor territories.

Because the meningioma invades both lateral walls, restoration by patch would not be possible. We would stage the operation in 2 steps: removal of the extrasinusal tumor leaving the intraluminal fragment in place, followed 15 days later by a venous bypass before removal of the remaining portion.

GENERAL CONSIDERATIONS

Classification

Our surgical experience, a series of 47 meningiomas involving the dural venous sinuses, led us to adopt the following attitude toward surgical treatment, according to the type of meningioma, based on a classification simplified from that of Bonnal and Brotchi.[2] Our classification has six types (Fig. 1).

Type I: The meningioma is attached to the outer surface of the sinus wall. The outer dural layer is resected and the site of attachment coagulated, leaving a clean and glistening dural surface.
Type II: The lateral recess is invaded. The intrasinusal fragment is removed and the dural defect repaired with either simple suture or a patch using dura mater, fascia temporalis, periosteum, or fascia lata.
Type III: The entire lateral wall is invaded. The invaded wall is resected and the sinus repaired with a patch.

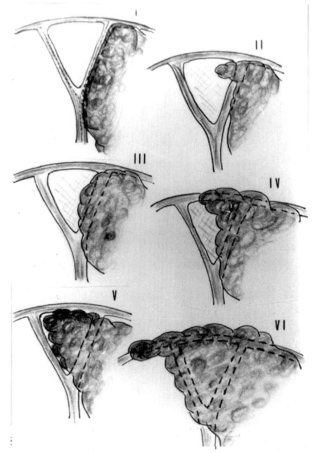

Fig. 1 Classification of parasagittal meningiomas. Type I: the meningioma is attached to the outer surface of the sinus wall; Type II: the lateral recess is invaded; Type III: the entire lateral wall is invaded; Type IV: both the lateral wall and roof of the sinus are invaded; Type V: the lateral wall and the roof of the sinus are invaded, and the lumen is occluded; Type VI: all sinus walls are invaded, and the sinus is totally occluded.

Type IV: The lateral wall and the roof of the sinus are both invaded. The sinus is kept patent through patch reconstruction (Fig. 2) or bypass.
Type V and VI: The sinus is totally occluded, one wall being free of tumor in type V. Although it is theoretically possible to remove the invaded portion of the sinus without re-establishing venous circulation, our preference is to restore venous circulation with a bypass. This bypass may be of an end-to-side type when realized before removal of the tumor and an end-to-end type when done after removal (Fig. 3).

For meningiomas of the posterior third of the superior sagittal sinus, of the torcular, or of the lateral sinus, sacrifice of the invaded portion can be preceded by a sinojugular bypass[11,12] (Fig. 4).

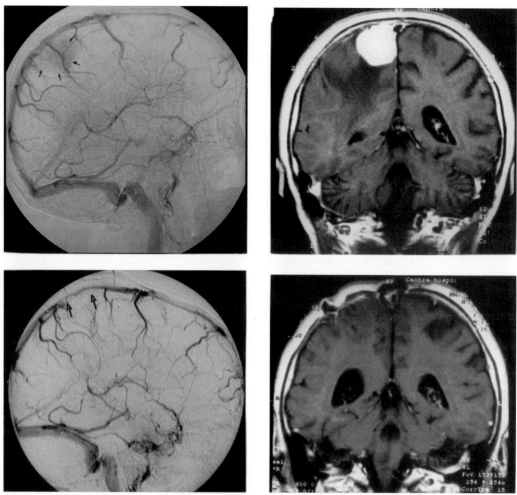

Fig. 2 Imaging studies of a 72-year-old woman with a history of 1 year of partial seizures of the left lower limb. She was diagnosed with a right parietal parasagittal meningioma, Type IV. (Upper left). Internal carotid angiogram, venous phase; lateral view. Note the tumor blush (arrows). (Upper right) T1-weighted coronal MRI after gadolinium injection. (Lower left) Postoperative angiogram showing patency of the superior sagittal sinus at the site of the patch made with periosteum (arrows). (Lower right) Postoperative MRI, coronal view, showing total removal of the meningioma, and patency of the lumen at the resection site of the invaded walls and reconstruction with a patch.

Technical Considerations

Surgery of meningiomas invading the dural venous sinuses is facilitated when the following technical considerations are respected. Good venous return is best obtained by placing the patient in a semi-sitting (lounging) position. The operative exposure should be as extensive as is allowed. The skin flap and craniotomy should extend across the midline to visualize both sides of the sinus, and some 3 cm in front of and behind the margins of the occluded sinus. If brain swelling occurs because of impairment of collateral venous pathways that are pericranium, diploic, or dural veins, the operative procedure should be stopped and further steps delayed for days or weeks. Because there are frequent discrepancies between images and anatomic operative findings, the sinus should be explored through a short incision to disclose an intrasinusal fragment. Temporary control of hemostasis is obtained rather easily by packing small pledgets of hemostatic material within the lumen and at the ostia of

afferent veins. Vascular clamps as well as aneurysmal clips may injure the sinus walls and afferent veins; balloons do not progress easily through sinus septa and may injure sinus endothelium. Venous reconstruction can then be done with patches or bypasses. This reconstruction is usually completed by placing 2 hemicontinuous sutures (prolene 8-0). Although autologous vein would appear to be the most suitable material for a patch, vein harvesting is disproportionate. Dura mater, fascia lata, fascia temporalis, or pericranium may be used as patches; they have a structure rigid enough to allow blood to flow inside. We have done 9 such patches; 5 of 6 angiographically controlled patches remained patent.

Bypass

Experimental studies have been undertaken by various authors to find the best material suitable for bypass in cerebral venous surgery. Late thrombosis of arterial grafts on the venous system

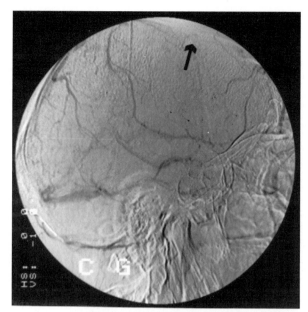
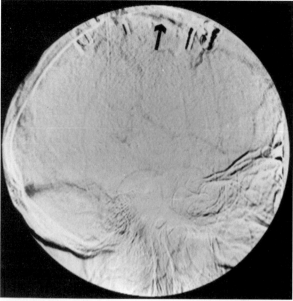

Fig. 3 Angiograms from a 63-year-old man with progressive right hemiparesis for 1 month. He was diagnosed with a left parasagittal Rolandic meningioma, Type V, and underwent a two-stage operation. The first step removed the extrasinusal portion of the meningioma, which was followed 3 weeks later by an end-to-side bypass before removal of the intrasinusal fragment. (Left) Preoperative angiogram, venous phase, lateral view. Note the occluded portion of the sinus (arrow). (Right) Postoperative internal carotid angiogram, venous phase, lateral view. The sinus was reconstructed with an end-to-side bypass using the saphenous vein. Note that the bypass is patent (arrow), although it did not pulsate after surgery because of low pressure within the superior sagittal sinus.

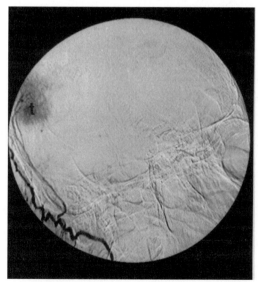
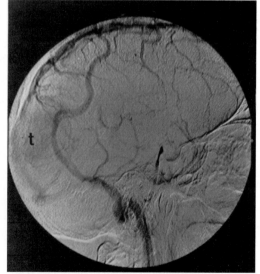

Fig. 4 Angiograms from a 33-year-old man who presented with a 3-week history of visual seizures. He was diagnosed with a right parasagittal occipital meningioma, Type VI. The extrasinusal portion of the tumor was removed, but the patient was lost to follow-up for 2 years. He was then referred for headaches, a decrease in visual acuity, and a meningocele. A sino-jugular bypass was done with a graft taken from the internal saphenous vein and placed between the superior sagittal sinus and the right external jugular vein. (Left) Preoperative angiogram, lateral view, occipital selective carotid injection. Note the tumorous vessels (t). (Right) Preoperative angiogram, lateral view, internal carotid injection, venous phase. Note the tumorous blush (t), complete occlusion of the posterior third of the sagittal sinus, and the collateral pathways that spontaneously developed between the superior sagittal sinus and the internal jugular vein. (Figure continued on the next page.)

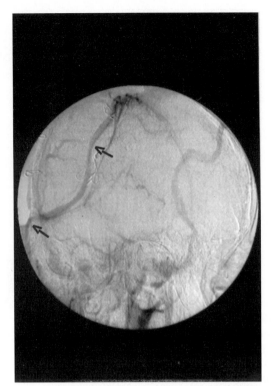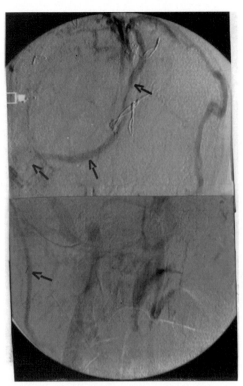

Fig. 4 (Continued). (Left and right) Postoperative angiograms, oblique views, internal carotid injection, venous phase. Note the patency of the venous bypass (saphenous vein, arrows) done between the superior sagittal sinus and the external jugular vein.

have been reported in experiments[3,10] and also in clinical assays. An autologous vein graft, taken either from the internal saphenous vein or the external jugular vein, is the most appropriate.[1,4–9,13] The harvesting technique has been described elsewhere.[14] Bypasses done with Gore-Tex® thrombosed in all cases in our series of 6 patients, asymptomatically in 5 patients and in 1 patient with acute but, fortunately, transient intracranial hypertension.

Of the 15 bypasses we carried out that were patent immediately after dural sinus reconstruction, 13 have been angiographically controlled. All 6 of the Gore-Tex® bypasses thrombosed. Four of 7 angiographically controlled autologous vein bypasses were patent 15 days after completion. In the 3 cases of graft thrombosis, there was no obvious clinical consequence of bypass occlusion. Long-term patency of venous flow with an autologous saphenous vein has not been tested. However, long-term patency may be of no real interest, in that progressive occlusion of the bypass allows time for compensatory venous pathways to develop.

The patency of the venous reconstruction is checked at the end of the procedure. The flow pattern reflects the equilibrium established between the preanastomotic outflow of the collateral veins and the newly created sinus. After surgery, patency of the bypass depends on maintaining blood volume and viscosity.

Heparin therapy is initiated for at least 12 days to avoid clotting within the new sinus and endothelization of the sinus walls (hypocoagulability equals twofold control). If the brain swells during tumor removal, it is better to delay sinus surgery (exploration and reconstruction) and stage venous reconstruction into 2, sometimes even 3, different operations.

CONCLUSION

We favor total removal of meningiomas to reduce their propensity to recur. Of 47 meningiomas involving the sagittal sinus, the transverse sinus or the torcular operated on in our series, tumors recurred in 2 patients (<5%, mean follow-up 5 years). We advocate venous reconstruction whenever it is possible. In our series, 3 patients died after total removal of a Grade VI meningioma; venous circulation had not been re-established in these 3 patients. Although dangerous, sinus surgery is most often technically affordable, even in the torcular area. The major constant danger is represented by impairment of afferent veins, in particular in the mid-third of the superior sagittal sinus; in our series, 5 permanent deficits resulted from surgery of meningiomas invading the midportion of the sinus. In any case, the strategy should be re-evaluated during the surgical procedure. In 5 of our patients, brain swelling occurred, but sinus surgery was completed later without any unfavorable consequences.

Conservative Treatment of Parasagittal and Falx Meningiomas Involving the Superior Sagittal Sinus

Robert G. Ojemann, M.D.

The sagittal sinus may be involved by both parasagittal and falx meningiomas. There are two general categories of parasagittal meningiomas. In the first category are those meningiomas that involve only the lateral edge of the sagittal sinus and the adjacent convexity dura. The second category includes those meningiomas that extensively involve the wall of the sinus, convexity dura and, in some patients, the adjacent falx. Meningiomas arising from the falx may grow into the sinus as they enlarge.

In considering both the symptoms and treatment of patients with parasagittal and falx meningiomas, it is useful to divide them into areas of occurrence: the anterior, middle, and posterior third of the sagittal sinus.[1-9] In general terms, the anterior third of the sinus extends from the crista galli to the coronal suture, the middle third from the coronal to the lambdoid suture, and the posterior third from the lambdoid suture to the torcular.

GENERAL ASPECTS OF TREATMENT

The indications for surgery in a patient with a parasagittal meningioma are worsening neurological symptoms at any age, a seizure in a younger patient or at any age, if there is significant edema in the adjacent brain, and regrowth after radical subtotal removal.[7] Observation is often recommended for older patients with only a seizure and little or no reaction in the surrounding brain. Radiation therapy has not been used as a primary treatment.

Conservative surgery is defined as a procedure that is planned to restore and preserve function, attempting to combine the lowest possible risk with the maximum benefit to the patient. In many patients this procedure will be resection of the entire tumor. However, in some patients it will be better judgment to leave a segment of tumor when there is a significant risk of causing neurologic disability by a complete removal.

Parasagittal and falx meningiomas involving the anterior third of the sagittal sinus can usually be totally removed, including the sagittal sinus and falx, even if the sinus is open. When the meningioma involves the middle or posterior third of the sinus, a total removal can be done if the sinus is occluded or if the meningioma only involves the edge of the sinus. In the latter case, the edge of the sinus may be opened to remove the tumor and closed with a continuous suture.[6-8] The controversy being discussed in this section is what to do when the sinus wall in the middle or posterior third is involved with the tumor and the sinus is still open. If this portion of the sinus is not kept open, there is a high probability that a severe venous infarction will occur.

DISCUSSION OF CASE PRESENTATION

The patient under discussion is a 40-year-old, right-handed woman who presented with headache and seizure. Her physical exam revealed mild left hemiparesis. This was surprising, because the MRI showed the maximum compression to be on the left cerebral hemisphere.

The MRI with gadolinium enhancement suggests that this is a large falx meningioma that is growing around the sagittal sinus from inferiorly. The falx origin is suggested by the rim of cerebral tissue that extends almost to the midline over the tumor on the left side, the bilateral growth seen on the MRI and the outline of the stain on the angiogram, which also suggests that the tumor has cerebral tissue over a portion of its superior surface. The angiogram also shows that the tumor includes the region of the middle third of the sinus, the sinus is still open, and important draining veins are centered over the tumor. We are not told if this is the venous phase of the right or left side. We should have angiograms of both sides available for review as well as a full set of the MRI studies.

SURGICAL TREATMENT

For the surgical approach, I prefer to place the patient in the semilateral, semi-sitting position with the head well elevated so the scalp over the area of the tumor is at the highest point.[6-8] A horseshoe incision is made starting on the left and extending about 2 cm across the midline with ample anterior and posterior exposure. A large bone flap is elevated. The dura is opened about 2 cm lateral and parallel to the midline on the left side, hinging a flap of dura as far medially as possible to visualize the tumor and adjacent falx. The dural opening may be limited by the adherence of the convexity veins. It may be good to determine the position of the motor cortex through stimulation to avoid a possible direct retraction on this area. I would probably expose the tumor anterior to the large convexity vein seen on the angiogram. Sometimes both anterior and posterior exposures are used. An extensive internal decompression would be done. The anterior falx would be opened to deal with the tumor growing on the right side. Initially, a plaque of tumor would be left along the sagittal sinus. The capsule would be brought into the area of decompression with retraction being used only to keep the overlying brain from falling into the area of tumor removal. It may be necessary to open the dura on the right side as well. Once the bulk of the tumor is removed, the area of the sagittal sinus is inspected. It is likely the tumor is growing into the wall of the sinus. I would remove the tumor down to as thin a layer as I thought was safe and then leave a plaque of tumor on the sinus.

The patient would then be followed with MRI. Subsequent treatment is based on the results discussed in the next section.

Results of Personal Series

My series of meningiomas treated through surgery from 1975 to 1992 included 45 patients with a parasagittal meningioma and 14 patients with a falx meningioma.[7] The group with parasagittal meningiomas consisted of 33 women and 12 men ranging in age from 25 to 81 years with 11 over 70 years of age. In 27 patients, only the edge of the sagittal sinus was involved and all had a gross total resection through opening the sinus and resuturing the wall. Twenty-four of these 27 patients had good results and 3 had a fair result because of significant preoperative deficits that did not fully resolve. Four patients had temporary weakness in one or both contralateral extremities. No patient had permanent worsening resulting from surgery. Most of the patients have been followed with scans. Two patients had recurrence 3 and 11 years after the first operation. In both, another gross total removal was done and the patients fully recovered.

In 18 patients, there was extensive involvement of the sagittal sinus. All 7 patients with tumors involving the anterior third of the sagittal sinus had complete removal, made a good recovery, and have not had a recurrence. Eleven patients had tumors involving the middle third. These patients frequently had neurological deficits preoperatively and a temporary increase in hemiparesis or sensory loss postoperatively. Six patients had a good result and 5 a fair result. Three of those with the fair results were the same or better than before the operation but still had residual preoperative disability; however, 2 had new postoperative neurological deficits. In 6 patients it was possible to remove the tumor totally because the sinus was occluded by tumor. In the other 5 patients, tumor was left in the wall of the sinus. Follow-up scans over 4 years have shown no change in the tumor in 3. One patient had documented slow regrowth of the tumor, but it was not symptomatic until 7 years after the operation, when seizures recurred. Angiography showed the sinus to be occluded and a total removal was done. The second patient showed more rapid regrowth of the tumor. Angiography 3 years later showed the sinus to be occluded and the tumor was removed. There has been no recurrence in either of these patients and both have a good result.

The series of falx meningiomas included 14 patients (9 females and 5 males) ranging in age from 10 to 90 years, with 3 over 70 years of age. Of the 14 patients, 13 had a good outcome and 1 was better but had residual deficits. A total removal was done in 12 patients, a subtotal removal in 1 patient because of involvement with the anterior cerebral artery, and a radical subtotal removal in 1 patient because of tumor in the inferior wall of the open sagittal sinus. There has been no evidence of regrowth of this tumor over 8 years.

RECOMMENDATION

In the patient with a parasagittal or falx meningioma, I have not seen an indication to undertake the risks of resecting the middle or posterior third of the sagittal sinus when it is open. When a plaque of tumor is left, the patients are carefully followed with MRI. Several have shown no regrowth. If regrowth occurs with a significant mass effect, another radical subtotal removal can be done. However, the sinus may gradually be occluded by the tumor and, when this occurs, the patient can be cured with a subsequent operation. The place of radiosurgery when regrowth is seen on the MRI remains to be determined. The one circumstance in which resection and graft of an open sagittal sinus might be indicated is when the patient has a malignant meningioma.

Aggressive vs. Conservative Treatment of Parasagittal and Falx Meningiomas Involving the Superior Sagittal Sinus

Edward R. Laws, Jr., M.D.

It has long been recognized that meningiomas originate from arachnoid cap cells in the arachnoid granulations. The nature of the neoplastic transformation is not known, but it is relatively common and frequently multiple. Sex differences in the frequency of occurrence of meningiomas and the presence of hormone receptors on the tumor cells themselves provide evidence for a genetic basis forming part of the pathogenetic mechanism, in at least some tumors. Spinal fluid is absorbed into the venous system through the arachnoid granulations and the superior sagittal sinus is a major route of spinal fluid absorption. It is therefore not surprising that arachnoid granulations are freely distributed along the sinus, and that parasagittal meningiomas make up the first or second most common location for meningiomas in most large clinical series. There are both descriptive and functional reasons for dividing the superior sagittal sinus into 3 segments when describing the location of parasagittal meningiomas. Obviously, the closer to the torcular one goes from anterior to posterior along the sinus, the more venous collaterals enter the sinus and the more robust is the venous flow. Additionally, the vein of Trolard, which tends to drain the motor cortex, usually enters the sinus at the junction between the middle and posterior thirds. The implications for brain function and for risks of surgery when these feeding veins or the sinus itself is interrupted as a result of surgery are evident.

CLINICAL PRESENTATION OF PARASAGITTAL MENINGIOMAS

The symptoms produced by parasagittal tumors depend on their location along the sinus, their size, and their ability to produce mass effect, either by direct compression of underlying brain or by inducing surrounding cerebral edema. They also depend on their ability to irritate underlying brain, producing episodic symptoms most commonly in the form of epileptic seizures.

Parasagittal meningiomas affecting the middle third of the superior longitudinal sinus most frequently present with symptoms relating to compression of the underlying brain. These include motor signs, such as progressive weakness, usually of the legs, but occasionally in the form of a hemiparesis. It has been well recognized that bilateral parasagittal meningiomas in this region can produce false localizing signs suggesting the presence of a spinal cord tumor, with bilateral weakness of the lower extremities. The typical Jacksonian epilepsy, a focal motor seizure with a march corresponding to the anatomic areas of the motor cortex, is most commonly seen in patients with parasagittal meningiomas. Farther back along the sinus, tumors may produce sensory symptoms, often in the form of sensory seizures. Sensory seizures can also occur with a similar march phenomenon and sensory changes involving half the body should alert the clinician to the possible presence of a parasagittal tumor. A pseudoParkinson syndrome may occur with tumors of the anterior two thirds of the sinus.

Vascular Considerations

Parasagittal meningiomas tend to be fed primarily from the blood supply of the dura, usually through the external carotid circulation. They can parasitize the pial blood supply of the brain and also the blood supply of the falx from the anterior cerebral arteries; these are less common arterial features that tend to occur with large tumors. The venous drainage is usually through small vessels directly into the sinus and most parasagittal meningiomas, because of their origin from arachnoid granulations, actually extend into the superior sagittal sinus. Their slow and progressive growth can lead to gradual occlusion of the major sinus with the development of collateral venous drainage, but this occurs very late in the evolution of these lesions. From the pathophysiological standpoint, patency of the superior longitudinal sinus and direction and pattern of venous blood flow from the cerebral cortex are among the most important facets of the diagnosis of these lesions.

EVALUATION OF PARASAGITTAL MENINGIOMAS

Virtually all patients will have imaging studies to evaluate their lesions. The current state of the art is magnetic resonance image (MRI) scanning with gadolinium contrast. Computed tomography occasionally is helpful because it may show the presence of calcification in some meningiomas, usually those of long standing. Gadolinium enhancement frequently shows evidence of multiplicity of involvement of the dura along a significant portion of the sinus and occasionally to the opposite side, occasionally in a multifocal fashion. These "tails" of enhancement seen with this technique are still the subject of some controversy, but probably should be considered as evidence of tumor involvement, until proven otherwise.

Angiography is generally recommended for all parasagittal meningiomas to delineate the arterial feeding pattern, the important veins around the tumor that may be draining into the sinus and, finally, the patency of the sinus itself. Standard angiography is useful and digital angiography with a submento-vertex view may show in exquisite detail the distribution of the venous tributaries into the superior longitudinal sinus, helping the surgeon plan the approach. Stereoscopic angiography can be done as well, and magnetic resonance angiography is rapidly developing and may ultimately replace standard contrast angiography as we know it today.

Positron emission tomography (PET) is another technique that has been applied to the assessment of meningiomas thought to be aggressive either because of their clinical presentation or their rate of evolution. It has been shown that glucose metabolism as measured by 2-deoxyglucose is higher in more aggressive tumors, and PET scanning can be used to characterize the aggressiveness of a tumor. It can also be used to follow its response to therapy, as successfully-treated tumors tend to show a decrease in glucose metabolism. PET scanning can be used to provide online measures of protein synthesis and may also be used for receptor studies.

Table 1 gives the results of surgery for parasagittal meningiomas in major reported series. Table 2 presents a number of different areas of controversy in the treatment of these lesions.

At present, the most significant areas of controversy include the following:

1. Methods for preoperative characterization of the arterial and venous anatomy of the tumor and the surrounding structures,
2. the advisability and need for preoperative embolization of the tumor,
3. techniques and methods for accurate placement of the craniotomy and tumor exposure,
4. methods for debulking the major portion of the tumor,
5. indications for and methods of resecting portions of the tumor involving the walls of the superior sagittal sinus,
6. techniques and methods for repairing and reconstructing the superior sagittal sinus,
7. methods of treating tumor residuals along the superior sagittal sinus and dural margins,
8. methods of dural closure,
9. indications for and types of postoperative radiation therapy or radiosurgery,
10. indications for and types of adjunctive hormonal- or chemotherapy,
11. the use of receptor studies and molecular markers for prognostic indicators,
12. the use of PET or SPECT scans to determine the metabolism of the tumor and prognosis.

As these controversies are gradually resolved, it will still remain important for patients with meningiomas to be diagnosed early in the stage of disease and to be followed carefully and periodically after successful treatment.

The specific case under discussion is that of a 40-year-old, right-handed woman who presents with a headache, a generalized seizure, and a mild left hemiparesis. The imaging studies show an extensive meningioma arising from the falx and involving the dural walls of the sagittal sinus, producing significant but incomplete occlusion of this structure. The tumor involves the middle third of the superior longitudinal sinus and has provoked only a modest degree of associated edema in the surrounding brain.

In this case, the indications for surgery are clear. This is a large lesion with a progressive neurological deficit in a young woman. The only acceptable therapeutic recommendation is one of excision of the tumor. From a surgical standpoint, the lesion is

Table 1. Relative Incidence and Distribution of Parasagittal Meningiomas[4]

Relative Incidence

Series	Number of cases	Percentage of cases	Operative mortality	5-year survival
Olivecrona[4]	292/902	32.3	12.3%	76%
Cushing and Eisenhardt[2]	51/294	29	11%	–
*Region of sinus**				
Anterior third	57	29		
Middle third	111	56		
Posterior third	32	15		

*Portion of longitudinal sinus involved.

Table 2. Controversies in the Treatment of Parasagittal Meningiomas

I. Utility and effectiveness of new technology:
    A. Magnetic resonance angiography (MRA) to delineate vascular supply, venous drainage and patency of longitudinal sinus
    B. Positron emission tomography (PET) for 2-deoxyglucose to detect malignant meningiomas
    C. Image-based stereotaxis to plan the surgical approach
    D. Lasers and ultrasonic aspirators for tumor resection
    E. Photodynamic therapy as an intraoperative adjunct

II. Surgical techniques:
    A. Total vs. subtotal excision
    B. Dural margins: 1. extent of resection
                            2. treatment of residual involved dura
    C. Handling of longitudinal sinus: 1. resection of sinus
                                            2. leave tumor involving wall
                                            3. open sinus—direct repair
                                            4. open sinus—graft repair
                                            5. resect sinus—bypass
    D. Dural closure
    E. Handling of bone flap

III. Adjunctive therapy:
    A. Preoperative embolization
    B. Postoperative radiation therapy/radiosurgery
    C. Receptor-based hormone therapy
    D. Chemotherapy for aggressive tumors

---

dangerous because of its size and location. The comments and recommendations of our two consultants represent different aspects of a difficult problem.

At one time, almost all meningiomas were considered to be benign and potentially curable lesions. With the advent of MRI for the diagnosis and follow-up of our patients, and with more sophisticated pathologic review incorporating modern techniques of molecular neuropathology, it is clear that many, if not most, meningiomas are much more extensive in origin than we had previously believed. It also seems true that most patients, if followed long enough, ultimately develop at least imaging evidence of recurrent or residual disease. Attempts have been made to alter the outcome for patients with ordinary meningiomas by using conventional radiation therapy, radiosurgery, and more aggressive resective surgery; each of these modalities has its enthusiasts. For aggressive meningiomas, many types of adjunctive therapy have been attempted, including radiotherapy, radiosurgery, and chemotherapy, but there is little evidence that the outcome for aggressive and malignant meningiomas can be altered in a significant fashion. The presence of hormone receptors on many of these tumors produced a wave of initial enthusiasm for adjunctive, hormonally based therapy; however, no truly effective therapy has been developed.

It is a fact that most ordinary meningiomas are slowly growing lesions, and it does not appear that an ordinary benign meningioma is likely to undergo more aggressive or malignant changes over time. These facts have been used to justify a conservative approach in patients who have meningiomas without significant progressive neurological deficit, and for those surgeons who take a more conservative posture with regard to the resection of lesions, such as the one under consideration here.

Is total resection of this lesion a realistic possibility? If the answer to this question is yes, then the neurosurgeon must consider various options for removing the tumor and maintaining the functional patency of the superior sagittal sinus. If the answer is no, then the treating neurosurgeon, after removing the bulk of the tumor, must make a sound recommendation with regard to how to deal with the residual tumor left in the walls of the sinus.

Let us consider the aggressive posture first. In this case, a recommendation is made for a staged procedure with the initial aspect being the removal of the bulk of the tumor and a subsequent procedure within 2 weeks to remove the remaining tumor tissue and to reconstruct the sinus. The various ways of dealing with involvement of the superior sagittal sinus by tumor are nicely discussed. When only a portion of the wall is removed, it is practical to resect that portion and repair it with a patch, preferably using autologous vein. The strategy of opening the sinus to evaluate the extent of involvement of the lumen is important in achieving a gross total removal. Creating a saphenous vein bypass of a completely resected segment of the superior sagittal sinus is a challenging technical exercise. It has been described both in situations of traumatic damage to the sinus and in the case of involvement of the sinus by tumor. Unfortunately, only a minority of these bypasses remain patent and they require anticoagulation, significantly increasing the risks involved. Although slowly progressive occlusion of the sinus by tumor occasionally allows adequate venous collaterals to develop, one can never be certain that this has occurred, just as one can never be certain about the patency of the sinus on angiography. Surely the development of cerebral edema related to temporary occlusion or surgical manipulation of the superior sagittal sinus is a clear danger sign, suggesting that the surgeon and the patient should settle for a more conservative approach.

In considering the more conservative approach advocated by the other consultant, it is worth re-emphasizing a number of points that have been made. The venous anatomy in the region of the tumor must carefully be evaluated with preoperative studies, so that the approach to the tumor can do minimal or no damage to the normal venous draining channels. Bilateral exposure and careful opening of the dura is an obvious requirement for successful resection. In a case such as this, it is both practical and necessary to remove the falcine origin of the tumor and, ordinarily, this can be accomplished without excessive difficulty. When it is necessary to leave tumor involving the edge of the superior sagittal sinus, it is possible and probably desirable to cauterize these remnants with either bipolar or monopolar cautery in a careful fashion. Some surgeons have advocated using laser thermocoagulation in this instance. In a tumor such as this one, the indications for postoperative radiotherapy or radiosurgery are not clear. The histology of the tumor is rarely a helpful guide. Further pathologic studies, including those of cell proliferation, are of interest but of little practical guidance; those aggressive and malignant tumors usually do not respond to radiation therapy, and tumors without these features may not need it.

For parasagittal meningiomas like the case reported here, a radical subtotal removal retaining patency of the parasagittal sinus is a philosophy that has a good track record and satisfactory results. A more aggressive posture with resection and grafting of the superior sagittal sinus may be justifiable in certain cases; however, it involves a high level of technical expertise and a risk to the patient that is significant. The question of whether to use adjunctive radiation therapy or radiosurgery is not settled, and at present we have no good guidelines. Meningioma surgery continues to require a great deal from the surgeon—good judgment, a sound philosophy of treatment, technical expertise, and careful follow-through for patients with these difficult lesions.

REFERENCES AND SUGGESTED READINGS

Marc Sindou, M.D., P. Hallacq, M.D.

1. Bonnal J: La chirurgie conservatrice et reparatrice du sinus longitudinal superieur (SLS). *Neurochirurgie* 1982; 28:147–172.
2. Bonnal J, Brotchi J: Surgery of the superior sagittal sinus of parasagittal meningiomas. *J Neurosurg* 1978; 48:935–945.
3. Bonnal J, Buduba C: Surgery of the central third of the superior sagittal sinus: Experimental studies. *Acta Neurochir* 1974; 30:207–215.
4. Hakuba A: Reconstruction of dural venous sinuses involved in meningiomas, in Al Mefty O (ed): *Meningiomas*. New York, Raven Press, 1991, pp 371–382.
5. Hakuba A, Huh CW, Tsujikawa S, et al.: Total removal of a parasagittal meningioma of the posterior third of the sagittal sinus and its repair by autogenous vein graft: Case Report. *J Neurosurg* 1979; 51:379–382.
6. Kapp JP, Gilchinsky I, Deardourff JL: Operative techniques for management of lesion involving the dural venous sinuses. *Surg Neurol* 1977; 7:339–342.
7. Kapp JP, Gilchinsky I, Petty C, et al.: An internal shunt for use in the reconstruction of dural venous sinuses: Technical note. *J Neurosurg* 1971; 35:351–354.
8. Lougheed WM, Marshall BM, Hunter M, et al.: Common carotid to intracranial internal carotid bypass venous graft: Technical note. *J Neurosurg* 1971; 34:114–118.
9. Sindou M, Daher A: Autogenous vein grafts for arterial and venous brain revascularization. *Neurosurgeons* 1987; 6:231–239.
10. Sindou M, Mazoyer JF, Pialat J, et al.: Microchirurgie veineuse intracranienne experimentale: Pontage du sinus sagittal par autogreffe arterielle ou veineuse et mesures per-operatoires de l'impedance cerebrale chez le chien. *Neurochirurgie* 1975; 21:177–189.
11. Sindou M, Mercier P, Bokor J, et al.: Bilateral thrombosis of the transverse sinuses: Microsurgical revascularization with venous bypass. *Surg Neurol* 1980; 13:215–220.
12. Sindou M, Mercier P, Brunon J, et al.: Hypertension intracranienne benigne par thrombose des 2 sinus lateraux, traitee par pontage veineux. *Nouv Presse Med* 1990; 9:439–442.
13. Steiger HJ, Reulen HJ, Huber P, et al.: Radical resection of superior sagittal sinus meningioma with venous interposition graft and reimplantation of the rolandic veins. *Acta Neurochir* 1989; 100:108–111.
14. Sundt TM Jr, Piepgras DG, Marsh R, et al.: Saphenous vein bypass grafts for aneurysms and intracranial occlusive disease. *J Neurosurg* 1986; 6:439–450.

Robert G. Ojemann, M.D.

1. Cushing H, Eisenhardt L: *Meningiomas: Their Classification, Regional Behaviour, Life History, and Surgical End Results.* Springfield, Charles C Thomas, 1938.
2. Giombini S, Solero CL, Lasio G, et al.: Immediate and late outcome of operation for parasagittal and falx meningiomas: Report of 342 cases. *Surg Neurol* 1984; 21:427–435.
3. Guthrie BL, Ebersold MJ, Scheithauer BW: Neoplasms of the intracranial meninges, in Youmans JR (ed): *Neurological Surgery.* Philadelphia, WB Saunders, 1990, pp 3250–3315.
4. Lanman TH, Becker DD: Falcine meningiomas, in Al-Mefty O (ed): *Meningiomas.* New York, Raven Press, 1991, pp 345–356.
5. Maxwell RE, Chou SN: Parasagittal and falx meningiomas, in Schmidek HH (ed): *Meningiomas and Their Surgical Management.* Philadelphia, WB Saunders, 1991, pp 211–220.
6. Ojemann RG: Meningiomas: Clinical features and surgical management, in Wilkins RH, Rengachary SS (eds): *Neurosurgery.* New York, McGraw-Hill, 1985, pp 635–654.
7. Ojemann RG: Management of cranial and spinal meningiomas. *Clin Neurosurg* 1993; 40:321–383.
8. Ojemann RG, Ogilvy CS: Convexity, parasagittal, and parafalcine meningiomas, in Apuzzo MLJ (ed): *Brain Surgery: Complication Avoidance and Management.* New York, Churchill Livingstone, 1993, pp 187–202.
9. Wilkins RH: Parasagittal meningiomas, in Al-Mefty O (ed): *Meningiomas.* New York, Raven Press, 1991, pp 329–344.

Edward R. Laws, Jr., M.D.

1. Al-Mefty O (ed): *Meningiomas.* New York, Raven Press, 1991.
2. Cushing H, Eisenhardt L: *Meningiomas: Their Classification, Regional Behaviour, Life History, and Surgical End Results.* Springfield, Charles C Thomas, 1938.
3. Hoessly GF, Olivecrona H: Report on 280 cases of verified parasagittal meningioma. *J Neurosurg* 1955; 12:614–626.
4. Olivecrona H: The parasagittal meningiomas. *J Neurosurg* 1947; 4: 327–341.

11

Surgical Approaches to Intradural Meningiomas of the Foramen Magnum: The Transoral Approach vs. the Far Lateral Transcondylar Approach

CASE

A 55-year-old woman came to medical attention for numbness in her arms, occipital headache, and spastic gait. A magnetic resonance image revealed a small lesion confined to the midline.

PARTICIPANTS

The Transoral Approach to Intradural Lesions of the Foramen Magnum–
H. Alan Crockard, M.D.

The Far Lateral Transcondylar Approach to a Foramen Magnum Meningioma–
Bernard George, M.D.

*Moderator–*Fernando M. Braga, M.D.

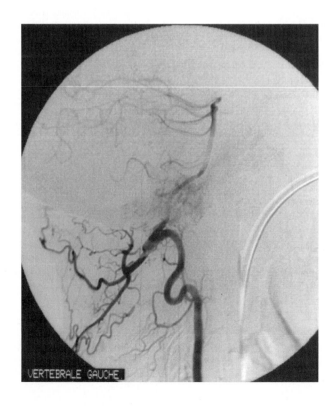

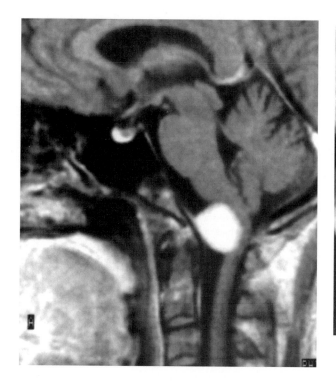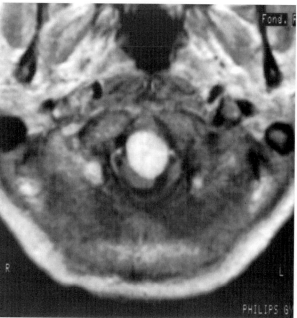

The Transoral Approach to Intradural Lesions at the Foramen Magnum

H. Alan Crockard, M.D.

The radiological investigations of this patient reveal an anteriorly placed extra-axial mass attached to and arising from the dura exactly at the craniovertebral junction, directly behind the arch of C1 at the tip of the odontoid peg.

The computed tomogram (CT) is a section taken through the upper part of the arch of C1 and the anterior rim of the foramen magnum. The appearance of the lesion exactly in the midline results from the imaging angle and is not because of any bone cyst in the area. Both vertebral arteries can be identified, displaced dorsally and laterally by the mass and lying on its surface. The left vertebral artery appears to be larger than the right.

On the MRI, the lesion is seen clearly arising from the dura and distorting the cervicomedullary junction. The uniform signal change between T1 and T2 and its position and relation to the dura make a diagnosis of meningioma in this area most likely. The transverse section reveals the neuraxis distorted dorsally and to the right. The left (dominant) vertebral artery is closely applied to the tumor surface, exposed to a left lateral approach.

The angiogram reveals tumor blush, again in keeping with the diagnosis. The left vertebral artery has been catheterized in the study. The right vertebral artery is probably outlined by the injection of the aortic arch. There is a tumor blush, probably supplied by dural vessels.

FREQUENCY AND TREATMENT

Foramen magnum meningiomas represent less than 2% of all intracranial meningiomas. They are 9 or 10 times more common in women than in men, are slow-growing, and are often present in patients over 50 years of age with vague symptoms such as neck pain, heaviness in the shoulders, and weakness of the hands.[4] Bulbar signs are usually very late, but the small muscles of the hands are often wasted. When bulbar signs are present, the patient may already have recurrent low-grade aspiration pneumonitis.

In the postoperative period, regardless of the surgical route taken, most of these patients have transient or prolonged difficulties in swallowing and, thus, great care of the airway and the prevention of aspiration pneumonitis is a most important part of their postoperative treatment. There is a strong argument for considering elective tracheostomy and an elective gastrostomy, if the patient has preoperative difficulties with swallowing.

SURGICAL APPROACHES

Any surgical approach to a lesion at the foramen magnum is technically demanding and potentially hazardous.

A pure *midline posterior approach* is definitely contraindicated because it risks an unnecessary hazard on the already stretched cervicomedullary junction and the lower cranial nerves—in particular, the accessory, hypoglossal, and vagal rootlets.

A pure *lateral approach*, as outlined by George and colleagues[2] could be used to good effect for this tumor. I also have considerable experience with this approach.[3] In this patient, the procedure would involve a hemilaminectomy of C1 and probably C2, and a small craniectomy on the posterolateral aspect of the foramen magnum. Part of the occipital condyle and lateral masses of the atlas and axis would be removed using the high speed air drill, and the vertebral artery would be mobilized. Because of the location of the tumor, a left-sided approach would be indicated, although it puts at risk the dominant vertebral artery; however, as the Circle of Willis is intact, this may not be a contraindication.

The particular disadvantage of the lateral approach in this patient is the risk to the accessory nerve and the lower cranial nerve rootlets, which are likely to be draped over the surface of the tumor. This approach, however, allows good control of the vertebral artery both proximally and distally, which can be achieved in the initial exposure and, thus, bleeding should not be a major problem. In any case, the tumor's blood supply is derived from anterior dural branches.

The *transoral approach* for intradural tumors has been used in less than 3% of patients treated at this institution.[4] In this particular patient, the tumor would be particularly amenable to the approach in that it is anteriorly placed on the midline, arises from the dura, separates the vertebral arteries, and all the cranial nerves are likely to be draped rostrally on its surface. The anterior spinal artery arising from the vertebral arteries is likely to be in the cleft between the tumor and the cervicomedullary junction, and is particularly at risk with the lateral approach. A further advantage of the transoral approach is the absence of any traction on the neuraxis or the lower cranial nerves. As the tumor is internally decompressed, it is likely that a plane of cleavage will develop between the ventral surface of the medulla and spinal cord and the dorsal capsule of the tumor. Thus, one is applying the same surgical principles to this part of the neuraxis as with, for example, a meningioma of the middle third of the sphenoidal wing approached through the zygomatico-orbital route extradurally in the first instance.[6] A further advantage of the transoral approach is that the blood supply of the tumor is derived from the dura and, thus, during the initial dissection to and through the dura, the tumor is devascularized, causing it to shrink. No major blood supply to the tumor comes from the intradural vertebral arteries.

In terms of exposure, the transoral approach is very simple. Assuming that the patient's mouth opens normally and head extension can be easily achieved, the tumor may be exposed by a vertical midline incision in the posterior pharynx with retraction of only the soft palate. If this exposure is not quite enough, a midline split of the soft palate allows access to the lower 1 cm of the clivus, the rim of the foramen magnum and down to the C2-C3 joint. Twenty of the anterior arch millimeters must be removed from the atlas (10 mm on each side of the midline; the vertebral arteries are 22 to 24 mm lateral to the midline at this point). The tip of the odontoid peg is removed but the transverse ligament, about 5 mm below the tumor, should be preserved to maintain stability. The anterior rim of the foramen magnum and the first 5 mm of the clivus can be removed with the high-speed air drill and the dura in that area exposed. Vigorous venous bleeding may well stem from the dura in the area because of tumor drainage and perhaps the marginal sinus; this bleeding can be controlled with the laser or monopolar diathermy.

The major disadvantage of transoral surgery is cerebrospinal fluid leakage and the danger of infection. Before the incision is made, a wide-bore lumbar drain is inserted and kept in position for at least 5 days postoperatively. This drain is then almost always converted to a lumboperitoneal shunt to maintain low cerebrospinal fluid pressure for about a month after surgery. Some of the dura is excised along with the tumor, resulting in a dural defect. Direct suturing of the dura in this area is difficult; instead, I concentrate on multilayer closure with a cellulose material, thrombin/fibrin glue, fat, and fascia. In such cases, there is an argument for choosing a laterally based square flap in the pharynx instead of the usual midline vertical incision, so that good tissue is available for closure. Some surgeons would also recommend the insertion of a bone graft from the lower clivus to the lower part of the second cervical vertebra to maintain stability and encourage a bony union across the craniovertebral junction, but the patient would lose lateral rotatory neck movement and be in a halo brace for 3 months. Other surgeons might reconstitute the ring of C1 with a titanium plate and screws and a bone graft rather than bridge the craniovertebral junction. The advantage of the latter is that normal craniovertebral movements are preserved. Our own simple approach of osteoplastic repair of the ring of the atlas using titanium miniplates[5] allows for the insertion of a bone graft behind the reconstituted arch. Our own long-term results with anterior bone grafting, however, are not as successful as those of the methods mentioned above. Without reconstituting the ring of C1 and having removed the alar and apical ligaments, late craniocervical instability may develop as a result of this surgical approach; long-term follow-up is required to ensure craniocervical stability.

Immediate Postoperative Care

After surgery, the elective tracheostomy is maintained for at least 5 days if there is good bulbar function. The nasogastric tube is used to empty the gastric contents for 36 hours after surgery to prevent soiling of the wound. Then, if the patient's bowel sounds are good, fluid replacement and nutrition can be administered in this way.

The patient should lie in bed with a slight head-up tilt while the lumbar drain is in position. Drainage of cerebrospinal fluid is rigorously maintained at 10 to 20 ml per hour for the first few days. When the blood staining has disappeared (at about 5 days) a lumboperitoneal shunt is inserted. Mouth care every 4 hours is absolutely essential and a nil oral food or drink regimen is instituted for 5 days. Buccal swelling is controlled with applications every 4 hours of 1% hydrocortisone ointment; with this regimen, the patient's need for systemic steroids can be reduced considerably. Nausea and vomiting are controlled with metoclopramide hydrochloride and a transdermal patch. Antibiotics, such as a cephalosporin and metronidazole, are given with the induction of anesthesia and for 48 hours after surgery. Long-term use of antibiotics may cause a fungal superinfection.

The Far Lateral Transcondylar Approach to a Foramen Magnum Meningioma

Bernard George, M.D.

My comments on this patient are based on my personal experience with 78 patients having tumors of the foramen magnum, including 28 meningiomas, as well as of a French cooperative study of 230 patients (106 meningiomas) observed between 1981 and 1992 whose cases have recently been collected and analyzed.[10–13] A comparison is also done with the literature, especially with several series published by the Mayo Clinic[7,17,24] and Guidetti and Spallone.[14]

CASE DISCUSSION

The patient presented here is a woman of 55 years with a 2-year delay between her first symptoms and diagnosis; this is what is usually observed in meningiomas of the foramen magnum (Table 1). The initial symptoms are posterior headaches and then paresthesias and numbness. Posterior headaches are the first symptom in 38% of patients in the French series[10–13] and in 77% of patients in the series of Guidetti and Spallone.[14] Paresthesias and motor deficit are the other usual initial symptoms.

This patient has no motor deficit, which is a little surprising for an anterior lesion with posterior displacement of the medulla oblongata. This displacement permits a long evolution of the tumor and allows the neuraxis to adapt to and tolerate such compression. Paresthesias and numbness suggest a dysfunction in the posterior columns, probably related to their compression against the bony structures (the posterior arch of the atlas). This point must be kept in mind when the patient is positioned for surgery and during the bone resection to open the foramen magnum. The lack of involvement of the lower cranial nerves suggests that they are not embedded in the tumor but that they

Table 1. Cases of Foramen Magnum Meningiomas Reported in the Literature

Series	Mean age of patients (years)	Sex	Duration of symptoms (months)
French series (n = 106)[10–13]	53.7	23F/1M	28.5
Literature (n = 158)[7,14,17,24]	46	3F/1M	36
Present case	53	1F	24

have slowly and progressively been displaced upwards and backwards.

The patient's imaging exams include a computed tomogram (CT), magnetic resonance imaging (MRI), and an angiogram. An MRI is certainly sufficient to assess the nature of this tumor and to define its localization and extent. A meningioma is the only diagnosis that can be proposed because the features do not indicate any other type of intradural lesion, such as a neurinoma, hemangioblastoma, melanoma, or any type of cyst (dermoid, epidermoid, arachnoid, or neurenteric). This tumor is entirely intradural. Extradural or the hour-glass form of meningioma were seen in 15 of the 106 patients with meningiomas in the French series.[10–13]

CLASSIFICATION OF TUMORS

The classification I use takes into account only the attachment of the tumor to any structure (for example, dura mater, nerves, or spinal roots). For meningiomas, the dural insertion is believed to define only the localization. The classification of the location of foramen magnum tumors must correspond to a particular difficulty in tumor removal; in so doing, an anterior localization should refer only to a meningioma taking insertion on both sides of the midline and, accordingly, displacing backwards the medulla oblongata and the spinal cord. Conversely, lateral localization is defined by an insertion between the midline and the dentate ligament, even if the tumor extends beyond the midline. The free portion of a foramen magnum tumor, meaning the portion without any attachment to any structure, is not to be considered because this part generally raises no problem in surgical extirpation. Lateral tumors generally displace the neuraxis not only posteriorly but also laterally. According to this way of analyzing the localization, any neurinoma is always lateral.

The tumor in the present case is classified as anterior. It has a slight predominance on the left side and pushes the medulla oblongata posteriorly but also a little laterally to the right side. In general, the delimitation of the true insertion of a foramen magnum meningioma is not easy; in many cases, the area where the meningioma is in contact with the dura overtakes the zone of real attachment and the vessels supplying the tumor. Around this zone, part of the tumor adheres to the dura but can be split from it. The differentiation between these two parts is not obvious, even on the MRI. This analysis is still more confusing when there is contrast enhancement of the dura around the meningioma. This feature was reported in other sites to correspond to either tumoral or nontumoral involvement.[1,4,18,22,23] In the present case, the base of insertion seems to be broad with some thickening of the dura surrounding it. If a complete removal with dural resection (grade I of Simpson[21]) is contemplated, this peripheral zone must certainly be resected.

THE VERTEBRAL ARTERY

The insertion of the tumor in this patient seems also to extend laterally and to come into contact with the vertebral artery. This relationship was frequently observed in our experience, but the vertebral artery raised a real problem and was freed from the tumor in only 4 patients. In most cases, the vertebral artery was in close relationship with the tumor, but with an arachnoid plane between the 2 structures making their separation rather easy. Angiography may be helpful to appreciate this point. In the patient under discussion, neither irregularities nor stenosis could suggest tumoral embedding of the vertebral artery. The 2 vertebral arteries are only shifted posteriorly, and both are of good and similar size. The posterior-inferior cerebral artery originates intracranially at the level of the tumor. The origin of this vessel has been found extracranially in up to 18% of patients.[6,9,13,15] This may be a supplementary difficulty in the exposure of the vertebral artery extracranially during the opening or intracranially during tumor removal. Finally, there is some vascular injection of the tumor by a branch of the vertebral artery at C3. Therefore, it is probably useful to begin the tumor removal at the inferior extremity to suppress the main vascular supply as soon as possible.

The computed tomogram could have been omitted as it provides only complementary information about the bony contours of the foramen magnum. There is no spina bifida or any other craniocervical malformation. The groove of the vertebral artery in the posterior arch of the atlas is normal, without calcification or ossification of the atlanto-occipital ligaments.[6,9,13]

SURGICAL APPROACH

The indications for surgical treatment are obvious; there is no other way to decompress the medulla oblongata and spinal cord. Any possible contraindications are related only to a poor general condition of the patient, which is not the case here. The surgical approach can be chosen from among 3 main routes: the anterior transoral, the posterior, and the posterolateral (also called the transcondylar, far lateral, and extreme lateral).

The anterior approach is not adequate for any intradural tumor because: (1) the subarachnoid space opens into a contaminated field (the mouth), (2) the surgical field is deep and narrow, (3) the most important structures, the medulla oblongata, spinal cord, cranial nerves, and vertebral artery, cannot be controlled, and (4) the dura around the area of insertion cannot be controlled. The few reported cases of intradural tumors treated through the transoral approach show that this technique gives a low rate of complete removal with a significant number of complications (meningitis, cerebrospinal fluid leakage, velopharyngeal incompetence, dehiscence of the soft palate, and spinal instability).[3,5,16]

The Posterior Approach

The posterior approach has been the standard technique since the first patient was successfully treated by Elsberg.[8] Its main drawback is the interposition of the neuraxis between the surgeon and the tumor, which requires retraction or twisting by a stitch passed through the dentate ligament. This problem is quite similar at any level of the spine and posterior fossa. Any maneuver that limits or, better, avoids this retraction and even contact between the instruments and the neuraxis must be employed. In fact, the best technique is to enlarge the bony opening as far laterally as possible to allow the instruments to reach the tumor directly, passing in front of the spinal cord.[2,11–13,19,20] Because the spinal cord and medulla oblongata are shifted posteriorly, it is not necessary to reach an angle of 90 degrees from the midline; an angle of 60 to 70 degrees is sufficient to be in a plane anterior to the spinal cord and medulla oblongata. This allows at least 20 degrees more than what is provided by the standard posterior approach. The lateral limit of the posterior approach is the vertebral artery. Therefore, the enlargement can be made only by exposing and displacing this artery out of its groove in the posterior arch of the atlas. The more the tumor is anterior, the more the opening must be extended laterally. At the maximum, the transverse process of C1 is unroofed and the vertebral artery transposed medially, allowing access above and lateral to it.[12] Accordingly, the joint C0-C1, that is, the lateral mass of the atlas and the occipital condyle, are more or less drilled out.

The first step in the control of the vertebral artery is to drill the arch of the atlas from the midline towards the transverse process at the level of the vertebral artery groove. It is safe to start at the inferior edge of the arch of the atlas and progress upwards. The important point is to stay subperiosteally; in so doing, the periosteal sheath surrounding the vertebral artery and its venous plexus is preserved, preventing venous bleeding while mobilizing the vertebral artery from its bony groove. The same technique is used if the transverse process is opened. The periosteal furrow around the vertebral artery proceeds along the course of the vertebral artery, including the segment between the groove of the atlas and the dural penetration. The bend of the vertebral artery as it leaves the groove is easily identified by the change in the height of the arch of the atlas, which increases medially. At its junction with the dura, the periosteal sheath invaginates the dura in such a way that the vertebral artery is enclosed in a double sheath for a few millimeters. To free the vertebral artery at this point, it is easier to cut the two sheaths at some distance around the artery.[11,13] In the present case, these principles of the posterolateral approach do not need to be carried to an extreme. Because the tumor is inserted a little laterally on the left side, the approach is to be done on this side. It is sufficient to mobilize the vertebral artery from its groove and to resect the medial part of the lateral mass of the atlas, the occipital condyle and the jugular tubercle (Fig. 1).

Another important point is the patient's head position and the bone resection on the posterior arch of the atlas. The patient's head must not be overly flexed; in flexion, the neuraxis projects anteriorly from 3 to 6 mm and, therefore would be compressed still more by the tumor.[10] The bone resection must never be limited to one side, especially if the spinal cord is pushed, not only posteriorly, but also laterally. Actually, it is useful to give as much space as possible to the neuraxis immediately; this is the first step of decompression. Moreover, it increases the tolerance of the spinal cord and medulla during manipulation of the tumor, which may transmit some pressure to the nervous structures. In the current patient, this point seems particularly important because the sensory disturbances probably result from the compression of the spinal cord on the posterior arch of the atlas. Similarly, cutting the dentate ligament and sometimes the first and second spinal roots may be useful to rapidly decrease the compression. These important goals cannot be attained through the anterior approach.

The last point to be discussed in a posterolateral approach is the operative position of the patient. One of 3 positions (sitting, prone, and lateral) can be used. The choice between the sitting and prone position is only a question of preventing air embolism. With the use of a G-suit and hypervolemia to raise the central venous pressure above 15 mmHg, there is almost no risk of air embolism. In these 2 positions, the skin incision follows the midline up to the occipital protuberance and then is curved laterally and extended more or less towards the mastoid process. The advantage of these 2 positions is to allow easy access to the posterior midline and towards the opposite side; this refers to the necessity of contralateral bone resection as mentioned above and, in some cases, to the need of working on both sides of the neuraxis. In the lateral position, the patient's head must be tilted down to the opposite side, which may have a deleterious effect on the spinal cord, especially in patients with lateral tumors. The skin incision is made along the anterior edge of the sternomastoid muscle and then curved medially on the mastoid process and more or less extended towards the occipital protuberance. With this approach, it is difficult to reach the posterior midline and the opposite side; conversely, it is possible to extend the opening on the anterior arch of the atlas. This is generally useful only for extradural tumors such as chordomas. Another advantage is the surgeon's more comfortable position for working, particularly when compared to the sitting position.

Surgical Technique

The tumor in the patient described herein should be handled as follows. The patient should be placed in the sitting position, and the surgeon should employ the posterolateral approach, opening the bone on both sides and drilling the internal part of the C0-C1 joint on the left side after mobilizing the vertebral artery out of its groove in the posterior arch of the atlas.

The dura is then opened in the usual Y-shape for the same reason as for the bilateral bone resection; however, the vertical part of this incision is made a little lateral to the midline on the side of the tumor. The dural flap on the opposite side is left in place to protect the spinal cord. On the side of the tumor, another incision is made following the direction of the vertebral artery up to its dural penetration. In this way, the exposure is done directly at the level of the tumor's insertion (Fig. 2). In this

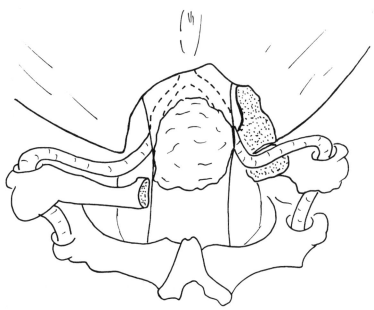

Fig. 1 Sketch of the localization of the tumor and of the exposure obtained through the posterolateral approach; notice the mobilization of the vertebral artery and the extent of bone resection.

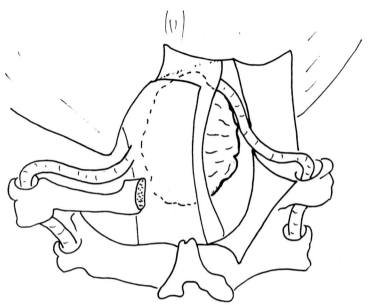

Fig. 2 Sketch of the exposure of the tumor after dural opening; the dural flap is kept in place to protect the spinal cord and the medulla oblongata.

patient, the intracranial vertebral artery is shifted posteriorly, and it is certainly useful to free the vertebral artery at the level of its dural penetration. This displaces the artery a little more posteriorly and laterally, enlarging the working space, which is below and medial to the vertebral artery. Control of the lower cranial nerves must be gained as soon as possible. These nerves are usually found at the superior aspect of the tumor after the cerebellar tonsil is retracted, and their displacement is usually parallel to the vertebral artery. They are left in place during most of the tumoral removal. The tumor is first removed piecemeal, starting at its inferolateral portion and progressing superiorly and medially; in this way, a superficial layer of tumor is kept against the medulla and the cranial nerves. Once the inferior and anterior portions of the tumor, including the zone of insertion, have been resected, the remaining part can be safely detached from the functional structures, that is, the medulla oblongata and the cranial nerves.

The arachnoid around the spinal cord and medulla must be preserved, not only to keep a safe plane of dissection at the periphery of the meningioma, but also to maintain these structures in position without retraction. Nevertheless, if the spinal cord and medulla oblongata tend to move anteriorly, they are kept in place by cottonoids or gelfoam, which is progressively laid to replace the space previously occupied by the tumor.[10,11] The final point is to resect the dura corresponding to the insertion and, if possible, the thickened dura surrounding it if it exists.

RESULTS

The French series[10] showed that the posterolateral approach provides a higher quality of tumoral resection with similar or better clinical results than the posterior approach (Table 2). In the patient presented here, the tumor can be completely resected and the vertebral artery and cranial nerves preserved with minimal risk to the spinal cord and medulla oblongata.

Table 2. Rate of Complete Removal and Good Results in the French Series[10–13]

	Anterior meningioma		Lateral meningioma	
Approach:	Posterior	Posterolateral	Posterior	Posterolateral
Complete removal	56%	81%	80%	86%
Good clinical results	81%	67%	86%	93%

Surgical Approaches to Intradural Meningiomas of the Foramen Magnum: The Transoral Approach vs. the Far Lateral Transcondylar Approach

Fernando M. Braga, M.D.

Intradural meningiomas of the foramen magnum can be located posteriorly, laterally, or anteriorly inside the spinal canal. An upper cervical laminectomy, associated with a posterior fossa

craniectomy (posterior approach) is still the best way to operate on posterior and lateral lesions. It is contraindicated, however, in cases of anterior localization, in which the cord and medulla oblongata are displaced backwards. Two very different ways are presented for this topography: the far lateral transcondylar and the transoral approach.

These tumors are so rare that, during their lifetime, most neurosurgeons have the chance to treat only 5 or 6 patients. Of course, those who acquire greater experience and publish more about this particular subject receive patients from other departments, other colleagues, and even from other countries; thus, they will have a greater number of cases. This certainly happened with the 2 excellent contributors, 1 of them stating that he treated 78 patients with foramen magnum tumors, 28 of them being intradural meningiomas.

DIAGNOSIS AND IMAGING

The experts emphasize the difficulty and delay in the diagnosis of these tumors, which are frequently misdiagnosed as arthrotic cervical myelopathy, multiple sclerosis, and amyotrophic lateral sclerosis, among other disorders. In the beginning, symptoms are vague and a great span of time passes between the initial and more defined signs. Today, with computed tomography and MRI, the diagnosis has become easier. Some years ago, we installed a ventriculoperitoneal shunt in a 65-year-old woman with a "typical" normal pressure hydrocephalus syndrome. She had a nice recovery, but developed tetraparesis 4 months later. At this time, computed tomography showed the presence of an anterolateral meningioma of the foramen magnum, previously overlooked because the image slices started higher in the posterior fossa.

Angiography is considered an important complement in the diagnosis because it shows the vascular aspects, chiefly of the vertebral arteries. Now, magnetic resonance angiography, a less-invasive technique, can produce vascular images related to the tumor and, in the near future, may take the place of angiography.

DIRECTION OF EXTENSIONS

Meningiomas located posteriorly usually expand laterally; those located laterally may also be anterior, and the anterior tumors are never restricted only to the midline but expand laterally, producing a posterior and lateral shift of the neuraxis.

The topography in the craniocaudal direction related to the level of the foramen magnum is also important. In this sense, the lesions may be craniospinal or spinocranial. Craniospinal lesions originate lower in the clivus, extend downward, and remain more cranial than cervical. The spinocranial tumors originate at C1-C2; they grow cranially but the bulk of the tumor remains in a spinal location. Craniospinal tumors present greater surgical difficulty. This also happens with petrosal meningiomas, in which those projecting anteriorly to the internal auditory canal require more difficult surgery than those projecting posteriorly. The patient herein presented, a 55-year-old woman, had an anterior intradural meningioma of the foramen magnum, shifting the upper cervical cord and mainly the medulla oblongata posteriorly and to the right. Thus, the tumor's location is craniospinal.

SURGICAL APPROACH

In relation to the posterolateral approach, many people criticize the denomination far lateral, extreme lateral, and even transcondylar. Far and extreme, it is said, is an exaggeration, as is transcondylar, which is not anatomical. The condylus is not crossed in the transcondylar route and no more than 10 to 30% must be drilled.

The Posterolateral Approach

The posterolateral route has been used for many decades. In this approach, the surgeon pursues the tumor laterally, removes C1 very laterally, does a posterior fossa craniectomy, exposes the vertebral artery epi- and intradurally, opens laterally the dura, and excises the tumor. After the tumor is removed, one can have a relaxed overview of the area, and the condylus is located anteriorly. This can be clearly seen in the postoperative computed tomogram. The condylus is only removed when it is infiltrated by the tumor. For spinocranial meningiomas, only rarely is there a need to perform a mastoidectomy, expose the sigmoid sinus and the jugular foramen, and drill the condylus. Only some craniovertebral tumors need the far lateral approach and can be easily excised through a normal posterolateral approach.

It is essential to expose the vertebral artery epidurally, removing the arch of C1, but there is no need to mobilize it in the epidural space. Actually, this portion cannot be mobilized because its intradural portion is fixed, embedded by the tumor and, only after a partial internal removal of the tumor, will it be more mobile. Extreme care must be taken to preserve small perforating vessels crossing and traversing the tumor, whose coagulation results in swallowing disturbances, and respiratory and motor deficits, leading to a longer stay in the intensive care unit.

Positioning the Patient

In the present case, one of the authors states that the opening does not need to be carried to the extreme because the tumor is a little lateral. Also emphasized is the compression of the nervous system against the bony structures during positioning. Actually, many patients experience a worsening of symptoms when the head is flexed or tilted and, chiefly, when flexed and tilted at the same time. It is advisable before surgery, in an alert patient, to try the same position he or she will be placed in during the long operative procedure (sitting, prone, or lateral). If the patient's symptoms worsen, that position must be avoided and the head fixed in the best asymptomatic position. Somatosensory potentials may be useful when positioning the patient. The lateral decubitus with the head a bit flexed but not tilted is a good position. The entire body can be posteriorly rotated about 30 degrees. In this position, the midline of the posterior fossa and the spinous process of C1 and C2 can be reached without difficulty. An initial laminectomy of C1 and C2 and a small lateral posterior fossa craniectomy allow partial decompression of the cord, even with the closed dura. At this stage, the opening of the dura of the cervical region laterally and then medially to the vertebral artery in the posterior fossa provides a good look at the region to analyze the existing difficulties. If necessary, it is possible to go more laterally, with the same proposed flap (medial incision, up to the inion, curved along the nuchal line, and down to the mastoid). After decompression of the nervous system, the head position can be modified to use the extreme approach, if necessary. Actually, the extreme lateral approach is not needed from the beginning, avoiding unnecessary surgery.

The Transoral Approach

The transoral approach is well accepted for extradural tumors, odontoid fractures, and some cases of basilar impression, but very rarely for these intradural meningiomas. Of course, this approach is being proposed by a very experienced neurosurgeon for very special cases, who mentions that in his own department, in the transoral unit, less than 3% of the intradural tumors were operated on through this approach.

For strictly anterior meningiomas, the transoral route provides the anatomic advantages discussed above, avoiding manipulation of the neuraxis. However, there are many controversies. In the present case, the tumor seems to expand a bit lateral and also has a broad insertion with thickening of the dura. A disadvantage is related to the narrow space in which to operate, where the lateral margins of the exposure are restricted by the occipital condylus and the jugular and hypoglossal foramina.

The excision of a richly vascularized dura in which the tumor is implanted, the complete extirpation of a mass that has some lateral expansion, the possibility of cerebrospinal fluid fistula with meningitis and, finally, possible instability of this region are the great disadvantages of this route. The necessity of posterior stabilization is common, causing the patient to have a stiff neck.

Actually, the transoral approach is a more invasive technique. The posterolateral approach, with or without the far and transcondylar extension, must be chosen as the first option in treating patients with these tumors.

REFERENCES

H. Alan Crockard, M.D.

1. Crockard HA, Johnston FG: The development of transoral approaches to lesions of the skull base and craniocervical junction. *Neurosurg Q* (in press).
2. George B, Dematons C, Cophignon J: Lateral approach to the anterior portion of the foramen magnum. *Surg Neurol* 1988; 29:484–490.
3. Kratimenos G, Crockard HA: The far lateral approach for ventrally placed foramen magnum and upper cervical spine tumours. *Br J Neurosurg* 1993; 7:129–140.
4. Miller E, Crockard HA: Transoral transclival removal of anteriorly placed meningiomas at the foramen magnum. *Neurosurgery* 1987; 20:966–968.
5. Rogers MA, Ransford AO, Crockard HA: Osteoplastic repair of the atlas. *J Bone Joint Surg* 1992; 74B:880–882.
6. Van Loveren HR, Keller JT, El-Kalliny M, et al.: The Dolenc technique for cavernous sinus exploration (cadaveric prosection): Technical note. *J Neurosurg* 1991; 74:837–844.

Bernard George, M.D.

1. Aoki S, Sasaki Y, Machida T, et al.: Contrast-enhanced MR images in patients with meningioma: Importance of enhancement of the dura adjacent to the tumor. *AJNR* 1990; 11:935–938.
2. Bertalanffy H, Seeger W: The dorsolateral, suboccipital, transcondylar approach to the lower clivus and anterior portion of the craniocervical junction. *Neurosurgery* 1991; 29:815–821.
3. Bonkowski JA, Gibson RD, Snape L: Foramen magnum meningioma: Transoral resection with a bone baffle to prevent CSF leakage. *J Neurosurg* 1990; 72:493–496.
4. Borovich B, Doron Y: Recurrence of intracranial meningiomas: The role played by regional multicentricity. *J Neurosurg* 1986; 64:58–63.
5. Crockard HA, Sen CN: The transoral approach for the management of intradural lesions at the craniovertebral junction: Review of 7 cases. *Neurosurgery* 1991; 28:88–98.
6. De Oliveira E, Rhoton AL Jr, Peace D: Microsurgical anatomy of the region of the foramen magnum. *Surg Neurol* 1985; 24:293–352.
7. Dodge HW, Love JG, Gottlieb CM: Benign tumors at the foramen magnum: Surgical considerations. *J Neurosurg* 1956; 13:603–617.
8. Elsberg CA, Strauss I: Tumors of the spinal cord which project into the posterior cranial fossa. *Arch Neurol Psychiatry* 1929; 21:261–273.
9. Francke JP, Di Marino V, Pannier M, et al.: The vertebral arteries (arteria vertebralis). The V3 atlanto-axoidial and V4 intracranial segments-collaterals. *Anatomia Clin* 1981; 2:229–242.
10. George B: Foramen magnum: Tumoral pathology and surgery. A cooperative study of 230 extra-medullary tumors observed over 10 years. *Neurochirurgie* 1993; 39 (Suppl 1):1–100.
11. George B: Meningiomas of the foramen magnum, in Schmidek HH (ed): *Meningiomas and Their Surgical Treatment*. Philadelphia, WB Saunders, 1991, pp 459–470.
12. George B, Dematons C, Cophignon J: Lateral approach to the anterior portion of the foramen magnum. *Surg Neurol* 1988; 29: 484–490.
13. George B, Laurian C: *The Vertebral Artery: Pathology and Surgery*. Vienna, Springer Verlag, 1987.
14. Guidetti B, Spallone A: Benign extramedullary tumors of the foramen magnum. *Adv Techn Standard Neurosurg* 1988; 16:83–120.
15. Margolis MT, Newton TH: The posterior-inferior cerebellar artery, in Newton TH, Potts DG (eds): *Radiology of the Skull and Brain*, vol. 2, book 2. St. Louis, CV Mosby, 1974, pp 1710–1774.
16. Menezes AH: Complications of surgery at the craniovertebral junction: Avoidance and management. *Pediatr Neurosurg* 1991–92; 17:254–266.
17. Meyer FB, Ebersold MJ, Reese DF: Benign tumors of the foramen magnum. *J Neurosurg* 1984; 82:313–334.
18. Schorner W, Schubeus P, Henkes H: "Meningeal sign." A characteristic finding of meningiomas on contrast-enhanced MR images. *Neuroradiology* 1990; 32:90–93.
19. Sen CN, Sekhar LN: An extreme lateral approach to intradural lesions of the cervical spine and foramen magnum. *Neurosurgery* 1990; 27:197–204.
20. Shucart WA: Lateral approach to the upper cervical spine. *Neurosurgery* 1980; 6:278–281.
21. Simpson D: The recurrence of intracranial meningiomas after surgical treatment. *J Neurol Neurosurg Psychiatry* 1957; 20:22–39.
22. Tokumaru A, O'uchi T, Eguchi T, et al.: Prominent meningeal enhancement adjacent to meningioma on Gd-DTPA-enhancement images: Histopathologic correlation. *Radiology* 1990; 175:431–433.
23. Wilms G, Lammens M, Marchal G: Thickening of dura surrounding meningiomas: MR features. *J Comput Assist Tomogr* 1989; 13: 763–768.
24. Yasuoka S, Okazaki H, Daube JR, et al.: Foramen magnum tumors: Analysis of 57 cases of benign extramedullary tumors. *J Neurosurg* 1978; 49:828–838.

12

Aggressive vs. Conservative Treatment of Sphenoid Wing Meningiomas Involving the Cavernous Sinus

CASE

A 50-year-old woman came to medical attention with complaints of facial pain and difficulty walking. A physical exam showed a decreased corneal reflex on the right and spasticity with upgoing toes bilaterally.

PARTICIPANTS

Sphenoid Wing Meningiomas Involving the Cavernous Sinus: Aggressive Treatment with Arterial Replacement–Laligam N. Sekhar, M.D., Donald C. Wright, M.D.

Conservative Treatment of Sphenoid Wing Meningiomas Involving the Cavernous Sinus–Armando Basso, M.D., Antonio Carrizo, M.D.

Moderator–Ossama Al-Mefty, M.D.

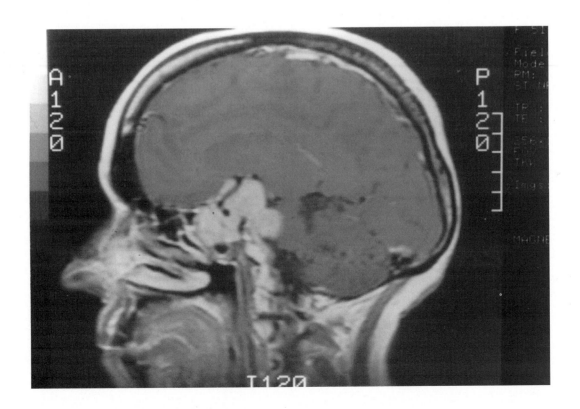

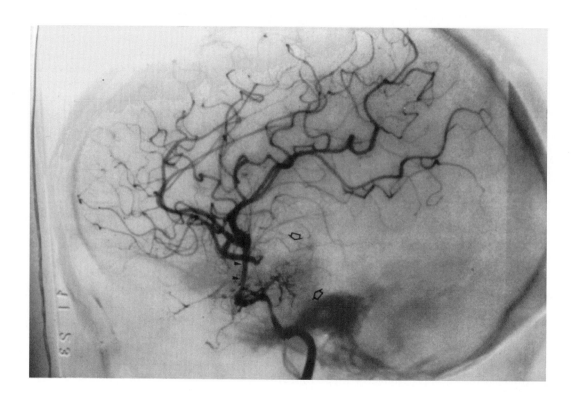

Sphenoid Wing Meningiomas Involving the Cavernous Sinus: Aggressive Treatment with Arterial Replacement

Laligam N. Sekhar, M.D., Donald C. Wright, M.D.

This 50-year-old woman is symptomatic with facial pain, gait ataxia, and spasticity.

CASE ANALYSIS

We are not provided with all of the magnetic resonance images, which are important in carefully evaluating extension into the sphenoid sinus, the tumor's arachnoid plane and consistency (low density on T2-weighted images indicates a soft tumor), and involvement of the cavernous internal carotid artery. The facial pain is presumably secondary to involvement of the trigeminal nerve, and the spasticity and ataxia stem from compression of the brain stem.

It is important to evaluate not only the arteriogram of the left internal carotid artery provided here, but also the circulation through the contralateral internal carotid artery, the ipsilateral external carotid artery, and the vertebrobasilar artery. These angiograms would provide further information about the collateral circulation, and also about the tumor's blood supply. According to the images provided, the tumor appears to encase and narrow both the cavernous and supraclinoid segments of the internal carotid artery. According to our classification system, this tumor can be classified as a grade IV cavernous sinus invasion (Table 1).

We also classify these tumors as:

1. Confined: Limited to the cavernous sinus and surrounding regions and less than 3.0 cm in maximal diameter.
2. Extensive: Extending to multiple areas of the skull base or larger than 3.0 cm in maximal diameter.

According to this scheme, this patient's tumor is extensive.

Table 1. Grading Meningiomas Involving the Cavernous Sinus (Based on Findings on Magnetic Resonance Images)

Grade	Intravenous internal carotid artery	Extent of cavernous sinus involvement
I	Not involved	One area only: anterior, posterior, lateral, or medial
II	Displaced or partially encased	Multiple areas
III	Totally encased	Multiple areas
IV	Encased and narrowed	Unilateral invasion
V	Encased with or without narrowing	Bilateral invasion

NATURAL HISTORY

The natural history of skull base meningiomas is variable and depends upon the intrinsic biology of the tumor and the influence of growth factors such as progesterone.

In this patient, the tumor will probably continue to grow, with further symptoms developing from brain compression and constriction of cranial nerves III through VI. Brainstem compression and intracranial mass effect would likely become marked well before the cranial nerves are totally paralyzed.

With respect to the internal carotid artery, we have followed the course of other patients with meningiomas, either operated or unoperated. When the tumor continues to grow, one sees progression from partial encasement to total encasement, to encasement and narrowing and, finally, to occlusion (Figs. 1, 2).

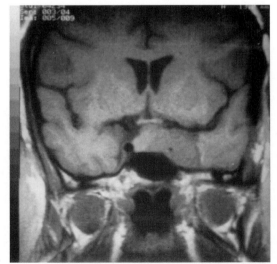
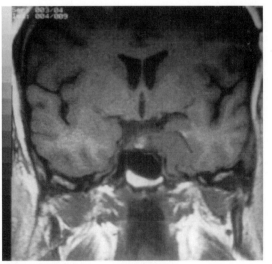

A   B

Fig. 1 *(A), (B)* **Coronal, nonenhanced, T1-weighted magnetic resonance images of a patient with a grade IV intracavernous meningioma.**

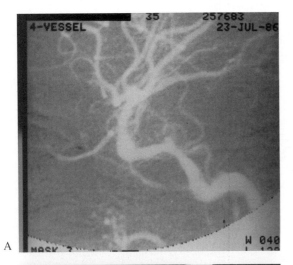

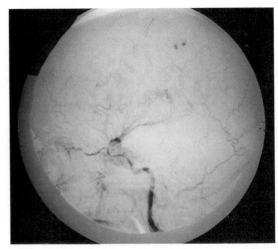

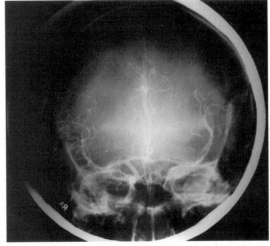

Fig. 2 (*A*), (*B*) Serial angiograms of the left internal carotid artery of the patient in Figure 1. Note that the artery is narrowed and a pseudoaneurysm has formed. In a few patients in these circumstances, the internal carotid artery has eventually been totally occluded. (*C*) Arteriogram of the right internal carotid artery after total occlusion of the left intracavernous internal carotid artery.

Spontaneous and gradual occlusion of the internal carotid artery rarely results in a stroke, unless the collateral circulation is markedly impaired.

INTERNAL CAROTID ARTERY: SURGICAL IMPLICATIONS

The pathologic correlates of carotid encasement by the tumor must be better defined in the future. In the subarachnoid space, the internal carotid artery is protected by the arachnoid membrane, such that even narrowed vessels can be dissected free of tumor. In the extradural space, however, the artery is only protected by the adventitia, which also contains the vasa vasorum of the blood vessel. While softer tumors can usually be peeled from the internal carotid artery, the firmer, more fibrous tumors cannot be peeled away without leaving tumor behind. The artery is often lacerated during such dissection, and requires repair. When multiple lacerations occur in an already narrowed vessel, the internal carotid artery may be occluded postoperatively.

In a retrospective pathologic study of 18 internal carotid arteries resected during cavernous sinus surgery, we found involvement of the artery wall in 7. In 5, the adventitia was invaded, and in 2, there was invasion up to the media. The study was not prospective, however, and the entire intracavernous internal carotid was not removed and examined in all the patients. Thus, we probably underestimated the involvement of the internal carotid artery.[1]

Resection vs. Preservation

During operations on meningiomas invading the cavernous sinus, if our intent is to carry out a gross total resection, we initially attempt to dissect the tumor away from the artery. This is successful in about 50% of patients with grade III lesions, and infrequently with grade IV lesions. It is easier in soft tumors than in firm tumors. If the tumor cannot be peeled away, what is done depends upon the patient's age and collateral circulation. We tend to act conservatively in patients older than 60 years, and in patients with medical problems. In younger patients, the tumor is resected after a saphenous vein graft is placed.

The patient's collateral circulation is assessed through a preoperative balloon occlusion test of the internal carotid artery with clinical and xenon cerebral blood flow studies. Patients who fail the test clinically are considered to be in a high-risk group; patients who pass the clinical test but have a reduction in cerebral blood flow in the range of 15 to 35 ml/100 g/min during occlusion of the internal carotid artery are considered to be in the moderate-risk group; and patients who pass the clinical test and have cerebral blood flow above 35 ml/100 g/min during test occlusion are considered to be in the low-risk group. When xenon blood flow studies are not available, single photon emission tomography (SPECT) may be used. This modality provides qualitative, but not quantitative, information. Transcranial Doppler appears to be too sensitive. Postocclusion stump pressure measurements are useful if they are considerably reduced, but

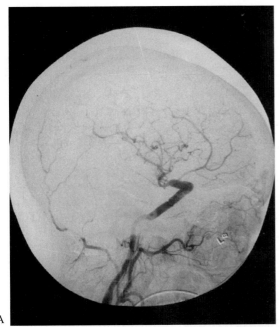

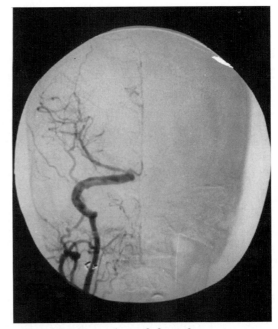

A   B

Fig. 3 *(A), (B)* **Arteriograms of a patient who underwent a long vein graft from the extracranial internal carotid artery to the M2 segment of the middle cerebral artery.**

not if they are normal. Positron emission tomography (PET) is the best test, but is available only as a research tool.

We originally used short vein grafts from the petrous to the supraclinoid segments of the internal carotid artery (Fig. 3). Because this requires a 60 to 90 minute occlusion of flow through the internal carotid artery mild hypothermia (34°C) and barbiturate-induced (burst suppression) coma were used for brain protection. Presently, our practice is to use a long vein graft from the cervical external or internal carotid artery to the M2 segment of the middle cerebral artery (Fig. 4). This requires

only about a 30-minute period of flow occlusion to a major branch of the middle cerebral artery and is well tolerated.

VEIN GRAFTS

Although we have treated about 270 neoplastic or vascular lesions involving the cavernous sinus, we used vein grafts in only 34 patients. The patency rate in our first 30 patients with vein grafts was only 85% but, in the recent group of 60 patients, there was only one occlusion (patency rate 98%).[3] The use of intraoperative arteriography practically eliminates postoperative

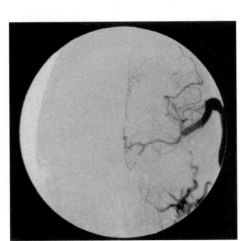

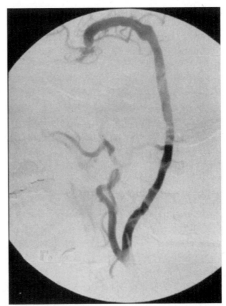

A   B

Fig. 4 *(A), (B)* **Arteriograms of a patient who underwent a short vein graft from the petrous to the supraclinoid segment of the internal carotid artery.**

occlusion by allowing the surgeon to recognize intraoperative technical problems. Since we started using long vein grafts for high-risk patients, brain protection with mild hypothermia and barbiturate burst-suppression anesthesia, and intraoperative arteriography, the risk of stroke has been greatly reduced.

Patients in the low-risk group may not need revascularization if the internal carotid artery is occluded surgically. From an analysis of 47 patients who underwent elective occlusion of the internal carotid artery, however, we concluded that occlusion of the internal carotid artery without revascularization is never totally risk-free,[2] despite good preoperative collateral circulation. This is particularly true in older patients.

RESULTS

Because meningiomas need a 5 to 10 year follow-up to assess recurrence rates, it is too early to compare patients who underwent resection of the internal carotid artery with those who did not. Our early results suggest that recurrence relates to the extent of resection and to tumor biology. Resecting the involved internal carotid allows a more complete removal of tumor, including removal from the medial cavernous sinus dura and the sphenoid bone. The surgeon can, perhaps, be conservative with slower growing tumors but must be more aggressive with faster growing lesions.

OPTIONS

In this patient, all extracavernous tumor should be removed. With respect to the intracavernous tumor, the options include observation only, radiosurgery of intracavernous tumor, partial resection (preserving the internal carotid artery), and radical resection (either preserving or excising the internal carotid artery). The options must be carefully discussed with the patient and her family so that they can make an informed decision about which procedure to choose. As always, the discussion is influenced by the surgeon's experience and philosophy.

Conservative Treatment of Sphenoid Wing Meningiomas Involving the Cavernous Sinus

Armando Basso, M.D., Antonio Carrizo, M.D.

This 50-year-old patient came to medical attention with facial pain and difficulty walking. Relevant findings at physical examination included a decreased corneal reflex towards the right, spasticity, and a bilateral Babinski sign. According to available data, there was neither diplopia, ophthalmoplegia or exophthalmos, nor alterations in visual acuity or fundus oculi.

COMPLEMENTARY EXAMINATIONS

The T1-weighted magnetic resonance image disclosed a large space-occupying mass in the basal frontotemporal region with a parasellar extension towards the sphenoid sinus and brain stem. This extension surrounded, elongated, and raised the supraclinoidal carotid segment and the horizontal portion of the sylvian artery. Intensity was roughly homogeneous and there was no evidence of perilesional edema. Angiography confirmed displacement of the vascular axes and narrowing of the intrapetrosal carotid artery. The angiogram also showed pathologic parasellar vascularization arising from the branches of the intracavernous carotid artery, and mainly affecting the meningohypophyseal and lower cavernous trunks.

The most likely diagnosis is a meningioma, as there are no findings suggestive of chordoma, lateralized hypophyseal adenoma, neurinoma, cavernous hemangioma, epidermoid cyst, hemangiopericytoma, metastasis, or any other lesion at this site.

ANATOMICO-CLINICAL CORRELATIONS

This voluminous, space-occupying lesion is not accompanied by evidence of intracranial hypertension, indicating slow development. The main manifestations were found in the trigeminal territory, namely, decreased corneal reflex towards the right and neuralgia in one or possibly more branches. These signs lead to a strong suspicion of compression of peripheral branches and the gasserian ganglion, but involvement of the greater retrogasserian root cannot be ruled out. The absence of diplopia, ophthalmoplegia, and proptosis seems to indicate that the oculomotor nerves have been spared, particularly along their cavernous and intraorbital pathways.

Signs of bilateral pyramidalism, hyperreflexia, and Babinski are attributable to compression of the pyramidal fascicles at the mesencephalic and pontine levels, perhaps directly along the side of the tumor and against the free tentorial border of the opposite side. Alternatively, these can stem from a medial or contralateral lesion extension, which cannot be ruled out on the basis of imaging evidence. In fact, the basal frontotemporal parenchyma and the sylvian and carotid arteries are displaced. Given the lack of supportive clinical manifestations, however, such as contralateral hemiparesia and seizures, among others (except for the pyramidal signs on the opposite side), bilateral involvement cannot be justified.

TREATMENT

Proposed surgical treatment for a lesion with the features described above starts with a basal frontotemporal approach that spares the superficial temporal artery, in case revascularization is necessary. Through microsurgical technique, the sylvian fissure is exposed, and the ipsilateral optic nerve and the supraclinoidal carotid and sylvian arteries identified. The tumoral mass is resected through conventional microsurgical technique or ultrasonic cavitation, followed by dissection of the tumoral capsule at the external cavernous sinus wall along the dural plane. If the sphenoid wing is severely compromised, it may be resected together with the involved dura mater.

Following Guiot and Derome's criteria,[4] every effort should be made to carry out the most complete resection possible for this tumor, followed by the reconstruction of excised structures. In the patient presented here, the apparent involvement of the intrapetrosal and intracavernous segments of the carotid artery limit the radical resection, in agreement with criteria advanced by Cophignon and colleagues.[3] In this patient, exposing the cavernous sinus and removing the carotid artery pose a high risk of altering uncompromised ocular motility in addition to increasing the morbidity of surgery with ischemic or thromboembolic complications.

Experience shows that such meningiomas resected as radically as possible have little tendency to recur, and the intracavernous remnant remains stationary for years. In contrast, intraorbital remnants exhibit an apparently higher index of recurrence at an earlier date.[1,2]

For a deeper understanding of tumoral biology that allows the surgeon to determine a realistic prognosis and evaluate alternative treatment modalities, the aggressivity of the tumor must be graded by means of cytogenetic and molecular genetic analyses, and by the determination of oncogenes, hormonal receptors, cell proliferation indices, and histopathologic features, including cellularity, mitotic number, size of cytoplasm and nucleoli, histological pattern, focal necrosis, cortical or bone invasion, and hypervascularity, among others. The proper characterization of atypical or anaplastic meningiomas allows a greater probability of recurrence to be anticipated, in spite of macroscopically complete resection.[5]

Through this treatment, symptoms arising from pyramidal and trigeminal compression may be expected to improve, or at least their progress may be arrested. On occasion, dysesthesia or neuralgia may appear due to deafferentation. If these complications prove refractory to medical treatment, the surgeon may resort to creating a stereotactic thermolesion of the descending trigeminal root at the bulbospinal junction. Alternatively, central neurostimulation techniques may provide relief.[7] Radiotherapy with the linear accelerator seems indicated in cases of intracavernous progression of a tumor remnant because it appears to arrest or delay tumoral growth.[6]

Our proposal cannot be termed conservative treatment, as it involves subradical resection that attempts to spare oculomotor nerves that are not clinically compromised. I believe this is the procedure of choice at most high-level neurosurgical services throughout the world, with reproducible and comparable results. Complex techniques of vascular and nerve reconstruction should be avoided; so far, they present highly variable results with a severe risk of irreversible oculomotor damage in patients who mostly seek advice because of pain or minor impairment of convergence.

Aggressive vs. Conservative Treatment of Sphenoid Wing Meningiomas Involving the Cavernous Sinus

Ossama Al-Mefty, M.D.

Meningiomas of the medial sphenoid wing that involve the cavernous sinus remain one of the most challenging lesions in neurosurgery. The tumor presented to the 2 groups of authors demands treatment because of the patient's age and neurological deficits. Considering the risk:benefit ratio for this patient, the authors took 2 opposing views with regard to the radicality of surgical removal. To avoid the risk of injury to the intracavernous carotid artery and ophthalmoplegia from dissecting the cranial nerve into the cavernous sinus space, Basso and Carrizo advocate removing the extracavernous portion of the tumor and leaving the intracavernous remnant untouched. They argue that the intracavernous portion could remain stable for years and, to arrest progression, radiotherapy can be used. Sekhar and Wright believe that the patient is best served through radical surgical removal in an attempt to achieve cure and minimize recurrence. In cases such as this, in which the carotid artery is involved, these authors find it necessary to resect and replace the carotid with a graft. The type of graft chosen and the timing of placement relates to the adequacy of collateral blood flow, which they have thoroughly studied preoperatively with balloon occlusion tests and studies of cerebral blood flow.

RADICAL REMOVAL

In my experience, which is supported by other reports, tumor recurrence is, above all, inversely related to the radicality of tumor removal; this is also true with regard to skull-base meningiomas. Hence, treatment should be aimed at achieving Simpson Grade I or II removal in quest of a cure and certainly to alleviate recurrence. This is best done at the first operation. The chance of attaining these goals in a repeated operation is much less and complications are much higher, particularly if radiation has been administered. Furthermore, the risk of cerebral ischemia arises,

not just from dissecting the cavernous carotid, but also from injury to the branches of the middle cerebral artery and supraclinoid carotid. Thus, although dissecting the cavernous carotid might add risk, stopping there does not eliminate the risk of vascular injury. I concur with Basso and Carrizo that tumor removal should include not only the intradural mass, but also the involved bone.

HANDLING THE CAROTID ARTERY

Having agreed with Sekhar and Wright concerning radical removal, which includes the tumor in the cavernous sinus, I differ with them about handling the carotid artery. Despite total encasement of the carotid, many intracavernous tumors can be dissected from the carotid because of the presence of an arachnoid membrane separating the tumor and the carotid. Three categories of clinoidal meningiomas have been distinguished based on the degree of surgical difficulty in their removal, the ability to achieve total removal, and the patient's outcome. The anatomic basis for this subclassification rests on the distinct differences in the site of origin of these 3 subgroups.[1]

After emerging from the cavernous sinus inferior and medial to the anterior clinoid process, the carotid artery enters the subdural space, where it lacks an arachnoidal covering over a distance of 1 to 2 mm. The carotid artery then enters the carotid cistern and is invested in arachnoid. Thus, if the meningioma's origin is proximal to the end of the carotid cistern (Group I), as is the case in a meningioma originating at the inferior aspect of the anterior clinoid process, the tumor enwraps the carotid artery, directly adhering to the adventitia and lacking an interfacing arachnoidal membrane. As the tumor grows, this direct attachment to the vessel wall continues to the carotid bifurcation and along the middle cerebral artery, advancing the arachnoid membrane ahead of it. This anatomic arrangement accounts for the inability to dissect the tumor from the carotid artery and middle cerebral branches.

Group II clinoidal meningiomas originate from the superior or lateral aspect of the anterior clinoid process above the segment of the carotid artery, which has already been invested in the arachnoid of the carotid cistern. As this tumor grows, an arachnoidal membrane of the carotid cistern and, more distally, of the sylvian cistern separates the tumor from the arterial adventitia. This plane allows the tumor to be dissected from the vessels, even though they may be entirely engulfed. In tumors of both Groups I and II, the optic chiasm and nerves are wrapped in the arachnoidal membrane of the chiasmatic cistern, allowing microsurgical dissection of these structures.

Group III clinoidal meningiomas originate at the optic foramen, and extend into the optic canal and to the tip of the anterior clinoid process. These tumors are generally small, appearing early with optic nerve compression and decreased visual acuity. The arachnoidal membrane investing the carotid artery is present. Because this tumor arises proximal to the chiasmatic cistern, however, there may be no arachnoidal investment between the optic nerve and the tumor.

Unfortunately, determining the type of tumor is possible only during surgical dissection. But, two thirds of these tumors can be separated from the carotid artery; thus, total removal can be achieved without sacrificing the carotid artery. A tear in the artery can be repaired with sutures.

For tumors in Group II, however, I try to avoid the additional complications stemming from attempts at grafting by leaving a small piece of tumor adhering to the artery. The treatment of this residual tumor depends upon its behavior and includes observation alone, stereotactic radiosurgery with the tumor now away from the optic nerve and the brain stem, or future surgery with carotid replacement. Carotid replacement with a short venous graft placed between the petrous carotid and the supraclinoid carotid arteries is appealing. Unfortunately, this bypass requires 120 minutes to carry out, and additional time may be required to remove and prepare the graft if this is not done before the craniotomy. In patients who can tolerate this prolonged period of occlusion, the benefits of the bypass are restricted to preserving ipsilateral vascularity and avoiding the potential long-term effects of carotid occlusion. However, these patients are at risk of induced complications related to establishing the graft that otherwise is not needed. Patients with absolute blood flow during test occlusion of less than 20 ml/100 g/min or intermediate cerebral blood flow of 20 to 40 ml/100 g/min during occlusion need arterial reconstruction. The mechanisms available for cerebral protection may not compensate for this prolonged period of interrupted flow. In such patients, if carotid sacrifice is planned or anticipated, a preoperative prophylactic extracranial-intracranial bypass is preferred, although it adds another operation. If a preoperative bypass was not done and the carotid is injured beyond repair, then the placement of a shunt should be considered. My colleagues and I have studied the use of an intraoperative shunt during the graft procedure.[2]

OTHER ISSUES

The issue of ophthalmoplegia is important. This patient had an ophthalmologic deficit (decreased corneal reflex) at the time of treatment. Extensive radical surgery in the cavernous sinus will most likely induce ophthalmoplegia. This is temporary, however, and in more than 90% of patients preoperative function returns. Thus, if one is willing to accept immediate postoperative ophthalmoplegia, the prospect for preserving ocular muscle function through curative radical removal is warranted. On the contrary, if ocular muscle function was deficient preoperatively, then, despite good surgical removal, the recovery is limited.[3]

The last and perhaps most definitive factor is the biologic behavior of the tumor. Despite having similar histopathologic structures, these tumors vary widely in their course. Both sets of authors emphasize this point. Unquestionably, one should know the likely behavior of the tumor before surgery; the treatment of this patient depends heavily upon this knowledge. Unfortunately, despite the availability of some indicators, radiologic or histochemical factors have not been reliable enough to predict the tumor's behavior accurately and influence its treatment.

In summary, I prefer to treat this patient through an attempt at radical curative removal of the entire tumor. I strongly believe in preserving the carotid artery and, if the tumor is of Group I and is so adherent to the artery that it cannot be dissected, leaving a small piece of tumor on the arterial wall for future treatment with follow-up or stereotactic radiation. Should sacrifice of the carotid artery be considered preoperatively in a patient with poor collateral, I believe that there is a need to establish a prophylactic preoperative bypass. If the carotid is injured beyond repair, I would establish an intraoperative interpositioned graft.

REFERENCES

Laligam N. Sekhar, M.D., Donald C. Wright, M.D.

1. Kotopka M, Kalia K, Martinez J, et al.: Infiltration of carotid artery by cavernous sinus meningiomas (abstract). *Skull Base Surg* (Suppl) 1993; 3:6.
2. Patel SJ, Sekhar LN, Linskey ME, et al.: Increased incidence of stroke in patients with elective ICA balloon occlusion followed by surgical sacrifice (abstract). *Skull Base Surg* (Suppl) 1993; 3:6.
3. Sen CN, Sekhar LN: Direct vein graft reconstruction of the cavernous and upper cervical internal carotid artery: Lessons found from 30 cases. *Neurosurgery* 1992; 30:732–743.

Armando Basso, M.D., Antonio Carrizo, M.D.

1. Basso A, Carrizo A: Sphenoid ridge meningiomas, in Schmidek HH (ed): *Meningiomas and Their Surgical Management*. Philadelphia, WB Saunders, 1991, pp 233–241.
2. Basso A, Carrizo A, Kreutel A, et al.: La chirurgie des tumeurs spheno-orbitaires. *Neurochirurgie* 1978; 24:71–82.
3. Cophignon J, Lucena J, Clay C, et al.: Limits to radical treatment of

spheno-orbital meningiomas. *Acta Neurochir* (Suppl) 1979; 28: 375–380.
4. Guiot G, Derome P: A propòs des méningiomes osseux hyperostosants. *Ann Chir* 1966; 20:1109–1127.
5. Maier H, Öfner D, Hittmair A, et al.: Classic, atypical and anaplastic meningioma: Three histopathologic subtypes of clinical relevance. *J*
Neurosurg 1992; 77:616–623.
6. Philippon J: Les méningiomas récidivants. *Neurochirurgie* 1986; 32(Suppl 1):40–49.
7. Schvarcz J: Stereotactic spinal trigeminal nucleotomy for dysesthesic facial pain. *Adv Pain Res Ther* 1979; 3:331–336.

Ossama Al-Mefty, M.D.

1. Al-Mefty O: Clinoidal meningiomas. *J Neurosurg* 1990; 73:840–849.
2. Al-Mefty O, Khalil N, Elwany MN, et al.: Shunt for bypass graft of the cavernous carotid artery: An anatomical and technical study.
Neurosurgery 1990; 27:721–728.
3. DeMonte F, Smith HK, Al-Mefty O: Outcome of aggressive removal of cavernous sinus meningiomas. *J Neurosurg* 1994; 81:245–251.

13

Treatment of Clival Meningiomas: Decompression and Radiotherapy vs. Radical Surgical Removal

CASE

A 50-year-old, right-handed man came to medical attention with acute visual loss in his left eye and a feeling of fullness in his left facial sinuses. Computed tomography (CT) and magnetic resonance images (MRI) showed a lesion.

PARTICIPANTS

Decompression and Radiotherapy of Clival Meningiomas–Charles B. Wilson, M.D., David A. Larson, M.D., Ph.D.

Radical Surgical Removal of Clival Meningiomas–Albino Bricolo, M.D.

Moderator–Shigeaki Kobayashi, M.D.

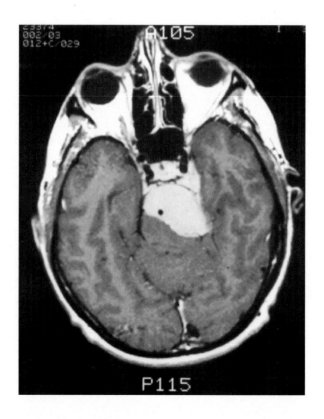

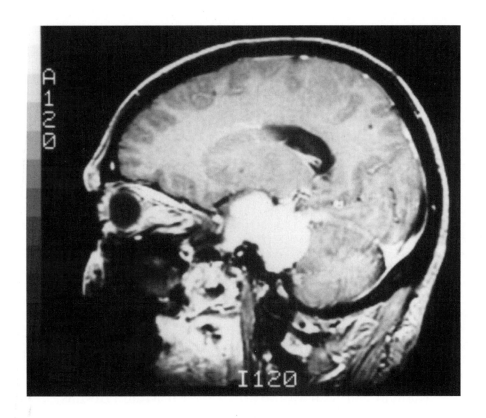

Decompression and Radiotherapy of Clival Meningiomas

Charles B. Wilson, M.D., David A. Larson, M.D., Ph.D.

Any therapeutic decision for this patient requires a critical appraisal of realistic objectives and the therapeutic risks involved in reaching these objectives. Lacking clinical information, the reader might assume that this patient had symptoms, although not necessarily, given the predictable relationship of a tumor's size to its secondary clinical manifestations. If symptomatic, a tumor such as this one might produce combinations of long tract and cranial nerve impairment. Assuming signs and symptoms, surgical decompression of the brain stem should have a beneficial effect on the impairment of long tract functions and, at the very least, an operation carries a limited risk of intensifying the problem. In our experience, however, cranial nerve malfunction would not be improved by an operation. In practice, an attempt to restore function to affected cranial nerves often either fails or worsens existing deficits.

In the patient presented here, is surgical cure a realistic expectation? No matter how radical the operation and the cost in terms of morbidity and potential mortality, surgical cure is out of the question. Our recent review of patients with subtotally removed meningiomas treated with postoperative irradiation has shown that, for benign meningiomas (85% of all meningiomas), subtotal removal followed by irradiation seems compelling. Although our data suggest that tumor volumes may be a factor, that is, a better outlook comes with smaller tumors, the size of the residual tumor after surgery has not emerged as a significant factor. We might add that the location of a meningioma, for example at the skull base or convexity, has little influence on the tumor's response to radiation therapy.

Recognizing the established effectiveness of irradiation after subtotal removal, the apparent insignificance of residual tumor volume and the probability that any radical operation will at the same time be noncurative and morbid, the logic of conservative removal and postoperative irradiation seems inescapable.

Radical Surgical Removal of Clival Meningiomas

Albino Bricolo, M.D.

The contrast-enhanced MRI image of this patient shows a large lesion of the skull base, extending more on the left, which is typical of a huge petroclival meningioma. In addition to the high and middle clival areas, the dural attachment of this tumor possibly involves the petrous apex, the tentorium, Meckel's cave, the parasellar region, and the petrous and cavernous sinuses. The tumor is wedged into the brain stem and seems to indent the ventral and lateral surface of the pons and pontomesencephalic junction, and the arachnoid plane between the mass and the brain stem may be absent. The basilar artery is at least partially encased by the tumor, as may be some of its branches, the arteries of the circle of Willis, and the left internal carotid artery. As Yasargil pointed out,[12] because these tumors originally arise from the dura along the petroclival line, they grow and expand medial to the intermediate cranial nerves, which are consequently stretched and sometimes embedded in the dorsolateral convexity of the mass.

CHOOSING THE APPROPRIATE TREATMENT

Two primary aspects of the meningioma in this patient plague the neurosurgeon confronted with its treatment:

1. A histologically benign tumor causes a mild neurological impairment with which the patient may comfortably live.
2. A major surgical procedure is needed to remove this meningioma, which entails a high risk of the patient's worsening after surgery.

Because the natural history of these tumors is characterized by progressive, inexorable deterioration, and radiation therapy offers precious little hope for patients with tumors of this size,[2] the indication for surgical removal should be taken for granted. This indication is supported by the hope that the lesion may be a soft meningioma, which is easier to debulk, and that the MRI picture of complete encasement of an important artery will, at the time of surgery, turn out to be only an engulfment, which often allows free dissection of the tumor from the encircling vessel with less risk.

The Rationale for Surgery

Often, the surgeon is, at first, pessimistic about surgery for this kind of tumor, but is then rewarded by the achievement of an easier and safer radical excision than is expected. In other words, to assume that the tumor is either inoperable or operable only at high, unacceptable risks may be the wrong attitude. A patient such as this one should have a primary attempt at radical removal by an experienced neurosurgeon. Many cranial base approaches can be used,[3,6,9,10] and the choice of the proper surgical avenue may be debated for a long time. In this difficult process, however, one must admit that the best approach is the one that provides the greatest exposure of the tumor and requires minimal retraction and manipulation of the surrounding brain tissue and nerves, but also one with which the neurosurgeon is confident.

THE SURGICAL APPROACH

For the patient presented in this case, my choice of the surgical route is the combined lateral supra-infratentorial transpetrous approach, originally designed in 1977 by Hakuba and colleagues[7] and refined in 1988 by Al-Mefty and colleagues.[1] This approach is the more elegant and less dangerous way to reach and possibly remove those petroclival meningiomas that involve a large portion of the skull base from the lower clivus to the parasellar areas.[4] The access afforded by the retromastoid-retrosigmoid or subtemporal routes is too restricted for tumors like these, unless one is willing to face a two-stage procedure, for which I feel no particular inclination. At the same time, I do not believe that wider approaches requiring a more extensive demolition of bone structures are, in the end, more favorable for the excision of the tumor.

In the combined temporal-suboccipital petrosal approach, as in the standard retromastoid-retrosigmoid, I prefer to place the patient in a semi-sitting position with the head turned slightly toward the side of the opening (the left, in this case) and bent over the opposite shoulder. A low posterior temporal craniotomy and a lateral retrosigmoid craniotomy are made to expose the lateral sinus and its junction with the sigmoid sinus. To improve the exposure, a zygomatic osteotomy, including the condylar fossa, may be added. A mastoidectomy is then done to allow skeletonization of the sigmoid sinus down to the jugular bulb. Drilling is continued along the pyramid to expose Citelli's angle and identify the position of the superior petrosal sinus, paying attention to keeping intact the facial canal and lateral and semicircular canals.

Once the retrolabyrinthine petrosectomy is completed, I favor the presigmoid route. In this, one must take great care opening the dura so as not to injure the vein of Labbé and to preserve its discharge into the sinuses. The dural incision is then carried downward along the anterior margin of the sigmoid sinus, crossing the superior petrosal sinus, which can be divided without any risk. The posterior portion of the temporal lobe is then gently lifted with a self-retaining retractor and the tentorium transected in a lateral-to-medial direction. A second retractor is placed anterior to the sigmoid sinus to keep both the posterior edge of the transected tentorium and the cerebellum posteriorly and medially. The complete division of the tentorium allows the cerebellum to spontaneously withdraw from the posterior surface of the pyramid. At this point, complete access to the lateral convexity of the tumor is obtained by pushing the sigmoid sinus and cerebellum dorsally and medially with one retractor and holding the posterior temporal lobe slightly elevated with a second retractor. Tumor removal is then initiated and continued through the use of microsurgical technique.

DISCUSSION

What remains the main problem is whether or not we should relentlessly pursue a radical exeresis of the tumor or, if some anatomic obstacles arise to preclude a safe resection (brainstem indentation, arterial or cranial nerve encasement, and epidural bone invasion), should we be satisfied with less drastic measures. In such circumstances, surgical removal done at all costs to pursue the ideal goal of radical removal at the risk of adding new, severe neurological deficits to those already existing does not seem to be the proper thing to do. We must admit that the complete excision of some petroclival meningiomas may be neither feasible nor justifiable because the tumor's behavior can be invasive and leave no room for a safe eradication, whichever approach is used.

If the procedure has allowed only a subtotal removal, my policy is to plan for stereotactic radiosurgery with the [201]Cobalt-60 source gamma knife as soon as the patient has recovered from the first surgery. I prefer this to waiting and documenting with serial neuroimaging studies the tumor's regrowth for 3 main reasons:

1. If a radical excision could not be done at the first operation because of involvement of the cranial nerves or vessels, excision is much more difficult at a second surgery;
2. when total resection of a benign meningioma is not feasible, subtotal resection combined with precise treatment planning for adjuvant radiosurgery can achieve results compatible to those of total resection;[5,8]
3. the efficacy of radiosurgery in controlling the tumor residual is greater if the volume of the mass is smaller.[8,11]

Finally, experience has shown that some meningioma residuals left only on the dura and bone may be stationary for long periods without evidence of regrowth. Therefore, once the subdural portion is removed, I prefer to adopt a wait-and-see strategy.

CONCLUSION

In summation, after a preoperative angiographic study and probable embolization, the treatment plan I would propose for this patient is direct surgery through the posterior subtemporal and presigmoid petrosal approach, and early stereotactic radiosurgery for the putative tumor remnant whenever radical removal is not achieved.

Treatment of Clival Meningiomas:
Decompression and Radiotherapy vs. Radical Surgical Removal

Shigeaki Kobayashi, M.D.

To determine the treatment options and indication for surgery of a clival meningioma, the patient's signs and symptoms must first be evaluated. This patient, a relatively young one, had an acute onset of unilateral visual loss and the feeling of fullness in the left facial sinuses. Whatever treatment is chosen, it must first aim to improve the patient's visual acuity. The left visual loss is likely vascular in nature, probably resulting from the tumor's affect on the ophthalmic artery or mechanical pressure on the left optic nerve; neither of these findings are certain from the given MRI. A fullness in the sinuses may mean a trigeminal sign. Points to be considered are that the tumor is located mainly in the petroclival region extending to the left cavernous sinus, and the basilar artery is encased in the tumor. To relieve the present symptoms or prevent the development of grave symptoms by future growth of the tumor, should the tumor be totally removed, preserving the basilar artery and the perforators, or should only the tumor in the cavernous sinus be removed?

DECOMPRESSION AND RADIOSURGERY

As Wilson and Larson mention, surgical decompression of the brain stem should have a beneficial effect on the impairment of long tract functions. It may be true that radical removal of the tumor may not improve cranial nerve function. I agree with these authors that surgical cure for this patient cannot be achieved even with a radical operation. The tumor extends into the cavernous sinus; more importantly, the basilar artery and probably the perforating arteries are encased in the tumor. Even if the tumor is easily dissected from the pontine surface, preserving those arteries is quite difficult. So it is acceptable not to attempt radical removal from the beginning. With this in mind, what approach should be taken to decompress the tumor with maximum effects and minimum deficits? Irradiation after surgery might be a good option if the tumor is not totally removed, although the definite effect of radiation on meningiomas has yet to be established.

RADICAL SURGICAL REMOVAL

Bricolo has analyzed the present case well. As he mentions, the indication for surgical removal should be taken for granted. Surgical removal (radical or just decompression), should be done because the patient had an acute onset of visual loss and because of the possibility of his developing devastating symptoms. The author mentions that the meningioma may be soft and therefore easier to debulk and that the MRI picture of complete encasement of an important artery may result at surgery to be only an engulfment, allowing free dissection of the tumor from the encircling vessel with the least possible risk. Even if the tumor is soft and easily dissected from the artery, however, complete removal might be difficult and some tumor might remain along the perforating artery and in the cavernous sinus. Small perforators are extremely difficult to preserve even in soft meningiomas; mechanical vasospasm may occur and lead to brainstem infarct. On the other hand, cranial nerves are gener-

ally easier to dissect from the meningioma. Furthermore, the patient has no signs related to the pons. Therefore, it may not be wise to attempt complete removal of the tumor from the brain stem, although the absence of perifocal edema in the brain stem might allow tumor dissection.

I agree with the author that the best approach is the one that provides the greatest exposure of the tumor while requiring minimal retraction and manipulation of the surrounding brain tissue and nerves, but also the one in which the neurosurgeon is most confident. The combined lateral supra-infratentorial transpetrous approach seems to be the best way to reach the tumor in this patient. As with meningiomas in general, this tumor's attachment must be separated at the initial stage of the operation. The operative approach should be designed with this principle in mind. Preoperative embolization is instrumental in reducing blood loss and facilitating tumor removal. If the surgeon is not accustomed to skull-base procedures, a two-stage operation might be a good choice. Because the tumor is located mostly in front of the pons, the surgical approach should be lateral rather than suboccipital, as in the presigmoid approach. The tumor in the cavernous sinus cannot be resected without causing cranial nerve deficits that are not present before the surgery.

In summary, total resection of the tumor is not recommended. If the tumor is soft, however, the main portion can be resected. Because of the patient's acute onset of visual loss without major deficits, debulking the tumor might be a realistic goal of surgery, followed by irradiation, as suggested by the authors.

REFERENCES

Albino Bricolo, M.D.

1. Al-Mefty O, Fox JL, Smith RR: Petrosal approach for petroclival meningiomas. *Neurosurgery* 1988; 22:510–517.
2. Al-Mefty O, Kersch JE, Routh A, et al.: The long-term side effects of radiation therapy for benign brain tumors in adults. *J Neurosurg* 1990; 73:502–512.
3. Al-Mefty O, Smith RR: Clival and petroclival meningiomas, in Al-Mefty O (ed): *Meningiomas.* New York, Raven Press, 1991, pp 517–537.
4. Bricolo A, Turazzi S, Cristofori L, et al.: Microsurgical removal of petroclival meningiomas: A report of 33 patients. *Neurosurgery* 1992; 31:813–828.
5. Goldsmith BJ, Wara WM, Wilson CB, et al.: Postoperative irradiation for subtotally resected meningiomas: A retrospective analysis of 140 patients treated from 1967 to 1990. *J Neurosurg* 1994; 80: 195–201.
6. Hakuba A, Nishimura S, Jang BJ: A combined retroauricular and preauricular transpetrosal-transtenorial approach to clivus menin-
giomas. *Surg Neurol* 1988; 30:108–116.
7. Hakuba A, Nishimura A, Tanaka K, et al.: Clivus meningiomas: Six cases of total removal. *Neurol Med Chir (Tokyo)* 1977; 17:63–77.
8. Lunsford LD: Contemporary management of meningiomas: Radiation therapy as an adjuvant and radiosurgery as an alternative to surgical removal? *J Neurosurg* 1994; 80:187–190.
9. Samii M, Ammirati M: The combined supratentorial presigmoid sinus avenue to the petroclival region: Surgical technique and clinical applications. *Acta Neurochir (Wien)* 1988; 95:6–12.
10. Sekhar LN, Jannetta PJ, Burkhart LE, et al.: Meningiomas involving the clivus: A six-year experience with 41 patients. *Neurosurgery* 1990; 27:764–781.
11. Steiner L, Lindquist C, Forster D, et al.: *Radiosurgery: Baseline and Trends.* New York, Raven Press, 1992.
12. Yasargil MG, Mortara RW, Curcic M: Meningiomas of the basal posterior cranial fossa. *Adv Tech Stand Neurosurg* 1980; 7:3–115.

14

Surgical Approaches to Clival Chordomas: The Transmaxillary vs. the Subtemporal and Preauricular Infratemporal

CASE

A 38-year-old woman came to medical attention for persistent headaches and diplopia. A physical exam revealed a left partial third nerve palsy with decreased vision in the left eye (20/100).

PARTICIPANTS

The Transmaxillary Approach to Clival Chordomas–Alfred P. Bowles, Jr., M.D., Ossama Al-Mefty, M.D.

The Subtemporal and Preauricular Infratemporal Approach to Clival Chordomas and Chondrosarcomas–Chandranath Sen, M.D.

Moderator–Takeshi Kawase, M.D.

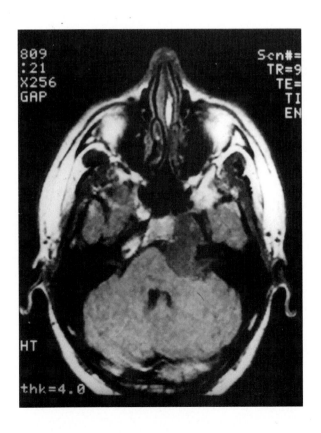
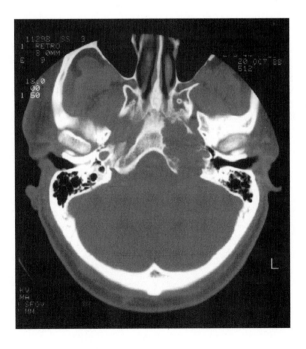

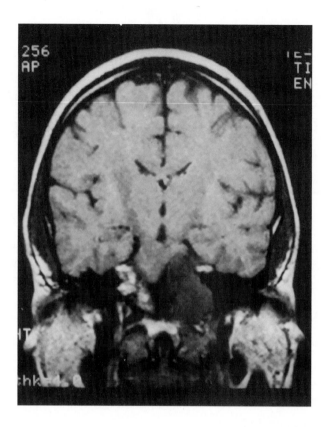

The Transmaxillary Approach to Clival Chordomas

Alfred P. Bowles, Jr., M.D., Ossama Al-Mefty, M.D.

In this case, the patient has a chordoma of the clivus that extends through both cortical surfaces and penetrates and compresses the brain stem. Although the overall prognosis for patients with chordomas is poor, surgery continues to be an integral part of the treatment and is certainly required if adjunctive therapy, including proton beam radiation, is to be effective.

The surgical approaches used for lesions of the clivus include a variety of techniques. Some of the craniotomies include subfrontal-transbasal routes and infratemporal-subtemporal approaches.[4–9,13,16] Both transcervical and transpharyngeal techniques have been used for these lesions.[10,11,17,18] We believe, however, that transmaxillary approaches are superior for clival tumors ventral to the neural axis, especially if the tumor remains extradural in location and encompasses the entire depth of the clivus.

Many of the craniotomies described are technically difficult and require excessive brain retraction with potential injury to cranial nerves and the carotid artery. Exposure for an anteriorly placed extradural lesion may be limited and complete removal of the tumor with drilling of the clivus, which is involved with the tumor, may be impossible. Transpharyngeal approaches allow only limited exposure and the larynx is sacrificed in the laryngopharyngectomy. Even though the transcervical approach allows better control of the carotid artery, exposure is limited to the upper cervical spine.

THE TRANSMAXILLARY APPROACH

Transmaxillary approaches have evolved from transoral routes with modifications, including various degrees of facial dismantling of the palate and maxilla to improve surgical access to the clivus. The transmaxillary approaches continue to evolve and currently include either a maxillotomy or subtotal maxillectomy, with or without splitting of the hard and soft palates. Although these approaches have the potential for complications, depending upon the extent to which the facial skeleton is dismantled, we believe that the overall operative exposure to the clivus is better.

The strongest argument for use of the transmaxillary approach is the provision of a direct and unobstructed route to the clivus. Within the limits of the maxillary osteotomy, the maxillary segments are retracted laterally and inferiorly, completely exposing the nasopharyngeal mucosa and pharyngeal muscles overlying the clivus. Through the transmaxillary route, the entire clivus can be exposed, extending superiorly to the sphenoid sinus and inferiorly to the level of the upper cervical spine. The lateral limits of exposure are defined by the fossa of Rosen-

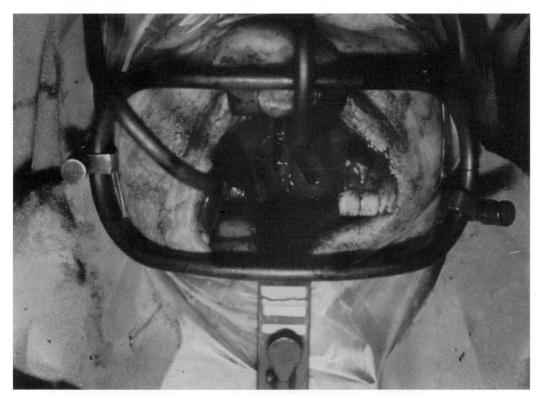

Fig. 1 Intraoperative photograph of the open door approach to a clival tumor. The operative exposure is provided with a Le Fort I osteotomy and paramedian-parasagittal split of the hard palate and entire soft palate. The nasopharyngeal mucosa and musculature overlying the clivus are exposed and readily dissected.

mueller, the medial edge of the foramen lacerum and the medial border of the occipital condyle, with minimal injury to the cranial nerves or carotid artery. The surgical techniques for the transmaxillary approach may vary, depending upon the surgeon, yet the overall review of results indicates that wide access to the clival region is provided with optimal view of the midline.

Previously, we have used an open door or Le Fort I maxillotomy approach for lesions of the clivus[1,15] (Fig. 1). In an attempt to minimize potential complications from the extensive osteotomies of the maxillary bone and palate, however, we continue to use a unilateral open-door approach,[2] which has been similarly described as a palatal hinge flap.[3] The unilateral open-door approach incorporates a unilateral Le Fort I osteotomy, a complete osteotomy of the hard palate, with cutting of only 1 or 2 cm of the soft palate. With the soft palate remaining intact, the maxillary segment is swung out and away inferiorly and laterally, completely exposing and providing an unobstructed view of the clivus.

SURGICAL TECHNIQUE

Before surgery, the patient's mouth and oral pharynx are closely inspected for either a planned sublabial or a Weber-Ferguson incision.

Incision

We generally begin the unilateral open-door maxillotomy with a transfixion incision in the nasal mucosa anterior to the septum. The mucoperichondria is elevated and dissected along the sides of the septum, and the septum is separated from the palate at the maxillary crest with an osteotome. A unilateral sublabial incision is made on the side of the maxillary osteotomy, with the incision placed above the dental roots of the alveolar ridge beyond the midline and continued to the maxillary tuberosity ipsilaterally (Fig. 2 **A**). The mucoperiosteum is then dissected superiorly, with exposure of the piriform apertures, infraorbital foramen and the floor of the nasal cavity (Fig. 2 **B**). The ipsi-

lateral inferior turbinate is sometimes removed to facilitate the operative exposure.

In preparation for the parasagittal palatal osteotomy, a vertical incision is made from the inferior margin of the sublabial mucosal incision and carefully placed between the canine and incisor, contralateral to the side of the maxillary osteotomy. The paramedian incision of the sagittal mucosa is then extended for the length of the hard palate to include 1 or 2 cm of the soft palate (Fig. 3). To ensure a proper dental occlusion upon reconstruction, compression plates with the holes drilled are then contoured over the maxillary buttresses and across the midline before the maxillary osteotomies are developed (Fig. 4).

Osteotomies

A unilateral Le Fort I osteotomy is done to extend medially from the floor of the nasal cavity septum and laterally across the maxilla. The osteotomy traverses the maxillary bone as a horizontal line from the floor of the nasal cavity and extends across the maxillary tuberosity, with the osteotomy placed above the supra-alveolar nerves in the upper alveolar ridge. The maxillary tuberosity is then detached from the pterygoid with a curved osteotome (Fig. 5). The paramedian palatal osteotomy is developed with a Gigli saw and begun by first passing the saw on top of the palate and then bluntly dissecting through the posterior incision in the soft palate. The hard palate is then cut in a posterior-to-anterior direction through the supra-alveolar ridge between the incisor and canine (Fig. 6).

The palatal osteotomy is then made in a paramedian sagittal plane and cut parallel to the midline to the contralateral canine and incisor, which increases the operative exposure for the unilateral maxillotomy. The maxillary segment is separated from the pterygoid plate, mobilized, and retracted inferiorly and laterally, with an intact soft palate and a little more than half of the maxilla detached (Fig. 7). An incision is then made through the mucosa and pharyngeal muscles of the nasopharynx and the soft tissues are then dissected subperiosteally along the entire

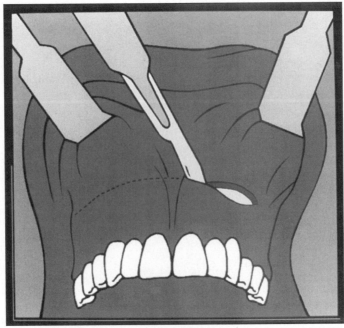

A

Fig. 2 (A) The sublabial incision placed above the dental roots for the unilateral open door approach. (Figure continued on the next page.)

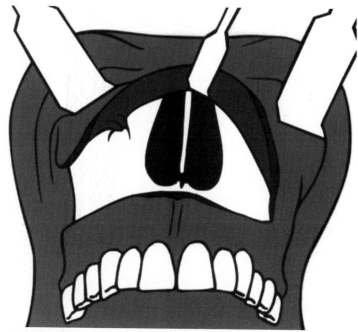

B

Fig. 2 (Continued). (*B*) **After the sublabial incision has been completed, the mucoperiosteum is subperiosteally dissected superiorly, exposing the piriform apertures, the infraorbital foramen, and the floor of the nasal cavity.**

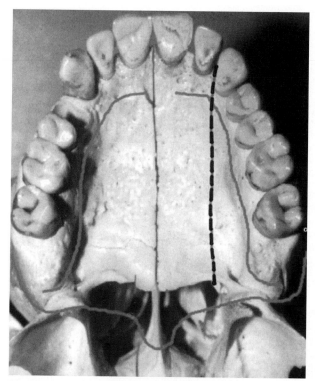

Fig. 3 The paramedian incision of the sagittal mucosa extends along the entire length of the hard palate and includes 1 or 2 cm of the soft palate.

length of the clivus. The vomer is exposed and removed, allowing entrance to the sphenoid sinus. This sinus is generally exenterated and the anterior cortical surface and cancellous portion of the clivus are then carefully drilled. The tumor may be encountered early with the initial drilling and dissection of the clivus. We generally remove the cortical surface last and facilitate bone and tumor removal with microsurgical techniques and surgical adjuvants including the ultrasonic aspirator and laser.

Closure

If the dura has been penetrated, dural closure is facilitated with a fascia lata graft, fat, and fibrin glue. The fat is sandwiched between two layers of the fascia lata graft. A lumbar drain is then placed and maintained for about 5 days. The pharyngeal muscles and mucosa are approximated and closed as a single layer. Titanium miniplates and screws are placed and secured in the previously drilled holes. The gingivobuccal mucosa is closed over the miniplates and the transfixion incision is closed with the septum and overlying mucosa held in place with nasal packing. The mucosa overlying the hard palate is not closed; however, a palatal splint measured preoperatively is placed, which will stay in place for at least 4 weeks after surgery.

DISCUSSION

We have used the unilateral open-door approach in several patients with clival tumors, with good results and no complications. The tumors have included chordomas and giant cell tumors, and lesions extending from the clivus, including basilar

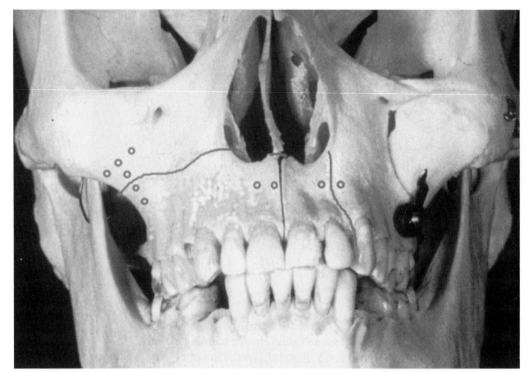

Fig. 4 Holes are drilled from the compression plates and contoured over the maxillary buttress and across the midline. The holes for the miniplates are placed before the osteotomies are done to ensure proper dental occlusion with reconstruction.

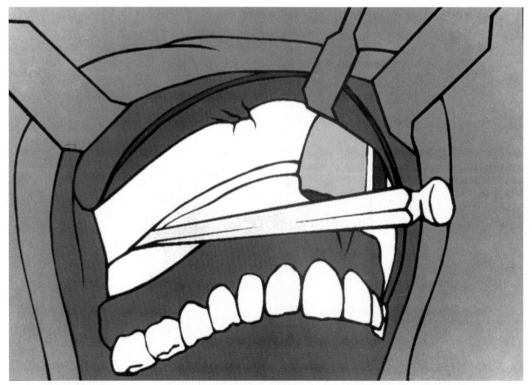

Fig. 5 The maxillary bone on one side is cut (unilateral Le Fort I osteotomy) with the osteotomy placed above the supra-alveolar nerves. The unilateral Le Fort I osteotomy is completed with the detachment of the maxillary tuberosity with a curved osteotome.

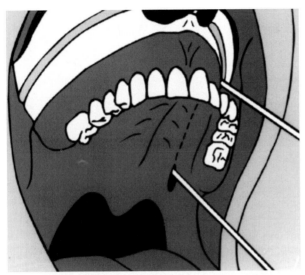

Fig. 6 The paramedian palatal osteotomy is cut with a Gigli saw and developed in an anterior-to-posterior direction between the contralateral incisor and canine.

impression with platybasia. All of our patients tolerated the open-door approach well. In one patient with an extensive clival chordoma (Fig. 8), the unilateral open-door maxillotomy exposed the clivus and tumor well. The clival region was exposed and the entire clivus with tumor was completely removed. The tumor penetrated through the dura into the brain stem but, with the direct visualization provided, we were able to meticulously remove all of the tumor. The patient had multiple cranial nerve palsies, long tract findings, and a lateral medullary syndrome.

Postoperatively, the patient's sensation and strength were immediately improved and, within a 2-month period, cranial nerve function returned to normal. There were no complications. Gross total resection of the tumor was achieved as shown radiographically (Fig. 8 **D**).

In another patient with a chondroid chordoma of the clivus, we used the unilateral open-door approach. As Figure 9 shows, the tumor was radiographically similar to the patient in the case discussed here, with the tumor extending from the clivus on the left. The tumor penetrated the dura and into the brain stem. The patient had headaches and a sixth-nerve palsy on the left. The tumor was completely removed and the patient's sixth-nerve palsy improved postoperatively.

With the approach described here, the obstruction imposed by the maxilla and palate is avoided and greater access to the clivus is provided with improved visibility. A little more than half of the maxilla is dismantled and swung out laterally and inferiorly, with the soft palate remaining intact. Reconstruction, therefore, is easily achieved and bony and vascular integrity improved, as compared to the other transmaxillary approaches, which require more bony dismantling and palatal disruption. An important point for reconstruction with this technique is the use of a palatal splint and miniplates for rigid fixation. The miniplates and palatal splint help stabilize the palate and improve healing. Furthermore, with an intact soft palate and use of the splint, nasopharyngeal reflux is avoided.

The unilateral open-door maxillotomy allows excellent access to the clivus through the shortest and most direct route with clear visualization of the lesion. In most patients with clival tumors, the entire depth of the clivus is involved, requiring that the it be completely removed with a drill. Again, the transmaxillary routes provide easy and direct pathways to the clivus,

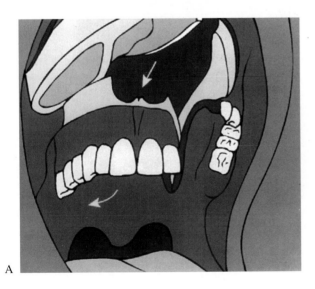

A

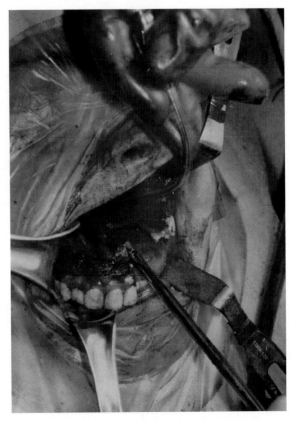

B

Fig. 7 The maxillary segment is separated from the pterygoid plates and mobilized and retracted inferiorly and laterally with an intact soft palate: (*A*) Illustration; (*B*) operative photograph.

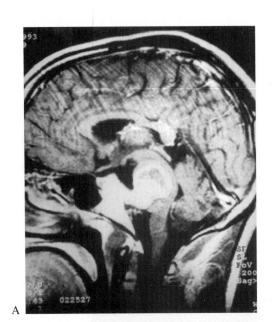

A

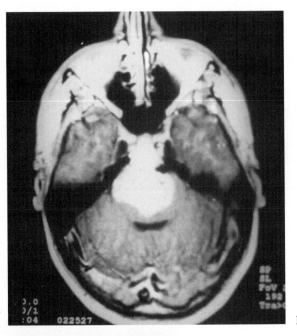

B

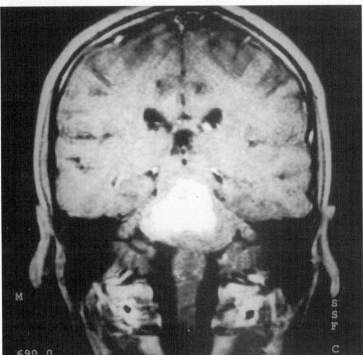

C

Fig. 8 Enhanced magnetic resonance images of a patient with a large clival chordoma: (*A*) The sagittal enhanced image shows that the tumor is extensive and penetrates the brain stem. (*B*) Axial enhanced image. (*C*) Coronal image. (Figure continued on the next page.)

so that the entire clivus can be removed. The direct visualization and surgical exposure for dissection provided by these approaches are not as easily achieved with a more posterolateral orientation.

As with all transmaxillary approaches, the midline view to the clivus is optimized. With our technique, and also as described in the other Le Fort I approaches,[1–3,12,15,19] the entire clivus can be exposed from the sphenoid sinus to the foramen magnum, with the lateral limits of the exposure defined by the fossa of Rosen-

mueller and medial edge of the foramen lacerum. In the patient described in this case, the chordoma has replaced and expanded the left side of the clivus and extended intradurally into the brain stem, and the lateral limits of the tumor are just beyond the foramen lacerum. Inferiorly, the tumor extends to the level of the foramen magnum. From a midline incision through the nasopharyngeal mucosa and pharyngeal muscles, both the open and unilateral open-door maxillotomies provide direct access to the left side of the clivus, as far inferiorly as the medial edge of

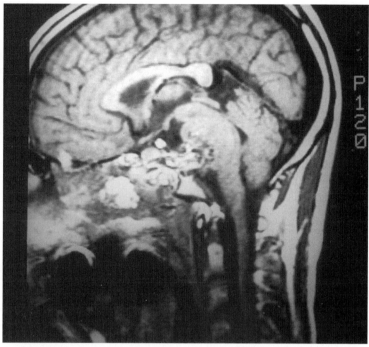

D

Fig. 8 (Continued). (*D*) The postoperative T1-weighted sagittal image shows that the tumor has been removed; the operative bed has been packed with fat.

the occipital condyle. Tumor and bone can be carefully removed laterally; however, the location of the carotid artery exiting the foramen lacerum should always be kept in mind. With the direct field of exposure provided, tumor and bone of the clivus can be carefully removed and the extension into the brain stem removed meticulously with direct visualization. Gross total resection can be achieved in this patient, leaving only a small amount of tumor behind. It would be difficult to reach the expansion of

tumor beyond the foramen lacerum, and the intradural extension along the petrous ridge would be difficult to remove completely, as well. Sufficient tumor, however, would be removed for adjuvant proton beam radiation therapy.

The most significant deterrent for the transmaxillary approach is that all transoral approaches involve surgery through a contaminated field, with the adherent risk of meningitis. We believe that the transmaxillary approach should be used for selected

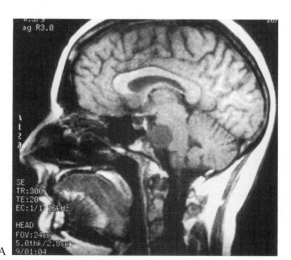

A

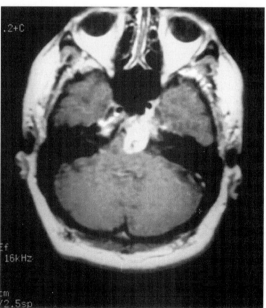

B

Fig. 9 Magnetic resonance image of a patient with a chondroid chordoma from the clivus on the left: (*A*) An unenhanced T1-weighted sagittal image shows the extensive involvement of the tumor with the brain stem. (*B*) Axial image. (Figure continued on the next page.)

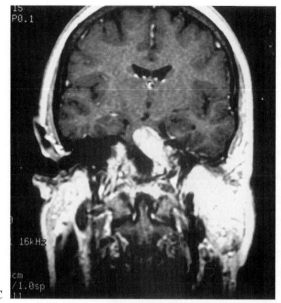

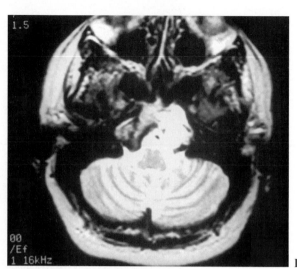

Fig. 9 (Continued). (*C*) **Coronal enhanced image.** (*D*) **A T2-weighted image shows that
the tumor has expanded and replaced the clivus on the left.**

patients, primarily those with extradural lesions or tumors. Even in our patients with clival tumors that penetrated the dura and impinged on the brain stem, we were able to achieve good reconstruction without the development of a cerebrospinal fluid fistula or meningitis with a sandwich of fascia lata, fat, and fibrin glue, lumbar drainage, and antibiotics for at least 5 days postoperatively. Roberson and Cocke[14] reported that their extended subtotal maxillotomy approach can provide direct and wide exposure of the clivus so that the dura can be reconstructed primarily with graft material. They also believed that intradural and extradural lesions of the clivus can be safely removed.

Surgical exposure for lesions of the clivus are challenging. A number of approaches that use transmaxillary routes have been developed to improve surgical access. A review of the results of transmaxillary approaches show their utility in gaining direct access to pathologic lesions of the clivus and, with this direct approach, there are generally no major vessels or cranial nerves at risk. Reconstruction is achieved without difficulty and most patients tolerate the transmaxillary routes well.

The Subtemporal and Preauricular Infratemporal Approach to Clival Chordomas and Chondrosarcomas

Chandranath Sen, M.D.

Chordomas and low-grade chondrosarcomas form a group of tumors involving the midline and paramedian region of the middle and posterior skull base. They share many common features, including a similar biologic nature, clinical presentation, radiographic features and, in some instances, histologic characteristics.[3,7] Thus, the 2 tumors must be considered together when discussing surgical approaches.

These tumors are both predominantly extradural, but invade the dura and extend intradurally in their advanced stages. Recurrent tumors that have been previously operated upon through a primarily intradural route also show intradural growth and involve the arachnoid mater and intra-arachnoid structures to varying degrees. In general, these tumors are soft and gelatinous, but extensively infiltrate the basal bony structures. Thus, the primary approach to these tumors should be extradural so that, in addition to tumor removal, the surgeon has access to the entire area of the involved bone, which is aggressively drilled away to prevent or delay recurrence. Radical resection is the treatment of choice, and radiation therapy should be reserved for recurrent or unresectable disease.[1,2] This chapter describes a lateral approach to these tumors through the temporal bone anterior to the labyrinth that displaces the petrous internal carotid artery to reach the clivus.[5]

RADIOGRAPHIC FEATURES OF THE CASE

The magnetic resonance image indicates that the tumor occupies the left side of the skull base, medial to the petrous segment of the internal carotid artery. The tumor descends almost to the foramen magnum; superiorly, it follows the internal carotid artery into the cavernous sinus. It approaches the midline but does not extend into the sphenoid sinus. It also projects into the posterior fossa, where it smoothly indents the ventral aspect of the brain stem. The radiographic images do not show whether the tumor has breached the clival dura to lie intradurally or if it is actually within the cavernous sinus. The high signal of the bone marrow of the clivus is in contrast with the low intensity of the tumor. This feature, in addition to the computed tomogram appearance of bone erosion, provides excellent information regarding the extent of bony involvement.

The computed tomogram shows an area of bone destruction at

the left side of the clivus and petrous bone in the vicinity of the petro-occipital synchondrosis. The area of bone destruction involves the carotid canal and foramen ovale and has irregular and finely scalloped margins. This area can be compared with the change in the bright marrow signal seen on the magnetic resonance image, indicating replacement by the tumor. An entire series of radiographic studies in thin sections would allow accurate delineation of soft tissue and bone.[4]

Although this type of tumor rarely invades the internal carotid artery, an arteriogram is essential because of the tumor's intimate relationship to the vessel. In most instances, these tumors are relatively avascular. Tumor removal necessitates manipulation of the internal carotid, with its potential risk of injury. Thus, a test balloon occlusion of the artery should also be done as part of the arteriographic evaluation. Although the test has inherent risks,[8] the information it provides about the circulatory reserve is important in formulating the treatment strategy.

SELECTING THE OPERATIVE APPROACH

Several points must be considered when selecting the appropriate operative approach to clival chordomas or chondrosarcomas.

1. The approach should allow access to the clivus extradurally from the petrous apex down to the foramen magnum and medially from the midline to the petrous internal carotid segment laterally.
2. When it is not clear whether the tumor has invaded the clivus intradurally or whether it is within the cavernous sinus, the approach must allow access to these areas (either at the same sitting or separately) without the risk of contamination through the paranasal sinuses and the pharynx.
3. The carotid artery must be moved out of the partially destroyed canal to safely drill away the involved bone. In the event of accidental injury, proximal control of the artery is essential for such maneuvers.
4. The status of the patient's hearing determines whether an approach through the labyrinth of the temporal bone may or may not be undertaken.
5. The surgeon must have experience with a particular approach.

THE SUBTEMPORAL AND PREAURICULAR INFRATEMPORAL APPROACH

Anesthesia and Intraoperative Electrophysiological Monitoring

General endotracheal anesthesia is used for the subtemporal and preauricular infratemporal approach to the clivus. Administration of long-acting muscle relaxants is generally avoided because the function of the facial nerve must be monitored during the approach and tumor removal. Electrophysiological monitoring of brainstem auditory evoked potentials to stimulation of the contralateral ear serves as a guide for retracting the temporal lobe. Somatosensory evoked responses are monitored during manipulation of the carotid artery. The anesthesiologist and the neurophysiologist must maintain a dialogue during the operation because of the effects of the anesthetic agents on the monitored modalities.

Patient's Position

The patient is placed supine with a bolster under the left shoulder. The patient's head is stabilized in a 3-point pin fixation, turned about 60 degrees to the opposite side and slightly extended. The head, neck, and ear, as well as the left thigh or abdomen (for a fat graft), are prepared. A lumbar spinal drain is inserted before the patient is positioned to relax the brain for this entirely extradural operation. If the drain is not used, the brain can be relaxed by formal opening of the dura and an arachnoidal cistern.

Incision

A unilateral question-mark-shaped incision is fashioned for a frontotemporal craniotomy, and the posterior limb is brought down in front of and close to the ear to slightly below the tragus to reach the neck of the mandible. A small cervical incision is made separately to control the carotid arteries proximally. The scalp flap is elevated superficial to the temporalis muscle with the frontalis innervation of the facial nerve carefully protected. The inferior limb of the incision is made to closely follow the cartilaginous external ear canal but not to extend into the main trunk of the facial nerve. The superior and lateral rims of the orbit and the entire zygomatic arch are exposed, including the mandibular condyle and its neck.

Craniotomy, Zygomatic Osteotomy, and Removal of the Mandibular Condyle

A unilateral frontotemporal craniotomy is done (Fig. 1) and the posterior limit of the bone flap is made just behind the root of the zygoma. The zygomatic arch is removed through an osteotomy, made with a reciprocating saw anteriorly at the lateral rim of the orbit, while the posterior cut at the root is made in a V-shape directed intracranially to include the mandibular fossa. This type of posterior osteotomy is used when the entire petrous segment of the internal carotid artery must be exposed. It allows the end of the zygoma to be properly reattached at the end of the operation. Before the posterior osteotomy is made, however, the temporomandibular joint capsule is opened and the condyle is dislocated inferiorly. Using the reciprocating saw, the mandibular neck is divided and the condyle and meniscus are removed after the pterygoid muscle attachments are divided. Excision of the mandibular condyle permits access to the upper cervical portion of the internal carotid artery.

Exposure and Displacement of the Petrous Internal Carotid Artery

After the zygomatic arch is removed, the temporalis muscle is further stripped from the greater sphenoid wing and the bone is drilled away to expose the foramina rotundum, ovale, and spinosum, which are completely unroofed. The middle meningeal artery is coagulated and divided. During this extradural-subtemporal dissection, cerebrospinal fluid is removed incrementally to relax the temporal lobe. The horizontal portion of the petrous internal carotid is identified by following the greater superficial petrosal nerve, which is anteromedial to the arcuate eminence, medial to V3 (Fig. 2). This portion of the artery may be devoid of bone on its superior aspect. With a diamond burr on a high-speed drill, the artery is completely unroofed superiorly, laterally, and inferiorly. The bone between the artery and V3 is also removed after the bony eustachian tube is divided. The anterior end of the tube leading into the pharynx must be obliterated at the end of the operation to avoid a cerebrospinal fluid leak. The subperiosteal plane between the artery and the bone allows clear separation of the vessel.

As the petrous internal carotid courses inferiorly, a fibrocartilaginous ring anchors the artery at its transition from the upper

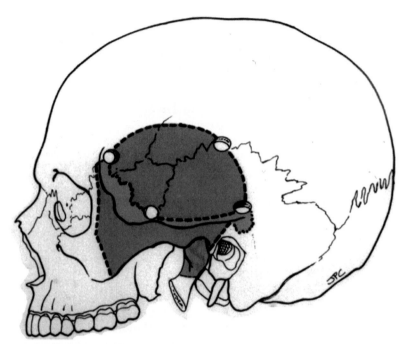

Fig. 1 The unilateral craniotomy, zygomatic osteotomy, and resection of the mandibular condyle. The posterior osteotomy of the zygomatic arch is modified to include the mandibular fossa with the zygoma in this case because the entire petrous segment of the internal carotid artery must be exposed.

cervical to the intrapetrous segments. This ring is divided sharply to completely elevate the artery out of its bony canal. During displacement of the internal carotid from the petrous bone, the relation of the carotid canal to the cochlea and the geniculate ganglion of the facial nerve must be kept in mind, to avoid injury to these structures. Both of these structures are immediately posterior to the genu of the petrous segment of the internal carotid artery; thus, drilling here must be avoided. Be-

cause the tumor destroys the bone medial to the internal carotid, the tumor should be visible as soon as the artery is displaced (Fig. 3).

Tumor Removal

The soft consistency of these clival tumors makes them relatively easy to excise once they are exposed. They are not very cohesive, however, and the removal must be carried out in a

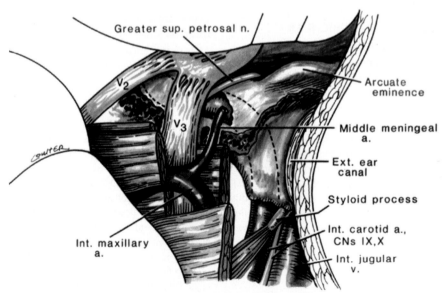

Fig. 2 The horizontal portion of the petrous internal carotid artery is identified medial to V3 by following the greater superficial petrosal nerve anteriorly; to a variable extent, this portion of the artery may be devoid of a bony covering.

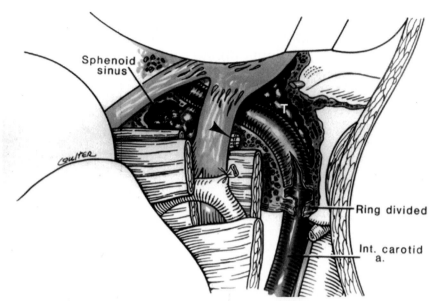

Fig. 3 **Exposure and mobilization of the entire petrous internal carotid artery requires removal of the bone anterior to the labyrinthine block, but the eustachian tube (arrow medial to V3) is transected. To completely mobilize the artery, the fibrocartilaginous ring around it at the transition from the upper cervical to the petrous portion must be completely divided. The greater superficial petrosal nerve is divided and the tumor (T) is exposed.**

systematic manner so as not to leave pockets of tumor behind in "blind" areas. The key areas in the patient described here are those parts extending toward the clivus and into the cavernous sinus. The clival dura between the internal auditory canal and Dorello's canal is clearly visible in this approach. Consequently, the surgeon can adequately assess this area for dural invasion and determine whether the tumor has advanced intradurally. In such situations, the involved dura and the intradural extension can be excised.[6] Larger intradural tumors require additional subtemporal intradural exposure with division of the tentorium, which can be done at the same time. The cavernous sinus portion of the tumor can be removed by following the tumor medial to the internal carotid artery and the gasserian ganglion. This route can be accomplished with the use of angled-ring curettes and the resection subsequently confirmed with the help of mirrors.

After the soft portion of the tumor is resected, the infiltrated bone is drilled down as aggressively as possible with a high-speed drill and a diamond burr until healthy, bleeding, cancellous bone of the clivus is seen. Drilling the bone medial to the jugular bulb can be difficult, especially if the bulb is patent, which can be determined by the preoperative arteriogram. If the occipital condyle and jugular and hypoglossal foramina appear to be involved on the preoperative studies, the transcondylar approach should be used at a separate sitting to achieve total resection.

Reconstruction

The clival and petrous defect is obliterated with autologous fat. This fat also occludes any clival dural defect. Fibrin glue may be used to achieve a better seal. The middle-ear portion of the divided eustachian tube is occluded with a small piece of fat, and the pharyngeal end is coagulated on the inside and packed with a small piece of muscle and sutured shut. The zygomatic arch is reapproximated with either sutures or titanium mini-plates and screws. Postoperative drainage of spinal fluid is not necessary.

Postoperative Care

A high-resolution computed tomogram is obtained in the immediate postoperative period to look for residual tumor and to assess the operative site. Any tumor remaining in the cavernous sinus is most likely to be within the sinus space. Formal entry into the cavernous sinus is necessary to remove the remaining tumor and should be done soon, before scarring distorts the anatomy. Because the mandibular condyle is resected, the patient will have to begin jaw exercises early to avoid difficulties with limited jaw opening. A maxillofacial surgeon may also be consulted if a prosthesis is required to realign the mandible.

If cerebrospinal fluid rhinorrhea or otorrhea occurs early after surgery, lumbar spinal fluid drainage is begun as the initial treatment. Persistent or profuse leakage must be investigated with a contrast cisternogram computed tomography and subsequently re-explored. The eustachian tube, middle ear, and sphenoid sinus are the most likely sites of a leak. Because the eustachian tube is transected during surgery, the patient will experience conductive hearing loss. If no cerebrospinal fluid accumulates in the middle ear after about 3 months, a permanent tympanostomy tube is inserted to restore hearing.

Surgical Approaches to Clival Chordomas:
The Transmaxillary vs. the Subtemporal and Preauricular Infratemporal

Takeshi Kawase, M.D.

This tumor is in one of the most difficult locations to be reached surgically, even with the highly developed techniques of skull-base surgery. The first point to consider when selecting the surgical approach is whether the lesion is medial or lateral to cranial nerves V through XII and to the petrous portion of the internal carotid artery. The tumor in this patient may arise from the left petroclival synchondrosis, is not on the midline, and extends from the posterior cavernous sinus to the jugular foramen. A large portion of the tumor, however, remains medial to those important structures. The cranial nerves are shifted more laterally than usual. The transmaxillary approach presented by Bowles and Al-Mefty allows access to the medial site without crossing the important structures. It is an excellent approach for midline lesions, but the lateral limitation of this approach must be recognized. The lateral view may be obstructed by the presence of the medial pterygoid process and the remaining petrous bone, as the authors point out. The contralateral transmaxillary approach may also be selected.

The second point to consider is the patient's symptoms. This patient does not have an abducens palsy. Instead, she has oculomotor palsy with decreased vision, suggesting that the parasellar tumor component, which is not clear from the limited data, may be a main symptomatic factor. The cavernous sinus lesion can be removed through the transmaxillary route, but this removal must be incomplete because of the presence of the abducens nerve in front. The subtemporal and preauricular infratemporal approach presented by Sen allows better access to remove a cavernous sinus lesion. In this approach, however, mobilization of the internal carotid artery with sacrifice of a unilateral mandibular joint, the eustachian tube, and the mandibular nerve is necessary because the tumor is located behind.

The third point is focused on the presence or absence of the subdural extension. On the axial magnetic resonance image, a tumor bulge toward the brain stem seems to be a sign of subdural tumor extension. However, an epidural extension may still be possible in this patient because a tumor narrowing, which is the presentation of a dural hole in chordomas (as shown in Fig. 8 **B** of Bowles and Al-Mefty), is not seen in this case.

I suppose total resection may be difficult through either approach with minimal surgical complications. A chordoma is a benign tumor, to be observed for many years. The purpose of surgery is to focus mainly on the prophylaxis of any subdural extension and the patient's neurological deterioration.

REFERENCES

Alfred P. Bowles, Jr., M.D., Ossama Al-Mefty, M.D.

1. Anand VK, Harkey HL, Al-Mefty O: Open-door maxillotomy approach for lesions of the clivus. *Skull Base Surg* 1991; 1:217–225.
2. Bowles AP, Suen J, Al-Mefty O: Unilateral open-door maxillotomy for lesions of the clivus (abstract). *Skull Base Surg* 1994; 4:26.
3. Catalano PJ, Biller HF, Sachdev V: Access to the central skull base via a modified Le Fort I maxillotomy the palatal hinge flap. *Skull Base Surg* 1993; 3:60–68.
4. Derome PJ: Surgical management of tumors invading the skull. *J Neurol Sci* 1985; 12:245–347.
5. Fisch U: Infratemporal approach to tumours of the temporal bone and base of the skull. *J Laryngol Otol* 1978; 92:949–967.
6. Fisch U, Pillsbury HC: Infratemporal fossa approach to lesions in the temporal bone and base of the skull. *Arch Otolaryngol* 1979; 105:99–107.
7. Holiday MJ, Nachlas N, Kennedy DW: Uses of modification of the infratemporal fossa approach to skull base tumors. *Ear Nose Throat J* 1986; 65:101–106.
8. House WF, Hitselberger WE, Horn KL: The middle fossa transpetrous approach to the anterior-superior cerebellar angle. *Am J Otol* 1986; 7:1–4.
9. James D, Crockard A: Surgical access to the base of the skull and upper cervical spine by extended maxillotomy. *Neurosurgery* 1991; 29:411–415.
10. Komisar A, Tabaddor K: Extrapharyngeal (anterolateral) approach to the cervical spine. *Head Neck Surg* 1983; 6:600–604.
11. Lesoin F, Jomin M, Pellerin P, et al.: Transclival transcervical approach to the upper cervical spine and clivus. *Acta Neurochir* 1986; 80:100–104.
12. Osterwold L, Samu M, Taiba M, et al.: Transethmoid-maxillary approach for tumors involving the clivus (abstract). *Skull Base Surg* 1994; 4:26.
13. Raffel C, Wright DC, Gooten PH, et al.: Cranial chordomas: Clinical presentation and results of operative and radiation therapy in 26 patients. *Neurosurgery* 1985; 17:703–710.
14. Roberson JH, Cocke EW: Extended subtotal maxillotomy for management of complex tumors of the clivus and craniocervical junction (abstract). *Skull Base Surg* 1994; 4:25–26.
15. Sasaki CT, Lowlicht RA, Astrachan DI, et al.: Le Fort I osteotomy approach for skull base tumors. *Laryngoscope* 1990; 100:1073–1076.
16. Sekhar LN, Schramm VL Jr, Jones NF: Operative exposure and management of the petrous and upper cervical internal carotid artery. *Neurosurgery* 1986; 19:967–982.
17. Southwick NO, Robinson RA: Surgical approaches to the vertebral bodies and cervical lumbar regions. *J Bone Joint Surg* 1957; 39A:631–643.
18. Stapleton SR, Wilkins PR, Archer DJ: Chondrosarcoma of the skull base: A series of cases. *Neurosurgery* 1993; 32:348–358.
19. Utley D, Moore A, Archer J: Surgical management of midline skull base tumors: A new approach. *J Neurosurg* 1989; 71:705–710.

Chandranath Sen, M.D.

1. Amendola BE, Amendola MA, Oliver E, et al.: Chordoma: Role of radiation therapy. *Radiology* 1986; 158:839–843.
2. Austin-Seymour M, Munzenrider J, Goitein M, et al.: Fractionated proton radiation therapy of chordoma and low-grade chondrosarcoma of the base of the skull. *J Neurosurg* 1989; 70:13–17.
3. Meyers SP, Hirsch WL Jr, Curtin HD, et al.: Chondrosarcomas of the skull base: MR imaging features. *Radiology* 1992; 184:103–108.
4. Oot RF, Melville GE, New PF, et al.: The role of MR and CT in evaluating clival chordomas and chondrosarcomas. *AJR* 1988; 151: 567–575.
5. Sekhar LN, Schramm VL Jr, Jones NF: Subtemporal preauricular infratemporal fossa approach to large lateral and posterior cranial base neoplasms. *J Neurosurg* 1987; 67:488–499.
6. Sen CN, Sekhar LN: The subtemporal and preauricular infratemporal approach to intradural structures ventral to the brain stem. *J Neurosurg* 1990; 73:345–354.
7. Sen CN, Sekhar LN, Schramm VL, et al.: Chordoma and chondrosarcoma of the cranial base: An 8-year experience. *Neurosurgery* 1989; 25:931–941.
8. Tarr RW, Jungreis CA, Horton JA, et al.: Complications of preoperative balloon test occlusion of the internal carotid arteries. *Skull Base Surg* 1991; 1:240–244.

15

Surgical Approaches to Acoustic Neuromas in Patients with Marginal Intact Hearing: The Retrosigmoid vs. the Translabyrinthine Approach

CASE

A 45-year-old man came to medical attention for tinnitus and hearing loss in his right ear. An audiogram showed normal hearing in the left ear and a hearing loss of 50 decibels in the right ear with 50% speech discrimination.

PARTICIPANTS

The Retrosigmoid Approach to Acoustic Neuromas in Patients with Intact Hearing–
   Stephen J. Haines, M.D.

The Translabyrinthine Approach to Acoustic Neuromas in Patients with Intact Hearing–
   Derald E. Brackmann, M.D.

Moderator–Kalmon D. Post, M.D.

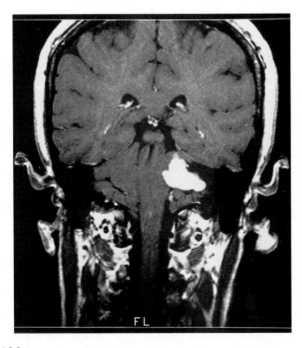
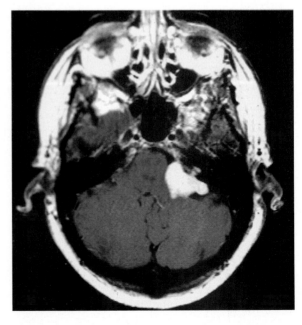

The Retrosigmoid Approach to Acoustic Neuromas in Patients with Intact Hearing

Stephen J. Haines, M.D.

This patient's clinical presentation creates an interesting and challenging exercise in clinical decision-making, for the factors that determine the choice of approach to this particular acoustic neuroma involve not just the size of the tumor and the patient's hearing status. Included also are factors that relate to the prior experience and philosophies of both surgeon and patient and to the patient's occupation, the need to localize sounds, and the future risk of contralateral hearing loss. These factors are fully and carefully discussed with each patient. I provide the information available from the literature and my experience when making a recommendation to the patient. However, I emphasize the varying importance of certain factors to different people and urge the patient to make his or her own decision. This results in a patient more fully prepared to accept the consequences, both planned and unexpected, of the operation.

CASE ANALYSIS

The information provided in the case report is sketchy. I have assumed that the patient is otherwise in good health, is not known to have a personal or family history of neurofibromatosis, and is gainfully employed in an occupation that poses neither unusual demands for hearing localization nor unusual risks of hearing loss. I have also assumed that the general physical and neurological examinations are entirely normal, with the exception of decreased hearing in the right ear. With this information in hand, I would discuss with the patient the relative advantages and disadvantages of the two standard procedures for removing this tumor—the retrosigmoid and translabyrinthine—focusing on the major factor that should determine the choice between the procedures, the desire to preserve hearing. The facts that underlie these discussions are detailed in the following paragraphs, along with my current scheme for selecting a surgical approach to an acoustic neuroma.

RECOMMENDATION

My current philosophy is to recommend a hearing-preservation operation for all patients with "serviceable" hearing according to the Gardner-Robertson classification, unless there is a strong patient preference that we not make such an attempt.[2] This preference has occasionally arisen when patients are experiencing unpleasant tonal distortion or severe tinnitus and would prefer deafness to preservation of the hearing they currently have. Therefore, assuming that this patient did not express a strong preference for deafness, I would recommend a retrosigmoid approach to this tumor through the posterior fossa with intraoperative electrocochleographic monitoring of auditory function and an attempt to preserve, not only the anatomic, but the functional status of the cochlear nerve.

TUMOR CLASSIFICATION

My scheme for selecting a surgical approach to an acoustic neuroma is outlined in Table 1. The selection depends on the size of the tumor, the patient's hearing status and, for intracanalicular tumors, the vestibular nerve of origin. Measuring the size of acoustic tumors has been complicated by gadolinium magnetic resonance imaging, which shows the irregularities, including the intracanalicular portion of the tumor, far better than any prior modality. It, therefore, becomes impossible to adequately assess the tumor's size with a single measurement. Attempts at using tumor volume are, likewise, prone to gloss over critical factors, such as the relationship of the tumor to the brain stem. Consequently, I have gravitated to a simple scheme that characterizes the tumors as intracanalicular if there is no extension into the posterior fossa, subarachnoid if the tumor extends out of the porus acusticus but does not touch the surface of the brain stem, and distorting if the brain stem is deformed by the tumor. This classification is useful because I consider the middle-fossa approach to be appropriate only for purely intracanalicular tumors and prefer the retrosigmoid approach when the brain stem is distorted, because of the superior exposure and control of the surface of the brain stem obtained through that route as opposed to the translabyrinthine route.

SELECTING THE SURGICAL APPROACH

Hearing status is an important factor for the obvious reason that the translabyrinthine procedure assures deafness and is, therefore, eliminated if hearing preservation is a consideration. My experience suggests that the middle fossa approach is most effective for tumors arising from the superior vestibular nerve and that those arising from the inferior vestibular nerve are significantly more difficult to remove through this approach. Therefore, intracanalicular tumors arising from the inferior ves-

Table 1. Choice of Surgical Approach for Acoustic Neuroma

Hearing	Size	Nerve of origin	Approach
Serviceable	Intracanalicular	Superior vestibular	Middle fossa
		Inferior vestibular	
		Lateral in internal auditory canal	Middle fossa
		Medial in internal auditory canal	Posterior fossa
	Subarachnoid	Either	Posterior fossa
	Deforming	Either	Posterior fossa
Nonserviceable	Intracanalicular	Either	Translabyrinthine
	Subarachnoid	Either	Translabyrinthine
	Deforming	Either	Posterior fossa

tibular nerve and located medially in the internal auditory canal are preferentially approached from the posterior fossa. Those located more laterally in the internal auditory canal are approached from the posterior fossa, if the relationship between the tumor and the labyrinth appears to be favorable. Lateral tumors, however, in which the labyrinth is medially placed, are best approached through the middle fossa.

This scheme for approaching acoustic neuromas requires facility with all 3 of the standard surgical approaches and, therefore, a cooperative neurosurgical/neuro-otologic surgical team. This strategy allows the surgeons to adapt to the tumor, rather than forcing the tumor to adapt to a single surgical approach. It also allows flexibility in dealing with constraints caused by the patient's individual situation and enhances the surgical team's ability to cope with unusual or previously unseen circumstances.

The Cochlear Nerve

Hearing preservation has become the benchmark of technical excellence for surgery on acoustic neuromas, displacing the facial nerve from that role, as acoustic neuromas have been diagnosed at an earlier and smaller stage. First brought to attention as a possibility by McKissick in the early 1960s,[8] held in abeyance by the dominance of the translabyrinthine approach through the 1960s and 1970s, preserving hearing has come into prominence during the past decade. Large reviews of attempted hearing preservation report variable results, with a central tendency suggesting that about one third of such operations are successful in preserving some degree of hearing function.[9] Some authors have relied solely on speech reception thresholds, although most use the scheme of Gardner and Robertson, which combines speech reception threshold and word recognition to classify the quality of hearing. With the benefit of modern diagnostic technology, which diagnoses lesions that are smaller in patients whose hearing is better preserved preoperatively, recent reports show a tendency toward increasing percentages of preservation. My own results with intracanalicular tumors currently approach 80% preservation of serviceable hearing. Tumor size and quality of preoperative hearing are clearly the best predictors of the likelihood of hearing preservation.

In the patient under discussion, the tumor distorts the brain stem and invaginates rather deeply into the middle cerebellar peduncle. This hearing is on the very margin of being "serviceable" and the prospects for preserving useful hearing must certainly be at the lower end of the reported range. Nonetheless, the ability to localize loud sounds can be life-saving in unusual circumstances, and progressive advances in cochlear stimulation technology may render the improvement of nonserviceable hearing to serviceable hearing a possibility in the future. In the event of unexpected loss of hearing in the currently normal ear, the preservation of even nonserviceable hearing on the side of the tumor could be of value. Therefore, the decision to undertake a hearing preservation operation in a patient such as this is heavily determined by answering the question, "Does attempted hearing preservation pose any additional risks to this patient?"

The Matter of the Facial Nerve

When one discusses hearing preservation in acoustic neuroma surgery, one almost assumes that facial nerve preservation is no longer an issue. For tumors that distort the brain stem, however, it is still a technical challenge and the surgeon who takes this matter lightly will develop facility in facial nerve reanastomosis, grafting, and hypoglossal-facial anastomosis. Proponents of the translabyrinthine approach have argued that this approach provides superior exposure of the facial nerve and thereby reduces the risk of facial nerve transection during surgery.[4] If true, this fact would weigh heavily against attempts to preserve hearing in patients with distorting tumors and marginal hearing. In my experience, however, the risk of facial nerve transection does not appear to be related to the surgical approach. Although it is true that the exposure of the facial nerve far laterally in the internal auditory canal is superior with the translabyrinthine as opposed to the retrosigmoid approach, the region where the nerve is thinnest and most adherent to the tumor, and therefore most likely to be injured, is not here but at the porus acusticus.[1,5] The facial nerve is compressed anterosuperiorly in the internal auditory canal but, as the tumor approaches the lateral aspect of the canal and begins to form its lateral dome, it pulls away from the nerve and a clear plane of separation develops.

Preserving the facial nerve laterally in the internal auditory canal is a relatively straightforward procedure and thousands of acoustic tumors have been successfully removed from the lateral portion of the internal auditory canal through the retrosigmoid approach, without direct visualization of the distal facial nerve. The point of maximum risk to the facial nerve is at the anterior margin of the porus acusticus. Here, the nerve, flattened against the bone of the internal auditory canal, makes a right-angle turn away from the surgeon and is flattened against the bone of the posterior fossa as the tumor spills out into the subarachnoid space. It then makes a rather more gradual turn around the anteroinferior surface of the tumor to head toward the brain stem. In the posterior fossa, the nerve may remain relatively robust, as it is not compressed against the hard surface. However, it is maximally compressed between unyielding bone and progressively enlarging tumor at that point where it enters the internal auditory canal.

None of the standard and effective approaches to acoustic neuromas provide the surgeon with direct visualization of the nerve in this location before substantial debulking and dissection of the tumor. With either the translabyrinthine or the retrosigmoid approach, we mobilize the tumor from both ends, progressively debulking and dissecting it and identifying the facial nerve as we close in on this most treacherous location. The visualization and management of the facial nerve in that location is essentially identical, regardless of the choice of approach, and our success in preserving the facial nerve is virtually identical regardless of approach. Intraoperative mapping of the facial nerve has improved its preservation with either approach, although it does not replace experience and anatomic knowledge. Skill with a given approach is probably more important than the specific choice of an approach. Therefore, preservation of the facial nerve is not a factor in choosing between these surgical approaches for our patient.

What About the Brain Stem?

It is clearly possible to remove large acoustic neuromas through the translabyrinthine approach.[3] The tumor is progressively debulked and dissected away from the surrounding structures in the same fashion that it is from the posterior fossa. However, the ability to visualize and control the superior and inferior poles of the tumor before the substantial amount of debulking and capsular dissection is, in my experience, superior with the retrosigmoid approach. The release of cerebrospinal fluid is accomplished early in the procedure and excellent relaxation of the contents of the posterior fossa is, thus, obtained. This promotes the reconstitution of the arachnoid plane between the tumor and brain stem during the operation. The lower cranial nerves are seen and protected early in the procedure and the interface between the brain stem and the tumor can be identified early. Venous and arterial structures can be followed from normal locations to their distorted locations in the region of the tumor more easily and at an earlier stage. Should an untoward hemorrhagic event occur, there is greater access to all of the structures in the posterior fossa to allow hemostasis to be obtained promptly. Therefore, I believe that the safety of the brain stem is a factor arguing in favor of the retrosigmoid over the translabyrinthine approach for tumors that distort the brain stem.

And the Cerebellum?

The translabyrinthine approach clearly results in less cerebellar retraction than the retrosigmoid approach. However, this factor is over-emphasized in the literature. With modern neurosurgical technique, the cerebellum is rarely retracted more than 1 cm from the petrous ridge during resection of even the largest acoustic neuromas. After 30 to 60 minutes of operating, one can actually remove the retractors and function quite satisfactorily, although I usually leave the retractors in place to protect the cerebellar surface. We have not had to resect the lateral cerebellar hemisphere to obtain exposure in our last 150 operations. Significant cerebellar injury is exceedingly uncommon and not a factor in deciding between surgical approaches.

OTHER ISSUES

Some have argued that headache and neck stiffness occur less frequently after the translabyrinthine approach. Although this is true for the first few postoperative days, since including a cranioplasty as part of the retrosigmoid procedure, I have found no long-term difference between the procedures in this regard. We have noticed no difference in the rate of cerebrospinal fluid leaks or other complications between the procedures.

SUMMARY

In this patient, and with the assumptions stated above, I would recommend the retrosigmoid approach to this tumor and an attempt to preserve hearing through the use of intraoperative electrocochleography to monitor hearing function. The attempt to preserve the cochlear nerve and its function might result in additional operating time of up to 1 or 2 hours, a factor that modern neuroanesthetic technique allows us to virtually ignore. This attempted hearing preservation does not add measurable risk to the patient's operation and may protect against future unexpected hearing loss on the opposite side. Although I would not be optimistic about the changes in preserved hearing and would so inform the patient, the continuing quest to improve the surgical treatment of acoustic neuromas, and the quality of life for patients who undergo surgery, demands aggressive efforts to preserve any function present preoperatively.[6,7]

The Translabyrinthine Approach to Acoustic Neuromas in Patients with Intact Hearing

Derald E. Brackmann, M.D.

The best method to remove acoustic neuromas is an ongoing controversy in neurotology and neurosurgery. Over the past 30 years, physicians of the House Ear Clinic have removed over 3000 acoustic neuromas, mostly through the translabyrinthine approach. This paper discusses the approaches currently employed at the House Ear Clinic for the treatment of acoustic neuromas. We still use the translabyrinthine approach for most of our patients. The reasons for this, particularly in those with intact hearing where the greatest controversy lies, are outlined. This discussion assumes a unilateral tumor with normal hearing in the opposite ear.

APPROACHES FOR ACOUSTIC TUMOR REMOVAL

We use 3 approaches to remove acoustic tumors at the House Ear Clinic; each has advantages and disadvantages.

The Middle-Fossa Approach

The major advantage of the middle-fossa approach is complete exposure of the internal auditory canal with preservation of the labyrinth. This exposure insures total tumor removal with the possibility of hearing preservation. This is the only approach that offers this advantage in all patients. Another advantage is identification of the facial nerve as it exits the internal auditory canal to begin its labyrinthine segment. One can dissect the tumor from the facial nerve under direct vision. It is advantageous to decompress the meatal foramen after acoustic tumor removal, which is possible with this approach.[3]

The major disadvantage of the middle-fossa approach is limited exposure of the posterior fossa. It is difficult to remove large tumors from the brain stem and identify the major vessels of the posterior fossa adherent to the tumor. A theoretical disadvantage of this approach is temporal lobe retraction. Even though it has been said that this retraction may lead to seizures and other complications, that has not been our experience. This has not occurred in our entire series of acoustic tumor removals, nor for many other indications in which the middle-fossa approach has been used.

The Retrosigmoid Approach

The advantage of the retrosigmoid approach is the ability to expose and remove larger tumors with the possibility of hearing preservation. One obtains excellent exposure of the posterior fossa, facilitating removal of tumor from the brain stem, as well as preservation of the major blood vessels. Drilling of the posterior lip of the internal auditory canal allows exposure of about half of the length of the internal auditory canal in most patients. If tumors do not extend to the fundus of the internal auditory canal, all tumor can be removed under direct vision.

Disadvantages of the retrosigmoid approach include more cerebellar retraction than in the other approaches. This is particularly so in cases of large tumors. Because of the overlying labyrinth, one is unable to expose the fundus of the internal auditory canal. This necessitates blind dissection of tumors that extend to the fundus. One must also, therefore, blindly dissect the facial nerve at the fundus of the internal auditory canal, and it is impossible to decompress the meatal foramen with this approach. There is a higher risk of cerebrospinal fluid leaks and headaches with this approach.[5] Finally, leaving the cochlear nerve opens the chance of leaving microscopic bits of tumor with the possibility of later recurrence.[4]

The Translabyrinthine Approach

The principle of skull-base surgery is to remove bone to spare brain retraction. The translabyrinthine approach is a prime example of this principle. It is the most direct route to the cerebellopontine angle and requires minimal cerebellar retraction. The origin of the tumor is exposed, allowing extensive intracapsular removal of large tumors without brain retraction. As large tumors collapse with intracapsular removal, the brain pushes the tumor into the surgical field.

The entire internal auditory canal is exposed, ensuring total removal. This is particularly important in tumors that expand into the temporal bone. Positive identification of the facial nerve in a constant anatomic location allows dissection of this nerve both from medial-to-lateral and lateral-to-medial directions to the area of the porus acusticus, where the facial nerve most often adheres to the tumor.

All of the eighth cranial nerve is removed, ensuring removal of all tumor. If the facial nerve cannot be preserved, a translabyrinthine approach facilitates rerouting and direct repair or insertion of a nerve graft.[2] Finally, this approach offers the lowest rates of morbidity and mortality (0.4% for the last 2300 patients and none in the last 750).

The only disadvantage of the translabyrinthine approach is total loss of hearing in the operated ear. It has been said that this approach compromises exposure of the tumor along the brain stem, complicating its removal. This has not been our experience in any size tumor.

HEARING PRESERVATION IN ACOUSTIC TUMOR SURGERY

What is useful hearing? Some would argue that the preservation of any hearing is useful. Another argument for hearing conservation procedures is that only with the routine use of such an approach will one develop the facility to improve the results of hearing conservation in patients with good intact hearing. There is no agreement, however, as to what constitutes useful hearing.

There are 3 major advantages of binaural hearing. The first is that hearing stereophonically allows one to localize the direction of sound. The second and main advantage is the improved ability to discriminate in the presence of background noise. The third advantage is in special situations, such as riding in a car, in which hearing in one good ear may be masked by road noise.

At what point does hearing become useful in these situations? To hear stereophonically, one must have hearing in the range of 50 decibels or better. Simple localization of sounds does not require good speech discrimination. The use of a hearing aid will, of course, improve pure tone thresholds and hearing aid use will improve stereophonic hearing, even with poor speech discrimination. In our experience, however, it is unusual for a patient to wear a hearing aid when speech discrimination is poor and hearing in the other ear is normal because the aided sound quality is inferior.

Discrimination of speech in noise is the most important aspect of binaural hearing. To achieve this advantage, hearing must be in the range of 25 to 35 decibels with good speech discrimina-

tion aided or unaided. Thus, if hearing cannot be aided to this level or if speech discrimination is poor, it is unlikely that the patient will achieve this advantage, even if some hearing is preserved. One must remember that hearing aids will not improve speech discrimination in and of itself. To understand speech in an automobile, one requires hearing within the normal range and normal speech discrimination. The requirements are essentially the same as for discrimination of noise.

Although it is not a substitute for normal hearing, a CROS hearing aid may be of distinct benefit in patients who have a profound loss in one ear with good hearing in the opposite ear. This device may offer more advantage than a hearing aid in an ear with poor hearing and speech discrimination.

SELECTING THE SURGICAL APPROACH

I have used all 3 approaches to remove acoustic tumors, and select the approach based upon the size and location of the tumor and the amount of residual hearing.

The Middle-Fossa Approach

We use the middle-fossa approach in patients with small tumors extending no more than 1 cm into the cerebellopontine angle. In general, we select patients who have hearing of at least 35 to 40 decibels with 70% or greater speech discrimination. An abnormal electronystagmography study (ENG) and good responses on auditory brain stem testing are favorable indicators for hearing preservation.[6]

The Retrosigmoid Approach

Larger tumors with up to a 2-cm extension into the cerebellopontine angle in patients with good hearing are approached through the retrosigmoid avenue. We use the same criteria for good hearing as for the middle fossa approach. Tumors that arise medially and do not expand into the internal auditory canal or reach the fundus are ideal candidates for this approach.

The Translabyrinthine Approach

Patients with tumors that expand into the temporal bone or have greater than a 2-cm extension into the cerebellopontine angle, and all patients with poor hearing are operated on using the translabyrinthine route. It has been said that large tumors cannot be removed in this way, but that is not our experience. The translabyrinthine approach is even more advantageous for large tumors for the reasons outlined above.

Selection of Approach for This Patient

Before discussing why I would select the translabyrinthine approach for this patient, I would like to point out that this is not a typical acoustic neuroma. Although centered on the internal auditory canal, it spreads along the face of the petrous pyramid. It does not, however, have a sessile attachment to the petrous pyramid, nor does it have an enhancing dural tail characteristic of a meningioma. I have seen several patients with metastasis to the cerebellopontine angle and a history for primary tumor should be carefully elicited in this case. Further studies are not indicated, however, for I believe that this tumor would best be approached through the translabyrinthine avenue regardless of its histology.

The reasons for selecting the translabyrinthine approach for this patient are several. First, the size of the tumor makes hearing preservation unlikely. In our experience, tumors with greater than a 2-cm extension into the angle and distortion of the brain stem are likely to intimately involve the cochlear nerve at its origin. The second reason is that there is an irregular expansion of the internal auditory canal. The tumor does not extend to the fundus of the canal, which would make it favorable for retrosigmoid removal. Nevertheless, with irregular expansion of the internal auditory canal, it is likely that the cochlear nerve will be extremely adherent, particularly at the porus. The final reason for selecting the translabyrinthine approach is the hearing level in this patient. Even if hearing could be preserved at the preoperative level, the patient would not have true binaural hearing even with the use of a hearing aid. This degree of preoperative cochlear nerve involvement also speaks poorly for the possibility of preserving hearing. With 50% speech discrimination, one knows that the cochlear nerve is severely affected by the tumor, decreasing the likelihood of any hearing preservation.

SURGICAL TECHNIQUE

The translabyrinthine approach is carried out with the patient under general endotracheal anesthesia without muscle relaxants, so that intraoperative facial nerve monitoring can be used. The patient is positioned supine on the operating table without head fixation.

A postauricular incision is made and the periosteum elevated from the mastoid cortex (Fig. 1). A complete mastoidectomy is then accomplished. It is important to remove bone far posterior to the sigmoid sinus to allow adequate retraction of this sinus. The dura of the middle and posterior fossa is skeletonized. Again, it is important to make as wide an opening as possible to allow easy entrance of instruments into the cerebellopontine angle. A labyrinthectomy is then completed (Fig. 2). The jugular bulb is skeletonized inferiorly and the descending segment of the facial nerve skeletonized anteriorly. Again, it is important to remove all of the bone to these normal structures to allow adequate exposure of the cerebellopontine angle.

Bone is then removed from three quarters of the circumference of the internal auditory canal, including the porus acusticus. The cochlear aqueduct is the anterior/inferior landmark. Limiting the dissection to the plane superior to the cochlear aqueduct avoids injury to the ninth cranial nerve lying in the

medial wall of the jugular foramen anteriorly-inferiorly. The lateral end of the internal auditory canal is dissected last to protect the facial nerve until all of the bone is removed. The facial nerve is decompressed through the meatal foramen.[3]

The dura of the posterior fossa is opened and the dural flaps retracted superiorly and inferiorly. The tumor is then separated from the cerebellum posteriorly, the ninth cranial nerve inferiorly, and from the tentorium, petrosal vein, and fifth nerve superiorly. The facial nerve is positively identified lying anteriorly or superiorly on the capsule of the tumor. Rarely, the facial nerve is displaced posteriorly so that positive identification is necessary before beginning tumor removal. The facial nerve stimulator is a great help in this identification.

For larger tumors, an extensive intracapsular removal is then done (Fig. 3). We prefer to use an Urban Rotary dissector for this, but it may be done with the ultrasonic aspirator or with cup forceps. The tumor is removed until only that portion lying along the facial nerve remains. The facial nerve is identified at the brain stem and also at the fundus of the internal auditory canal. Usually, the tumor dissects from the facial nerve readily in the internal auditory canal. In the area of the porus acusticus, it is often adherent. The tumor is then rolled either anteriorly-inferiorly or posteriorly-superiorly to identify the entire course of the facial nerve lying on the remaining tumor capsule. Then, working both from lateral-to-medial and medial-to-lateral directions, the tumor is removed from the facial nerve (Fig. 4).

The dural flaps are closed with silk sutures, and abdominal fat is then packed into the cavity in strips to obliterate the mastoid defect. The incus is removed and the attitus ad antrum packed with temporalis muscle. A standard mastoid head dressing is applied.

DISCUSSION

We have used the translabyrinthine approach to remove about 2800 acoustic neuromas. The last in-depth review of all parameters was a series of 216 patients operated on in 1980 to 1981.[1] Small tumors with less than a 5-mm extension into the cerebellopontine angle comprised 9% of the series. Medium tumors with 5 to 20 mm extension into the cerebellopontine angle

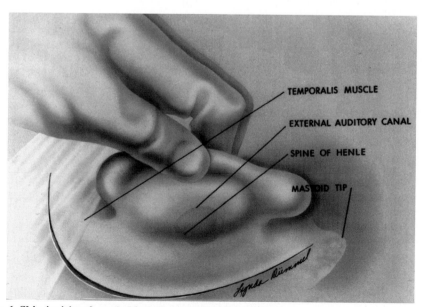

Fig. 1 Skin incision 2 cm behind the postauricular sulcus.

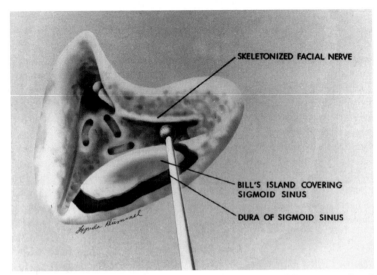

Fig. 2 The labyrinth is progressively removed, and an island of bone over the sigmoid sinus is created.

comprised 51%. Thirty-one percent of tumors had a 2 to 4 cm extension into the cerebellopontine angle, and 9% were giant tumors with a greater than 4-cm extension into the cerebellopontine angle.

The average length of surgery was 3 hours and 12 minutes. One death occurred in this series (0.4%). This patient had a postoperative hemorrhage and, despite early evacuation of the clot, sustained brain stem infarction and died.

Facial nerve function was studied 1 year after surgery. At that time, 83% of patients had grade I or II facial function. Partial paralysis occurred in 16%. In 4 patients, the facial nerve was divided during tumor removal and an immediate facial anastomosis was done in the cerebellopontine angle.[2] All patients had

satisfactory recovery of facial function (grade III or IV). Two patients had total facial paralysis 1 year after surgery and underwent hypoglossal facial anastomosis with satisfactory recovery.

More recently, we have studied the facial nerve function in 1014 patients operated on over a 7-year period (1982 to 1989). The facial nerve was anatomically preserved in 97.6% of these patients.

CONCLUSION

The translabyrinthine approach is the preferred method for removal of all sizes of acoustic tumors, when the patient has nonserviceable hearing, and for larger tumors when the likelihood of hearing preservation is small.

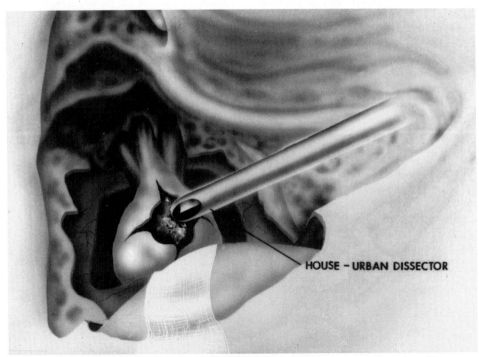

Fig. 3 The bone is completely removed; the tumor is packed away from surrounding structures and the rotating vacuum dissector guts the tumor within its capsule.

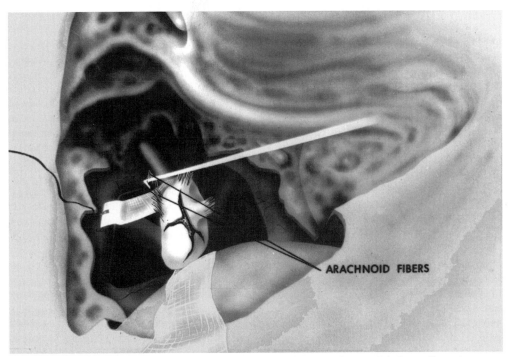

Fig. 4 The tumor capsule is separated from the facial nerve by careful sharp dissection of the arachnoid sheath.

Surgical Approaches to Acoustic Neuromas in Patients with Marginal Intact Hearing: The Retrosigmoid Approach vs. the Translabyrinthine Approach

Kalmon D. Post, M.D.

The authors of both approaches have several points in agreement that must be stressed:

1. A team effort is best for removing acoustic tumors through all 3 approaches, the middle fossa, the translabyrinthine, and the retrosigmoid-posterior fossa.
2. The facial nerve must be preserved in the greatest number of patients possible.
3. The involved structures must be visualized to allow safe and complete removal.
4. A classification must exist to standardize both the size of tumor and the patient's level of hearing; without these, a meaningful discussion of the various approaches and results would be impossible.
5. The tumor size and preoperative hearing level are most important in predicting hearing preservation; patients with tumors larger than 2 cm and poor preoperative hearing are unlikely to have useful hearing preserved.

AREAS OF CONTROVERSY

The authors have some differences in philosophy about many other areas.

The Middle-Fossa Approach

Both authors agree that the middle-fossa approach is ideal for tumors that are intracanalicular and laterally placed in patients with good preoperative hearing. This approach allows complete removal of the tumor and spares the cochlear nerve. A criticism

of the transmeatal approach has been that complete removal of the most lateral portion of the tumor cannot be achieved while attempting hearing preservation. Larger tumors with posterior fossa extensions should not be approached through the middle fossa. The authors have some disagreements about this approach. One believes that tumors arising from the inferior vestibular nerve, rather than the superior vestibular nerve, cannot be as safely removed this way. The other makes no distinction between the nerve of origin. A point is made that the middle fossa is a better approach than the transmeatal if the labyrinth is medially placed; this point is well-taken. The authors also disagree as to the risks of elevating the temporal lobe; one author claims no complications from this, while the other is more concerned. The reader should be cognizant of the potential complications of manipulating the temporal lobe. The middle-fossa approach is also a more technically challenging operation requiring considerable experience.

The Facial Nerve

Both authors agree that the facial nerve is thinnest, most adherent, and at greatest risk at the porus acusticus. It, therefore, needs to be dissected from both medial and lateral directions at this point. Both authors believe their approach allows this. Early claims that facial nerve preservation, both anatomical and functional, are better with the translabyrinthine approach, however, are not borne out in the literature. The use of stimulating dissectors for the facial nerve was raised by one author and is extremely valuable and should be stressed. Facial nerve preservation should not be a factor in choosing between these surgical approaches for any particular patient. The point is made that, if the facial nerve cannot be preserved, then the translabyrinthine approach exposes the facial nerve better for a primary anastomosis. I believe this is true, but find the incidence of facial nerve loss to be so low now that this is not a primary consideration. A standard grading system, most commonly the House-Brackmann, must be used. During the translabyrinthine discussion of technique, a point is made of rolling the residual tumor either anteriorly-inferiorly or posteriorly-superiorly to identify the entire course of the facial nerve on the remaining capsule. Caution should be great with this type of maneuver as the anatomy can be distorted, altering the appearance of the interface between the nerve and the tumor with subsequent injury to the facial nerve.

The Brain Stem

The proponent for the posterior fossa approach makes the point that the tumor can be dissected away from the brain stem and major vessels more safely under direct vision than can be done through the translabyrinthine operation. The lower cranial nerves can also be protected better. Should a complication such as hemorrhage arise, it can best be handled through the posterior fossa under direct vision. The proponent for the translabyrinthine operation states that even large tumors can be adequately debulked internally so that the tumor capsule lying against the brain stem will be delivered into the operative field. Whether this occurs is questionable. One of the major areas of controversy between the advocates of these 2 approaches is whether a large tumor that distorts the brain stem can be as safely removed consistently. As a general rule, neurosurgeons have preferred maximum exposure of the brain stem and vessels.

Cerebellum

Claims are made as to the amount of cerebellar retraction necessary with the posterior fossa approach and its potential complications. The proponent of the posterior approach notes that the supine or lateral positions do not require more than 1 cm of cerebellar retraction, and that injury to or resection of the cerebellum is extremely rare. There is no difference in cerebellar complication rates with either procedure.

Other Complications

The proponent of the translabyrinthine approach claims that the occurrence of cerebrospinal fluid leaks and other causes of morbidity and mortality are lower with this approach. This is contradicted by the other author, who claims that the morbidity and mortality rates are no different, even for headaches, if a cranioplasty is done during closure. Modern medical literature does not show any significant differences.

Other Pathologic Processes

The author advocating the translabyrinthine approach notes that it is not entirely clear that this patient has an acoustic neuroma. He believes, however, that the translabyrinthine approach is best for this patient regardless of the histologic characteristics of the tumor. This is not a generally accepted principle. I find it easier and safer to deal with the blood supply of meningiomas and metastatic tumors through the posterior fossa. The tumors can often be devascularized before resection, making removal safer with less blood loss.

The Cochlear Nerve

The major difference of opinion focuses on hearing preservation and what constitutes useful hearing. The point is very well taken from both authors that a classification of hearing is mandatory, but there are differences as to what is considered useful. The 50/50 rule (SRT <50 decibels and discrimination >50%) is used by one author, while the other prefers hearing in the range of 35 to 40 decibels with 70% or greater speech discrimination. A point is made that preoperative ENG and auditory brain stem testing may yield favorable indicators for hearing preservation. It is important to discuss the preferred outcome with the patient. The tinnitus may be such that he may prefer deafness to annoying hearing. Tinnitus may persist, despite translabyrinthine removal or section of the eighth nerve. Neither author discusses the outcome in regard to tinnitus other than to infer that it will probably remain. The results at my institution do not support that inference.

A point is made that the patient's occupation may be such that even poor hearing with the ability to localize sounds is important. Consideration must also be given to the potential for future hearing loss in the contralateral ear. If the cochlear nerve is left intact with poor function, it may at least keep the door open for new technology to aid hearing. The argument against attempting to preserve hearing is that it is very unlikely to preserve useful hearing, and the most lateral portion of the tumor cannot be directly visualized and, therefore, may not be completely removed. The true rate of recurrence for hearing preservation procedures is not yet known. Additionally, the claim is made that, if the cochlear nerve is left intact, bits of tumor may remain on the surface of the nerve, causing a recurrence. The same argument, however, is not presented for the facial nerve. The question of true intimacy of the vestibular and cochlear branches of the eighth nerve are, thus, raised. The proponent for hearing preservation claims that good planes exist between the vestibular and cochlear branches, and that practicing this dissection in every patient improves the results when hearing preservation is more likely. It may also improve the overall preservation rates for the facial nerve.

RECOMMENDATIONS

I believe acoustic tumor surgery should be carried out as a team involving both neurosurgeons and otolaryngologists. Such a team offers the ability to approach these tumors through all avenues and to select the most appropriate procedure for any particular patient. Surgeons must employ a standardized classification system for both hearing and facial nerve function to evaluate the results in comparison to the experience of others. For patients with intracanalicular tumors and useful hearing—a simple gross test is the ability to use the telephone with the affected ear—either a middle-fossa or a posterior suboccipital transmeatal resection allows for hearing preservation. If the tumor is very lateral in the canal or the jugular bulb is high, the middle-fossa approach has advantages.

For patients with tumors smaller than 2 cm and no useful hearing, the translabyrinthine or the suboccipital approach will do well. For patients with tumors larger than 2 cm, I prefer the suboccipital transmeatal approach, as it offers excellent exposure and control of the brain stem, lower cranial nerves, and major vessels. If useful hearing is present preoperatively (I use the 50/50 rule), then I believe it is worthwhile to attempt to preserve the patient's hearing. The limitation is that some of the tumor may be left in the lateral portion of the canal if the drilling is not carried far enough. Measurements must be made from the computed tomogram to assess the extent of drilling necessary to reach the lateral portion of the tumor without injury to the cochlea.

In my own experience with tumors less than 2 cm in patients with useful preoperative hearing, there is a 59% chance of maintaining this hearing. For patients with tumors of less than 1.5 cm and good hearing preoperatively, the success rate for hearing preservation is 70%. In 56 consecutive patients undergoing hearing preservation procedures with tumors up to 4 cm, 96.4% had facial nerve function of House-Brackmann Grades I or II postoperatively.

Intraoperative monitoring is extremely helpful. Facial nerve monitoring is mandatory to maximize results. The use of auditory evoked potentials or electrocochleography are more debatable. If the information is close to on-line, then it may be helpful. If the averaging time is significantly delayed, they are less helpful.

Half of our patients who had tinnitus preoperatively complained of it postoperatively, and only 14% developed tinnitus as a result of surgery when hearing preservation was attempted. If hearing was preserved, no patient developed tinnitus and 60% complaining of tinnitus preoperatively had it resolve postoperatively. If the pathology of the tumor is questionable, a suboccipital exposure may offer more control of the resection, especially for meningiomas.

REFERENCES

Stephen J. Haines, M.D.

1. Brackmann DE, Green JD: Translabyrinthine approach for acoustic tumor removal. *Otolarnygol Clin North Am* 1992; 25:311–329.
2. Gardner G, Robertson JH: Hearing preservation in unilateral acoustic neuroma surgery. *Ann Otol Rhinol Laryngol* 1988; 97:55–66.
3. Giannotta SL: Translabyrinthine approach for removal of medium and large tumors of the cerebellopontine angle. *Clin Neurosurg* 1992; 38:589–602.
4. Hardy DG, Macfarlene R, Baguley D, et al.: Surgery for acoustic neurinoma: An analysis of 100 translabyrinthine operations. *J Neurosurg* 1989; 71:799–804.
5. Jackler RK, Pitts LH: Acoustic neuroma. *Neurosurg Clin North Am* 1990; 1:199–223.
6. Jannetta PJ, Møller AR, Møller MB: Technique of hearing preservation in small acoustic neuromas. *Ann Surg* 1984; 200:513–523.
7. Samii M, Torker KE, Penkert G: Management of seventh and eighth nerve involvement by cerebellopontine angle tumors. *Clin Neurosurg* 1985; 32:242–272.
8. Walsh L: The surgery of acoustic neuromas. *Proc R Soc Med* 1965; 58:1073–1076.
9. Whittaker CK, Luetje CM: Guest editorial: Vestibular schwannomas. *J Neurosurg* 1992; 76:897–900.

Derald E. Brackmann, M.D.

1. Brackmann DE, Hitselberger WE, Beneche JE, et al.: Acoustic neuromas: Middle fossa and translabyrinthine removal, in Rand RW (ed): *Microneurosurgery*. St Louis, CV Mosby, 1985, pp 311–334.
2. Brackmann DE, Hitselberger WE, Robinson JV: Facial nerve repair in cerebellopontine angle surgery. *Ann Otol Rhinol Laryngol* 1978; 87:772–777.
3. Kartush JM, Graham MD, LaRouere MJ: Meatal decompression following acoustic neuroma resection: Minimizing delayed facial palsy. *Laryngoscope* 1991; 101:674–675.
4. Neely JG: Is it possible to totally resect an acoustic tumor and conserve hearing? *Otolaryngol Head Neck Surg* 1984; 92:162–167.
5. Schessel DA, Nedzelski JM, Rowed D, et al.: Pain after surgery for acoustic neuroma. *Otolaryngol Head Neck Surg* 1992; 107:424–429.
6. Shelton C, Brackmann DE, House WF, et al.: Acoustic tumor surgery: Prosgnostic factors in hearing conservation. *Arch Otolaryngol Head Neck Surg* 1989; 115:1213–1216.

16

Approaches to Acoustic Tumors
in Patients with a Single Hearing Ear:
Surgery vs. Radiosurgery vs. Conservative Treatment

CASE

A 30-year-old woman with neurofibromatosis II underwent resection of a large left acoustic tumor 1 year ago. At that time, she had no functional hearing in the left ear and a loss of 30 decibels with 80% speech discrimination in the right ear. Now, a repeated audiogram reveals a 40-decibel hearing loss with 70% speech discrimination in the right ear.

PARTICIPANTS

The Retrosigmoid Approach to Acoustic Tumors in Patients with a Single Hearing Ear–
   Madjid Samii, M.D.

Stereotactic Radiosurgery for Patients with Bilateral Acoustic Tumors–
   L. Dade Lunsford, M.D., John C. Flickinger, M.D.

Conservative Treatment of Acoustic Tumors in Patients with a Single Hearing Ear–
   Donlin M. Long, M.D.

Moderator–Stephen J. Haines, M.D.

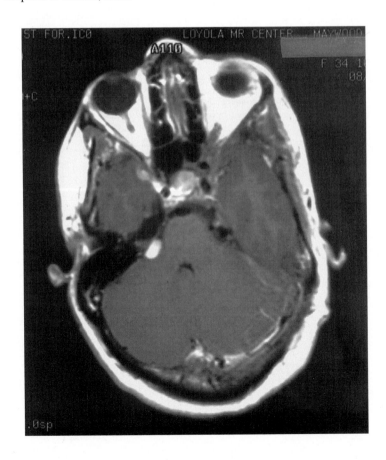

The Retrosigmoid Approach to Acoustic Tumors in Patients with a Single Hearing Ear

Madjid Samii, M.D.

I believe that the only chance to remove this still relatively small tumor and, eventually, to preserve hearing in this patient is through operative treatment with monitoring of acoustic evoked brain stem potentials. As the patient's ability to hear decreases, the chance of preserving the hearing function worsens. I have operated on 80 patients with bilateral acoustic neurinomas.

When the hearing deficit was under 30 decibels and speech discrimination was better than 70% preoperatively, I could preserve the hearing function in 50% of patients. If it is discovered intraoperatively that the cochlear nerve itself is affected by the tumor, the operative treatment is limited to a partial resection, whereby monitoring will help reduce the risk of hearing loss.

Stereotactic Radiosurgery for Patients with Bilateral Acoustic Tumors

L. Dade Lunsford, M.D., John C. Flickinger, M.D.

Patients with neurofibromatosis type 2 have bilateral acoustic tumors (vestibular schwannomas) that provide a continuing challenge to surgeons specializing in their treatment.[1] Although bilateral acoustic tumors cannot be distinguished histologically from unilateral acoustic tumors, they are often associated with a different surgical anatomy. Small unilateral acoustic tumors tend to displace the facial and cochlear nerves, a feature that facilitates tumor resection and facial and hearing preservation. The auditory nerve of patients with neurofibromatosis type 2 frequently either enters the tumor directly or is engulfed by multiple tumor lobules.[2] In addition, acoustic tumors in these patients may invade the cochlea and temporal bone; occasionally, they reach considerable size yet are still associated with preserved hearing. Because symptoms may first be recorded during the patient's teenage years, over the patient's lifetime the risk of cumulative morbidity becomes significant, because of the subsequent development of other multiple central nervous system tumors. Conservative treatment of the tumor in many patients with neurofibromatosis type 2 is appropriate until progressive neurological symptoms force therapeutic intervention.

THE CHALLENGE OF THE PRESENT CASE

Various treatment options can be presented to this 30-year-old woman who underwent resection of a moderately sized acoustic tumor 1 year previously. The status of her hearing before microsurgery was not disclosed; after microsurgery no functional hearing was noted in the left ear. The current bilateral status of her facial nerve function is also not revealed. Over the observation interval of 1 year, the contralateral tumor has not grown significantly, but the possibility of some deterioration in hearing function in the only hearing ear has been raised. This case provides the prototypical treatment quandary presented by these patients:

1. The tumor is located in the only ear with hearing.
2. Hearing preservation for as long as possible is critical to this patient, who still has very useful hearing (which is probably associated with 100% sentence recognition). The change in hearing tests reported are probably within the range or variation noted between 2 separate testing dates and does not necessarily reflect significant deterioration in hearing in the 1-year interval.

3. The unoperated tumor is small, a feature associated with the best results in terms of hearing preservation, regardless of the surgical option selected.
4. The tumor is probably likely to grow over the course of several years if treated conservatively.

In our recently published experience evaluating bilateral acoustic tumors in 17 patients who underwent unilateral stereotactic radiosurgery with the multisource gamma unit,[6] the untreated tumor progressed in 79% of patients who had a median neuroimaging follow-up of only 1.4 years (Fig. 1). The rate of growth of acoustic tumors that were treated conservatively is variable. Although many tumors show relatively slow growth, in a series of conservatively treated patients observed before radiosurgery, virtually all patients showed signs of tumor growth if followed for up to 4 years.[8] A single neuroimaging study is unable to successfully predict the growth rate; some tumors

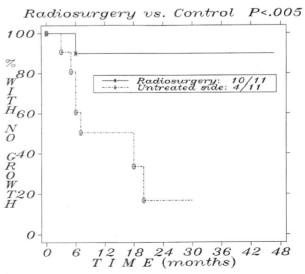

Fig. 1 Comparison of tumor growth rates in patients with bilateral acoustic tumors—tumors undergoing radiosurgery vs. untreated contralateral control tumors; 79% of patients had progressive growth of the untreated tumor within a median follow-up of 1.4 years.

remain dormant for years and then grow rapidly and others grow continuously.

TUMOR CONTROL WITH SUCCESSFUL RADIOSURGERY

Three levels of evidence support the concept that absence of delayed tumor growth represents long-term tumor control. First, in long-term follow-up studies exceeding 20 years, tumor size stabilization has been permanent in 80 to 85% of patients.[9] Second, radiosurgery provides statistically significant tumor control compared with a historical series of untreated acoustic tumor patients.[5] Third, in comparison to contralateral untreated tumors, stereotactic radiosurgery achieves tumor control.[6] Stereotactic radiosurgery achieves tumor control with an incidence of delayed facial and trigeminal neuropathy that compares favorably with the best results reported after microsurgical removal (Fig. 2). In addition, stereotactic radiosurgery is associated with preservation of useful hearing (Gardner-Robertson Class I or II, pure tone average < 50 decibels, speech discrimination ≥ 50%) in a significant number of patients with useful preoperative hearing. Some degree of hearing can be preserved in up to 70% of patients (Fig. 3).

RELATIONSHIP OF RESULTS TO PREOPERATIVE TUMOR SIZE

Our experience suggests that the length of the cranial nerve (as best estimated by the overall pons-petrous tumor diameter) helps to predict the risk of developing delayed neuropathies after acoustic tumor radiosurgery.[4] Preservation of hearing is clearly related to tumor size and probably to tumor anatomy. In our combined experience with unilateral and bilateral tumors, the actuarial rates for preserving pretreatment hearing levels (Gardner-Robertson Class I or II) were 34% ± 6% and, for useful hearing preservation (Gardner-Robertson Class I or II), 35% ± 10%, respectively. Hearing preservation rates were greater in patients who had smaller tumors and those who were treated

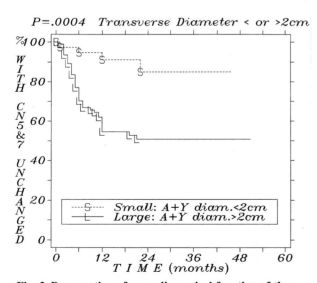

Fig. 2 Preservation of preradiosurgical function of the facial and trigeminal nerves appears to be related to the tumor's size. For patients with a pons-petrous tumor diameter (A+Y) < 2 cm, function of the facial and trigeminal nerves was preserved in more than 85%; facial and trigeminal neuropathies were usually transient.

with multiple stereotactic radiation isocenters, which provided enhanced stereotactic conforming radiation. In our multivariant analysis, a significant increase in hearing loss was seen in patients with neurofibromatosis (p = 0.003).

Current concepts as to what is useful hearing (using the Gardner-Robertson hearing classification) generally reflect the assessment of patients with unilateral acoustic tumors; most such patients have normal hearing in their contralateral ear. Ipsilateral useful hearing for patients with neurofibromatosis type 2 is quite different from what we consider useful hearing in a patient who has poor contralateral hearing or is contralaterally deaf. Preservation of some Class III hearing (speech discrimination score <50%) may be functional for these patients (especially for sentence recognition) if properly augmented with hearing amplification. Even Class IV hearing may be useful to detect localized sound, thereby helping to direct lip reading in patients who are contralaterally deaf. Fifty percent of our patients with neurofibromatosis type 2 had preservation of some hearing, tested by pure tone audiometry after radiosurgery. Hearing loss after radiosurgery was usually gradual, unlike the immediate deafness detected after microsurgery.[6,7] For some of these patients, this gradual hearing loss provided additional time to learn other forms of communication and to adjust emotionally and psychologically to impending deafness.

MODERN MULTIMODALITY TREATMENT

Patients with neurofibromatosis type 2 who have bilateral acoustic tumors (before and after microsurgery) have a significantly higher risk of cumulative morbidity than patients with unilateral tumors, regardless of the therapeutic modality used. These patients should be evaluated and treated at major centers with experienced surgical and radiosurgical teams. Modern treatment goals include a reduction in patient morbidity and provision of all therapeutic options that reflect individual patient needs.

Patients with small to moderate extracanalicular acoustic tumors should consider gamma knife stereotactic radiosurgery as a primary surgical modality. In our experience, the natural history of untreated tumors is not benign (80% actuarial growth rate in 2 years). Because morbidity is greater in patients with larger acoustic tumors, a significant delay in performing radiosurgery is not warranted. Successful stereotactic radiosurgery requires dose-planning technology for narrow-beam (4 to 8 mm) multiple isocenter conforming. Radiosurgery eliminates the need for delayed microsurgical removal (89.5% tumor control rate) in most patients (Fig. 4). Useful hearing preservation is rarely possible after microsurgery (except perhaps in patients with intracanalicular tumors). Hearing preservation remains a worthwhile goal that may be enhanced by early surgery. Our ability to preserve speech discrimination scores greater than 50% in patients with neurofibromatosis type 2 is still unsatisfactory, although some hearing was preserved in one third of our patients.

Even now, the rates of hearing preservation in these patients has been enhanced by a radiosurgery dose reduction or treatment of tumors when they are small (intracanalicular). Staged bilateral radiosurgery can also be considered for those patients with bilateral tumors. Delayed dysfunction of the facial and trigeminal nerves after radiosurgery is usually minimal and improves over time. After radiosurgery, the facial nerve remains anatomically intact. If paresis develops, subsequent recovery is the rule rather than the exception. Only 8% of our patients had residual facial nerve function greater than House Grade III[3] after radiosurgery alone.

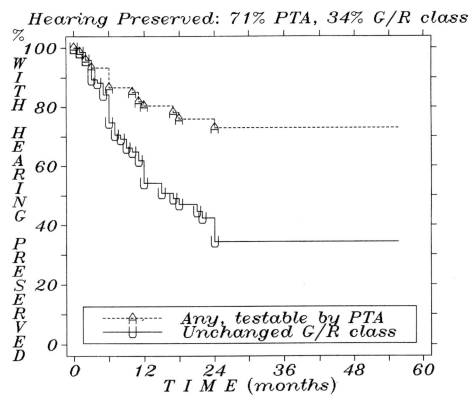

Fig. 3 Preradiosurgical hearing levels were preserved in more than 30% of patients; 70% of patients had some hearing preserved after radiosurgery. PTA, audiogram; G/R, Gardner-Robinson.

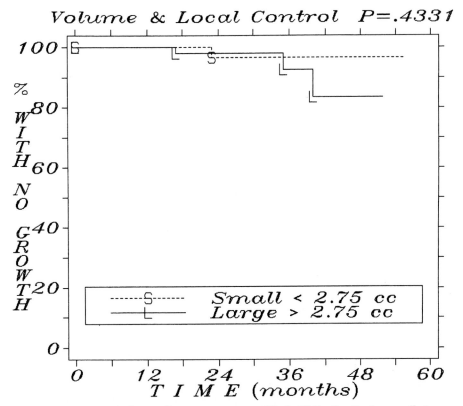

Fig. 4 Tumor control after radiosurgery was possible in 89% of patients overall; tumor size did not significantly affect tumor control rates.

RECOMMENDATIONS

Stereotactic radiosurgery using a multiple isocenter gamma knife technique should have been offered to the patient before resection of the initial contralateral microsurgical tumor. In the 1990s, failure to do so probably constitutes lack of informed consent. The patient should immediately undertake comprehensive training in lip reading or an alternative means of communication while useful hearing is maintained. Stereotactic radiosurgery for the current tumor should be performed without further delay. The unoperated tumor has a high likelihood of growth over the course of 2 more years. Although the risks of radiosurgery are lowest with small tumors and the benefits greater (increased chance of hearing preservation and tumor control), hearing preservation is not the only criterion of success. Regardless of the therapeutic treatment selected (conservative treatment, microsurgery, or radiosurgery), the patient has a relatively high risk of eventual hearing loss and complete deafness over time. Facial nerve function is also a very important goal because a unilateral or bilateral facial palsy often proves to be a physical and psychological disaster for patients with neurofibromatosis type 2.[8] In the 10% likelihood that tumor growth continues despite radiosurgery, delayed microsurgical removal is unlikely to be more difficult for a patient who underwent prior radiosurgery.

CONVENTIONAL FRACTIONATED EXTERNAL BEAM RADIATION THERAPY

In contrast to stereotactic radiosurgery, conventional external beam fractionated radiation has no role in the treatment options for this patient. External beam fractionated radiation has been used in relatively few patients, most of whom have growing tumors despite one or more microsurgical attempts at removal; in this clinical context, fractionated radiation may enhance tumor control rates.[10] Recently, stereotactic fractionated narrow-field irradiation of small acoustic tumors has been suggested as one technique to reduce cranial nerve deficits in patients with acoustic neuromas. Such investigative efforts should be restricted to established centers for stereotactic linear accelerator therapy that evaluate the longitudinal risk benefit over the course of many years. Radiobiologic extrapolations that compare tumor control rates obtained after radiosurgery with estimated control rates after fractionated radiation therapy are tenuous, at best.

SUMMARY

Stereotactic radiosurgery is not associated with any of the other potential risks associated with microsurgery: spinal fluid leaks, meningitis, cerebellar infarction, or death. It should be considered as a primary treatment option for patients with unilateral and bilateral acoustic tumors who are unwilling to undertake the risks of either conservative treatment or microsurgical removal. Stereotactic radiosurgery has been used in more than 1200 patients with acoustic tumors since 1968. Radiosurgery should be offered to patients only at experienced centers whose technology permits the delivery of extremely accurate, single-fraction irradiation that anatomically conforms the dose to the three-dimensional volume of the tumor defined by high-resolution magnetic resonance imaging.

Conservative Treatment of Acoustic Tumors in Patients with a Single Hearing Ear

Donlin M. Long, M.D.

The treatment of the patient with bilateral acoustic neuromas is one of the most perplexing conundrums existent in neurosurgery. To understand various possibilities for treatment and the rationale of my thinking, it is worthwhile to review the preservation of hearing in patients undergoing surgery for acoustic neuroma.

PRESERVING HEARING

I recently reviewed the world's literature comprising more than 10,000 reported cases of the so-called acoustic neuromas. Of the 10,000 cases, hearing preservation was deemed possible in about one quarter and successful in only about 10%. However, this general observation requires a more detailed analysis. Hearing preservation in patients with larger tumors, certainly those above 3 cm, is extremely unusual; only a few such cases have been reported. Lost hearing has been restored so infrequently that, based upon any material available in the literature, it cannot be considered a goal with larger tumors.

On the other hand, the successful preservation of hearing in patients with smaller tumors is now recognized and this success is gradually being reported in the literature. It appears that intracanalicular tumors can be removed with hearing preservation approaching 50%. A few surgeons are reporting success rates in the 80% range. Although these reports are encouraging, this level of hearing preservation has not yet been documented with rigorous studies of preserved high-level hearing threshold and speech discrimination. Certainly, this success does not reflect the general experience and remains the province of a few of the most experienced surgeons.

With extracanalicular tumors greater than 1 cm, but less than 3 cm, the success rate falls dramatically. The current experience available for review suggests that no more than one third of these patients will have satisfactory hearing. The chance of preservation is apparently directly related to the tumor size. Stereotactic radiosurgical techniques have been equally unsuccessful; the tumors are cured less often. Tumors larger than 3 cm cannot be radiated effectively and hearing is preserved in no more than one third.

My review of the current literature, including the results presented at the First International Congress on this subject held in 1992, leads me to believe that, currently, in the hands of the most accomplished surgeons hearing preservation is predictable only with small tumors. If the tumor is within the canal or less than 1 cm in size, the success rate for hearing preservation may be as high as 80%, but is probably closer to 50%. The higher success rate of some surgeons suggests that, with greater experience, the 80% level may be achievable. Preserving hearing in patients with these small tumors is currently the greatest challenge of acoustic neuroma surgery. Preserving hearing in those with larger tumors (from 1 to 2.5 or 3 cm) occurs in no more than

30 to 50%, and is probably lower than either of these figures for tumors at the upper end of this range. Beyond 3 cm, the chance of hearing preservation is extremely small, certainly no greater than 10% at present. Stereotactic radiosurgical techniques are competitive with, but no better than, the suboccipital approach with attempted hearing preservation in patients with medium tumors, and less satisfactory than direct surgery in those with small tumors.

TREATMENT OPTIONS

To discuss treatment, it must be emphasized that the most optimistic surgical reports indicate hearing preservation in no more than 80% of patients with acoustic tumors. This means a 20% failure rate as the best that can be envisioned currently and, with all but the most favorable circumstances, this figure falls precipitously.

The goal of surgery with these tumors is threefold. First, we wish to cure the tumor. Second, we wish to preserve all possible neurological function and, third, we wish to preserve functional hearing for as long as possible. But, other factors must also be considered. Most patients with neurofibromatosis type 2 are prone to develop additional neoplasms: meningiomas, neurofibromas, schwannomas, and intrinsic gliomas. Tumors at the cerebellopontine angle may be multiple and may be on cranial nerves other than the vestibular portion of the acoustic nerve. Neurofibromas on these nerves are rare, but certainly not unknown. Therefore, the surgeon who decides to operate upon one of these tumors cannot automatically assume that the tumor is a simple schwannoma of the vestibular nerves. All of these factors must be considered in planning a therapeutic course.

Treatment Strategy

When the only visible tumors are the bilateral acoustic tumors, I make my decisions based upon the size of the tumors and the state of the patient's hearing. If both threshold and discrimination are normal bilaterally and the tumors are small, the patient can be followed safely. However, rapid loss of hearing is not infrequent; regular evaluations are required. Because the growth potential of the tumors is not known when they are first found, I use the following strategy. Images of the tumors are taken every 3 months during the first year using magnetic resonance with gadolinium enhancement. I obtain a complete hearing evaluation every 3 months, so that the patient is undergoing imaging hearing tests every 6 weeks during that year. If no growth has occurred during the second year, I reduce the imaging studies to 2, but continue hearing examinations every 3 months. If no changes occur, I reduce the imaging examinations to yearly and reduce the hearing tests to every 6 months, but I tell the patient to consciously alternate ears when using the telephone and to notify me if he or she has any difficulty using the telephone with either ear. I have one elderly patient whom I have followed for nearly 20 years who has had no apparent change in tumor size or in hearing function. On the other hand, I have seen patients whose tumors have changed rapidly over 6 to 9 months. Therefore, all patients need to be assessed regularly. The need for reevaluation in the event of any apparent change should be made clear to the patient.

With these patients and with all others with bilateral acoustic tumors, I make the assumption that eventually the worst will happen and deafness will occur. Therefore, as soon as the diagnosis is made, I insist that the patient begin to learn sign language and take advantage of this period of good hearing to do so.

The next scenario is usually the patient with bilateral small tumors but significant hearing loss on one or both sides. In my experience, once hearing loss begins, it is usually progressive and, therefore, I wish to act to preserve hearing. If the hearing is still functional on both sides, I choose the smallest tumor and operate using either the middle fossa or the suboccipital approach, making every attempt to preserve hearing. This includes monitoring throughout surgery. If the hearing is preserved, even at a level that allows the use of a hearing aid, I wait 6 to 12 weeks and operate on the opposite side, again making every effort to preserve hearing. I still insist that the patient begin to learn sign language even before the first procedure. I discuss the use of stereotactic radiosurgery below, but I believe hearing preservation as documented to date is best with the surgical procedure. If hearing is lost at the first procedure, I then procrastinate with the second while the patient becomes proficient in sign language and, then, offer either stereotactic radiosurgery or direct surgery, choosing the latter if the patient's hearing can be salvaged when the educational process is complete.

CASE ANALYSIS

The case in point illustrates a common situation. One tumor is larger and the brain stem is compressed. The other tumor is smaller and represents a threat only to hearing. I would remove the larger tumor in this patient first, and would make every effort to preserve hearing, expecting that it would be lost. I would have the patient begin learning sign language and wait to operate upon the smaller tumor until that educational process is complete. My indications for surgery with the smaller tumor are growth demonstrated on an imaging study or declining hearing function. In this situation, the patient had satisfactory hearing when first seen, with a 30-decibel hearing loss and 80% retained speech discrimination. The patient's hearing has clearly worsened in 1 year. The patient now has a 40 decibel hearing loss and 70% speech discrimination. This is still satisfactory hearing function.

In my experience, once this hearing loss begins, it progresses steadily. When hearing has declined below the level of 50 decibels/50% speech discrimination, it is probably no longer functional. We need to do something to preserve hearing before that time, but we hope for the patient to be proficient in sign language before running the risk of deafness. Hopefully, this patient began the educational process shortly after the previous left-sided tumor was removed. If not, I would begin that process immediately and institute an evaluation program that would include repeated hearing studies in 6 weeks, 3 months, and then at 3-month intervals while sign language is being learned. If rapid deterioration occurs, I would operate upon this patient through the suboccipital route and attempt to preserve hearing. If it does not, I would stage the surgery to proceed as soon as the patient is proficient in sign language. I do not believe that stereotactic radiosurgery is as good as direct surgery for preserving hearing in a patient with a tumor of this size and I would not employ it.

DELAYING SURGERY

An argument can be made for simply procrastinating surgery until functional hearing is lost, in this way guaranteeing the patient the longest possible period of hearing preservation. Those who champion this view are pessimistic about the reported preservation of hearing, and point out that most of the reports do not clearly document hearing preservation at a functional level. The more optimistic will say that hearing can be preserved at least one third of the time in patients with tumors like this, and that some report 50 to 80% rates of hearing salvage. Because the eventual outcome of not treating this tumor will almost certainly be deafness, they argue that even the 30% chance is better than the virtual certainty of deafness and that preserving hearing in the interim is less important than the chance of preserving lifelong hearing.

Another phase of the argument is introduced by the studies currently being undertaken with implanted devices that restore at least some hearing function. A study involving patients with neurofibromatosis type 2 is ongoing. It is too early to state whether any implant will be satisfactory, but it seems probable that adequate devices will be devised at some point in the future.

CHOOSING THE CONSERVATIVE APPROACH

At present I still take a relatively conservative role with these patients. The first goal must be to protect the patient's life and vital neurological function. When these are not at risk, preserving hearing is the most important factor in decision-making. I want to plan treatment so that the patient has been given adequate time to learn sign language and the tumors are treated at a time when preserving functional hearing is still a possibility. This approach means that tumors involving nonfunctional ears can be removed immediately. Hearing should be preserved for as long as possible to allow the patient to become proficient in sign language and begin the rest of the education that a potential life of deafness requires. Suboccipital surgery currently offers the best chance to cure the tumor and preserve hearing, and should be undertaken whenever progressive hearing loss or

growth of the tumor is documented. Otherwise, I prefer to be conservative and watch these tumors for as long as possible to give the patient the greatest period of functional hearing without risk of deafness.

Treating Giant Tumors

One other situation that is extremely difficult and requires attention is that a few of these patients have giant bilateral tumors. In these circumstances, the issue is preservation of life and general function. The surgeon can rarely take a conservative approach in these patients. Most of these giant tumors have already caused deafness. If they have not, I routinely operate on the side in which hearing is least satisfactory and hope that surgery will not be required on the opposite side until the patient learns sign language. No one has presented data indicating that hearing can be preserved in patients with larger tumors and, at present, deafness must be considered the virtually certain consequence of the removal of bilateral large tumors. For that reason, I remove the tumor on the side with the least adequate hearing or the one producing the most significant symptoms, and hope to leave the other until the patient can be prepared for deafness.

CONCLUSION

Preserving hearing is our greatest challenge in patients undergoing acoustic tumor surgery. It is now possible in some patients, which is a considerable step forward. It is to be hoped that continued improvements in surgical technique will make the preservation of hearing in functional ears the rule, rather than the exception.

Approaches to Acoustic Tumors in Patients with a Single Hearing Ear: Surgery vs. Radiosurgery vs. Conservative Treatment

Stephen J. Haines, M.D.

This patient has the misfortune of suffering from a condition for which there is no consensus regarding the most appropriate treatment, but for which each form of treatment offers the tantalizing prospect of success. She has obtained a bewildering array of opinions from internationally recognized experts with great experience in the treatment of her condition and my task is to help her choose among 4 mutually exclusive treatment options.

The choice cannot be made on the basis of data comparing the treatment options, for no such data exist. We will have to rely on the far less accurate method of interpreting the existing experience with the proposed methods of treatment in the light of logic, our own experience, and the patient's preference with regard to the likely outcomes. While this is not a highly satisfactory way of resolving controversy, it is our only option in the absence of good data comparing treatments.

It will help if we separate the 2 primary goals that a patient in this situation has: cure of her tumor and preservation of her hearing. We will also assume that we wish to minimize the morbidity of whatever form of treatment is undertaken.

Our experts have proposed 3 forms of treatment: immediate microsurgical resection with attempted hearing preservation, delay of microsurgical resection until such time as the tumor shows growth on an imaging study or progressive hearing loss is demonstrated, and immediate stereotactic radiosurgery. An im-

plicit fourth option is present: to defer surgery until such time as the tumor has completely destroyed hearing and is beginning to impinge on the brain stem.

THE FIRST GOAL

The first goal is maximal preservation of hearing. There is little doubt that, for short-term preservation of hearing, the most conservative approach has the best outcome. On any given day, the probability that hearing will be preserved at its present level for the next 24 hours is highest if no therapeutic intervention is undertaken. Each of the authors has acknowledged the clinically important risk of hearing loss associated with his or their proposed therapeutic intervention. It is more difficult to assess the lifetime benefit of preserved hearing associated with each course of action. I do not know of a good method for comparing the value of 3 years of slowly progressive hearing loss with 15 years of Gardner-Robertson Class III hearing, and so on. With each of the proposed treatment regimens, the probability of preserving useful hearing appears to be directly related to the size of the tumor, producing an argument in favor of early intervention if the long-term preservation of diminished auditory acuity is of greater value to the patient than short-term preservation of hearing at its present level. Unfortunately, the very long-term prognosis for hearing in patients whose hearing is preserved at some useful level after any of the proposed interventions is not well known. I have seen a patient with progressive hearing loss in the absence of tumor recurrence several years after hearing was preserved through microsurgical excision of the tumor. I agree with all 3 experts that the possibility of intervention with hearing preservation must be presented to the patient, and I think that the estimates of the likelihood of hearing preservation they have provided are consistent with existing data. However, the uncertainties in our knowledge of the future prognosis for hearing, with and without treatment, must also be presented; the patient's own preference must play an important role in the decision-making process, especially when we cannot produce data that clearly answer the question.

THE SECOND GOAL

The second goal is cure of the tumor. Microsurgical excision of vestibular schwannomas, when thought to be complete by the operating surgeon, is associated with a very low rate of tumor recurrence, in the range of 1 to 2%. One worries that attempts to preserve hearing may lead to less aggressive tumor resection, particularly in the lateral end of the internal auditory canal, thereby increasing tumor recurrence rates. It is unclear whether this is true, particularly for smaller tumors. Stereotactic radiosurgery does not claim as its goal a complete removal of the tumor. Control of tumor growth is the goal, and lack of growth over a prolonged period of follow-up is considered to be successful treatment. While radiosurgeons have argued that long-term tumor control is equivalent to cure, I do not think this position is supported on either a logical or factual basis. The tumor is still present and, in most cases, can be imaged throughout follow-up. In my opinion, the existing long-term follow-up data are not of sufficient quality, rigor, or duration to document this assertion. Therefore, with respect to the goal of tumor cure, radiosurgery is best compared to nontreatment. Here it may well have an advantage, as Lunsford's prospective comparison of treated and untreated bilateral tumors suggests. For cure, logic still requires us to turn to microsurgical excision. Here, I think it unlikely that the cure rate is much different between early or delayed microsurgical excision. In theory, excision after hearing

has been allowed to decline to clinically undetectable levels might allow for a more aggressive resection, but I suspect that the slight increase in morbidity associated with removal of the larger tumor would counteract this theoretical slight decrease in tumor recurrence rate. Neurofibromatosis type 2 is one situation in which the concept of tumor control being equivalent to cure may be most applicable. The propensity of these patients to develop other intracranial tumors is sufficiently high that their treatment is, indeed, one of tumor control rather than tumor cure. Even if both acoustic tumors are totally removed and never recur, other intracranial tumors may well supervene; the very long-term follow-up data that we need so desperately for patients with an isolated acoustic neuroma are less relevant in the setting of neurofibromatosis type 2.

THE PATIENT'S CHOICE

But what about this patient? Have I helped her to make a decision? If she is a professional musician at the height of her career, preserving the highest quality of hearing for the next year or 2 may be of extreme importance and override all of the considerations. If she works in a high-noise environment where most communication is done through hand signals, the inevitability of her deafness without treatment and the desire for permanent cure of this particular tumor may push her toward immediate microsurgical excision. Most patients will find themselves between these extremes. To some, avoiding hospitalization and surgery outweighs the long-term uncertainties associated with radiosurgery. To others, Long's deliberate approach to delaying microsurgical excision, without unnecessarily compromising the possibility of an operation to preserve hearing or losing the benefits of actual tumor removal, will have the greatest appeal. Most patients will be best served when an experienced surgeon with access to and a willingness to use each of these treatment options spends enough time with the patient to provide full information about each option and help the patient understand how each will combine with his or her unique circumstances. At the end of that process, both the patient and the surgeon should be comfortable, if not satisfied, with the decision.

REFERENCES

L. Dade Lunsford, M.D., John C. Flickinger, M.D.

1. Baldwin D, King TT, Chevretton E, et al.: Bilateral cerebellopontine angle tumors in neurofibromatosis Type 2. *J Neurosurg* 1991; 74:910–915.
2. Hitselberger WE, Hughes RL: Bilateral acoustic tumors and neurofibromatosis. *Arch Otolaryngol* 1985; 88:146–147.
3. House JW, Brackmann DE: Facial nerve grading system. *Otolaryngol Head Neck Surg* 1985; 93:146–147.
4. Linskey ME, Flickinger JC, Lunsford LD: Cranial nerve length predicts the risk of delayed facial and trigeminal neuropathies after acoustic tumor stereotactic radiosurgery. *Int J Radiat Oncol Biol Phys* 1993; 25:227–233.
5. Linskey ME, Lunsford LD, Flickinger JC: Neuroimaging of acoustic nerve sheath tumors after stereotactic radiosurgery. *AJNR* 1991; 12:1165–1175.
6. Linskey ME, Lunsford LD, Flickinger JC: Tumor control after

stereotactic radiosurgery in neurofibromatosis patients with bilateral acoustic tumors. *Neurosurgery* 1992; 31:829–839.
7. Linskey ME, Lunsford LD, Flickinger JC, et al.: Stereotactic radiosurgery for acoustic tumors. *Neurosurg Clin North Am* 1992; 3: 191–205.
8. Norén G, Greitz D: The natural history of acoustic neurinomas. *Proceedings of the First International Conference on Acoustic Neuroma, Copenhagen, Denmark, August 25–29, 1991*, pp 191–192.
9. Norén G, Greitz D, Hirsch A, et al.: Gamma knife radiosurgery in acoustic neurinomas. *Proceedings of the First International Conference on Acoustic Neuroma, Copenhagen, Denmark, August 25–29, 1991*, pp. 289–292.
10. Walner KE, Shelene GE, Pitts LH, et al.: Efficacy of radiation for incompletely excised acoustic neurilemmomas. *J Neurosurg* 1987; 67:858–863.

17

Treatment of Malignant Diseases of the Paranasal Sinus with Transcranial Extension: Radical vs. Conservative

CASE

A 50-year-old man came to medical attention with progressive loss of vision in his left eye and rhinorrhea. A transethmoid biopsy revealed an adenocarcinoma in the paranasal sinus. An eye exam revealed total blindness in the left eye. A systemic workup revealed no other primary site.

PARTICIPANTS

Radical Treatment of Malignant Diseases of the Paranasal Sinus with Transcranial Extension–Franco DeMonte, M.D., John R. Austin, M.D., Steven E. Benner, M.D., Adam S. Garden, M.D.

Conservative Treatment of Malignant Diseases of the Paranasal Sinus with Transcranial Extension–Oren Sagher, M.D., Gregory K. Meekin, M.D., James F. Reibel, M.D., Steven A. Newman, M.D., John A. Jane, M.D., Ph.D.

Moderator–Jatin P. Shah, M.D.

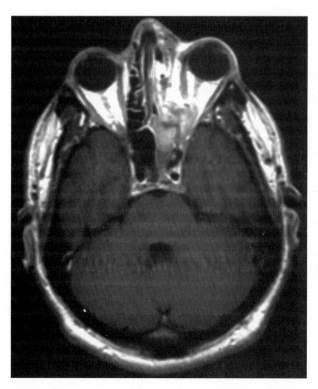 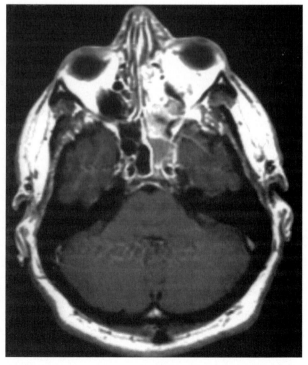

Radical Treatment of Malignant Diseases of the Paranasal Sinus with Transcranial Extension

Franco DeMonte, M.D., John R. Austin, M.D., Steven E. Benner, M.D., Adam S. Garden, M.D.

Neoplasms of the paranasal sinuses are an uncommon occurrence, having an annual incidence in the general population of about 0.3 to 1 in 100,000. They account for 0.2 to 0.8% of all cancers and for 2 to 3% of head and neck cancers.[3,9,19] Most of the tumors in the paranasal sinuses are malignant. The area most commonly involved is the maxillary antrum (55 to 63%); less commonly, the sites are the frontal and sphenoid sinuses (1 to 2%) and the ethmoid sinus (10 to 15%).[14,15] When they involve the frontal, ethmoid or sphenoid sinuses, these lesions generally require combined surgical approaches. In most series, the predominant pathologic process is squamous cell carcinoma.[3,9,14] Other common pathologies include anaplastic or undifferentiated carcinoma, nonkeratinizing (transitional) carcinoma, adenocarcinoma, and sarcoma. Table 1 shows the breakdown of pathologic processes encountered in our patients undergoing anterior craniofacial resection over a 13-year period. The unusually high incidence of olfactory neuroblastoma likely reflects a referral bias.

The treatment philosophy at The University of Texas MD Anderson Cancer Center is aggressive, both surgically and medically. A complete range of surgical, chemotherapeutic, and radiotherapeutic options are available. Each patient is evaluated by an interdisciplinary team from the departments of neurosurgery, head and neck surgery, reconstructive and plastic surgery, diagnostic radiology, radiotherapy, and medical oncology. Every attempt is made to maintain the patient's normal function.

Table 1. Anterior Skull Base Resections, MD Anderson Cancer Center, 1981–1994

Type of lesion	No. of patients
Olfactory neuroblastoma*	16
Adenocarcinoma	14
Squamous cell carcinoma	12
Adenoid cystic carcinoma	6
Melanoma	6
Osteosarcoma	4
Undifferentiated carcinoma	4
Chondrosarcoma	4
Rhabdomyosarcoma	2
Meningioma	2
Schneiderian carcinoma	2
Undifferentiated sarcoma	2
Fibrosarcoma	2
Inverting papilloma	2
Other**	9
TOTAL	87

* Includes esthesioneuroblastoma and neuroendocrine carcinoma.

**Myoepithelial carcinoma, osteoblastoma, small cell carcinoma, renal cell carcinoma, plasmacytoma, mucoepidermoid carcinoma, teratocarcinosarcoma, ossifying fibroma, and mucocele.

The orbit is conserved whenever it is deemed oncologically sound. Bilateral blindness is not considered an acceptable deficit, either surgically or radiotherapeutically.

TREATING THE CONTROVERSIAL PATIENT

In the case of the 50-year-old man with a blind left eye and an adenocarcinoma of the ethmoid sinus that extends to the orbital apex, our head and neck and cranial base teams determined that the most efficacious treatment is surgical excision followed by external beam radiotherapy. If this patient's left eye were functional, then an alternative plan of initial chemotherapy followed by radiation therapy or surgical resection could be considered, with the goal of preserving the organ. Such an approach cannot be considered standard. This strategy is limited by the low response rate of adenocarcinoma to chemotherapy.[20] There are, however, certain circumstances in which a trial of therapy may be warranted, such as in a patient in whom orbital salvage is attempted or in a patient in whom surgery is not deemed an option. Good response rates have been reported.[12]

Chemotherapy agents that can be incorporated into this treatment include adriamycin, cisplatin, and taxol. At our institution, external beam radiotherapy is generally reserved for postoperative treatment or for palliation. Treatment consists of delivering 60 Gy to the tumor bed, with an adjustment as needed to limit the dose to the optic chiasm to 54 Gy. The treatment fields are constructed to spare the lacrimal gland if an orbital exenteration has not been done; this plan avoids exposure keratitis and the subsequent need for enucleation. The cervical lymphatics are not treated in patients with tumors arising from the ethmoid, sphenoid, or frontal sinuses, or in the nasal cavity. Therefore, we would not treat these areas in the patient presented here. The ipsilateral lymphatics are treated in patients with advanced squamous cell carcinoma of the maxillary sinus; a high incidence (38%) of failures in the neck occur when these lesions are left untreated.[6]

The surgical treatment of the patient presented here consists of an *en bloc* removal of the left maxilla and anterior and posterior ethmoid sinuses with the cribriform plate, and a radical orbitectomy to the level of the optic canal and anterior cavernous sinus area. If the hard palate is not involved and the tumor has not penetrated the anterior maxillary sinus wall, the palate can be preserved. The tumor does not appear to extend into the cavernous sinus, but it does abut the most proximal portion of the orbital apex. The proximal osteotomy through the skull base is through the optic canal into the sphenoid sinus just anterior to the sella and pituitary gland (Fig. 1).

In this patient, surgical access to the anterior skull base and paranasal sinuses is through a bicoronal incision and a bifrontal craniotomy with a left supraorbital osteotomy, and a typical Weber-Ferguson incision with an additional circumorbital incision. A subfrontal, extradural approach allows sectioning of the dural sleeves around the olfactory tracts, the extradural removal of the anterior clinoid process, and the opening of the optic canal. The dura propria of the optic canal is then opened, the optic nerve and ophthalmic artery cut, and the basal dura re-

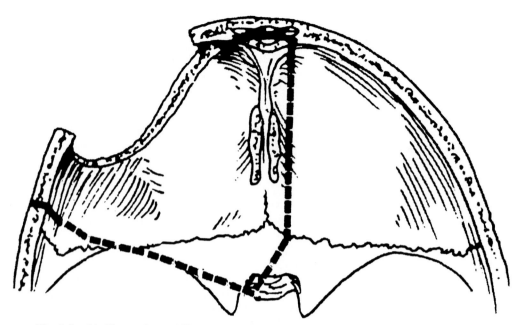

Fig. 1 In this illustration, a bifrontal craniotomy and a left supraorbital osteotomy have been done; the heavy dotted line shows the location of the osteotomies of the skull base. These osteotomies are required for *en bloc* resection of the adenocarcinoma in the patient described in this case.

flected further posteriorly, thus, transposing the anterior cavernous sinus. The dura is primarily repaired. The intracranial osteotomies are made with a high-speed drill and developed with fine osteotomes. The contents of the superior orbital fissure are divided just anterior to the anterior genu of the cavernous internal carotid artery.

Through the transfacial approach, the nasal bone is separated from the frontal process of the maxilla with an osteotome. This cut is continued posteriorly into the orbit to meet the anterior cut through the cribriform plate. Care is exercised to prevent violation of the tumor in this region. The zygomatic arch is sectioned. A Le Fort I osteotomy is cut to transect the anterior maxilla and pterygoid plate, and the medial wall of the maxilla is transected through the inferior meatus. The soft-tissue attachments to the pterygoid plates, the posterior maxilla, and the posterior choana are cut with heavy scissors. This frees up the specimen, thereby allowing *en bloc* removal. Modification of the extent of orbital resection or inclusion of a palatal excision depends upon the extent of disease in these regions. Repair requires a free rectus abdominis flap to obturate the large defect. Postoperative external beam radiotherapy is given as described above to deal with any microscopic disease that remains.

The cavernous carotid artery must be manipulated in this patient. Therefore, preoperative cerebral angiography and temporary balloon occlusion testing of the internal carotid artery with single photon emission computed tomography (SPECT) helps define the vascular anatomy and possibly allows an estimate of vascular reserve and the risk of ischemia if vascular occlusion should occur.

DISCUSSION

Malignant tumors of the paranasal sinuses have a poor prognosis, especially when the dura is involved.[24] Early reports of traditional maxilloethmoidectomy and postoperative external beam radiotherapy noted a 5-year survival rate of only 25 to 35%.[18] The development of combined craniofacial resection has raised the survival rates. The early series of Ketcham and Van Buren[8] reported a 5-year survival rate of 53%, whereas Terz and colleagues[23] reported a 3-year survival rate of 72%. More recent surgical reports have maintained these numbers, with reported 5-year survival rates of 40 to 77%.[2,4,5,13,21,22] Reporting on a series of 48 patients with malignant disease of the paranasal sinuses, Parsons and colleagues[16] found a 5-year survival rate of 52% with radiation alone (with curative intent). If the 22 patients in the series with intracranial extension are considered separately, however, a 5-year survival rate of only 30% is noted.

Of concern to everyone involved in the treatment of patients with these lesions is the complication rate attending the proposed treatments. Certainly, craniofacial resection is not without risk. Various authors report complication rates ranging from 30 to 50% and mortality rates of 0 to 4%.[10,11,13,17,21,24] The surgical complications encountered at our institution are listed in Table 2. About 30% of the patients suffered a complication. The overall mortality rate was 1% and the permanent morbidity rate was 4.7%. In the 20 patients treated most recently (during the past 18 months), no mortality and no permanent morbidity occurred. Complications related to postoperative radiation therapy also occurred,[1,6] and included visual loss, brain necrosis, bone necrosis, trismus, pituitary insufficiency, and hearing loss. With current techniques, treatment planning with computed tomography, and a better understanding of the dose tolerance of the optic pathways, complications can be minimized.[6]

The delivery of external beam radiation therapy with curative intent can be considered an alternative to surgical excision and postoperative radiotherapy. Parsons and colleagues[16] were able to achieve an overall actuarial 5-year survival rate of 52%. The disease-free survival at 10 years for patients with stage III disease (destruction of skull base or pterygoid plates, or intracranial extension) was 22%. In this series, there was a 33% incidence of unilateral blindness (16/48) and an 8% incidence of bilateral

Table 2. Anterior Skull Base Resections, MD Anderson Cancer Center, 1981–1994

Complications	No. of patients
Hematoma	6
Tension pneumocephalus	5
Cerebrospinal fluid leak	3
Superior sagittal sinus thrombosis with bilateral frontal venous infarction	2
Dysrhythmia	2
Transient diplopia	2
Wound infection	1
Transient unilateral blindness	1
Deep venous thrombosis	1
Spinal low-pressure headache	1
Parotitis	1
Pseudomembranous colitis	1
TOTAL	26 (30%)
Operative mortality 1%	
Permanent morbidity 4.7%	

blindness (4/48). Of concern is that none of the 4 patients who were left totally blind had orbital invasion and most, but not all, of the patients with unilateral blindness had orbital invasion. When the data were examined actuarially, these rates increased to 63% for unilateral blindness and 15% for bilateral blindness. Other complications encountered in this series were leakage of cerebrospinal fluid, oral-antral fistula, acute sinusitis that required drainage, and meningitis.[16] Karim and colleagues[7] fared better, with only 7 of their 45 patients losing vision. There were 2 instances of bilateral visual loss, and 5 patients developed unilateral visual loss. These authors achieved a 5-year recurrence-free survival rate of 68% in their group of patients treated with complete, but piecemeal, tumor removal and external beam radiation therapy (mean dose 65 Gy) or external beam radiotherapy with brachytherapy (mean dose 82 Gy).

The complication rates for both craniofacial resection followed by external beam radiotherapy and for radiotherapy alone (at curative doses) underscore the degree of aggressiveness with which the treatment of paranasal sinus malignancy must be pursued. It is only with aggressive therapy that survival rates can be increased from the traditional levels of 30 to 40% to the current rates of 50 to 70% achieved with multimodality treatment.[2,4,5,13,21,22]

Conservative Treatment of Malignant Diseases of the Paranasal Sinus with Transcranial Extension

Oren Sagher, M.D., Gregory K. Meekin, M.D., James F. Reibel, M.D., Steven A. Newman, M.D., John A. Jane, M.D., Ph.D.

The treatment of malignant tumors of the paranasal sinuses poses a unique surgical challenge. Involvement of the anterior skull base and invasion of the adjacent brain are not uncommon, and attempts to resect these tumors are fraught with complications. Consequently, surgical treatment falls short of total gross resection, leaving behind disease that has been variably responsive to chemotherapy or radiotherapy. Overall, response rates to this method of treatment have been poor, relegating the role of surgery to the realm of palliation rather than cure.

The development of craniofacial surgery, in which access to tumors of this region is simultaneously through the intracranial route and the nasal sinuses, has permitted a much more aggressive surgical approach to malignant disease in this region. Described by Smith and colleagues[3] and later by Ketchum and associates,[2] the combined craniofacial approach allows resection of paranasal tumors extending into the cranial cavity. Invasion of the sinuses, orbit, and brain may be dealt with, and an *en bloc* resection can be achieved safely. When used in combination with radiation therapy and chemotherapy, this method of treatment may prolong the patient's survival, and in many cases provide disease-free survival.

A number of malignant tumors of the paranasal sinus region may invade the skull base and brain. These include esthesioneuroblastoma, adenoid cystic carcinoma, sinonasal undifferentiated carcinoma, melanoma, and squamous cell carcinoma. The following is a description of the evaluation and treatment protocol used at the University of Virginia Health Sciences Center for patients with malignant paranasal sinus tumors involving the skull base.

DIAGNOSIS

Malignant tumors involving the paranasal sinuses and skull base are frequently discovered and evaluated through otolaryngological examination. The initial pathologic diagnosis is commonly made through a biopsy. A complete head and neck examination, as well as thorough neurological and ophthalmologic evaluations, are then carried out. Radiological evaluation with magnetic resonance imaging and high-resolution computed tomography is imperative, as these tumors tend to be more extensive than initially suspected.

A staging system developed by Kadish and colleagues[1] is used to classify the degree of involvement in patients with both esthesioneuroblastomas and other types of tumors. Briefly, these tumors are classified as follows:

Stage A, nasal cavity involvement only;
Stage B, nasal cavity and paranasal sinus involvement;
Stage C, involvement outside the nasal cavity (e.g., the orbit, skull base, intracranial cavity, cervical lymph nodes, or distant metastases).

Disease in stage A does not require neurosurgical attention and is, therefore, beyond the scope of this discussion. Patients with stage C disease, on the other hand, require a combined approach and represent the bulk of our experience. Stage B disease, indicating tumor involvement of the paranasal sinuses, is approached in the same manner as stage C disease because there is a high propensity for such tumors to extend into the skull base.

TREATMENT

The best treatment of malignant disease, which calls for *en bloc* resection of all tumor, presents special difficulties in this region. The frequent involvement of the skull base and intracranial contents, where the functional implications of wide resection may be unacceptable, forces the surgeon to compromise in the general principles of cancer surgery. Therefore, the treatment protocol for malignant disease of the paranasal sinuses and skull base calls for an effort to provide cure while minimizing morbidity.

Because it is not possible to resect wide margins around a tumor in the skull base region, we have used a treatment protocol in which surgical removal is preceded by a course of chemotherapy and radiation therapy. Although the choices of chemotherapeutic agents and irradiation dosages are based on the pathologic process and the extension and natural history of the tumor, the general scheme of treatment is the same. Patients initially undergo 2 cycles of chemotherapy. If there is evidence of tumor response, another cycle is administered. Then, all patients undergo external beam radiation treatment. Four to 6 weeks later, the patients undergo a craniofacial resection with *en bloc* removal of all gross tumor. Figure 1 illustrates this scheme, with our treatment protocol for esthesioneuroblastoma as an example.

The rationale for preoperative adjuvant chemotherapy and radiation therapy is twofold. First, it may reduce the tumor bulk, allowing subsequent surgery to be less extensive. Second, preoperative therapy may sterilize the tumor margins; this is particularly important in areas in which wide margins cannot be obtained without prohibitive morbidity. We have, for example, been able to avoid sacrificing the orbit even for patients in whom the tumor involved its medial wall, without compromising the adequacy of resection.

SURGICAL PROCEDURE

Successful treatment of malignant disease in the paranasal sinuses and skull base requires a combined craniofacial approach. To address the different regions invaded by these tumors, the surgical team must include a neurosurgeon, an otolaryngologist—head and neck surgeon, and a neuro-ophthalmologist. The craniofacial resection involves the *en bloc* removal of the cribriform plate in conjunction with both ethmoid complexes and involved structures in the nasal and paranasal sinuses.

Preparation and Positioning

The patient undergoes endotracheal intubation and placement of the appropriate monitoring lines. A throat pack is placed to keep blood from entering the stomach during the procedure. A lumbar cerebrospinal fluid drain is placed at this time, but it is not opened until the craniotomy is carried out. The patient is then placed supine with the head in a vertical, if somewhat extended, position to reduce retraction on the frontal lobes. The abdomen is exposed to facilitate harvesting of abdominal fat.

Neurosurgical Procedure

The approach to tumors in this region consists of a frontal craniotomy, with resection of intracranial tumor and removal of the cribriform plate. The pericranium must be preserved during the opening, as it is used later to close the defect in the floor of the anterior fossa. A pericranial flap is pedicled laterally, and may include the superior portion of the contralateral temporalis muscle (Fig. 2). In addition, an anterior pericranial flap is developed over the supraorbital region.

The neurosurgical approach is modified, based on the size of the paranasal sinus and the pattern of tumor extension. In general, the approach is classified into one of the following groups:

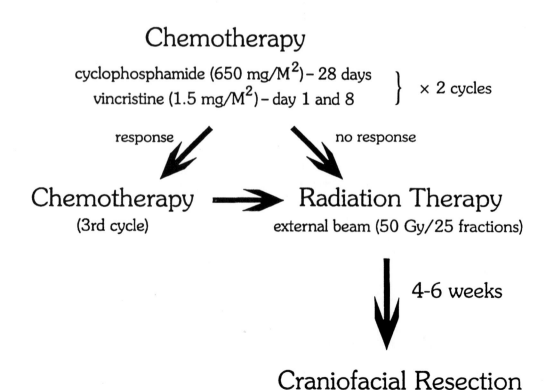

Fig. 1 Schematic representation of the treatment protocol for esthesioneuroblastomas.

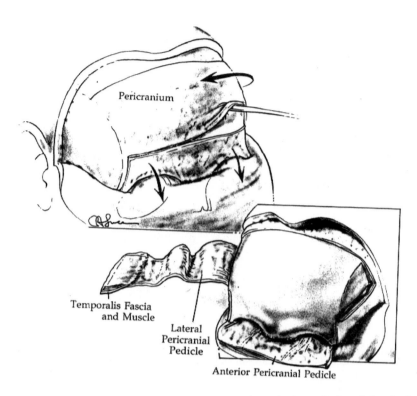

Fig. 2 The creation of pericranial flaps during opening; the laterally based flap includes the superior portion of the contralateral temporalis muscle. This flap is used to close the defect in the anterior skull base at the end of the resection. An anterior-based pericranial flap is also developed; this flap is also used to augment the closure.

I No radiological evidence of intracranial extension.

II Extension of tumor into the intracranial compartment in a patient with a large paranasal sinus.

III Extension of tumor into the intracranial compartment in a patient with a small paranasal sinus.

In patients with group I tumors, the resection may be done through a paranasal sinus exposure. An anteroposterior skull X-ray is used as a template of the paranasal sinus, allowing removal of the anterior wall of the paranasal sinus (Figs. 3, 4). The opened paranasal sinus then serves as a point of entry to the intracranial cavity, which can later be closed without cosmetic defect (Fig. 4). The olfactory tracts are sacrificed and the frontobasal dura oversewn (Figure 5 **A**, **B**). A biopsy is done of any suspicious areas and intraoperative pathologic analysis is carried out. The cribriform plate is then fractured in a controlled fashion with osteotomes (Figure 5**C**).

In patients with group II tumors, a more extensive intracranial resection must be done. With the presence of a large, aerated paranasal sinus, however, it is still possible to do this strictly through a paranasal sinus opening (Fig. 6). The dural opening is frequently extended over the midline and the intracranial portion of the tumor is resected. The cribriform plate is then disconnected, as described above. The lateral osteotomies may extend to the medial orbital walls, and the posterior margin may extend to the planum sphenoidale. We have not found it necessary to exenterate the orbit, but should the tumor obviously extend into the orbital muscle cone, the orbit can be exenterated later.

Group III tumors are approached in the same manner as those in group II, although the paranasal sinus in these patients is too small to allow adequate intracranial exposure. In these patients,

the opening in the paranasal sinus is used as an entry point for an otherwise standard bifrontal craniotomy (Fig. 7). Tumor removal and resection of the cribriform plate proceeds in a similar manner.

Otolaryngological Procedure

A lateral rhinotomy is typically used to expose the tumor in the nasal cavity and paranasal sinuses. An ethmoidectomy, septectomy, and maxillectomy may be done through this incision, as dictated by the extension of the tumor (Fig. 8). The sphenoid sinus is often entered during the procedure, and wide visualization of this region allows removal of any tumor within it (Fig. 9). Once the tumor is freed from all of its attachments, it can be delivered *en bloc* from below. Margins are then inspected, and any suspicious areas are sent for intraoperative analysis by a pathologist. An example of the bony resection possible with this combined approach is illustrated in Figure 10.

Closure

Dural closure is an extremely important aspect of this operation. All involved dura must be removed during the tumor resection. Should a primary closure then be impossible, it is augmented with either cadaveric human dura or tensor fascia lata. The defect in the floor of the anterior fossa is then covered with the lateral pericranial flap created at the beginning of the operation. The pericranial flap is secured with a number of anchoring sutures placed in the periphery of the defect (Fig. 11). This combined closure is augmented with fibrin glue and thrombin. The paranasal region is generously packed with abdominal fat to buttress the skull base closure (Fig. 12). Gauze packs are placed in the nasal cavity at the end of the procedure. The anterior

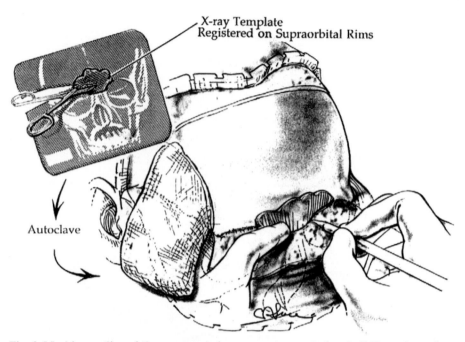

Fig. 3 Marking outline of the paranasal sinus; an anteroposterior skull X-ray is used as a template for the paranasal sinus. The film may be safely autoclaved and placed on the calvarium to obtain an accurate outline of the sinus.

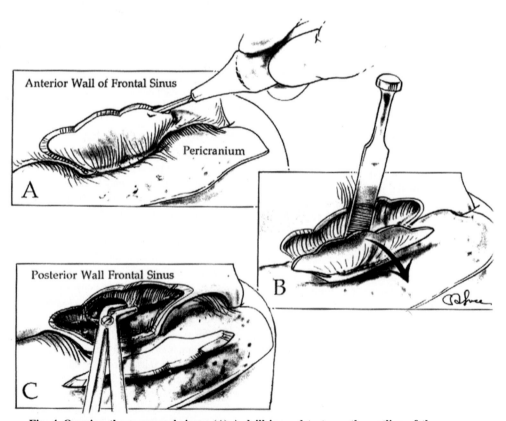

Fig. 4 Opening the paranasal sinus: (*A*) A drill is used to trace the outline of the paranasal sinus to remove the anterior paranasal sinus wall. (*B*) An osteotome may be used to fracture the septa and assist in the opening. (*C*) A burr hole is placed in the posterior wall. The dura is carefully separated from the bone, and the opening in the posterior wall is enlarged with rongeurs. As the inferior portion of the paranasal sinus curves posteriorly, a radical removal of the posterior wall allows excellent visualization of the floor of the anterior fossa.

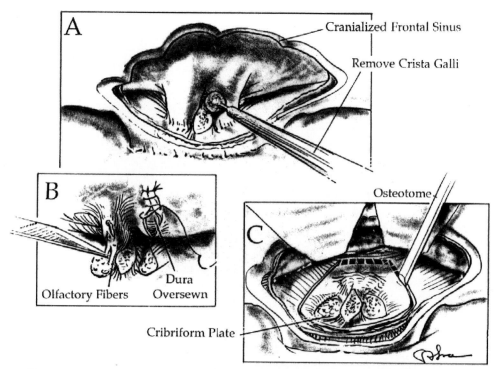

Fig. 5 **Resection of the cribriform plate:** (*A*) **The crista galli is removed.** (*B*) **When no intracranial tumor is visible, the olfactory fibers are sacrificed, and the frontobasal dura is oversewn. Biopsies of the olfactory bulb and dura may be obtained to ascertain the absence of microscopic tumor.** (*C*) **The cribriform plate is fractured with a circumferential osteotomy.**

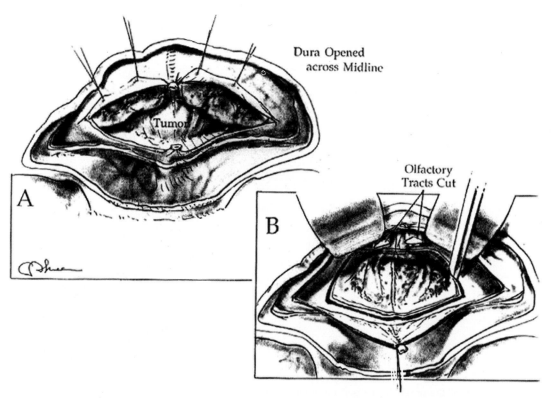

Fig. 6 **Intracranial tumor resection in a large paranasal sinus:** (*A*) **The paranasal sinus is frequently large enough to permit access to tumors extending intracranially.** (*B*) **Removal of the cribriform plate is tailored to the degree of tumor extension.**

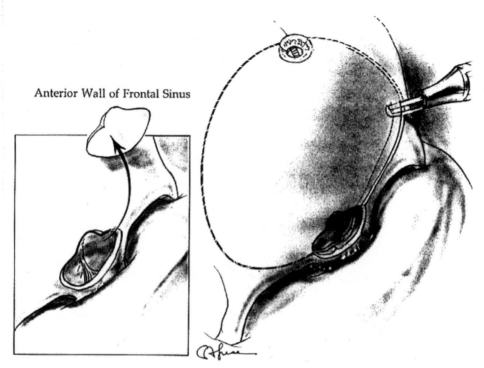

Anterior Wall of Frontal Sinus

Fig. 7 The bifrontal extension of the paranasal sinus opening; in patients in whom the paranasal sinus is too small to permit adequate intracranial exposure, the sinus serves as an entry point for a bifrontal craniotomy.

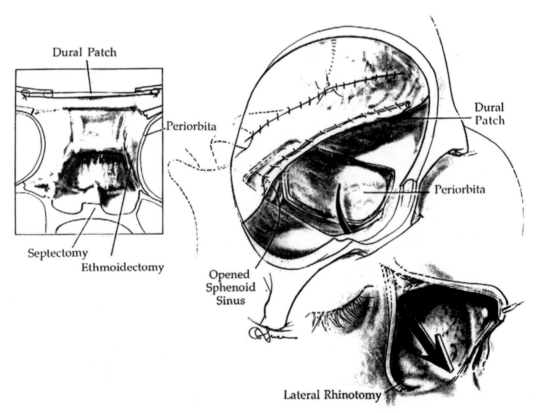

Dural Patch

Periorbita

Septectomy

Ethmoidectomy

Dural Patch

Periorbita

Opened Sphenoid Sinus

Lateral Rhinotomy

Fig. 8 Overview of the combined exposure; after the cribriform plate is resected, the portion of the tumor in the paranasal sinuses is addressed. The entire tumor may be removed through a lateral rhinotomy (note that the sphenoid sinus has been opened in this case). Inset: A coronal view of the cribriform plate region, showing the resected ethmoid sinuses, medial orbital walls, and septum.

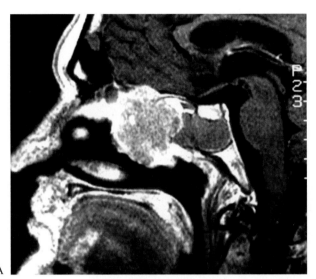
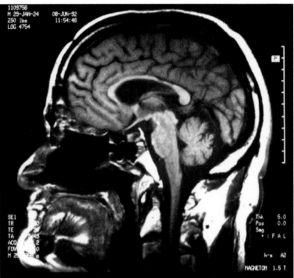

Fig. 9 Removal of tumor from the sphenoid sinus: (*A*) Preoperative gadolinium-enhanced magnetic resonance image of a 67-year-old man with an esthesioneuroblastoma extending into the sphenoid sinus. (*B*) Follow-up gadolinium-enhanced magnetic resonance image done 1 year later, showing no recurrent tumor. The sphenoid sinus can be visualized widely during the procedure, from both above and below.

pericranial flap is placed on the floor of the anterior fossa to enhance the closure of the defect. The bone flap is replaced and secured to the calvarium with sutures through matching drill holes (Fig. 13). Recently, we have used titanium microplates to secure the bone flap, and have been impressed with the rigidity of this fixation method.

Postoperatively, the patient is monitored in an intensive care unit for 24 to 48 hours. The spinal drain is removed on the second or third postoperative day, and nasal packs are removed

between days 7 and 10. Patients are usually discharged on the fourteenth postoperative day.

CONCLUSION

The treatment of tumors involving the facial sinuses and skull base poses a number of difficulties. Even those tumors that involve paranasal sinuses, but do not appear to have intracranial extensions, cannot be cured by resection through the nose alone. A cancer operation that includes resection of the cribriform plate

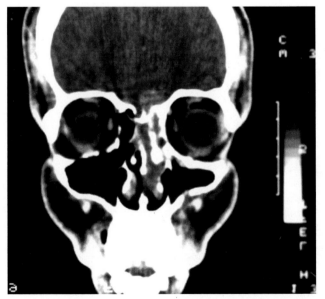
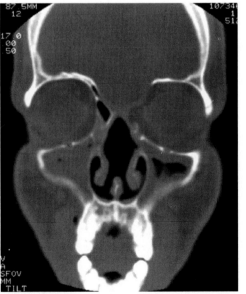

Fig. 10 The extent of bony resection during the craniofacial approach: (*A*) Preoperative coronal computed tomogram of a 36-year-old man with an esthesioneuroblastoma showing an intracranial extension, as well as tumor within the nose and paranasal sinuses. (*B*) Postoperative coronal computed tomogram illustrating the extent of bony removal achieved.

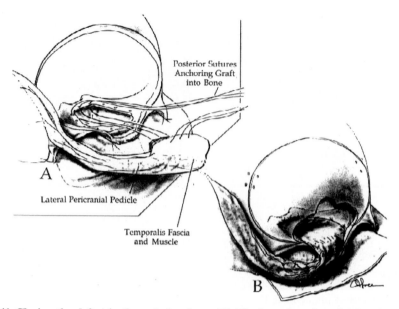

Fig. 11 Closing the defect in the anterior floor: (*A*) **The lateral pericranial flap is anchored to the posterior margin of the defect with sutures through holes in the bone.** (*B*) **The closure is completed with lateral and anterior sutures and augmented with fibrin glue and thrombin.**

must be done to achieve local control of the disease. The treatment regimen of smaller tumors must also include adjuvant chemotherapy and radiotherapy to help decrease tumor bulk and sterilize tumor margins.

Resection of large tumors presents additional difficulties related to their intracranial extension. Often, wide margins cannot be obtained during resection of these tumors without unacceptable morbidity. Therefore, initial treatment with chemotherapy and radiotherapy is imperative in these cases, as it often allows the surgery to be less radical without compromising the on-cologic adequacy of the resection.

The development of the craniofacial resection and advances in surgical techniques have enabled us to treat malignancies once relegated to palliative therapy. The use of adjuvant chemotherapy and radiation therapy has improved the success of such treatment to the point that long disease-free survival and cure can be achieved in many patients. However, only by individualizing the treatment protocol to the particular anatomy and pattern of involvement in each patient can one hope to achieve a good oncologic result while minimizing morbidity.

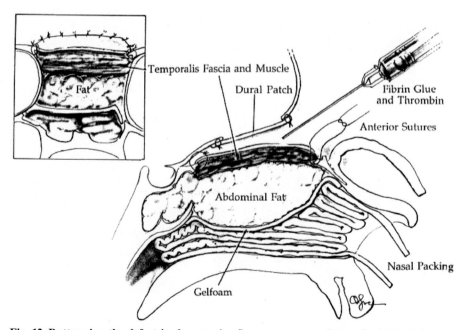

Fig. 12 Buttressing the defect in the anterior floor: a generous fat graft obtained from the abdominal subcutaneous region is placed under the pericranial flap closure. Gelfoam is placed under the fat graft, separating it from the intranasal gauze packing. Inset: A coronal overview of the region.

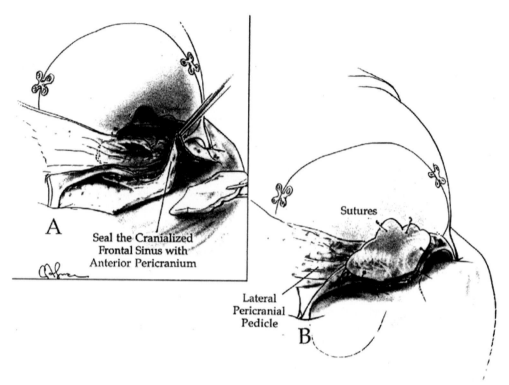

Fig. 13 Replacing the wall of the anterior paranasal sinus wall: (*A*) The anterior pericranial flap is placed under the bone and is laid into the operative site. (*B*) The anterior wall of the paranasal sinus is then secured to the surrounding bone.

Treatment of Malignant Diseases of the Paranasal Sinus with Transcranial Extension: Radical vs. Conservative

Jatin P. Shah, M.D.

The role of craniofacial surgery in the treatment of malignant tumors of the paranasal sinuses extending intracranially, or approaching the cranial base, is well established. Although minor technical variations are reported in the literature, the basic surgical approach is standard. Adequate surgical exposure through a generous craniotomy, appropriate facial exposure to provide a monobloc resection and retain the aesthetic appearance of the patient, a three-dimensional monobloc resection, and satisfactory repair of the dura and soft tissue support at the skull base remain the hallmarks of successful craniofacial surgery for malignant disease. The availability of microvascular free tissue transfer has further enhanced our ability to achieve these goals.

The surgical techniques described by both groups of authors are consistent with the contemporary surgical approaches for skull base lesions. Although the lateral pericranial flap described by Sagher and associates is often satisfactory, consideration should be given to the applicability of a microvascular free tissue transfer to support the skull base defect, particularly when an orbital exenteration is undertaken. In the patient discussed here, clearly the use of a rectus abdominis free flap, as advocated by DeMonte and colleagues, or any other composite microvascular free flap is appropriate. Obliterating the orbital defect provides satisfactory soft-tissue support at the skull base and avoids the need for maintenance and care of the defect left by orbital exenteration. The approach advocated by Sagher and his

colleagues with the use of preoperative chemotherapy is not supported by improved results in their own experience.

THE ROLE OF CHEMOTHERAPY

As rightfully pointed out by DeMonte and his colleagues, the role of chemotherapy in the treatment of malignant diseases of the paranasal sinuses is still investigational. Observations from other sites in the head and neck area indicate that survival is not improved for patients receiving neoadjuvant chemotherapy before local treatment with surgery alone or surgery and radiotherapy. On the other hand, the concept of "organ preservation" can be employed in this clinical setting. The experience with larynx preservation through induction chemotherapy followed by radiotherapy has shown that the organ in question can be preserved in a significant number of patients, without any adverse impact on prognosis, although long term survival remains unchanged with this approach.

This observation regarding the role of chemotherapy for "organ preservation" can be extended to preserving the eye, particularly when a functioning eye forms a margin of a malignant tumor of the paranasal sinuses. Clearly, sacrifice of the eye in that setting is not justified. Whether chemotherapy adds anything to survival after surgery and postoperative radiation therapy remains to be proven. In the patient discussed here, however, this is not an issue because he was already blind at the time of initial presentation. The results of surgery followed by post-operative radiation therapy advocated by DeMonte and his colleagues are comparable to others reported in the literature.

PROGNOSIS

The prognostic factors for patients undergoing craniofacial surgery for malignant tumors of the paranasal sinuses are related to the histologic type and grade of the primary tumor, its extension to and through the dura to involve the brain, and the ability of the surgeon to resect the entire tumor. Admittedly, surgical margins are close in many instances and, therefore, postoperative radiotherapy is warranted in most patients. Complications of surgery and postoperative radiation therapy, particularly as they relate to preserving vision, are important. In their argument, DeMonte and colleagues allude to the high incidence of eye complications in patients treated with radiotherapy alone. Employment of three-dimensional conformal radiotherapy techniques can reduce the incidence of blindness because of the ability of such techniques to spare adjacent normal structures while delivering high-dose radiation to the target volume. Other complications, such as cerebrospinal fluid leakage and local, wound-related problems, can be reduced with the generous application of microvascular free tissue transfer when local and regional tissues are not satisfactory for primary repair.

LOOKING TO THE FUTURE

The concept of reduction in tumor volume with preoperative chemotherapy appears attractive, but has not resulted in improvement in overall survival or locoregional control. I believe that a multi-institutional cooperative trial to further define the role of chemotherapy, particularly with the concept of organ preservation, is warranted at this juncture. Observations from studies that used simultaneous chemotherapy and radiotherapy, particularly in patients with advanced or unresectable disease, are encouraging. Local control is achieved in a large proportion of patients, improving the quality of their lives and altering the patterns of treatment failure. Perhaps the response to chemotherapy reflects the biologic behavior of a more favorable tumor. Further work in assessing the natural history of the tumor should be directed at biologic parameters of tumor assessment to predict its behavior and allow clinicians to select appropriate treatment.

REFERENCES

Franco DeMonte, M.D., John R. Austin, M.D., Steven E. Benner, M.D., Adam S. Garden, M.D.

1. Ang KK, Jiang GL, Frankenthaler RA, et al.: Carcinomas of the nasal cavity. *Radiother Oncol* 1992; 24:163–168.
2. Bridger GP, Mendelsohn MS, Baldwin M, et al.: Paranasal sinus cancer. *Aust NZ J Surg* 1991; 61:290–294.
3. Carrau RL, Myers EN, Johnson JT: Paranasal sinus carcinoma: Diagnosis, treatment, and prognosis. *Oncology* 1992; 6:43–50.
4. Irish JC, Gullane PJ, Gentili F, et al.: Tumors of the skull base: Outcome and survival analysis of 77 cases. *Head Neck* 1994; 16:3–10.
5. Jackson IT, Bailey MH, Marsh WR, et al.: Results and prognosis following surgery for malignant tumors of the skull base. *Head Neck* 1991; 13:89–96.
6. Jiang GL, Ang KK, Peters LJ, et al.: Maxillary sinus carcinomas: Natural history and results of postoperative radiotherapy. *Radiother Oncol* 1991; 21:193–200.
7. Karim AB, Kralendonk JH, Njo KH, et al.: Ethmoid and upper nasal cavity carcinoma: Treatment, results and complications. *Radiother Oncol* 1990; 19:109–120.
8. Ketcham AS, Van Buren JM: Tumors of the paranasal sinuses: A therapeutic challenge. *Am J Surg* 1985; 150:406–413.
9. Kraus D, Roberts JK, Medendorf SV, et al.: Non-squamous cell malignancies of the paranasal sinuses. *Ann Otol Rhinol Laryngol* 1990; 99:5–11.
10. Kraus DH, Shah JP, Arbit E, et al.: Complications of craniofacial resection for tumors involving the anterior skull base. *Head Neck* 1994; 16:307–312.
11. Levine PA, Scher RL, Jane JA, et al.: The craniofacial resection—Eleven year experience at the University of Virginia: Problems and solutions. *Otolaryngol Head Neck Surg* 1989; 101:665–669.
12. LoRusso, Tapazoglou E, Kish JA, et al.: Chemotherapy for paranasal sinus carcinoma. *Cancer* 1988; 62:1–5.
13. Lund VJ, Harrison DF: Craniofacial resection for tumors of the nasal cavity and paranasal sinuses. *Am J Surg* 1988; 156:187–190.
14. Lyons BM, Donald PJ: Radical surgery for nasal cavity and paranasal sinus tumors. *Otolaryngol Clin North Am* 1991; 24:1499–1521.
15. Osguthorpe JD: Sinus neoplasia. *Arch Otolaryngol Head Neck Surg* 1994; 120:19–25.
16. Parsons JT, Mendenhall WM, Mancuso M, et al.: Malignant tumors of the nasal cavity and ethmoid and sphenoid sinuses. *Int J Radiat Oncol Biol Phys* 1988; 14:11–22.
17. Richtsmeier WJ, Briggs RJS, Koch WM, et al.: Complications and early outcome of anterior craniofacial resection. *Arch Otolaryngol Head Neck Surg* 1992; 118:913–917.
18. Robin PE, Powell DJ: Treatment of carcinoma of the nasal cavity and paranasal sinuses. *Clin Otolaryngol* 1981; 6:401–414.
19. Roush GC: Epidemiology of cancer of the nose and paranasal sinuses. *Head Neck* 1979; 2:3–11.
20. Roux FX, Brasnu D, Menard M, et al.: Les abords combines des tumeurs malignes de l'ethmoïde et autres sinus paranasaux. *Ann Oto-Laryng (Paris)* 1991; 108:292–297.
21. Shah JP, Kraus DH, Arbit E, et al.: Craniofacial resection for tumors involving the anterior skull base. *Otolaryngol Head Neck Surg* 1992; 106:387–393.
22. Sisson GA, Toriumi DM, Atiyah RA: Paranasal sinus malignancy: A comprehensive update. *Laryngoscope* 1989; 99:143–150.
23. Terz JJ, Young HF, Lawrence W: Combined craniofacial resection for locally advanced carcinoma of the head and neck. II: Carcinoma of the paranasal sinuses. *Am J Surg* 1980; 140:618–624.
24. VanTuyl R, Gussack GS: Prognostic factors in craniofacial surgery. *Laryngoscope* 1991; 101:240–244.

Oren Sagher, M.D., Gregory K. Meekin, M.D., James F. Reibel, M.D.,
Steven A. Newman, M.D., John A. Jane, M.D., Ph.D.

1. Kadish S, Goodman M, Wang CC: Olfactory neuroblastoma: A clinical analysis of 17 cases. *Cancer* 1976; 37:1571–1576.
2. Ketchum AS, Chretien PB, Van Buren JM, et al.: The ethmoid sinuses: A re-evaluation of surgical resection. *Am J Surg* 1973; 126:469–476.
3. Smith RR, Klopp CT, Williams JM: Surgical treatment of cancer of the paranasal sinus and adjacent areas. *Cancer* 1954; 7:991–994.

18

Surgical Approaches to the Basilar Bifurcation: The Pterional Approach vs. Skull Base Approaches

CASE

A 47-year-old, right-handed woman came to medical attention with a sudden onset of severe headache and a momentary loss of consciousness, after which she awoke with nausea, vomiting, and mild confusion. Computed tomography (CT) showed a subarachnoid hemorrhage with some blood in the interpeduncular cistern. The ventricles were not enlarged. A cerebral angiogram showed an aneurysm at the basilar bifurcation, pointing upward and measuring 13 mm. The neck of the aneurysm was 2 mm below the posterior clinoids.

PARTICIPANTS

The Pterional Approach to an Aneurysm at the Basilar Bifurcation–John L. Fox, M.D.

Skull Base Approaches to the Basilar Bifurcation–T.C. Origitano, M.D., Ph.D.,
   Ossama Al-Mefty, M.D

Moderator–Duke Samson, M.D.

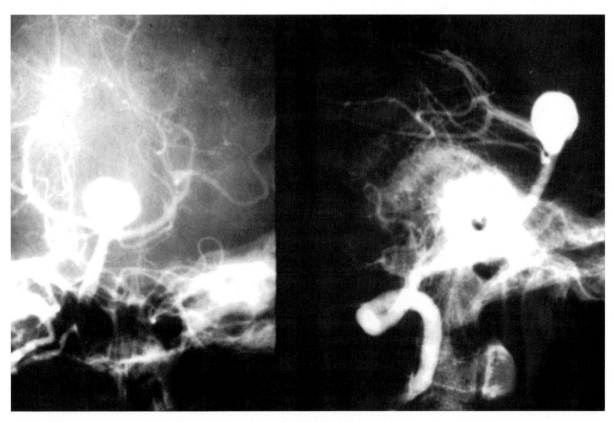

The Pterional Approach to an Aneurysm at the Basilar Bifurcation

John L. Fox, M.D.

Over the past few years, the pterional, or frontolateral, approach to the interpeduncular cistern has gained increasing acceptance.[3–6,9,12]

SURGICAL APPROACH

To visualize any targeted lesion in this cistern between the upper clivus and the midbrain, the surgeon must open a pathway between the sphenoid wing and the base of the sylvian fissure. Failure to drill the sphenoid wing and insufficient opening of the sylvian fissure under good magnification have been common causes of a surgeon's disappointment in using the pterional approach. Figure 1 (**A**) illustrates the relationship of the aneurysm to cerebral structures as seen through a right pterional approach. Figures 1 (**B**) and (**C**) show the opening of the sylvian fissure. Figure 1 (**D**) emphasizes the lysis of the arachnoid and adhesions between the optic nerve and the base of the frontal lobe.

In Figure 2, we see the pathway taken caudally. The wide separation of the right frontal and temporal lobes with visualization of the middle cerebral artery is evident. The exposure is developed between the internal carotid artery and the oculomotor nerve; the posterior communicating artery is followed, Figures 2 (**A**) and (**B**). Occasionally, the exposure is between the optic nerve and the internal carotid artery (rare in my experience). As illustrated in Figures 2 (**C**) and (**D**), the rostral pons, the superior cerebellar artery, the origin of the oculomotor nerve, and the junction of the posterior communicating artery with the P1 and P2 portions of the posterior cerebral artery are evident.

At times, the posterior clinoid process is in the visual field. In such uncommon cases, I use a small high-speed diamond drill to remove this projection. Figure 3 (**A**) reveals the aneurysm at the tip of the basilar artery coming into view between the retracted right internal carotid artery and the oculomotor nerve. Often, the posterior communicating artery must be severed between small malleable clips (avoiding perforators) to gain an adequate view of the aneurysm, Figure 3 (**B**). After the aneurysm is separated from the posterior thalamic perforators, the neck is clipped, Figures 3 (**C**) and (**D**). A large aneurysm, such as that seen in the patient under discussion, often requires a long clip to be placed across the equator of the dome to collapse the aneurysm before clipping the neck. Otherwise, the clip on the neck will slip and occlude the P1 arteries.

DISCUSSION

Samson and colleagues[8] and Wright and Wilson[11] have emphasized the importance of appreciating the relationship of the posterior clinoid process to the neck of the aneurysm on the lateral arteriogram. They concluded that the frontolateral approach is too difficult if the neck of the aneurysm lies below the level of the posterior clinoid process. With wide opening of the sylvian fissure, however, and excellent brain relaxation, I believe it is still usually possible to deal with these low-lying basilar tip aneurysms.

Yasargil and colleagues[12] preferred the frontolateral to the subtemporal route for the following reasons:

- There is less retraction pressure on the temporal lobe.
- The anatomy of the interpeduncular cistern is better seen (both P1 arteries and perforators) with a more frontal view of the aneurysm.
- The oculomotor and trochlear nerves are less disturbed.
- The surgeon can better treat additional aneurysms on the anterior circle of Willis at the same time.

The disadvantages of the frontolateral route may include the following:

- The internal carotid or M1 arteries must often be retracted (this is dangerous if the patient has atherosclerosis or if blood pressure drops very low).
- The posterior communicating or P1 artery must often be ligated and sectioned.
- The posterior clinoid process may be in the way of low-lying aneurysms at the basilar bifurcation.
- Aneurysms high up in the interpeduncular cistern that project backward are more difficult to visualize.
- Perforators between the posterior aspect of the aneurysm and the brain stem may be less easily seen in some cases.
- The working space between the internal carotid artery and the oculomotor nerve is confining, requiring expert microtechnique.

Some surgeons have used a modified approach, that combines the pterional exposure with the subtemporal, usually resulting in posterior retraction of the temporal lobe rather than a true transsylvian exposure.[7,10] The supraorbital-pterional approach of Al-Mefty[1] provides further low, basal exposure to these lesions.

Early in my neurosurgical career, I operated on aneurysms at the basilar bifurcation through the standard subtemporal approach described by Drake.[2] After observing the techniques of Yasargil (who first used the pterional approach for those aneurysms),[12] I changed to using the pterional approach because many patients had multiple aneurysms that could not all be clipped through the subtemporal approach during the same surgery. As I gained experience, I found myself more comfortable with the pterional approach and now rarely use the subtemporal approach to aneurysms in the interpeduncular fossa. In the patient described in this case, I would use the right pterional approach, operating after the patient is in good condition and after the phase of vasospasm has passed.

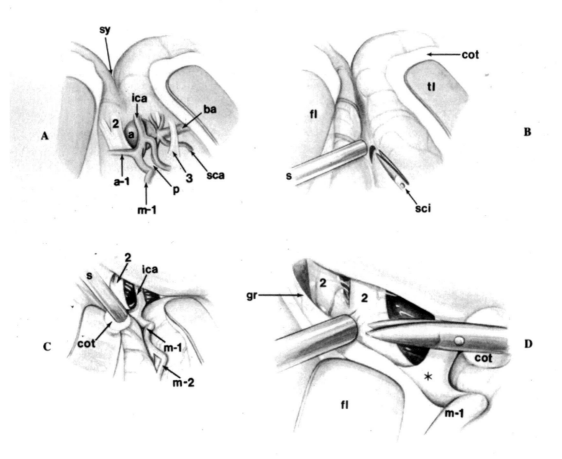

Fig. 1 (*A*) This diagram illustrates the projected relationship of an aneurysm at the basilar bifurcation to (a) arteries and nerves as seen in the right frontotemporal or pterional approach after the sylvian fissure (sy) is opened. Note the right A-1 artery (a-1) crossing the chiasm behind the optic nerve (2); the internal carotid artery (ica) continuing toward the surgeon as the M-1 artery (m-1); the right oculomotor nerve (3) arising from the midbrain and flanked by the posterior cerebral artery rostrally and the superior cerebellar artery (sca) caudally (seen on left side also); the termination of the basilar artery (ba); and the junction (p) of the right posterior communicating, P-1, and P-2 arteries. (*B*) The arachnoid in the sylvian fissure is incised with microscissors (sci). The surgeon holds the suction tube (s) in the left hand. Self-retaining retractors support and separate the frontal lobe (fl) and temporal lobe (tl). cot, cotton ball. (*C*) The sylvian fissure has been opened widely, exposing M-1 (m-1) and M-2 (m-2) and the internal carotid artery (ica), as well as the optic nerve (2). The tip of the suction tube (s) rests on a small dental cotton ball (cot). (*D*) The retractor (fl) is used to elevate the right frontal lobe and its gyrus rectus (gr) off the optic nerves (2) and chiasm. Arachnoid adhesions between the chiasm and frontal lobe are severed. The middle cerebral artery (m-1) and bifurcation of the internal carotid artery (*) are in view. (Reproduced with permission from Fox JL: Microsurgical exposure of vertebrobasilar aneurysms, in Rand RW (ed): *Microneurosurgery*, ed. 3. St Louis, CV Mosby, 1985, pp 589–599.)

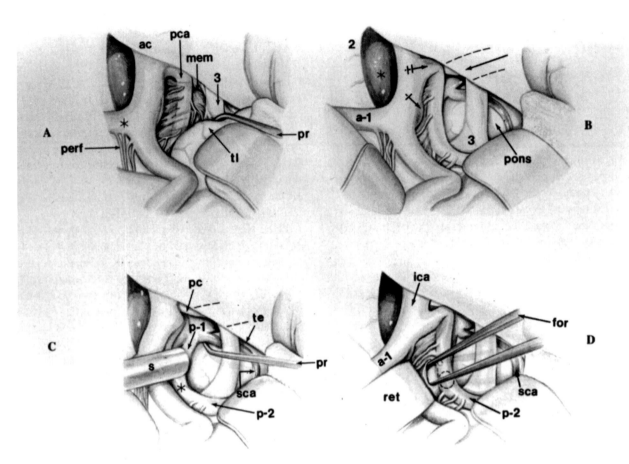

Fig. 2 (*A*) The posterior communicating artery (pca) is followed back, and the uncus of the temporal lobe (tl) is dissected off the oculomotor nerve (3) with a microprobe (pr). In the background is the arachnoid membrane (mem) of Liliequist separating the chiasmatic and interpeduncular cisterns. Note the anterior clinoid process (ac) and the bifurcation of the internal carotid artery (*) and its perforators (perf). (*B*) The same view after the membrane of Liliequist and arachnoid adhesions have been cleared away. The origin of the right oculomotor nerve (3) is seen. The optic nerve (2), A-1 artery (a-1), origin of the posterior communicating artery (double-crossed arrow), origin of the anterior choroidal artery (single-crossed arrow), rostral border of the pons, and tip of the basilar artery (uncrossed arrow shows its direction) are seen. The pituitary stalk and dome of this rostrally projecting aneurysm are hidden behind the arachnoid (*) between the optic nerve and the carotid artery. (*C*) The suction tube (s) is used to retract the internal carotid and posterior communicating arteries, exposing the right P-1 artery (p-1), the right P-2 artery (p-2), and their junction (*) with the posterior communicating artery. The posterior clinoid process (pc) hides part of the tip of the basilar artery in this view. A probe (pr) is used to lift the origin of the superior cerebellar artery (sca). Note the edge of the superior cerebellar artery (sca) and the edge of the tentorium (te). (*D*) The bipolar forceps (for) is used to dissect arachnoid off the posterior communicating artery and its anterior thalamoperforators. Care must be taken not to perforate the adjacent dome of the aneurysm with the tips of the forceps. A narrow, self-retaining retractor (ret) is used to draw back the M-1 artery and the internal carotid bifurcation. Also seen are the internal carotid artery (ica) and the A-1 artery (a-1). The P-2 artery (p-2) and the superior cerebellar artery (sca) flank the oculomotor nerve. (Reproduced with permission from Fox JL: Microsurgical exposure of vertebrobasilar aneurysms, in Rand RW (ed): *Microneurosurgery*, ed. 3. St Louis, CV Mosby, 1985, pp 589–599.)

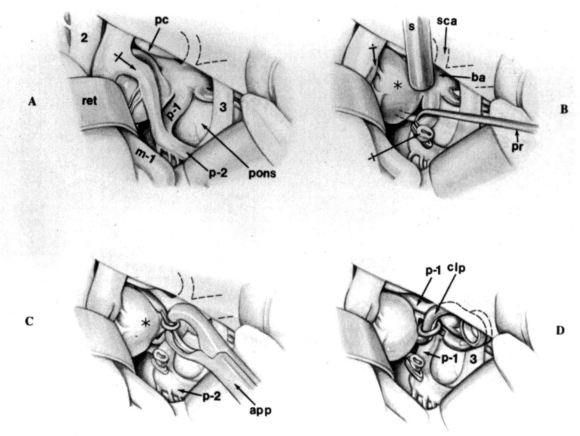

Fig. 3 (*A*) A narrow retractor (ret) is used to displace the internal carotid bifurcation and M-1 (m-1). The crossed arrow points to the posterior communicating artery lying lateral to the dome of the aneurysm. The optic (2) and oculomotor (3) nerves are seen. The posterior clinoid process (pc) hides part of the left P-1 artery. The right P-1 (p-1) and P-2 (p-2) arteries and the rostral pons are seen. (*B*) The posterior communicating artery (single-crossed arrows) has been clipped with small, malleable, tantalum clips and severed to better expose the aneurysm (*). The suction tube (s) hides the junction of the left P-1 and the aneurysm. The tip of the basilar artery (ba) is seen. The left superior cerebellar artery (sca) is hidden. A probe (pr) is used to retract the right P-1 artery to expose the posterior thalamoperforators. (*C*) A Yasargil clip straddles the neck of the aneurysm (*) before closure. The clip is in its applicator (app). The right P-2 artery (p-2) is seen. (*D*) The clip (clp) has been closed. Both P-1 arteries (p-1) and their perforators are preserved. The shank of the clip touches the oculomotor nerve (3). (Reproduced with permission from Fox JL: Microsurgical exposure of vertebrobasilar aneurysms, in Rand RW (ed): *Microneurosurgery*, ed. 3. St Louis, CV Mosby, 1985, pp 589–599.)

Skull Base Approaches to the Basilar Bifurcation

T.C. Origitano, M.D., Ph.D., Ossama Al-Mefty, M.D.

Aneurysms of the basilar bifurcation remain a formidable surgical challenge, and the subtemporal[3] and pterional approaches[5,9,11,13,14] have been established as the classic surgical treatment for these lesions. We, however, have adopted the cranio-orbital zygomatic approach for vascular lesions of the upper basilar trunk. The advantage of this approach is in the geometry of the corridor, which is described below.

THE CRANIO-ORBITAL ZYGOMATIC APPROACH

For the cranio-orbital zygomatic approach, the patient's neck is slightly extended, and the head is placed in a three-point head rest and rotated 45 degrees away from the side of the lesion. A spinal drain is placed. The scalp is incised beginning from in front of the tragus and continuing behind the hairline to the contralateral temporal line. Care is taken not to injure the underlying pericranium. The pericranial flap, a large rectangular vascularized flap, is lifted, preserving the supraorbital arterial vascular supply. If the neurovascular bundle appears in a distinct foramen, a small notch of bone is removed to allow the bundle to move with the flap. The temporalis fascia is split to preserve the frontal branch of the facial nerve, and the temporal muscle is cut to the zygomatic squamous junction. The muscle is then elevated, exposing the pterion and allowing access to the zygoma.

The zygoma is cut obliquely with a saw at its attachment to the zygomatic bone and at its base on the temporal bone. With this maneuver, the temporal muscle is moved completely out of the temporal fossa. Holes are then placed at the base of the zygoma and in the frontal bone (the keyhole). The notch produced by moving the complex of the supraorbital nerve and artery is carried through the back wall to the frontal sinus. The sinus is then exenterated and packed with Gelfoam® soaked in antibiotics. The orbital roof is notched and the keyhole is connected with the lateral orbit through the zygomatic process of the frontal bone. To make these cuts safely, the periorbitum is gently dissected free and protected with a malleable brain spatula. The burr holes are connected with a craniotome, producing a free bone flap that includes the supraorbital rim, the pterion, and a portion of the orbital roof. The bone over the temporal tip is rongeured away. This exposure can be carried out in less than 1 hour.

The dura is opened in a curvilinear fashion from the frontal lobe across the sylvian fissure to the temporal tip. A second T-shaped incision is made over the sylvian fissure. Extradural removal of the orbital bone to the base of the clinoid process opens the proximal carotid cistern when the dura is opened. The arachnoid is then opened to expose the optic nerve and carotid artery, and the veins at the tip of the temporal lobe are divided with the bipolar. These two maneuvers permit the temporal lobe to fall away from the frontal lobe and out of the middle cranial fossa, yielding an unobstructed view of the tentorial edge from the anterior clinoid to the petrous tip. The arachnoid is opened over the third nerve and the entire course of the posterior communicating artery, from its origin on the carotid to its junction with the posterior cerebral artery, is seen from the side. From this angle, the posterior communicating artery can be gently retracted, rather than sectioned, if greater working room is necessary.[4]

The third nerve is followed back to the brain stem and the origins of the posterior cerebral and superior cerebellar arteries are seen. The basilar trunk below the superior cerebellar artery can be reached for placement of a temporary clip. For further exposure, the tentorium behind the third nerve can be split and the third nerve mobilized from its insertion in the cavernous sinus. With the temporal lobe out of the anterior portion of the middle cranial fossa and the temporal muscle retracted downward, the surgeon's fingers are brought into the middle cranial fossa, shortening and widening the working distance (Fig. 1). This, in combination with a lateral approach below the carotid, facilitates drilling of the posterior clinoid when low-lying basilar aneurysms are encountered.[1,12] The surgeon may then view the aneurysm from multiple angles, which incorporate and exceed those offered by the pterional and subtemporal approaches

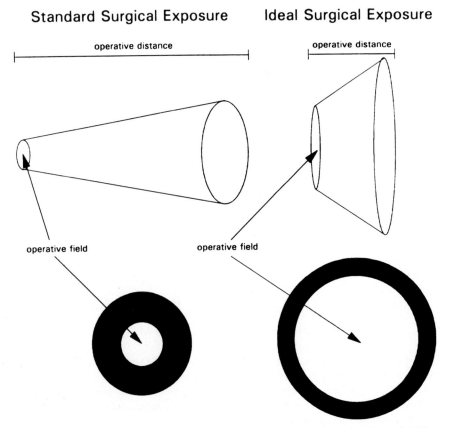

Standard Surgical Exposure   **Ideal Surgical Exposure**

operative distance

operative distance

operative field

operative field

Fig. 1 The overall differences between skull base and traditional approaches; skull base approaches shorten and widen the operating field.

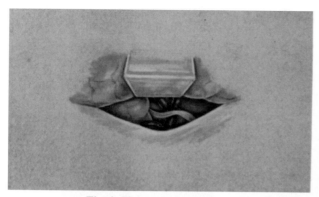

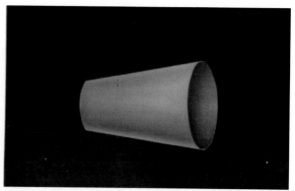

Fig. 2 The geometry of the subtemporal approach to the basilar apex; the corridor, a long narrow cylinder, is opened by increasingly retracting the temporal lobe.

either alone or in combination. The multiple viewing and working angles can accommodate a variety of aneurysms and variations in the parent vessel. The basal nature of this approach with emphasis on removal of bone obviates the necessity to resect the brain for additional exposure.[7]

OTHER APPROACHES

The subtemporal approach is made through a narrow elliptical cone (Fig. 2). In this approach, viewing the contralateral cerebral artery is difficult and the working space at the neck of the aneurysm is limited. The pterional approach is made through a long narrowing pyramid (Fig. 3). The working space at the level of the aneurysmal neck is limited, and may require retraction of the carotid or middle cerebral artery to improve exposure. In contrast, the cranio-orbital zygomatic approach has a wide opening, a shortened operative distance, and a large base (Fig. 4). This approach allows early proximal and distal control of vessels and multiple viewing and dissection angles, affording visualization of both ipsilateral and contralateral P1 perforators. Brain retraction is minimized, and the parent vessels do not need to be retracted for additional working space.

DISCUSSION

Many other authors have described similar approaches to lesions in the area of the upper basilar trunk.[2,6,8,10] In our experience, the major complication of the cranio-orbital zygomatic approach is transient third-nerve palsy stemming from manipulation of this nerve during dissection. Closure time is about 1 hour, and cosmetic results are good.

In this particular patient, the many advantages of the cranio-orbital zygomatic approach can be employed to their fullest. The aneurysm is large; its neck lies below the posterior clinoid. The basal approach facilitates drilling of the clinoid, and the drill does not pass between the carotid artery and the third nerve. Rather, drilling is carried out anterolaterally without an extended drill attachment. A temporary clip can be applied above the superior cerebellar arteries, if necessary, to decompress without obstructing the view. Both the anterior and posterior aspects of the basilar aneurysm are visualized, and a clip can be applied through a lateral or anterolateral vector.

The pterional and subtemporal approaches are widely used and time-proven—as are their limitations. The cranio-orbital zygomatic approach addresses these limitations and facilitates overall surgical treatment of aneurysms at the basilar bifurcation.

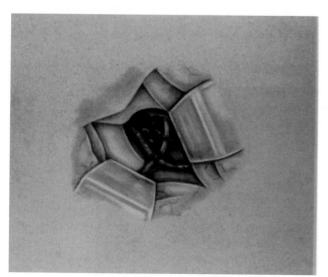

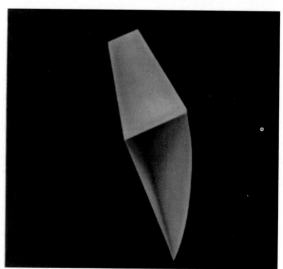

Fig. 3 Geometry of the pterional approach to the basilar apex; the corridor, a long, rapidly narrowing pyramid with limited distal space, is opened by retracting the carotid or middle cerebral artery.

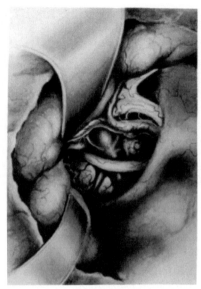 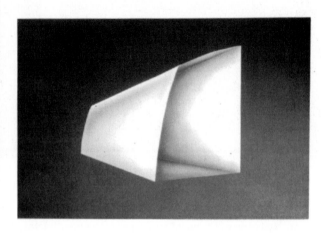

Fig. 4 Geometry of the cranio-orbital zygomatic approach; the corridor is basal and wide, both distally and proximally.

Surgical Approaches to the Basilar Bifurcation: The Pterional Approach vs. Skull Base Approaches

Duke Samson, M.D.

The surgical treatment of distal basilar aneurysms is most successful when the surgeon, operating from a generally accepted set of cerebrovascular surgical principles, applies these general tenets to the specific aneurysm in question and, from that application, develops an operative approach adequately tailored to respond to the unique surgical challenges posed by any distal basilar aneurysm.

ESTABLISHING CRITERIA

For the sake of the discussion surrounding this patient, let's designate the following cerebrovascular principles as being of significant importance in the treatment of aneurysms at the basilar bifurcation:

- Minimal brain retraction.
- Excellent visualization of all afferent and efferent arterial vasculature.
- Maintenance of multiple options for aneurysmal dissection and clip orientation.
- Preservation of an unimpeded view of the aneurysm and perforating vessels during clip placement.

Admittedly, a different list of operative principles might be selected as being of prime importance. I believe most surgeons and, certainly, the authors writing here, however, would concur that not only are these factors a major concern, but also that their recognition and achievement determine in a significant fashion the technical success of an operative procedure directed at distal basilar aneurysms. Let's then examine the rationale each of our authors uses to assure the maintenance of these principles as applied to this patient's case.

Minimize Retraction of Brain Tissue

Preliminary reduction of brain volume through the use of spinal or ventricular drainage and osmotic diuretics is standard therapy in treating patients with basilar aneurysms and would, presumably, be used in any approach. The authors here have adopted exposures based on varying degrees of removal of components of the skull base, and seek to avoid the deep and often injurious elevation of the temporal lobe (especially dangerous in the patient with acute subarachnoid hemorrhage), which forms the basis of the subtemporal exposure. Wide opening of the sylvian fissure after radical removal of the bony sphenoid ridge is a critical feature of all variations of the transsylvian approach, and will suffice without additional bone or brain resection to expose most distal basilar aneurysms, including the one in this patient.

This aneurysm is located at an optimal height in relationship to the dorsum sellae for exposure through the classic transsylvian exposure. This avenue does not require the extremes of brain retraction necessary to see aneurysms at great altitudes above the posterior clinoid processes; it is in the surgery of these latter lesions that removal of the orbital portion of the frontal bone and transection of the zygoma are of benefit. Similarly, aneurysms that arise from a low basilar bifurcation (>10 mm below the posterior clinoid process) are seen only with great difficulty through the routine transsylvian approach; removal of the zygoma and alteration of the exposure to a more anterior subtemporal orientation provides optimal visualization of these aneurysms. Furthermore, when used for low-lying aneurysms, this combined exposure minimizes the retraction of brain tissue by employing a posterior, rather than a superior, retraction of the temporal lobe.

Good Visualization of Afferent and Efferent Vasculature

One of the significant advantages of the transsylvian or pterional exposure of aneurysms at the distal basilar segment is the operator's ability to easily identify and completely visualize the major arterial components of the basilar termination, to include the basilar trunk itself, both superior cerebellar arteries and, perhaps most importantly, the P1 segments of both posterior cerebral arteries. This exposure permits early and definitive access to proximal arterial control and provides an unparalleled view of not only the P1 segments, but also of the important perforating arteries that originate from these segments lateral to the neck of the aneurysm. The trade-off for this excellent exposure of the anterior and anterolateral aspect of the basilar apex is the surgeon's inability to see the posterior portion of the neck of the aneurysm and the critical perforating branches. These, having originated from the dorsal surface of the distal basilar trunk, now course superiorly and are inevitably bound by arachnoidal adhesions to the hidden portion of the aneurysm's neck and fundus. Placing the clip before these small arteries are identified and liberated from the aneurysm's neck causes severe neurological morbidity, or even mortality, secondary to mesencephalic and diencephalic infarction. The safest and most efficacious method to effect this exposure involves anterior mobilization of the aneurysmal sac and gentle separation of the perforating arteries posteriorly, a maneuver best performed with the fullness of the aneurysm reduced with a temporary clip on the distal basilar artery. Both of the approaches described above suffice in achieving this end, and neither is to be preferred over the other for this specific reason.

Maintaining Options for Dissection and Clip Placement

Routinely, small anteriorly and anteriorly-superiorly projecting aneurysms at the basilar bifurcation can be dissected and clip-ligated through the corridor provided by a wide opening of the cistern of the posterior communicating artery, the route of exposure used in the classic transsylvian or pterional approach. Larger aneurysms, those with calcified or thrombosed components, and those with more complicated projections almost always require more extensive dissection and frequently necessitate the use of 2 clips for complete closure. Additionally, the routine pterional approach does not often allow optimal orientation for placement of one or both clips. It is in dealing with these more complex situations, which are not always predictable on the basis of preoperative X-rays, that the diversity of options for dissection and clip placement provided by the more extensive (combined) approaches is of greatest value. For example, a large fenestrated clip may be introduced into the interpeduncular cistern through the low anterior temporal approach, placing the right P1 origin within the fenestration and allowing observation of the contralateral P1 origin and aneurysmal neck through either a retrocarotid or opticocarotid triangle exposure. This combination of exposures provides maximum certainty that the clip will be well-placed, obliterating the aneurysm and preserving all arterial components. The increased visibility and subsequent multiple therapeutic options provided by aggressive and focused bone removal, wide opening of the sylvian fissure, and appropriate gentle retraction of both frontal and temporal lobes are persuasive arguments favoring the carefully chosen combined approach to most large aneurysms, such as the one in the patient presented here.

Unimpeded View of the Aneurysmal Neck and Perforating Arteries

Ergometric drawings and author protestations aside, all exposures of the distal basilar artery within the interpeduncular cistern result in a deep, narrow field that is easily obscured by the overlying neural and vascular structures. The necessary additions of a surgical suction tip and clip applier/clip combination further impair the surgeon's ability to see critical structures during definitive clip placement. The additional light and, more importantly, the added access for introduction of the clip applier offered by a low anterior temporal exposure can significantly improve the operator's ability during final dissection and clip placement. These additions represent a real advantage of the combined transsylvian-anterior temporal approach, with or without removal of the orbital roof and resection of the zygoma.

SUMMARY

In the hands of an experienced microvascular surgeon, both of the approaches described by these authors provide more than adequate exposure of the lesion in question and permit its uncomplicated obliteration. Because of this aneurysm's location, the classic transsylvian approach demands no more brain retraction than the skull base exposure, allows adequate visualization of the vascular anatomy, and is to be recommended because of its speed, lack of complexity, and ease of both opening and closure. However, the size of the aneurysm in this patient, our lack of information regarding its consistency and content, and recognition of the often-unforeseen problems with clip positioning and visualization during clip placement, suggest that the greater flexibility provided by the combined exposure might well prove advantageous. When treating these difficult aneurysms, it is generally better to have extensive exposure and not need it than to need good exposure and not have it.

REFERENCES

John L. Fox, M.D.

1. Al-Mefty O: Supraorbital-pterional approach to skull base lesions. *Neurosurgery* 1987; 21:474–477.
2. Drake CG: The surgical treatment of aneurysms of the basilar artery. *J Neurosurg* 1968; 29:436–446.
3. Fox JL: *Atlas of Neurosurgical Anatomy*. New York, Springer, 1989, pp 165–200.
4. Fox JL: *Intracranial Aneurysms*. New York, Springer, 1983, pp 771–787, 1024–1069.
5. Fox JL: Microsurgical exposure of vertebrobasilar aneurysms, in Rand RW (ed): *Microneurosurgery*, ed. 3. St Louis, CV Mosby, 1985, pp 589–599.
6. Ito Z: *Microsurgery of Cerebral Aneurysms*. Amsterdam, Elsevier, 1985, pp 180–201.
7. Peerless SJ, Drake CG: Management of aneurysms of the posterior

circulation, in Youmans JR (ed): *Neurological Surgery* ed. 3. Philadelphia, WB Saunders, 1990, pp 1764–1806.

8. Samson DS, Hodosh RM, Clark WK: Microsurgical evaluation of the pterional approach to aneurysms of the distal basilar circulation. *Neurosurgery* 1978; 3:135–141.

9. Sugita K: *Microneurosurgical Atlas.* Berlin, Springer, 1985, pp 62–81.

10. Sundt TM Jr: *Surgical Techniques for Saccular and Giant Intra-* *cranial Aneurysms.* Baltimore, Williams and Wilkins, 1990, pp 213–233.

11. Wright DC, Wilson CB: Surgical treatment of basilar aneurysms. *Neurosurgery* 1979; 5:325–333.

12. Yasargil MG, Antic J, Laciga R, et al.: Microsurgical pterional approach to aneurysms of the basilar bifurcation. *Surg Neurol* 1976; 6:83–91.

T.C. Origitano, M.D., Ph.D., Ossama Al-Mefty, M.D.

1. Batjer HH, Samson DS: Causes of morbidity and mortality from surgery of aneurysms of the distal basilar artery. *Neurosurgery* 1989; 25:904–916.

2. Dolenc VV, Skrap M, Sustersic J, et al.: A transcavernous-transsellar approach to the basilar tip aneurysms. *Br J Neurosurg* 1987; 1:251–259.

3. Drake CG: Treatment of aneurysms of the posterior cranial fossa. *Prog Neurol Surg* 1988; 9:122–194.

4. Fox JL: The ambient and interpeduncular cisterns, in Fox JL (ed): *Atlas of Neurosurgical Anatomy: The Pterional Perspective.* New York, Springer, 1989, pp 165–200.

5. Fox JL: Technique of aneurysm surgery: V. basilar artery aneurysms, in Fox JL (ed): *Intracranial Aneurysms*, vol. 2. New York, Springer, 1983, pp 1024–1069.

6. Fujitsu K, Kuwabara T: Zygomatic approach for lesions in the interpeduncular cistern. *J Neurosurg* 1985; 62:340–343.

7. Heros RC: Brain resection for exposure of deep extracerebral and paraventricular lesions. *Surg Neurol* 1990; 34:188–195.

8. Ikeda K, Yamashita J, Hashimoto M, et al.: Orbitozygomatic temporo-polar approach for a high basilar tip aneurysm associated with a short intracranial carotid artery: A new surgical approach. *Neurosurgery* 1991; 28:105–110.

9. Samson DS, Hodosh RM, Clark WK: Microsurgical evaluation of the pterional approach to aneurysms of the distal basilar circulation. *Neurosurgery* 1978; 3:135–141.

10. Sano K: Temporo-polar approach to aneurysms of the basilar artery at and around the distal bifurcation: Technical note. *Neurol Res* 1980; 2:361–367.

11. Sugita K, Kobayashi S, Shintani A, et al.: Microsurgery for aneurysms of the basilar artery. *J Neurosurg* 1979; 51:615–620.

12. Wilson CB, U HS: Surgical treatment for aneurysms of the upper basilar artery. *J Neurosurg* 1976; 44:537–543.

13. Wright DC, Wilson CB: Surgical treatment of basilar aneurysms. Neurosurgery 1979; 5:325–333.

14. Yasargil MG, Antic J, Laciga R, et al.: Microsurgical pterional approach to aneurysms of the basilar bifurcation. *Surg Neurol* 1976; 6:83–91.

19

The Treatment of Giant Aneurysms
of the Carotid Ophthalmic Artery:
Coils vs. the Decompression Clipping Technique

CASE

This 48-year-old, right-handed woman came to medical attention with a gradual visual loss in her right eye over the past 18 months. Over the past 2 months, she has had some minor loss of vision in her left eye as well. Computed tomography (CT) showed a large mass in the area of her left carotid artery. Upon examination, she had 20/80 vision in the left eye and was able to count fingers with the right. She had a left homonymous hemianopsia, a right afferent pupillary defect, and bilateral optic atrophy on the right greater than on the left. Angiograms with a right carotid injection and compression of the left carotid artery showed a large aneurysm of the left carotid artery. No A-1 was seen on the left and the aneurysm did not fill. With a catheter in the vertebral artery and compression of the left carotid artery, there was no filling of the posterior communicating artery. The patient had a balloon placed in the petrous carotid on the left. After 2 minutes of left carotid occlusion, she developed a right hemiplegia with aphasia. With reperfusion, she rapidly resumed her usual neurological function.

PARTICIPANTS

Treatment of Giant Aneurysms of the Carotid Ophthalmic Artery: The Use of Coils–
   Fernando Viñuela, M.D.

Treatment of Giant Aneurysms of the Carotid Ophthalmic Artery: The Decompression Clipping Technique–H. Hunt Batjer, M.D.

Moderators–Evandro de Oliveira, M.D., Helder Tedeschi, M.D., Albert L. Rhoton, Jr., M.D., David A. Peace, M.S., M.A.

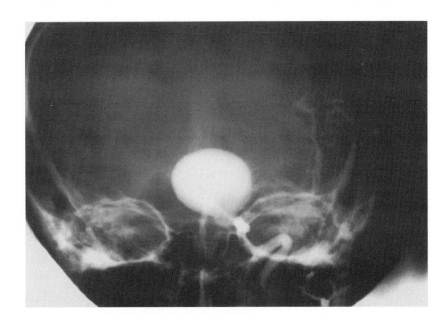

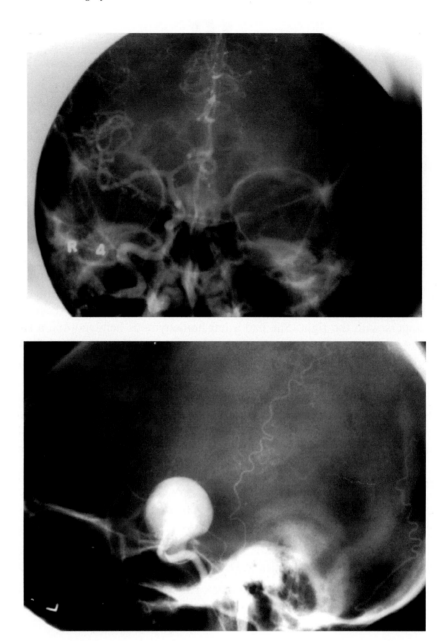

Treatment of Giant Aneurysms of the Carotid Ophthalmic Artery: The Use of Coils

Fernando Viñuela, M.D.

The role of intravascular techniques in the therapeutic treatment of this giant aneurysm of the left carotid-ophthalmic artery include: (1) internal carotid occlusion with balloons immediately below the neck of the aneurysm after extracranial-intracranial bypass, and (2) embolization of the aneurysm with balloons or coils, sparing the left internal carotid artery.

CAROTID OCCLUSION

For internal carotid occlusion with balloons after extracranial-intracranial bypass, the patient should be brought immediately after surgery to the angiography suite. A temporary balloon occlusion of the internal carotid artery (30 minutes), with the patient fully awake, and electroencephalographic (EEG) monitoring should be carried out. Intravenous injection of xenon before and during temporary balloon occlusion should also be done to assess blood flow to the brain. If the patient tolerates the temporary balloon occlusion and the intravenous blood flow study shows normal cerebral blood flow in the left hemisphere, the left internal carotid artery can be permanently occluded with 2 detachable balloons. This procedure may produce massive thrombosis of the aneurysm, even if some reconstitution of the aneurysm from the ophthalmic artery remains. The patient may be followed with magnetic resonance angiography (MRA) and a final complete cerebral angiogram should be done when the MRA shows no aneurysm. If the patient's vision does not progressively improve in the following week or her visual defect suddenly worsens because of the thrombosis, surgical explora-

tion with decompression of the aneurysm should be strongly considered.

COILS

Embolization of the aneurysm with balloons or coils, sparing the left internal carotid artery, aims to pack the aneurysm with embolic material. In my experience with aneurysms presenting with mass effect, the patient had a 20% chance of clinical worsening before improvement. Therefore, the patient in this case may become completely blind without the certainty of recovery. In my experience using Guglielmi detachable microcoils in one patient with a giant carotid-ophthalmic aneurysm, the mass effect worsened after embolization and the patient required surgical decompression of the aneurysm. In that case, the patient tolerated temporary balloon occlusion of the internal carotid artery, and the surgeon had to permanently occlude the artery because there was no clippable neck. The patient was discharged 5 days later with marked improvement of vision (Fig. 1). The possibility of untoward migration of balloons and coils in this wide-neck aneurysm is also possible. This technical complication may rupture the aneurysm or cause untoward embolization of the intracranial circulation. This complication occurs in about 2% of giant aneurysms with a wide neck, but it has been dramatically reduced with the use of the detachable microcoil system. The coils appear to adhere to the dome of the aneurysm, even in giant aneurysms with a very wide neck. I have been able to treat a giant fusiform aneurysm with asymmetrical dilation of

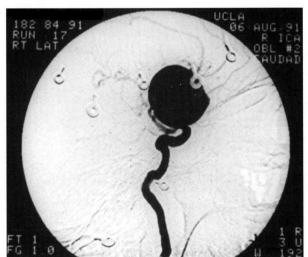
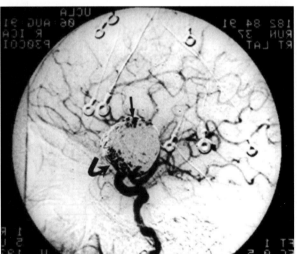

Fig. 1 These figures show the postembolization increase in mass effect: (*A*) A right internal carotid angiogram shows a giant aneurysm of the carotid-ophthalmic artery measuring 35 mm in diameter; its neck could not be clearly identified. (*B*) The postembolization angiogram of the right internal carotid artery shows that the aneurysm has been obliterated with detachable microcoils. Evidence of stagnant contrast material remains in the dome (straight arrow) and neck (curved arrow) of the aneurysm. After embolization, the aneurysm was surgically decompressed because the patient's vision deteriorated.

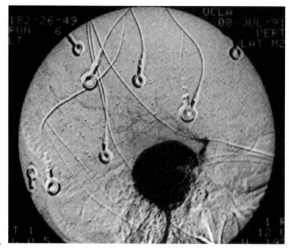
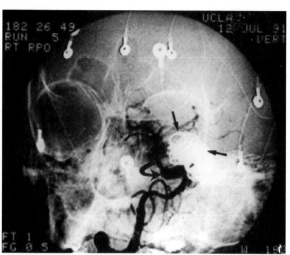

Fig. 2 A giant aneurysm of the carotid-ophthalmic artery arising from the inferomedial wall of the internal carotid artery: (*A*) Preoperative right digital carotid angiogram. (*B*) The postoperative right digital carotid angiogram shows complete obliteration of the aneurysm and reconstruction of the internal carotid artery with multiple fenestrated clips.

the basilar artery, thrombosing most of the aneurysm and leaving a tunnel to reconstitute the trunk of the basilar artery distal to the aneurysm (Fig. 2). Based upon recent experience with the detachable microcoil system, the possibility of occluding the aneurysm while sparing the lumen of the internal carotid artery may also be considered. If the patient's vision deteriorates after embolization, an extracranial-intracranial bypass followed by an attempt to clip with decompression of the aneurysm should be

done immediately. If the aneurysm is successfully occluded using coils, it is imperative to obtain 3- and 6-month follow-up angiograms. In giant aneurysms with a wide neck, reconstitution of the aneurysm has resulted from the packing of coils into the dome by turbulent flow (Fig. 3). In this particular patient, reconstitution of the aneurysm should be followed by surgical exploration and not by re-embolization because of the risk of severe compromise of vision.

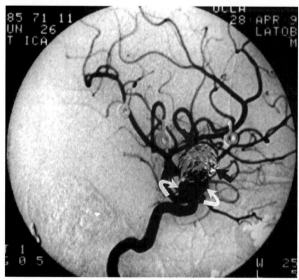
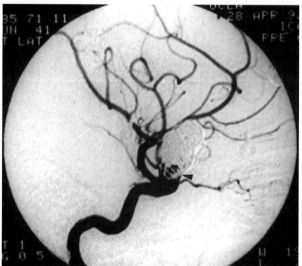

Fig. 3 Recanalization of an aneurysm after embolization with coils: (*A*) An internal carotid angiogram taken 3 months after embolization shows the packed microcoils in the dome of the aneurysm (straight arrows) and recanalization of its base (curved arrows). (*B*) The angiogram taken immediately after re-embolization shows packed coils in the base of the aneurysm (arrow), sparing the lumen of the internal carotid artery.

Treatment of Giant Aneurysms of the Carotid Ophthalmic Artery: The Decompression Clipping Technique

H. Hunt Batjer, M.D.

This patient presents with progressive visual failure, which is actually more pronounced contralateral to her giant paraclinoidal aneurysm. The anatomic and physiological circumstances in her situation highlight a number of unsolved and controversial aspects of vascular neurosurgery.

CASE ANALYSIS

This woman's predominantly contralateral visual deficits are informative from 2 perspectives. First, the relative preservation of the left optic nerve and optic tract (20/80 vision) suggests that these structures were distorted laterally by the expanding aneurysm. With directly superior and medial displacement by a lesion of this size, one would anticipate profound ipsilateral visual loss. This point is pertinent anatomically as the surgeon plans therapy because it is likely that this aneurysm actually has a superior hypophyseal origin from the medial and inferomedial carotid wall, and not the typical superomedial origin of a carotid-ophthalmic aneurysm. Careful scrutiny of the anteroposterior angiogram also supports this hypothesis, as the proximal aspect of the neck appears to project initially inferomedially. This seemingly subtle distinction has direct relevance when one contemplates direct clipping.

The second important issue arising from the patient's clinical presentation is that, if a direct approach to the aneurysm is planned from the left side, extreme care must be exercised to avoid damaging the left optic nerve and tract by manipulation or trauma to the vascular supply of the optic apparatus. I am thinking primarily about the perforating vessels from the internal carotid artery, but one also has to keep in mind the relatively rare but not unheard-of complication of retinal ischemia related to sacrifice of the ophthalmic artery. Any significant worsening of this patient's left visual deficit might well render her functionally blind. With successful therapy, one would hope for, but certainly not guarantee, improvement of the right-sided visual deficits. These neurological and anatomic features suggest clearly that any direct approach to this aneurysm should include temporary deflation of the sac to facilitate clipping with minimal manipulation of the left optic nerve. It should have as its goal the ultimate deflation of the aneurysm to maximize the patient's chances for improved visual function.

TRIAL OCCLUSION

According to angiographic criteria, this woman has an isolated left middle cerebral artery circulation. She did not tolerate trial occlusion of the internal carotid. My recent experience with giant petrous and cavernous aneurysms has suggested that 80 to 85% of patients tolerate acute sacrifice of the parent artery. In addition to awake neurological monitoring, as was done for this patient, I have found a significant benefit to the use of cerebral blood flow measurement and transcranial Doppler recordings during the occlusion trial. Patients who remain neurologically well but develop hemodynamic abnormalities during the trial, appear to be at significant risk of developing delayed ischemic deficits. For those who cannot tolerate carotid occlusion, either clinically or hemodynamically, a number of options are available. If asymmetry developed in only the cerebral blood flow but neurological function remained stable, graded and progressive occlusion with a clamp often gives the collateral bed time to dilate and makes the loss of the vessel tolerable. Alternatively, a low-flow bypass graft followed by a repeated trial occlusion or graded occlusion is reasonable. For the patient who develops an immediate neurological deficit with an isolated middle cerebral circulation, however, one would anticipate the need for a higher flow conduit to increase the immediate availability of collateral flow.

Occasionally, if an extremely robust superficial temporal artery is present, either a routine cortical or distal sylvian bypass, with either the scalp artery itself as donor or the use of a short venous interpositioned graft, will suffice. More commonly, however, a long saphenous vein graft from the common or external carotid artery is needed to achieve adequate flow volumes in these patients with neurological deficits during trial occlusion. While hemodynamically attractive, these procedures carry a much higher risk of postoperative hemorrhage or ischemia during temporary occlusion of the middle cerebral branch during the anastomosis. The patient presented in this case has a relatively small superficial temporal artery, which would not be of much help. If a large vein graft were carried out, it should be followed quickly by carotid occlusion, as the increased resistance in the distal runoff bed would risk distention and rupture of the aneurysm.

LIGATION

Hunterian ligation procedures have been shown to result in delayed improvement in cranial neuropathy, even if no real decompression of the mass is accomplished. Presumably, this results from elimination of pulsations and perhaps subtle absorption of the aneurysm's contents over time. This maneuver, however, is dangerous in patients with a subarachnoid aneurysm and visual compromise. As lesions thrombose over the hours after vessel occlusion, the sac may actually expand somewhat because of the thrombotic process. This complication could be visually devastating and, perhaps, life-threatening in this patient. Therefore, if vessel sacrifice were planned with distal revascularization, the aneurysmal segment should be trapped and the sac deflated. It must be kept in mind that trapping in this setting is accomplished at the expense of an additional source of middle cerebral supply, the ophthalmic artery.

Endovascular methods should be mentioned as potential alternatives. Although the newly developed platinum coils are relatively effective at obliterating the angiographically patent aneurysm, they do not offer the potential to eliminate mass effect, which is important for this particular patient. Because of this problem, I would not consider this option unless the patient was not medically suitable for a general anesthetic.

CLIPPING

It is my strong opinion that the aneurysm in this patient can be and should be definitively clipped, and the internal carotid and ophthalmic arteries preserved. This procedure must be designed

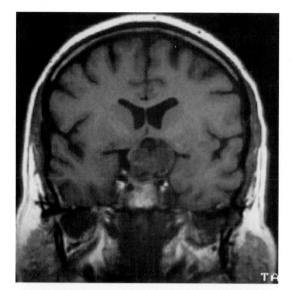

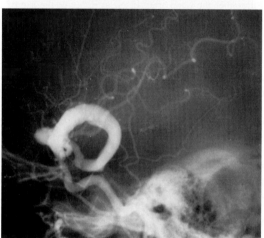

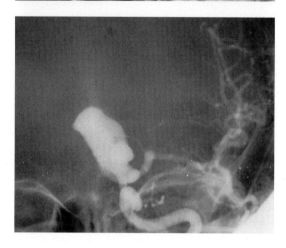

A

B

C

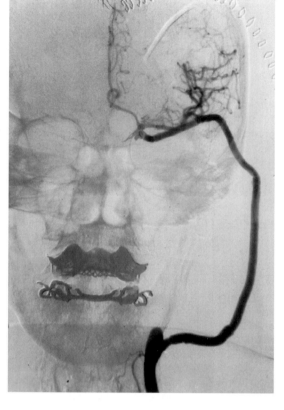

D

Fig. 1 This 50-year-old man presented with a several-year history of blindness in his left eye and newly progressive visual loss in his right eye. (*A*) A magnetic resonance image shows a large suprasellar mass eccentric to the left. (*B*) A lateral angiogram of the left carotid artery shows a giant paraclinoidal aneurysm that is thrombotic and partially canalized. (*C*) An angiogram in the anteroposterior projection shows reconstitution of the normal but inferiorly displaced supraclinoidal carotid. (*D*) At surgery, no attempt was made to reconstruct the thrombotic carotid. A long saphenous graft was employed from the external carotid (end-to-end) to the supraclinoidal carotid (end-to-side). Normal internal carotid perfusion was allowed during proximal anastomosis. The internal carotid was then ligated in the neck and the aneurysm trapped and evacuated to depress the optic apparatus. The patient awakened well and regained visual function.

with the assumptions that temporary arterial occlusion is necessary, that temporary deflation of the sac decreases the duration of occlusion and minimizes visual trauma, and that, because of this patient's poor collateral potential, the period of iatrogenic ischemia must be brief.

I will address the issue of ischemic protection first. It has been my experience that almost all patients tolerate temporary occlusion intervals of under 15 minutes with metabolic suppression by etomidate (Abbott Laboratories, North Chicago, IL) or pentothal

if used in suppressive doses. The protocol I originally used for brain protection[1] has been modified. I currently use a balanced general anesthetic in a normovolemic and normotensive patient. The EEG is monitored throughout the procedure. Before temporary clipping is begun, etomidate is administered with a loading dose of 1.0 mg/kg until burst suppression is documented, and then a drip of 10 micrograms/kg/minute is instituted and continued throughout the ischemic period. Recently, mild hypothermia (32° Celsius) has been added as a means of further decreasing the cerebral metabolic rate in high-risk patients. Because this woman could not tolerate trial occlusion, I would add hypothermia to her regimen. I should mention that profound hypothermia and circulatory arrest in this context facilitates aneurysm deflation and provides about 45 minutes of safe ischemia time. I would not opt for this technique for this patient as the procedure is clearly not without risk and her lesion can be adequately deflated and quickly clipped through more conventional measures. I currently reserve circulatory arrest primarily for patients with giant thrombotic aneurysms of the basilar circulation.

SURGICAL TECHNIQUE

The patient is placed supine with her head rotated about 30° to the right. Before the craniotomy, a cervical incision is made to isolate the first 2 or 3 cm of the cervical internal carotid artery. This exposure is the safest and quickest means to assure early proximal control and facilitates decompression of the aneurysm.[2] Although exposure of the clinoidal segment of the internal carotid allows proximal control, decompression of the aneurysm is not feasible without direct puncture and the technical sacrifice of the surgeon's nondominant hand. After the cervical internal carotid is isolated, a routine left pterional craniotomy is done, with resection of the lateral aspect of the sphenoid ridge. The medial sylvian fissure is then microsurgically dissected, allowing entry into the carotid cistern. Clear control of the internal carotid should be achieved just proximal to the posterior communicating artery, which may be vestigial in this patient. The distal aspect of the aneurysmal neck is then defined and the left optic nerve gently elevated from the distal neck and aneurysmal segment of the carotid. Attention is then focused proximally.

The dural component of the optic canal is opened sharply just lateral to the nerve. Occasionally, this simple maneuver allows the surgeon access to the proximal neck, as well as to the ophthalmic artery. In this patient, however, significant bone resection is necessary. In many patients with superior hypophyseal aneurysms, fenestrated angled clips are necessary to reconstruct the proximal carotid artery. Not infrequently, these clips do not seem to lie comfortably without some bony resection. If bone of the anterior clinoid must be removed, the dura is deflected over the aneurysm and carotid artery and a high-speed air drill is used to remove all necessary bone to expose the healthy carotid wall proximal to the neck. This exposure should also allow easy access to the ophthalmic artery.

Before excessive manipulation of the aneurysm, the neuro-anesthesiologist achieves burst suppression by administering etomidate, and the patient's temperature is cooled to 32° Celsius. A temporary clip is then applied to the ophthalmic artery, if this is feasible. The assistant places a vascular clamp across the cervical internal carotid artery. The surgeon then applies a temporary clip intracranially, just proximal to the posterior communicating artery. The assistant inserts an 18-gauge angiocatheter distally into the cervical carotid and, once good retrograde flow is established, the angiocatheter is attached to an extension tube with a three-way stopcock. A number 7-French neurosurgical suction tube is inserted into the stopcock[2] and suction applied. This maneuver decompresses the aneurysm sac retrograde by removing collateral flow from the cavernous branches and the ophthalmic artery, if this artery is not clipped. It is surprising how turgid an aneurysm, such as this one, remains despite trapping. This retrograde suction maneuver immediately deflates the sac, allowing the surgeon bimanual access for dissection and clipping. One or more fenestrated clips, possibly in tandem, may be required in this case.

After definitive clipping, the temporary clip is removed from the intracranial carotid, followed by slow release of the cervical clamp. The carotid is carefully inspected for signs of clip-induced stenosis and the aneurysm examined for evidence of refilling. If the result is satisfactory, the ophthalmic temporary clip is removed and the etomidate drip stopped. If concern about stenosis arises, the cervical exposure can be used for intraoperative angiography. The puncture site usually becomes hemostatic by distal pressure, but a single 7-0 suture is sometimes necessary.

This aneurysm should be treatable with this technique, with about 10 minutes of temporary occlusion. My experience has been excellent with lesions of this type, particularly if no mural thrombus is present. A remarkable case (Fig. 1) represents the unusual situation in which the parent vessel must be sacrificed. The retrograde suction techniques can be used when the aneurysm must be opened to evacuate thrombus, but the ophthalmic artery should be temporarily clipped to minimize troublesome bleeding.

The Treatment of Giant Aneurysms of the Carotid Ophthalmic Artery: Coils vs. The Decompression Clipping Technique

Evandro de Oliveira, M.D., Helder Tedeschi, M.D., Albert L. Rhoton, Jr., M.D., David A. Peace, M.S., M.A.

Large and giant aneurysms arising from the ophthalmic segment of the carotid artery still represent a formidable challenge, even to the most experienced neurosurgeon. Many of these aneurysms arise from the superomedial aspect of the internal carotid artery, and are in close relationship with the origin of the ophthalmic artery. They may project superiorly or superomedially, and usually displace the optic nerve superomedially (Fig. 1). In other circumstances, the aneurysm may originate from the inferior or inferomedial aspects of the carotid artery (Fig. 2), and project inferiorly to the parasellar region or medially beneath the optic chiasm. Because these aneurysms can reach considerable size before diagnosis, and many of them may present with large necks, identifying their site of origin from the parent artery is difficult.

ANATOMIC CONSIDERATIONS

The ophthalmic segment of the internal carotid artery maintains an intimate relationship with the optic nerve and the anterior clinoid process. Aneurysms arising from this segment are best termed *paraclinoid* as, regardless of their projection, the neck of such an aneurysm is often hidden by the anterior clinoid process.[5] The ophthalmic segment of the carotid artery extends

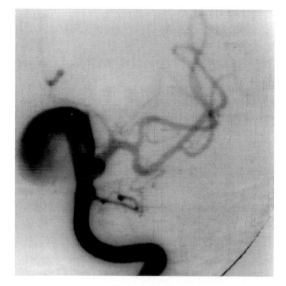

A

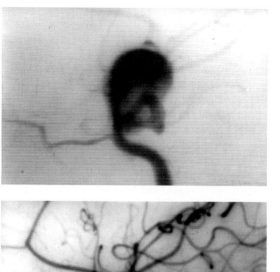

B

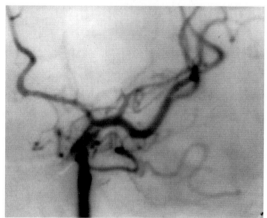

C

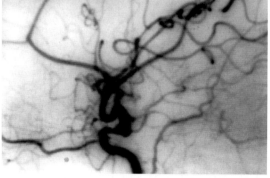

D

Fig. 1 A giant aneurysm of the carotid-ophthalmic artery arising from the superomedial wall of the internal carotid artery: (*A*), (*B*) Preoperative left digital carotid angiogram, anteroposterior and lateral views (*C*), (*D*). The postoperative left digital carotid angiogram in both anteroposterior and lateral views shows complete obliteration of the aneurysm with the use of a single clip.

from the point where the internal carotid artery penetrates the dura, usually at the level of origin of the ophthalmic artery, to the origin of the posterior communicating artery. The ophthalmic segment is the site of origin of several perforating branches that arise from the inferior or inferomedial walls of the carotid artery and supply the optic nerve, the pituitary stalk, and the optic chiasm. The ophthalmic artery originates from the superomedial wall of the internal carotid artery and courses laterally, below the inferior aspect of the optic nerve, to penetrate the optic canal, Figure 3 (**C**), (**D**). Several perforating branches also originate from the communicating and choroidal segments of the internal carotid artery. Along with the posterior communicating and anterior choroidal arteries, these branches can be displaced by large or giant carotid-ophthalmic aneurysms, and usually are closely related to the wall of such aneurysms. Although it is difficult, their dissection and preservation should always be attempted because their sacrifice is responsible for high morbidity rates in the postoperative period.

The anterior clinoid process is situated at the medial end of the lesser sphenoid wing, in the anterior part of the roof of the cavernous sinus, and forms the lateral wall of the intracranial end of the optic canal, Figures 3 (**A**) to (**D**). The anterior clinoid process is usually solid, but it may be pneumatized and communicate with the sphenoid sinus at the medial wall of the cavernous sinus. It may be united to the posterior clinoid process by a fibrous or osseous bridge that can make its removal more

difficult. The anterior and the middle clinoid processes may also be connected by a bony bridge forming a true osseous foramen around the internal carotid artery.[3] Removal of the anterior clinoid process unveils a unique segment of the internal carotid artery that is continuous with the anterior vertical segment of the artery. Lying medial to the anterior clinoid process, it is situated neither in the cavernous sinus nor in the subarachnoid space. This so-called clinoidal segment of the internal carotid artery is surrounded by two distinct rings. The more proximal one, the carotid-oculomotor membrane,[3] Figures 3 (**C**), (**D**), a tenuous connective membrane that surrounds the anterior vertical segment of the internal carotid artery, forms the actual roof of the cavernous sinus. It extends from the oculomotor nerve to the lateral side of the carotid artery, across the interval between the artery and the oculomotor nerve and, finally medial to the oculomotor nerve to the posterior clinoid process. This membrane separates the venous contents of the cavernous sinus from the virtual space occupied by the anterior clinoid process. Laterally, the carotid oculomotor membrane is continuous with the inner reticular layer that envelops the nerves running on the lateral wall of the cavernous sinus.

The dura covering the base of the skull extends anteriorly to the anterior clinoid process and tightly envelops the internal carotid artery at its entrance, to the subarachnoid space to form the distal ring. The supraclinoid internal carotid artery enters the subarachnoid space medial and inferior to the anterior clinoid

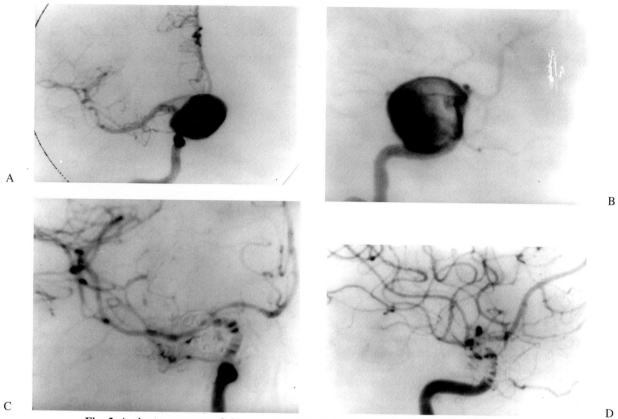

Fig. 2 A giant aneurysm of the carotid-ophthalmic artery arising from the inferomedial wall of the internal carotid artery: (*A*), (*B*) Preoperative right digital carotid angiogram, anteroposterior and lateral views. (*C*), (*D*) The postoperative right digital carotid angiogram in both anteroposterior and lateral views shows complete obliteration of the aneurysm and reconstruction of the internal carotid artery with multiple fenestrated clips.

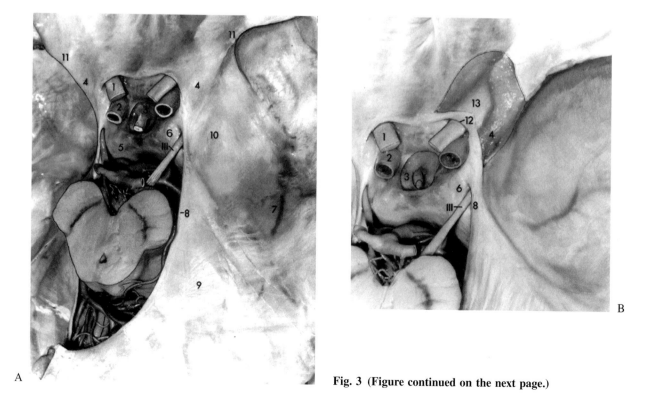

Fig. 3 (Figure continued on the next page.)

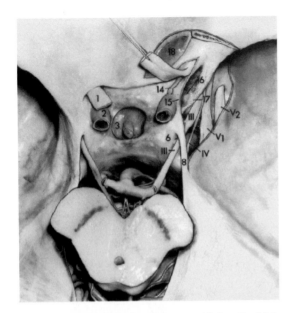

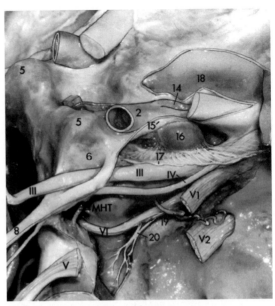

C

D

Fig. 3 Stepwise dissection of the clinoidal segment of the internal carotid artery:
(*A*) The brain has been exposed to the level of the cerebral peduncles, revealing the anterior and middle cranial fossae, the tentorium cerebelli and the sellar and parasellar regions. 1, optic nerve; 2, carotid artery; 3, pituitary gland and stalk; 4, dura over the anterior clinoid process; 5, posterior clinoid process; 6, oculomotor trigone; 7, middle fossa; 8, tentorial edge; 9, tentorium; 10, lateral wall of the cavernous sinus; 11, sphenoid ridge; Ill, oculomotor nerve. (*B*) The dura has been removed over the anterior clinoid process and planum sphenoidale and the superior aspect of the optic canal has been exposed. 1, optic nerve; 2, carotid artery; 3, pituitary gland and stalk; 4, anterior clinoid process; 6, oculomotor trigone; 8, tentorial edge; 12, falciform ligament; 13, optic canal; Ill: oculomotor nerve. (*C*) The anterior clinoid process has been removed, exposing the clinoidal space and the clinoidal segment of the carotid artery, the dural ring, and the carotid-oculomotor membrane. The lateral wall of the cavernous sinus has been opened and the course of the oculomotor and trochlear nerves, and of the ophthalmic and maxillary divisions of the trigeminal nerve, can be seen. The optic sheath has been opened and the optic nerve elevated to expose the origin of the ophthalmic artery from the superomedial aspect of the intradural internal carotid artery. 1, optic nerve; 2, carotid artery; 3, pituitary gland and stalk; 6, oculomotor trigone; 8, tentorial edge; 14, ophthalmic artery; 15, distal ring; 16, clinoidal segment of the internal carotid artery; 17, carotid-oculomotor membrane; 18, bone drilled over the sphenoid sinus; Ill, oculomotor nerve; IV, trochlear nerve; V1, trigeminal nerve, ophthalmic division; V2, trigeminal nerve, maxillary division. (*D*) Lateral view of the cavernous sinus. The anterior clinoid process, the lateral wall of the cavernous sinus, and the dura covering the middle fossa have been removed. The gasserian ganglion and the ophthalmic and maxillary divisions of the trigeminal nerve have been cut, exposing the abducens nerve, the carotid sympathetic fibers, and the horizontal portion of the intracavernous carotid artery. The clinoidal space, the clinoidal segment of the carotid artery, the dural ring, and the carotid-oculomotor membrane can be seen. 2, carotid artery; 5, posterior clinoid process; 8, tentorial edge; 14, ophthalmic artery; 15, distal ring; 16, clinoidal segment of the internal carotid artery; 17, carotid-oculomotor membrane; 18, bone drilled over the sphenoid sinus; 19, artery of the inferior cavernous sinus; 20, sympathetic nerve fibers; Ill, oculomotor nerve; IV, trochlear nerve; V, trigeminal nerve; V1, trigeminal nerve, ophthalmic division; V2, trigeminal nerve, maxillary division; Vl, abducens nerve; MHT: meningohypophyseal trunk.

process. The dura forming the distal ring is contiguous medially with the dura of the diaphragma sellae and laterally with the dura that envelops the anterior clinoid process, Figures 3 (**A**) to (**D**). Removal of the anterior clinoid process and section of the distal ring are important steps to providing a site for temporary clipping and proximal control of arterial bleeding, and to allow for better visualization of the proximal part of the neck of the aneurysm during dissection. From the level of the optic chiasm, each optic nerve projects anterolaterally towards the planum sphenoidale to enter the optic canal medial to the anterior clinoid process and superomedial to the internal carotid artery. At its point of entrance into the optic canal at the edge of the planum sphenoidale, the optic nerve is covered superiorly by a dural fold called the falciform ligament, Figure 3(**B**). Aneurysms of the ophthalmic artery tend to push the optic nerve against the falciform ligament as they project superomedially.

DIRECT SURGICAL APPROACH

Because angiographic examinations can give only indirect indications about the anatomic aspects of the internal carotid artery and the aneurysmal neck, the probabilities of direct clipping of the aneurysm are difficult to predict before surgery. At times, large lesions have surprisingly small necks that are not depicted on the angiograms (Fig. 1). We believe that, with the use of microsurgical techniques and extensive knowledge of the anatomy of the region, most large and giant aneurysms of the ophthalmic artery can be approached directly with acceptably low morbidity.

Exposing the Aneurysm

We favor an extradural approach to aneurysms in this location with removal of the anterior clinoid process as described by Dolenc.[1,2] Through a classic fronto-temporal sphenoidal craniotomy, the superior and lateral walls of the orbit are removed to completely expose the superior orbital fissure. With the aid of a high-speed drill, the superior and medial walls of the optic canal and the anterior clinoid process are carefully removed. This maneuver exposes the clinoidal segment of the internal carotid artery and allows medial mobilization of the optic nerve. The extensive bony resection of the extradural approach provides a better three-dimensional anatomic perspective of the course of the internal carotid artery and its clinoidal segment in relation to the intradural structures; it also gives a much wider operative field than that provided by the intradural approaches. Before the craniotomy, the common, internal, and external carotid arteries are exposed in the neck and prepared for temporary occlusion. To gain early proximal control of arterial bleeding, we expose the carotid artery in the neck rather than in the petrous bone, as the anatomical variants implicated in such a procedure are difficult to predict.

The extradural approach for large or giant aneurysms of the carotid-ophthalmic artery is now standard in our practice, and it can be tailored to specific aneurysms. For true ophthalmic aneurysms (Fig. 1), that is, those with superior or superomedial projections, the extradural approach can be combined with intradural resection of the anterior clinoid process under direct visualization of the aneurysm, as sometimes a broad neck can penetrate the clinoidal space. In aneurysms that project laterosuperiorly, the dome can partially indent the anterior clinoid process, making its extradural removal particularly risky.

After the anterior clinoid process is removed and the optic canal unroofed, the dura mater is opened. The dural incision follows the superficial sylvian vein towards the superior orbital fissure, progressing then to the clinoidal space, where it changes direction to proceed medially, exposing the extra- and intradural portions of the optic nerve and the extra- and intradural course of the internal carotid artery. After the dura is opened, the sylvian and basal cisterns are dissected widely to minimize brain retraction. The dural sheath that envelops the optic nerve is then carefully incised along the lateral aspect of the nerve, care being taken not to injure the ophthalmic artery as it adheres closely to the optic sheath in its lateral course beneath the inferior aspect of the optic nerve. The optic nerve can then be displaced medially, allowing for positive identification of the ophthalmic artery and the proximal neck of the aneurysm.

The clinoidal segment of the internal carotid artery is denuded from its covering by the carotid-oculomotor membrane and prepared for temporary clipping. At this point, any bleeding from the cavernous sinus can be controlled by packing; however, excessive packing should be avoided as it can produce inadvertent stenosis of the carotid artery within the cavernous sinus. The distal dural ring around the carotid artery is then completely incised to allow free mobilization of the anterior vertical segment. This maneuver is extremely important to individualize the proximal part of the neck of the aneurysm and to insure proper placement of the aneurysmal clip. For those aneurysms projecting superiorly or superomedially, the complete incision of the dural ring avoids narrowing of the parent vessel after the clip is applied, as would be expected if the inferior wall of the artery is still fixed to the dura of the base of the skull. A similar situation relative to sectioning of the dural ring occurs with those aneurysms having inferior or inferomedial projections (Fig. 2). These aneurysms usually present with broad necks that extend to the level of the dural ring, making its incision mandatory for correct clip placement and complete obliteration of the aneurysm neck. If the proximal and inferior aspects of the neck are not freed from the attachments to the dural ring and if the inferior aspect of the anterior vertical segment of the internal carotid artery is not properly isolated, the clip blades cannot be completely closed without causing stenosis or kinking of the parent vessel.

Clipping the Aneurysm

After enough space is obtained from proximal exposure of the aneurysmal neck, we frequently place a fenestrated right-angled clip, moving from a proximal to distal direction to first occlude the proximal part of the neck. Then, according to the situation, the artery is reconstructed with the use of clips of various types. Temporary clipping of the clinoidal segment and of the distal internal carotid artery below the level of the posterior communicating artery permits deflation of the aneurysmal sac and even evacuation of its contents before definitive clips are applied.

Before temporary occlusion of the internal carotid artery, the brain is protected through suppression of the cerebral metabolism using 3 to 7 mg/kg of thiopental. Monitoring is carried out with repeated blood samples taken from a catheter placed at the level of the jugular bulb, where the arterial-venous difference of oxygen consumption is continuously measured and kept at normal levels. Mild hypothermia (32° Celsius) and osmotic agents, such as mannitol are also used. For patients who show a high risk of permanent occlusion of the internal carotid artery after four-vessel angiography or insufficient collateral circulation, we favor a high-flow bypass procedure using a long saphenous vein graft from the external carotid artery to the sylvian middle cerebral artery before direct intervention (Fig. 4). This graft

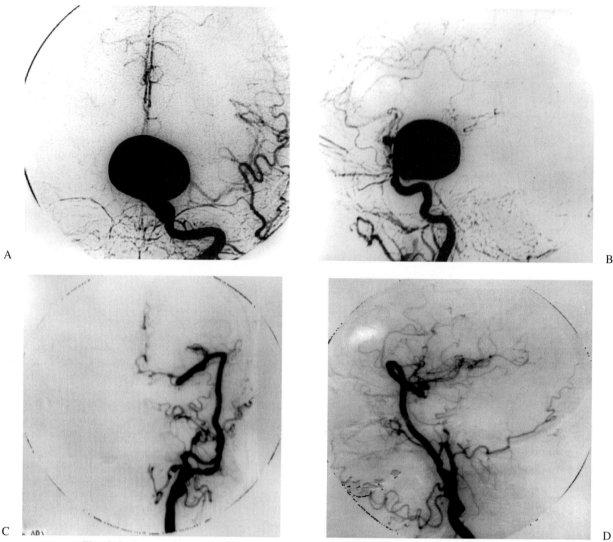

A

B

C

D

Fig. 4 A giant aneurysm of the carotid-ophthalmic artery arising from the inferomedial wall of the internal carotid artery: (A), (B) Preoperative left digital carotid angiogram, anteroposterior and lateral views. (C), (D) The postoperative left digital carotid angiogram in both anteroposterior and lateral views shows complete obliteration of the aneurysm with a long saphenous vein bypass from the external carotid to the middle cerebral artery, followed by ligation of the internal carotid artery.

should probably be the initial method of treatment for the patient presented in this discussion, followed by direct intervention through the extradural approach. With the neuroanesthesiologic, cardiovascular, and neurosurgical teams working in perfect co-ordination, the use of profound hypothermia and circulatory arrest to increase cerebral protection to safe periods of up to 50 minutes[4] could also be considered for this patient.

VISUAL DETERIORATION

The issue of progressive visual deterioration is still controversial. Even though untreated aneurysms tend to grow and compress the optic apparatus, surgery or alternative methods of treatment do not guarantee visual recovery or improvement. Nevertheless, direct surgery remains the only treatment that eliminates the mass effect, offering the possibility of visual recovery or the arrest of visual deterioration. Other methods of treatment, such as endovascular procedures, are promising and have developed rapidly in the past few years. Although these

procedures are elegant, they carry a significant risk of major complications, primarily because of thromboembolic events. These alternative methods can be used to obliterate even the largest lesions, but they still lack the capability of dealing with the mass effect.

CONCLUSION

When there are no clinical contraindications for surgery, the treatment of choice for patients with large or giant aneurysms of the carotid-ophthalmic artery should be direct clipping of the aneurysmal neck with reconstruction of the carotid artery and decompression of the optic apparatus. This kind of treatment should be attempted whenever the aneurysm is amenable to clipping, in either symptomatic or asymptomatic patients, regardless of whether the aneurysm has ruptured, as these lesions tend to grow and impair neurological function. Patients whose clinical conditions contraindicate surgery should be carefully considered for alternative methods of treatment.

REFERENCES

H. Hunt Batjer, M.D.

1. Batjer HH, Frankfurt AI, Purdy PD, et al.: Use of etomidate, temporary arterial occlusion, and intraoperative angiography in surgical treatment of large and giant cerebral aneurysms. *J Neurosurg* 1988; 68:234–240.

2. Batjer HH, Samson DS: Retrograde suction decompression of giant paraclinoidal aneurysms. *J Neurosurg* 1990; 73:305–306.

Evandro de Oliveira, M.D., Helder Tedeschi, M.D., Albert L. Rhoton, Jr., M.D., David A. Peace, M.S., M.A.

1. Dolenc V: Direct microsurgical repair of intracavernous vascular lesions. *J Neurosurg* 1983; 58:824–831.

2. Dolenc V: A combined epi- and subdural approach to carotid-ophthalmic artery aneurysms. *J Neurosurg* 1985; 62:667–672.

3. Inoue T, Rhoton AL Jr, Theele D, et al.: Surgical approaches to the cavernous sinus: A microsurgical study. *Neurosurgery* 1990; 26: 903–932.

4. Lundar T, Froysaker T, Nornes H: Cerebral damage following open heart surgery in deep hypothermia and circulatory arrest. *Scand J Thorac Cardiovasc Surg* 1983; 17:237–242.

5. Nutik S: Carotid paraclinoid aneurysms with intradural origin and intracavernous location. *J Neurosurg* 1978; 48:526–533.

20

Treatment of Symptomatic Vasospasm: Angioplasty vs. "Triple-H" Therapy vs. Early Clipping

CASE

A 46-year-old, right-handed woman had a subarachnoid hemorrhage that did not cause a coma. Two weeks later, she re-bled, required intubation, and gradually began to follow a few commands but had bilateral sixth-nerve palsies. In the operating room on that same day, her right pupil became fixed and dilated during the induction of anesthesia. A computed tomogram (CT) showed hydrocephalus and a probably recurrent subarachnoid hemorrhage. Because of the likelihood of a tight brain, coils were placed within the aneurysm to prevent rebleeding and to incite thrombosis. The patient improved with a left frontal ventriculostomy and, 4 days later, was oriented and moving all her extremities. After another 4 days, she abruptly became stuporous and was decerebrate on the left. An immediate angiogram showed severe vasospasm in the left vertebral artery, the basilar artery, and the right carotid artery.

PARTICIPANTS

Balloon Angioplasty for Treatment of Symptomatic Vasospasm–Mazen H. Khayata, M.D., John G. Golfinos, M.D., Ajay K. Wakhloo, M.D., Y. Pierre Gobin, M.D., Robert F. Spetzler, M.D.

"Triple-H" Therapy for Treatment of Symptomatic Vasospasm–T.C. Origitano, M.D., Ph.D., O. Howard Reichman, M.D.

Early Clipping for the Treatment of Symptomatic Vasospasm–Bryce K. Weir, M.D., Daniel Yoshor, M.D.

Moderator–Robert R. Smith, M.D.

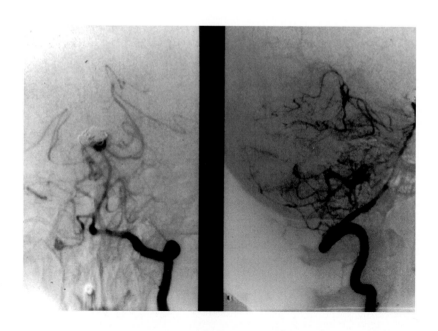

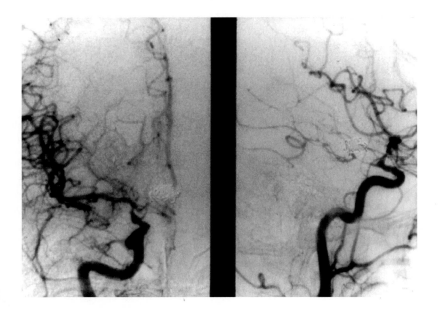

Balloon Angioplasty for Treatment of Symptomatic Vasospasm

Mazen H. Khayata, M.D., John G. Golfinos, M.D., Ajay K. Wakhloo, M.D.,
Y. Pierre Gobin, M.D., Robert F. Spetzler, M.D.

Vasospasm is observed in about one third of all patients with intracranial subarachnoid hemorrhage resulting from the rupture of cerebral aneurysms. Until recently, the methods available for treating vasospasm have had limited efficacy. Vasospasm can affect any segment of the arterial tree: the distal small cerebral vessels, the intermediate vessels, such as the A2 portion of the anterior cerebral artery, and the proximal trunks, such as the A1 portion of the anterior cerebral artery and the vertebrobasilar system. Its long-term effects are usually devastating. About one third of patients eventually have a stroke with major morbidity, another one third have neurological deficits of a more moderate nature, and the remaining group recovers without any evident residual symptoms. Despite an apparent clinical recovery, follow-up magnetic resonance imaging often reveals many diffuse areas of infarction that are apparently asymptomatic.

Four new modalities have recently come to the forefront for treating cerebral vasospasm after subarachnoid hemorrhage: cerebral protection through calcium-channel antagonists, hyper-volemic hemodilutional hypertensive (Triple-H) therapy, balloon angioplasty, and intra-arterial infusion of papaverine (Eli Lilly Co., Indianapolis, IN, and others). All patients with conditions that may be associated with vasospasm benefit from the cerebral protective effects of calcium-channel blockers and routinely receive these when they are admitted to the hospital. This therapy seems to be especially important for patients with vasospasm of distal small vessels that cannot be reached through other methods. Proximal vasospasm involving the internal carotid or vertebrobasilar arteries, such as the A1, M1, or P1 portions of the cerebral vasculature, that does not respond to medical treatment can be treated with balloon dilation, as described in this section (Fig. 1). Vasospasm of vessels of intermediate diameter may be treated either with Triple-H therapy, superselective papaverine injection or, in certain cases, with balloon dilation according to the particular vascular anatomy and the clinical condition of the patient.

INDICATIONS FOR ANGIOPLASTY

The indication for angioplasty is symptomatic vasospasm that does not respond to medical therapy. Clinical and transcranial Doppler monitoring should be helpful in making the decision. Other existing disorders that may be related to the neurological symptoms, such as metabolic disturbances, recurrent hemorrhage, hydrocephalus, or infection, must be excluded. Good results may be achieved if the endovascular procedure is undertaken within 24 hours after the onset of neurological deficits.[7,10] Although the delayed results of angioplasty are less satisfactory, the procedure should nonetheless be considered in neurologically critical patients. A few patients may benefit even if angioplasty is done as late as 48 hours after neurological deterioration.[7]

Focal spasm affecting 1 or more vessel segments is easier to treat and the results may be better than those obtained with treatment for spasm of multiple vessels. Diffuse spasm affecting multiple arteries, however, should not be considered as an absolute contraindication to angioplasty.

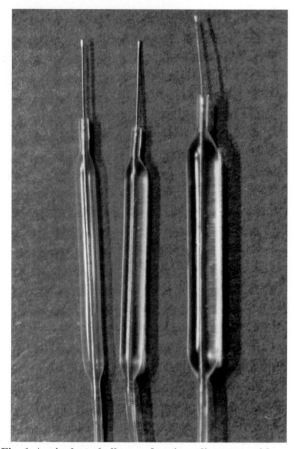

Fig. 1 Angioplasty balloons of various diameters with 0.014-inch steerable guidewires.

No acute infarction should be visible on the magnetic resonance image or a computed tomogram (CT) scan of the treated vascular area. Because systemic anticoagulation with heparin is required during the procedure, acute hemorrhage within the first hours must be considered as a relative contraindication, or the procedure must be done without anticoagulative protection.

Because a significant risk of recurrent hemorrhage has been observed after reperfusion, an aneurysm in the treated vascular area should be clipped before angioplasty.[7,13] In patients with severe generalized atherosclerosis, angioplasty—especially of the basilar artery—may be hazardous because of the danger of vessel dissection, dislodging plaques, and occlusion of perforators.[1,20] The decision must be made case by case. If, in tortuous vessels, percutaneous placement of the angioplasty catheter is not feasible, an intraoperative endovascular approach, either of the vertebral or carotid artery, should be considered.

The indications for angioplasty are highlighted in the following illustrative case of an aneurysm causing subarachnoid hemorrhage. At our institution, surgery for aneurysms is undertaken early, with clipping within 24 hours whenever possible. The patient is then treated according to a protocol that includes Swan-Ganz monitoring of cardiac parameters and fluid status.

All patients are given calcium-channel blockers; colloid substitutes are used liberally as needed to support intravascular volume, and 3% sodium chloride solution is infused as needed in patients with hypovolemia. At the first signs of delayed ischemic deficits, the intravascular volume is aggressively increased and pressors are used as needed to drive the mean arterial pressure upward until symptoms abate. Initially, a CT scan is obtained to exclude other causes of neurological deterioration, including hydrocephalus, recurrent hemorrhage, parenchymal hemorrhage or established infarction. All patients are maintained on nimodipine from the time of admission. If ischemic deficits persist beyond 8 hours of adequate therapy, or if symptoms worsen despite therapy, angiography with angioplasty of affected arteries is considered. Transcranial Doppler monitoring is used routinely to monitor the patient's response to both conventional and endovascular treatment.

Illustrative Case

A 44-year-old woman was admitted with a severe headache and was found to have subarachnoid hemorrhage (Fisher's grade II, Hunt and Hess grade I). A four-vessel arteriogram revealed an aneurysm on the tip of the basilar artery (Fig. 2). The aneurysm was explored, but could not be clipped easily because of its particular anatomic configuration. The patient was returned to the neurosurgical intensive care unit. On the third day of hospitalization, the patient was suddenly found stuporous in her bed. She had been taking nimodipine since the day of admission. Hypertensive hypervolemic therapy was instituted. Because the patient was still stuporous after 4 hours of treatment and was becoming less responsive, we did a second angiogram. The angiogram of the vertebral artery revealed focal distal stenosis of the basilar artery with decreased distal flow (Fig. 2). Because of the patient's deteriorating medical condition, we decided to try balloon dilation of the distal basilar artery to relieve the vasospasm and occlude the aneurysm.

The patient underwent transfemoral catheterization of the left vertebral artery. A 3.5-mm balloon angioplasty catheter was coaxially introduced and then navigated according to a "road map" (Fig. 1). The guidewire was first advanced across the area of stenosis and the balloon was placed into the area of stenosis. A 1-ml syringe was used to inflate the balloon manually 2 to 3 times to dilate the area of stenosis. After dilation, a control vertebral arteriogram revealed patency of the distal basilar circulation (Fig. 3). Within 20 minutes of the procedure, the patient became responsive and alert. The aneurysm was then treated through implantation of transluminal microcoils (Figs. 4 and 5). The patient continued to improve over the next 3 days and returned to baseline status. She was discharged 1 week later and continued to do well at the 6-month follow-up.

ANGIOPLASTY TECHNIQUE

There are essentially 2 ways of dilating the mid or upper portion of the basilar artery. One is simply to use a nondetachable balloon, passing it across the stenosis and then inflating it to dilate the area of stenosis up to a pressure of 3 atmospheres (atm), which usually requires 2 or 3 dilations. The second technique, which we prefer, uses guidewire-associated balloon dilation. The guidewire is first passed into the basilar artery through the area of stenosis. However, a proximal severe spasm with insufficient distal filling may limit the definition of vasospasm on the angiogram. The guidewire stabilizes the balloon, which otherwise has a tendency to flip forward or backward instead of dilating the area of stenosis. By anchoring the balloon to a specific area, it can be dilated with small injections of diluted

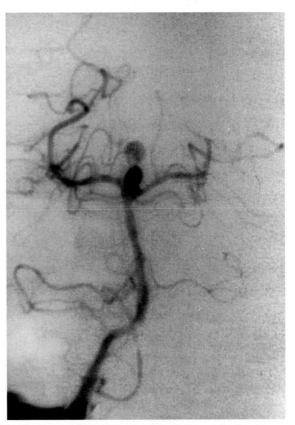

Fig. 3 A control angiogram of the left vertebral artery (Towne projection) shows the dilated basilar artery with improved perfusion.

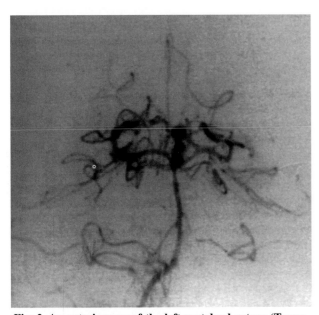

Fig. 2 An arteriogram of the left vertebral artery (Towne projection) shows an aneurysm of the tip of the basilar artery and stenosis of the distal vessel segment; this stenosis was dilated through the use of a balloon with a guidewire.

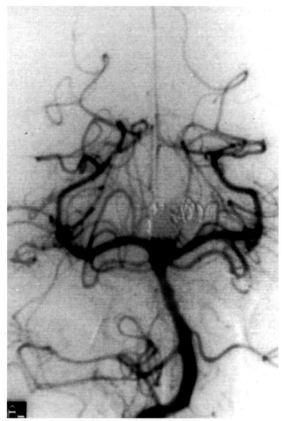

Fig. 4 An arteriogram of the left vertebral artery after endovascular treatment of the aneurysm at the basilar tip with complete patency of the distal basilar circulation.

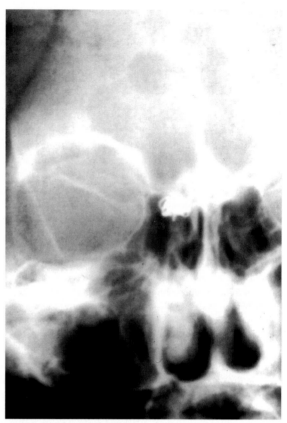

Fig. 5 A skull roentgenogram (anteroposterior projection) shows the tuft of tightly packed coils inside the aneurysm.

contrast material. The balloon is inflated 2 or 3 times for a few seconds until the stenosis resolves.

Great care should be taken to choose a balloon of the appropriate diameter. For the basilar artery, a diameter of 3 to 4 mm should never be exceeded; otherwise, there is a risk of vessel rupture. Because recent experimental studies with a silicone balloon showed that angioplasty with 1 atm over an interval of 10 seconds done 10 times repeatedly did not rupture the intima and has good clinical results,[13] higher inflation pressure should be avoided. Even after using a higher inflation pressure of 3 atm, scanning electron microscopy revealed compression of the intima without fragmentation and stretching of the media. This may explain why, in contrast to the effects of angioplasty in patients with atherosclerotic disease, no secondary fibrosis occurs in the long term follow-up after endovascular treatment of vasospasm.

Other experimental studies in vitro showed that the long-lasting effect of balloon dilation may be caused by the disruption of the connective tissues that proliferate in the medial layer of the vessel wall after a subarachnoid hemorrhage.[23] Scanning electron microscopy showed stretching of collagen fibers with a loss of complex appearance stemming from mechanical damage to the medial layer. In in vitro studies of canine cerebral vessels, angioplasty of preconstricted vessels resulted in endothelial desquamation, damage to the internal elastic membrane, thinning of the muscle layer with rupture of the medial layer and no response to pharmacological stimulation.[18] This is consistent with clinical studies that showed no evidence of stenotic recurrence angiographically if there was no rebleeding.

Silicone balloons (Fig. 1) require an inflation pressure of 0.5 atm, thus reducing the risk of endothelial damage and vessel rupture. Polyethylene microballoons require a higher inflation pressure of 5 atm. This increases the danger of vessel rupture and intimal disruption. A normal vessel diameter or a cosmetically good angiographic result is not necessary. Improved circulation is generally achieved with restoration of 50% of the original vessel diameter.

ENDOVASCULAR STEPS

Angioplasty is performed with the patient under local mild sedative anesthesia. The groin is shaved, prepared with betadine, and draped in the usual sterile fashion. An 18-gauge needle is used to gain access to the femoral artery, and a No. 6-French femoral sheath is placed in the iliac artery. This sheath is connected to a heparinized pressurized saline drip. A No. 5.5-French Royal flush catheter is then navigated, under fluoroscopic control and road-map, into the left dominant vertebral artery with the help of a 0.035-inch angle-tipped guidewire. This catheter guide is also connected to a heparinized pressurized saline drip to avoid clot formation. The Stealth® angioplasty balloon microcatheter (Target Therapeutics, Fremont, CA) (Fig. 1) is then coaxially introduced into the catheter guide with a Y-valve connector, and is navigated with its own 0.014-inch diameter guidewire. The guidewire, followed by the balloon, are advanced across the area of stenosis. The balloon is then inflated by hand 2 or 3 times with a 1-ml syringe. After dilation, arteriography is repeated to confirm the patency of the circulation and the catheter is withdrawn.

The Stealth® balloons are available in 2-, 2.5-, 3-, 3.5- and 4-mm diameters (Fig. 1). The 0.014-inch guidewire is similar to the Seeker® guidewire of that diameter, but has a valve that closes off the distal end of the balloon to permit inflation. The guidewire has an extended tip distally of 1, 2, or 4 cm. For the intracranial circulation, the 1- or 2-cm distal tip is generally the only one required.

DISCUSSION

Vasospasm with delayed ischemic deficits remains an unsolved problem in patients with aneurysmal subarachnoid hemorrhage. Before nimodipine was available for use, permanent delayed ischemic deficits occurred in almost 30% of patients not receiving calcium-channel blockers.[17] Even with the routine use of calcium-channel blockers in patients with subarachnoid hemorrhage, delayed deterioration from vasospasm continues to be a significant cause of morbidity and mortality.[22] Hypertensive hypervolemic hemodilutional therapy has also proved beneficial in combating vasospasm.[2] Despite these recent advances in the care of the aneurysm patient, vasospasm can be expected to cause permanent deficits in at least 7% of patients treated with nimodipine. The clinical outcome of vasospasm is even worse in patients with a poor-grade aneurysm.[17]

The Evolution of Angioplasty

Facing this problem, Zubkov and colleagues[24] were the first to successfully dilate cerebral arteries mechanically in the presence of aneurysmal subarachnoid hemorrhage. In a series of 33 patients, they were able to dilate 105 arteries using an inflatable balloon. The angiographic dilations were long-lasting and improved the ischemic deficits in many patients. This early experience marked transluminal angioplasty as a promising means of reversing vasospasm. About 5 years later, transluminal angioplasty for vasospasm was used for the first time in the United States.[3,16] There are now more than 124 cases of angioplasty treatment for vasospasm reported in the English-language medical literature.[3–6,10,13–15,19,21,24]

The largest series of cases have been reported by Zubkov and colleagues,[24] Higashida and associates,[10] Takahashi and colleagues,[21] and Eskridge and co-workers.[7] In their first report, Higashida and colleagues[8] had 5 patients (40%) with excellent results and 4 (30%) with good results after angioplasty. Four patients (30%) had no clinical improvement and died; three of those patients were moribund and comatose. One patient with a spastic middle cerebral artery died of a hemorrhagic infarct in the basal ganglia after initial improvement after angioplasty; this was considered a complication of the reperfusion of infarcted brain tissue. Thus, the importance of magnetic resonance imaging or CT scanning before the procedure cannot be overemphasized in making the decision to proceed. In a larger series published subsequently, Higashida and colleagues[9] observed immediate neurological improvement 24 hours after angioplasty. Spasm did not recur during the follow-up period of several days to 2 weeks after the procedure. In about 40% of patients, no clinical improvement was seen, although angioplasty had been successful. Good results occured in 60% even over a long-term follow-up period of 2 years.[10] Two patients died of technical complications.

In general, transluminal angioplasty has effectively reversed angiographic vasospasm and, more importantly, ischemic deficits in patients after subarachnoid hemorrhage. To date, the treated populations have been somewhat heterogeneous, encompassing patients with aneurysmal hemorrhage of both good and poor clinical grades. Moreover, angioplasty has been used in patients awaiting aneurysmal clipping and in patients postoperatively.[4,24] Stable xenon CT cerebral blood flow studies document improved perfusion of the microcirculation after angioplasty of proximal vessel segments.[19] Interestingly, use of xenon blood flow measurements before the angioplastic procedure predicts the brain tissue that would be irreversibly damaged. Above the critical flow rate of 12 ml/100 g/min, however, the reperfusion time may determine the outcome.

Timing of Angioplasty

Because the decrease in microcirculation may differ in each patient, the proper time for the performance of angioplasty is difficult to predict. Experience shows, however, that better results are achieved if angioplasty is done while the patient is still in an early stage of clinical deterioration. The perioperative treatment protocols for subarachnoid hemorrhage have also differed in the aggressive use of adjunctive therapy, with 70 to 80% of patients achieving neurological improvement.[7,21] In all patients, angioplasty resulted in immediate angiographic improvement in vasospasm with sustained dilation of the treated arteries on follow-up angiograms 2 or more weeks later. Several reports document immediate and persistent improvement in transcranial Doppler flow studies after angioplasty as well.[4,16]

The time course of neurological improvement after angioplasty varies and is probably related to the duration of the deficit. In patients in whom vasospasm has been iatrogenic during endovascular aneurysmal occlusion and treated with virtually no delay, the neurological improvement has immediately coincided with the successful dilation of the affected artery.[8] When ischemic symptoms have been present for more than 24 hours, clinical improvement after angioplasty may take from a few to as many as 48 hours.[3,4] Some authors believe that such delayed improvement should not be attributed to the effects of angioplasty but may, in fact, reflect the natural improvement in the effects of vasospasm. This view no longer seems tenable, however, given the significant number of patients now reported in whom improvement has occurred within less than 24 hours and in whom all other therapeutic measures failed to arrest a progressive neurological decline. Most groups now advocate undertaking angioplasty as soon as possible, once it becomes clear that more conventional measures have failed to reverse ischemic symptoms. The reasons are manifold: to limit the duration of ischemia, to improve the chances of success, and more rapid recovery, and because the intracranial arteries are reportedly more easily dilated during the early stages of vasospasm.[7,8] Angioplasty done within 12 hours of the onset of ischemic symptoms seems to be the most effective.[16]

The poorest results have been in patients with poor-grade aneurysms (Hunt and Hess grades IV and V).[8] In these patients, vasospasm may be so severe and diffuse that angiographic improvement is accompanied by little or no clinical improvement.

Equipment

The technical details of the procedure vary from operator to operator. All operators, however, have had success with soft silicone microballoons.[5,9] The major stem arteries of the anterior and posterior circulations have been successfully dilated.[5,8] Initial difficulties cannulating the anterior cerebral arteries have been overcome with the use of steerable tapered guidewires.[5] The use of digital road-mapping fluoroscopy has proved important in navigating spastic arteries and in placing the microcatheter exactly, as well as in monitoring during inflation of the balloon to avoid overdilation and, thus, to reduce the danger of rupture. Underdilation is preferred to overdilation, which, although it may produce a good angiographic result, may be linked with arterial occlusion from intimal damage or with possible rupture or development of an aneurysm.

Complications

Complications of angioplasty have so far been infrequent. The initial mortality rate after angioplasty was related to aneurysmal rupture from either improved perfusion or rupture at the clipped part of the aneurysm itself.[7,14] Aneurysm surgery should be carried out before angioplasty; rupture of unclipped aneurysms has occurred on a delayed basis after angioplasty.[7,16] This most logically resulted from the change in perfusion dynamics subsequent to dilation. One group of investigators reported delayed occlusion of a dilated artery that they believed had been subjected to trauma from use of a stiff guidewire.[16] Arterial rupture has been reported in only one case of treatment for aneurysmal subarachnoid hemorrhage.[14] The operators believed that a small area of unclipped aneurysmal neck ruptured after angioplasty of the supraclinoid internal carotid artery. In restoring flow to ischemic tissue, the great fear is either exacerbation of the reperfusion injury or injury from conversion of the bland infarction to a hemorrhagic infarction. Hemorrhagic infarction resulting in death has been reported in one patient.[8]

Concerns about hemorrhagic infarction and reperfusion injury have prevented most operators from attempting angioplasty when ischemic symptoms are of long duration, and when established large areas of infarction are visible on magnetic resonance images or CT scans. Diffuse spasm may still be a challenge for this technique, and the decision in favor of angioplasty may be difficult. Brothers and Holgate[5] observed persistent narrowing of distal vessel segments after proximal dilation in 3 patients with diffuse vasospasm. Nevertheless, 2 patients had neurological recovery, probably because of improved microcirculation.

Use of Papaverine

Recently, intra-arterial infusion of papaverine has been discussed for the treatment of cerebral vasospasm after sub-arachnoid hemorrhage.[11,12] Papaverine is a strong nonspecific vasodilator. This technique was applied after angioplasty of a proximal vasospasm to treat segmental, as well as diffuse, vasospasm. Papaverine is injected just proximal to the affected vessel through a superselectively placed microcatheter. However, the total amount of papaverine differs in both studies. Kaku and colleagues[11] used 6 to 20 mg, whereas Kassell and associates[12] injected 100 to 300 mg over a period of 30 to 60 minutes. No systemic effect was noticed, except a 10 to 20% acceleration of the heart rate. In most of the patients, no recurrence was seen. When vasospasm recurred, it was successfully treated with a repeated papaverine infusion. Although the therapeutic experience is limited, this treatment may be a further option for patients with hemorrhage-induced vasospasm and should be considered, especially in treating the diffuse type of spasm involving distal branches not accessible for balloon angioplasty. Compared with angioplasty, injection of papaverine has no technical hazards and, thus, the procedure may be practical in centers with less interventional experience.

CONCLUSION

Angioplasty using the protocol described in this section cannot be considered controversial. All other measures are used first to combat ischemia and, in most patients, are adequate. Only in those in which ischemia persists is angioplasty considered a treatment option. In these patients, the alternative to angioplasty is to do nothing further. The literature confirms our experience that better results can be obtained with angioplasty than with reliance on hypervolemic hypertensive therapy in the presence of progressive deficits.

We stress that aggressive medical treatment is the cornerstone of good treatment of patients with aneurysmal subarachnoid hemorrhage. Angioplasty serves to help those who do not respond to more conventional therapy. It should be undertaken as early as possible, once it becomes clear that ischemic deficits are not improving. Great care should be exercised in considering angioplasty for patients harboring unprotected or partially protected aneurysms. Similarly, angioplasty is not indicated for patients who have already suffered a large established infarction.

"Triple-H" Therapy for Treatment of Symptomatic Vasospasm

T.C. Origitano, M.D., Ph.D., O. Howard Reichman, M.D.

This patient illustrates the complexity of the natural history of aneurysmal subarachnoid hemorrhage and the pitfalls inherent in its overall treatment. *Triple-H* therapy aims to address the pathophysiological changes that occur after subarachnoid hemorrhage. By definition, Triple-H therapy consists of a graded prophylactic protocol of hypovolemic hemodilution, augmented with hypertension and guided by serial measurements of cerebral blood flow combined with prompt surgery (within 24 hours of admission).

CASE ANALYSIS

This patient suffered the malignant triad of subarachnoid hemorrhage: rebleeding, hydrocephalus, and delayed ischemia secondary to vasospasm. True to its reported propensity,[6,11] rebleeding took place within 2 weeks of the initial hemorrhage (25% risk). Hydrocephalus requiring the placement of a shunt occurs in 14% of patients having subarachnoid hemorrhage, and is often associated with significant vasospasm.[2] Generally, the morbidity and mortality after rebleeding is exceptionally high, often exceeding 70%.[11] Angiographic and symptomatic clinical vasospasm develop over a 2-week course, generally beginning 4 days after the bleeding and reaching a peak between days 10 and 12.[17] Conversely, cerebral blood flow declines over the same 2-week period, reaching its nadir on day 12.[9]

As a high-grade patient (according to Hunt-Hess grades I–II),[5] this woman survived her initial hemorrhage, which is presumed to be minor (Fisher Class I).[3] Her rebleed on day 14 set off a series of events rendering her a low-grade patient at high risk for developing significant diffuse vasospasm and delayed ischemia. The patient's presentation and the timing of the vasospasm shown by an angiogram on day 12 after the bleed is a classic scenario.

While the anatomic changes on the angiogram are impressive, the pathophysiological decline in cerebral blood flow to below an ischemic threshold is responsible for the patient's clinical picture. Many studies have shown that hypovolemic hemodilution augmented with hypertension can improve cerebral blood flow and a patient's clinical status.[1,4,7,10,12,13,15,16] Cerebral blood flow is elevated with hypervolemic hemodilution alone, providing a buffer against ischemia.

RESULTS OF TRIPLE-H THERAPY

Our service has now treated more than 100 patients using Triple-H therapy in a prophylactic fashion, as described above. We have experienced no surgical mortality associated with prompt surgery. Delayed ischemia leading to infarction occurred in 10% of our patients. Although some authors have reported systemic complications, increased cerebral edema and hemorrhagic infarction with this treatment,[8,14] this has not occurred in our patients. These complications may be caused by implementing hypovolemic hemodilution late in the ischemic course, when the patient is symptomatic and the changes documented by CT have already occurred. Once the ischemic cascade has progressed to an irreversible point, increased volume and hypertension can, indeed, lead to edema or hemorrhagic infarction. We believe the improved outcome in our patients is associated with prompt surgery, which obviates rebleeding and permits aggressive rheological treatment. Routine serial measurements of cerebral blood flow guide the intensity and duration of therapy, allowing us to anticipate impending clinical changes, and directly measure end-organ responses to therapy.

Applying this philosophy (with 20/20 hindsight) to this patient illustrates the utility of our approach. Initial early surgery would have eliminated rebleeding and avoided the associated sequelae in this patient. Once the aneurysm was surgically obliterated, the options for and aggressiveness of treatment could expand.

Here, however, we are now faced with a poor-grade patient. Because the short- and long-term benefits of incomplete endovascular coiling are not known, 2 treatment options exist: Triple-H therapy or multiple-vessel endovascular angioplasty. The angiogram shows severe diffuse narrowing of many vessels and, if used, angioplasty of the left vertebral, basilar, bilateral posterior cerebral, and right carotid arteries would be necessary. To date, no large series reporting on the efficacy, timing, outcome, and complications associated with multiple-vessel angioplasty exist. In light of the diffuse nature of this patient's spasm, we would opt for initial treatment with Triple-H therapy.

TREATMENT TECHNIQUE

To initiate Triple-H therapy, a baseline measurement of cerebral blood flow is obtained and hypervolemic hemodilution begun. Serial monitoring of cerebral blood flow values then follows. In our experience, a decline in cerebral blood flow is a harbinger of impending clinical change. At this point in the patient's course, augmentation with hypertension is initiated. As illustrated by her neurological deficit, this patient has already crossed the ischemic threshold, and the angiogram indicates a global ischemic process. Triple-H therapy can be started at this juncture. Measurements of cerebral blood flow become even more critical in guiding therapy and avoiding intracranial complications. In addition, a Swan-Ganz catheter is placed to follow and optimize cardiac performance and fluid status.

After treatment is begun and the clinical and cerebral blood flow responses are monitored, a decision as to whether to augment with hypertension can be made. A decline in cerebral blood flow can be stabilized and even increased; systolic pressures of 180 to 200 mmHg may be necessary to achieve improvement. In light of this patient's clinical status and widespread diffuse signs seen on the angiogram, the risk of rerupture of the aneurysm is considered secondary to impending global ischemic infarction. Hypertension is initiated and maintained until the patient improves clinically. Once the patient's clinical status stabilizes, definitive clipping of the aneurysm is undertaken.

CONCLUSION

In patients with aneurysmal subarachnoid hemorrhage, early aggressive surgical treatment coupled with prophylactic optimization of cerebral blood flow can improve the outcome and limit complications. Although still beneficial, delayed treatment is limited and prone to complications. The role of angioplasty has yet to be defined, and serious questions as to the timing of its application, the number of vessels involved, and the overall complication rate must be answered before its widespread application in these patients.

Early Clipping for the Treatment of Symptomatic Vasospasm

Bryce K. Weir, M.D., Daniel Yoshor, M.D.

A patient of this status would have to be accurately assessed with respect to her circulating blood volume state, serum electrolyte and osmolality, blood gases, and cerebral anatomy as shown by a computed tomography (CT) scan. Was there any evidence of sepsis? What was her blood pressure? Has she received antifibrinolytic agents, antihypertensive medication, or other vasoactive drugs? The aneurysm can be assumed to be partly protected (most ruptures are from the dome) and it shows only residual patency of the neck and proximal body.

IMMEDIATE TREATMENT

We would start off by elevating the patient's blood pressure and assuring that the patient had adequate circulating blood volume through the use of a Swan-Ganz catheter and fluid replacement, if required. The blood pressure would be elevated to at least 200 systolic, assuming that the patient did not improve at a lower level. If the patient did not improve after an hour or so of hypertension, consultation would be sought with an interventional radiologist to carry out balloon angioplasty of the spastic vessels. The various factors that must be weighed in treating such patients are discussed below.

Dealing with Vasospasm

Cerebral vasospasm, or delayed ischemic neurological deficit, remains a vexing and difficult problem for neurosurgeons to face, and the morbidity and mortality of this "second stroke" remains significant. Prophylactic maneuvers that have been shown to reduce the incidence and severity of vasospasm after subarachnoid hemorrhage and the associated ischemic injury are critical to improve the patient's condition. At present, the administration of calcium antagonists, such as nimodipine or nicardipine, and avoidance of hypovolemia should be a part of the treatment plan for any patient with subarachnoid hemorrhage that results in visible blood on the CT scan. The value of prophylactic nimodipine in decreasing the incidence of infarction caused by vasospasm and improving overall clinical outcome has been amply shown in prospective, randomized, placebo-controlled, double-blind trials.[1,29,31,34–36] Recently, similar trials have shown that two other calcium antagonists, nicardipine and AT877, effectively reduce the incidence of angiographically demonstrable vasospasm.[18,42]

Managing Fluid Losses

Hypovolemia with decreased red cell mass and total blood volume are frequently present after subarachnoid hemorrhage.[22,25,44] This depleted volume status increases the risk of cerebral ischemia and should be promptly and vigorously corrected.[13,44] It is controversial as to whether aggressive overcorrection of fluid deficits, as in hypertensive hypervolemia or hypertensive hypervolemia with hemodilution, provides benefits that outweigh their risks (most commonly pulmonary edema and catheter complications) and costs if applied to all patients with subarachnoid hemorrhage even before the onset of neurological deficits. Whether or not hemodilution confers an added prophylactic benefit to hypertension and hypervolemia is especially problematic. The advantage of these maneuvers in comparison to the maintenance of euvolemia and prophylactic nimodipine alone has not been rigorously shown.[16,27,32,43] Further clinical trials are necessary to elucidate this point. We keep the routine patient suffering subarachnoid hemorrhage well hydrated, using clinical criteria to guide the generous replacement of fluid losses. Invasive monitoring and aggressive volume expansion are reserved for the few patients who do develop delayed ischemia after subarachnoid hemorrhage.[10,36]

Other Methods of Treatment

Several other treatments have been shown to reduce the risk of vasospasm after subarachnoid hemorrhage in preliminary trials, but most require large-scale controlled studies to establish their validity before they become a part of standard clinical practice. Of particular interest is clot lysis with recombinant tissue plasminogen activator (rtPA) to prevent vasospasm. Subject to the results of the ongoing randomized clinical trials, its use may be strongly considered as a prophylactic measure in patients with thick clots on CT who are at high risk of severe vasospasm and delayed ischemia.[7–9,12,40]

To date, no pharmacological agent has proven routinely effective in reversing established vasospasm.[49] Recently, Nakagomi and colleagues[28] showed pharmacological reversibility of vasospasm using a potent, but deadly, vasodilator "cocktail" in an animal model. This creates hope for benefits from intra-arterial vasodilator therapy. Preliminary clinical evidence of the efficacy of intra-arterial papaverine infusions is now available (Kassell, personal communication). Current treatment of established vasospasm relies on the prompt application of 2 techniques: (1) induced hemodynamic alterations to raise blood pressure and increase cardiac output and, if this fails, (2) percutaneous transluminal angioplasty-mechanical dilation of narrowed arteries with balloon-tipped catheters.

HYPERVOLEMIA, HYPERTENSION, AND HEMODILUTION

In spite of the absence of randomized, controlled clinical trials, hypervolemic, hypertensive therapy, with or without hemodilution, is widely employed as a therapy for symptomatic vasospasm. An abundance of anecdotal clinical evidence has shown its value in rapidly reversing delayed ischemic neurological deficits after subarachnoid hemorrhage.[2,4,19,21,32,38,43] Increased cerebral blood flow to ischemic brain after both hypertension-hypovolemia therapy and hypertension, hypervolemia, hemodilution therapy has been shown in animal studies and in humans.[5,26,32,39] Whether or not increased blood flow is necessarily accompanied by increased oxygen delivery to the ischemic brain remains moot.

Hypervolemia is thought to increase blood flow to ischemic brain that has lost cerebral autoregulation (the ability to maintain consistent flow in the presence of changing arterial pressure). In dysfunctional ischemic regions, local flow may become directly proportional to alterations in cardiac output (direct coupling between cardiac output and cerebral blood flow) in the presence or absence of similar changes in blood pressure.[5,20,47] Although blood pressure can alter cerebral blood flow by changing cerebral perfusion pressure, cardiac output changes alone and independent of perfusion pressure changes can cause direct changes in blood flow in the brain of primates with focal ischemia.[47] The resultant increased blood flow to acutely ischemic areas is believed to rescue acutely and reversibly ischemic and malfunctioning brain tissue from infarction and permanent deficit.[17] Experimental evidence supports the clinical impression that hypervolemia leading to increased cardiac output alone (independent of blood pressure) can rapidly reverse or ameliorate acute ischemic deficits.[22,38,44,48] This evidence has led us to choose an approach to hemodynamic alterations in therapy of vasospasm similar to that taken by Kassell and colleagues in the largest hypertension-hypervolemia series.[19] After the diagnosis of clinical deterioration from vasospasm is confirmed, we rapidly begin hypertension with dopamine if the patient's aneurysm has been secured. The pressure is raised until the systolic is in at least the range of 160 to 180 mm. Simultaneously, an albumin bolus is given and the crystalloid infusion rate is increased. Depending upon the patient's clinical response, the hypertension is titrated. If the patient's condition does not improve, a Swan-Ganz catheter is inserted to raise pulmonary wedge pressure to a level that provides the highest cardiac output.[37] The documented risks of insertion complications, ventricular arrhythmias, and catheter-associated infections has led us to avoid routine use of Swan-Ganz monitoring in treatment of patients after subarachnoid hemorrhage in the early period before vasospasm is likely to occur (Day 3). Such monitoring, however, is of great value in determining which pulmonary artery wedge pressure generates the greatest cardiac output in a given patient and, thus, should be employed in the seriously ill patient with severe symptomatic vasospasm.[37,41]

Colloid solutions may present a significantly lower risk of inducing cerebral edema than crystalloids. In experimental isovolemic hemodilution in a canine model of focal cerebral ischemia, albumin was ideal in maintaining long-term hypervolemia (1 day) and may have had additional value as a scavenger of oxygen-free radicals.[6,14] In postoperative patients with secured aneurysms, Kassell and colleagues[19] used dopamine, dobutamine or, occasionally, phenylephrine to gradually increase the systolic blood pressure up to 220 torr or until the ischemic deficits began to reverse. In patients with recently ruptured, unsecured aneurysms, systolic blood pressure was only increased to a target level of 160 torr to avoid aneurysmal rebleeding. With this protocol, a 19% incidence of rebleeding in patients with unsecured, previously ruptured aneurysms occurred. All the patients whose aneurysms re-bled had a systolic blood pressure greater than 160 torr at the time.

A great amount of controversy regarding the relative contribution of hemodilution to the efficacy of hypertension and hypervolemia exists. Hemodilution is generally an incidental effect of combined hypertension and hypervolemic therapy; however, some investigators believe that the improved blood flow results primarily from the decreased viscosity that hemodilution causes. From the Hagen-Poiseuille equation, blood flow is inversely proportional to blood viscosity, particularly at low velocity gradients present in the microcirculation during cerebral ischemia.[14,51] Thus, theoretically, the decrease in viscosity that results from a decreased hematocrit should increase cerebral blood flow to the ischemic brain. Whether the increased blood flow actually increases oxygen and glucose delivery probably varies according to a multitude of other factors.

Clinically, this variance usually is not an issue as the drop in blood volume after subarachnoid hemorrhage, combined with the appropriate prophylactic correction of hypervolemia, usually results in a hematocrit of less than 40 even before aggressive hypervolemia is begun.[23] The hematocrit that balances optimal viscosity and maximal oxygen delivery is 33% in normal patients, but the ideal is unknown in pathologic situations, such as ischemia or vasospasm after subarachnoid hemorrhage. Thus, any target hematocrit in a hemodilution protocol is more or less a guess.[16] The only clear clinical evidence of the efficacy of hemodilution in treating cerebral ischemia is in cases of polycythemia.[45,46] The results of clinical trials conflict with regard to the benefit of hemodilution in patients with acute ischemia.[11]

Experimental evidence exists to support both increased cardiac output and hemodilution as crucial factors in the success of hypervolemia. Whole blood infusions did not increase cerebral blood flow in an animal model of cerebral ischemia.[50] On the other hand, isovolemic hemodilution did not affect cerebral blood flow to ischemic areas in a similar experimental model. Subsequently, in a more relevant primate model of focal ischemia, cerebral blood flow changes in ischemic regions were found to be directly proportional to changes in cardiac output.[20,47]

An elegant series of positron emission tomography (PET) studies showed that unintended decreases in hematocrit in patients with vasospasm after subarachnoid hemorrhage led to a significantly decreased oxygen supply to tissue throughout the brain. The decreased oxygen delivery that hemodilution caused may be a stimulus for increased cerebral blood flow, and hemodilution may actually aggravate delayed ischemia.[16] The balance of evidence has led us to avoid actively inducing hemodilution. Hypervolemic therapy alone places patients' hematocrits within the generally targeted range without any need for additional withdrawal of blood.[23] In the largest series of hypertension-hypervolemia therapy (without deliberate hemodilution), sustained neurological improvement occurred in 74% of patients with no hemorrhagic infarction or cerebral edema.[19]

BALLOON ANGIOPLASTY

In the past 10 years, 3 published series of 10 or more patients have shown the efficacy of balloon catheter angioplasty in producing long-lasting, angiographically demonstrable dilation of vasospastic arteries after subarachnoid hemorrhage and rapid amelioration and, often, resolution of deficits believed to result from vasospasm-induced ischemia.[15,30,52] Combined data from the 2 most recently published series reveals significant post-angioplasty improvement in 18 of 23 patients, with good or excellent long-term outcome in 15. In these patients, the only reported complications of the technique included a hemorrhagic infarct 24 hours after angioplasty, which led to death, rebleeding from an unclipped aneurysm 1 week after angioplasty, and occlusion of the middle cerebral artery branch 6 weeks after angioplasty, which led to stroke and was believed to be related to endovascular trauma. A subsequent case report described a fatal rupture of the intracranial carotid artery during angioplasty, which was believed to result from the balloon exerting excessive transmural pressure at a small portion of the weak wall of the aneurysm that lay proximal to the clip.[24] However, complications may have been underreported.

In spite of these impressive results, more clinical research is needed before balloon angioplasty can be widely accepted as the initial treatment of patients having cerebral vasospasm. At present, it remains an important potential therapy whose role should be limited to use in selected centers with expertise in interventional neuroradiology, and where it can be applied expeditiously before established infarction. Even in these centers, it should only be used as a final heroic measure in patients with vasospasm refractory to aggressive medical therapy. Although several reports cite successful results of angioplasty performed more than 24 hours after the onset of delayed ischemic deficits, success has been greatest when it was done early.[3,15,52] The presence of substantial infarction on CT or magnetic resonance images should contraindicate angioplasty, as there is an added risk of hemorrhagic conversion of ischemic infarction. Although there is a theoretical risk of rebleeding of an unsecured aneurysm secondary to the sudden increase in transmural pressure from increased flow through the dilated artery, a number of the patients reported as having been treated with angioplasty have had unsecured aneurysms. Until a scientific study of this risk is available, one should consider an unsecured aneurysm as only a relative contraindication to angioplasty.

We do not advocate any strict protocol in treating cerebral vasospasm in clinical practice. We assume that the patient described in this report has received standard prophylactic treatment with calcium-channel blockers and maintenance of normovolemia, the hematocrit is less than 40, and work-up has ruled out other concurrent contributing causes of neurological deterioration. The angiogram shows diffuse severe vasospasm. The security of the aneurysm is unsure; it has been coiled and not clipped. The volume status of the patient is unknown. The presence of a ventriculostomy may be essential to decreasing intracranial pressure and improving cerebral perfusion pressure, although one must be cautious because this also increases trans-mural pressure and the risk of rebleeding.[33] Patients usually improve with the hypervolemia and hypertension. If so, we maintain the blood pressure at a level at which the ischemic symptoms are absent or at least stable. After 24 hours or so, we would successively try to end the induced hypertension. If pulmonary edema develops, we would use controlled ventilation and furosemide and insert a Swan-Ganz catheter to guide fluid therapy.

CONCLUSION

In summary, we believe the balance of clinical and experimental evidence indicates that hemodynamic alterations of hypervolemia and hypertension, individually and in combination, have a beneficial effect in treating patients with cerebral isch-emia from vasospasm. We do not believe that a protocol of targeted hemodilution is clearly supported by the clinical evidence unless the hematocrit is greater than 40. Balloon angioplasty now has a role in cases of vasospasm refractory to more standard medical therapy, but should only be applied in centers with such expertise, after hemodynamic manipulation has failed and before infarction has developed.

The patient described in this case illustrates the complex interplay of risks and benefits that must be considered in treating anyone with symptomatic cerebral vasospasm. In light of these considerable risks and unsure benefits of all the therapies for vasospasm, we must develop effective prophylactic measures. Early clipping prevents rebleeding, permits clot removal and instillation of fibrinolytic agents, and is compatible with vigorous hypertension/hypervolemia.

Treatment of Symptomatic Vasospasm: Angioplasty vs. "Triple-H" Therapy vs. Early Clipping

Robert R. Smith, M.D.

Some recent rhetoric has noted a reduced incidence of vasospasm resulting from our better treatment protocols. As the patient in this case shows, however, the condition still exists and significantly affects our overall outcome. In almost every patient studied with the use of transcranial Doppler sonography, flow velocity is elevated toward the end of the first week after hemorrhage, indicating arterial narrowing. Unfortunately, no single parameter allows us to identify the patient who will become symptomatic and develop infarction from vasospasm. In 9 of every 10 of my patients, a velocity change of 25% or more on any single day was associated with a deteriorating neurological status that occurred within 24 hours.

NEUROLOGICAL DEFICITS

The patient in this case also gives us an opportunity to discuss the differential diagnosis of the abrupt onset of neurological deficits after subarachnoid hemorrhage. The symptoms from cerebral vasospasm may occur suddenly, but this is seen in only a few patients. When it happens, it probably is associated with vasospasm of large arterial trunks from which short arteries arise, such as lenticulostriates or perforators from the basilar apex. The areas of the brain giving rise to consciousness are deep and supplied by short penetrating branches. In this particular patient, the P1 and basilar trunk are both compromised by constriction and, therefore, the percheron arteries from P1, the thalamoperforators, and the superior mesencephalic arteries that arise from the dorsal surface of the basilar artery are probably affected. The purpose of the coil is to create thrombus, thus occluding the aneurysm. I have seen acute infarction in one patient caused by embolic material from an aneurysm treated with coils. Therefore, embolization must be included in the differential diagnosis in patients with abrupt onset.

APPROPRIATE TREATMENT

Each group of authors has presented a discussion of treatment protocols and, as Weir and Yoshor emphasize, no single regimen seems appropriate for all patients. Several of the authors infer that calcium-channel blockade is effective, but many still question the efficacy and especially the rationale of this form of treatment. If the treatment works, the mechanism by which it does so is unknown. Even the industry-supported and sponsored trials have not shown release of constricted arteries. Likewise, if the effect is upon distal vessels, this treatment could be detrimental rather than helpful. The free radical reaction from lipid peroxidation may play a role in the patient's deteriorating condition, and the radical scavenging compound may prove effective over the long term.

Triple-H Therapy

In the meantime, we are left with several protocols that have never been adequately tested. The Triple-H regimen has gained some enthusiasm among neurosurgeons. Neurological deficits abate and patients improve when this therapy is instituted and vigorously applied. It probably is best applicable to the patient with mild vasospasm. Once cerebral blood flow has been critically reduced and infarction has taken place, the theoretical value of this form of treatment decreases. The addition of hemodilution to hypertension and hypervolemia is of questionable value. Weir and Yoshor raise serious concerns about using hemodilution unless the patient is frankly polycythemic.

Early Clipping and Angioplasty

Recently, many surgeons have turned to an aggressive operative treatment plan, such as that advocated by Origitano and Reichman. In fact, it is currently difficult to argue rationally for delaying the operative clipping of a recently ruptured cerebral aneurysm. Perhaps the less-experienced surgeon operates on some patients who otherwise, because of their poor neurological condition, would not benefit from surgery but, more importantly, overall salvage probably improves. Khayata and associates attack the root of the problem. Their treatment produces immediate results, provides lasting relief, and agrees with the concept that this disease is actually a constrictive vasculopathy. The disadvantages are the risks involved in its application, its availability at only selected centers and, of course, the issue of timing. When should it be done?

Khayata and colleagues argue that this treatment entails risk and should only be used after symptoms develop. Zubkov and his colleagues in St. Petersburg have suggested that vasospasm should be treated when it is recognized. In their established angioplasty center, only one ruptured artery was described in more than 100 patients who underwent angioplasty. There are other complications of angioplasty, however, especially in the patient whose blood flow is already considerably compromised. Treatment must be delivered quickly; otherwise, ischemia may result from even a brief period of balloon inflation. Perhaps some common ground must be found between the patient *in extremis* and the one who might remain asymptomatic from this disease. We must learn to identify the patient who will become symptomatic. The Doppler shift, the Fisher CT grading system of subarachnoid hemorrhage, or the diameter of the vessel as measured from high-quality cerebral angiograms may provide the answer. An individual who is comatose with infarction seen on CT is the poorest candidate for this form of treatment.

The question of which type of balloon or which configuration is best is unresolved. Endovascular neurosurgeons outside the United States continue to favor the soft and pliable latex balloons, which tend to become sausage-shaped when inflated in the constricted artery, rather than the harder silicone balloons, which take a globular shape when inflated. The Food and Drug Administration has consistently taken the attitude that the naturally occurring substance, latex, is difficult to quantify. Perhaps the foreign data will eventually be accepted. An opinion regarding the efficacy and dosage of papaverine has not been standardized. The dose recommended by Kassell and associates is actually tenfold greater than that used by Kaku and colleagues. Perhaps active vasospasm accompanies each case of angiopathy and papaverine causes some release.

CONCLUSION

The authors together have presented a cohesive set of options concerning the treatment of a patient with vasospasm. We must continue to work aggressively to identify an agent responsible for vasospasm because, as shown, its treatment remains only partly successful. Access to certain parts of the cerebral arterial tree will remain a problem for those employing angioplasty. Intracranial hemorrhage, cerebral edema, and even cardiac failure complicate the Triple-H regimen. Perhaps the best hope for the patient with an aneurysm is to find it and obliterate it from the arterial tree before it ruptures.

REFERENCES

Mazen H. Khayata, M.D., John G. Golfinos, M.D., Ajay K. Wakhloo, M.D., Y. Pierre Gobin, M.D., Robert F. Spetzler, M.D.

1. Ahuja A, Guterman LR, Hopkins LN: Angioplasty for basilar artery atherosclerosis. *J Neurosurg* 1992; 77:941–944.
2. Awad IA, Carter LP, Spetzler RF, et al.: Clinical vasospasm after subarachnoid hemorrhage: Response to hypervolemic hemodilution and arterial hypertension. *Stroke* 1987; 18:365–372.
3. Barnwell SL, Higashida RT, Halbach VV, et al.: Transluminal angioplasty of intracerebral vessels for cerebral arterial spasm: Reversal of neurological deficits after delayed treatment. *Neurosurgery* 1989; 25:424–429.
4. Bracard S, Picard L, Ducrocq JCMX, et al.: Role of angioplasty in the treatment of symptomatic vascular spasm occurring in the postoperative course of intracranial ruptured aneurysms. *J Neuroradiol* 1990; 17:6–19.
5. Brothers MF, Holgate RC: Intracranial angioplasty for treatment of vasospasm after subarachnoid hemorrhage: Technique and modifications to improve branch access. *Am J Neuroradiol* 1990; 11:239–247.
6. Dion JE, Duckwiler GR, Viñuela F, et al.: Pre-operative microangioplasty of refractory vasospasm secondary to subarachnoid hemorrhage. *Neuroradiology* 1990; 32:232–236.
7. Eskridge JM, Newell DW, Pendleton GA: Transluminal angioplasty for treatment of vasospasm. *Neurosurg Clin North Am* 1990; 1:387–399.
8. Higashida RT, Halbach VV, Cahan LD, et al.: Transluminal angioplasty for treatment of intracranial arterial vasospasm. *J Neurosurg* 1989; 71:648–653.
9. Higashida RT, Halbach VV, Dormandy B, et al.: New microballoon device for transluminal angioplasty of intracranial arterial vasospasm. *AJNR* 1990; 11:233–238.
10. Higashida RT, Halbach VV, Dowd CF, et al.: Intravascular balloon dilatation therapy for intracranial arterial vasospasm: Patient selection, technique, and clinical results. *Neurosurg Rev* 1992; 15:89–95.
11. Kaku Y, Yonekawa Y, Tsukahara T, et al.: Superselective intra-arterial infusion of papaverine for the treatment of cerebral vasospasm after subarachnoid hemorrhage. *J Neurosurg* 1992; 77:842–847.
12. Kassell NF, Helm G, Simmons N, et al.: Treatment of cerebral vasospasm with intra-arterial papaverine. *J Neurosurg* 1992; 77:848–852.
13. Konishi Y, Maemura E, Shiota M, et al.: Treatment of vasospasm by balloon angioplasty: Experimental studies and clinical experiences. *Neurol Res* 1992; 14:273–281.
14. Linskey ME, Horton JA, Rao GR, et al.: Fatal rupture of the intracranial carotid artery during transluminal angioplasty for vasospasm induced by subarachnoid hemorrhage. *J Neurosurg* 1991; 74:985–990.
15. Mayberg M, Eskridge J, Newell D, et al.: Angioplasty for symptomatic vasospasm, in Sano K, Takakura K, Kassell NF, et al. (eds): *Cerebral Vasospasm: Proceedings of the IVth International Conference on Cerebral Vasospasm.* Tokyo, University of Tokyo Press, 1990.
16. Newell DW, Eskridge JM, Mayberg MR, et al.: Angioplasty for the treatment of symptomatic vasospasm following subarachnoid hemorrhage. *J Neurosurg* 1989; 71:654–660.
17. Petruk KC, West M, Mohr G, et al.: Nimodipine treatment in poor-grade aneurysm patients: Results of a multicenter double-blind placebo-controlled trial. *J Neurosurg* 1988, 68:505–517.
18. Pile-Spellman J, Berenstein A, Bun T, et al.: Angioplasty of canine cerebral vessels (abstract). *Am J Neuroradiol* 1987; 8:938.
19. Pistoia F, Horton JA, Sekhar L, et al.: Imaging of blood flow changes following angioplasty for treatment of vasospasm. *AJNR* 1991; 12:446–448.
20. Sundt TM Jr, Smith HC, Campbell JK, et al.: Transluminal angioplasty for basilar artery stenosis. *Mayo Clin Proc* 1980; 55:673–680.
21. Takahashi A, Yoshimoto T, Mizoi K, et al.: Transluminal balloon angioplasty for vasospasm after subarachnoid hemorrhage, in Sano K, Takakura K, Kassell NF, et al. (eds): *Cerebral Vasospasm: Proceedings of the IVth International Conference on Cerebral Vasospasm.* Tokyo, University of Tokyo Press, 1990.
22. Wilkins RH: Cerebral Vasospasm, in Wilkins RH, Rengachary SS (eds): *Neurosurgery Update II: Vascular, Spinal, Pediatric, and Functional Neurosurgery.* New York, McGraw-Hill, 1991.

23. Yamamoto Y, Smith RR, Bernanke DH: Mechanism of action of balloon angioplasty in cerebral vasospasm. *Neurosurgery* 1992; 30:1–6.

24. Zubkov YN, Nikiforov BM, Shustin VA: Balloon catheter technique for dilatation of constricted cerebral arteries after aneurysmal SAH. *Acta Neurochir (Wien)* 1984; 70:65–79.

T.C. Origitano, M.D., Ph.D., O. Howard Reichman, M.D.

1. Awad IA, Carter LP, Spetzler RF, et al.: Clinical vasospasm after subarachnoid hemorrhage: Response to hypervolemic hemodilution and arterial hypertension. *Stroke* 1987; 18:365–372.

2. Black PMcL: Hydrocephalus and vasospasm after subarachnoid hemorrhage from ruptured intracranial aneurysms. *Neurosurgery* 1986; 18:12–16.

3. Fisher CM, Kistler JP, Davis JM: Relation of cerebral vasospasm to subarachnoid hemorrhage visualized by computerized tomographic scanning. *Neurosurgery* 1980; 6:1–9.

4. Geraud G, Tremoulet M, Geull A, et al.: The prognostic value of non-invasive CBF measurement in subarachnoid hemorrhage. *Stroke* 1984; 15:301–305.

5. Hunt WE, Hess RM: Surgical risk as related to time of intervention in the repair of intracranial aneurysms. *J Neurosurg* 1968; 28:14–19.

6. Kassell NF, Drake CG: Timing of aneurysm surgery. *Neurosurgery* 1982; 10:514–519.

7. Kassell NF, Peerless SJ, Durward QJ, et al.: Treatment of ischemic deficits from vasospasm with intravascular volume expansion and induced arterial hypertension. *Neurosurgery* 1982; 11:337–343.

8. Medlock MD, Dulebohn SC, Elwood PW: Prophylactic hypervolemia without calcium channel blockers in early aneurysm surgery. *Neurosurgery* 1992; 30:12–16.

9. Meyer CHA, Lowe D, Meyer M, et al.: Progressive change in cerebral blood flow during the first three weeks after subarachnoid hemorrhage. *Neurosurgery* 1983; 12:58–76.

10. Muizelaar JP, Becker DP: Induced hypertension for the treatment of cerebral ischemia after subarachnoid hemorrhage: Direct effect on cerebral blood flow. *Surg Neurol* 1986; 25:317–325.

11. Nishioka H, Torner JC, Graf CJ, et al.: Cooperative study of intracranial aneurysms and subarachnoid hemorrhage: A long-term prognostic study. II. Ruptured intracranial aneurysms managed conservatively. *Arch Neurol* 1984; 41:1142–1146.

12. Origitano TC, Wascher TM, Reichman OH, et al.: Sustained increased cerebral blood flow with prophylactic hypertensive hypervolemic hemodilution ("Triple-H" Therapy) after subarachnoid hemorrhage. *Neurosurgery* 1990; 27:729–740.

13. Rosenstein J, Suzuki M, Symon L, et al.: Clinical use of a portable bedside cerebral blood flow machine in the management of aneurysmal subarachnoid hemorrhage. *Neurosurgery* 1984; 15:519–525.

14. Shimoda M, Oda S, Tsugane R, et al.: Intracranial complications of hypervolemic therapy in patients with a delayed ischemic deficit attributed to vasospasm. *J Neurosurg* 1993; 78:423–429.

15. Solomon RA, Fink ME, Lennihan L: Early aneurysm surgery and prophylactic hypervolemic hypertensive therapy for the treatment of aneurysmal subarachnoid hemorrhage. *Neurosurgery* 1988; 23:699–704.

16. Solomon RA, Fink ME, Lennihan L: Prophylactic volume expansion therapy for the prevention of delayed cerebral ischemia after early aneurysm surgery: Results of a preliminary trial. *Arch Neurol* 1988; 45:325–332.

17. Weir B, Grace M, Hansen J, et al.: Time course of vasospasm in man. *J Neurosurg* 1978; 48:173–178.

Bryce K. Weir, M.D., Daniel Yoshor, M.D.

1. Allen GS, Ann HS, Preziosi TJ, et al.: Cerebral arterial spasm—A controlled trial of nimodipine in patients with subarachnoid hemorrhage. *N Engl J Med* 1983; 308:619–624.

2. Awad IA, Carter LP, Spetzler RF, et al.: Clinical vasospasm after subarachnoid hemorrhage: Response to hypervolemic hemodilution and arterial hypertension. *Stroke* 1987; 18:365–372.

3. Barnwell SL, Higashida RT, Halbach VV, et al.: Transluminal angioplasty of intracerebral vessels for cerebral arterial spasm: Reversal of neurological deficits after delayed treatment. *Neurosurgery* 1989; 25:424–429.

4. Brown FD, Hanlon K, Mullan S: Treatment of aneurysmal hemiplegia with dopamine and mannitol. *J Neurosurg* 1978; 49:525–529.

5. Davis DH, Sundt TM Jr: Relationship of cerebral blood flow to cardiac output, mean arterial pressure, blood volume, and alpha and beta blockade in cats. *J Neurosurg* 1980; 52:745–754.

6. Emerson TE Jr: Unique features of albumin: A brief review. *Crit Care Med* 1989; 17:690.

7. Findlay JM, Macdonald RL, Weir BKA: Current concepts of pathophysiology and management of cerebral vasospasm following aneurysmal subarachnoid hemorrhage. *Cerebrovasc Brain Metab Rev* 1991; 3:336–361.

8. Findlay JM, Weir BKA, Kanamaru K, et al.: Intrathecal fibrinolytic therapy after subarachnoid hemorrhage: Dosage study in a primate model and review of the literature. *Can J Neurol Sci* 1989; 16:28–40.

9. Findlay JM, Weir BKA, Kanamaru K, et al.: The effect of timing of intrathecal fibrinolytic therapy on cerebral vasospasm in a primate model of subarachnoid hemorrhage. *Neurosurgery* 1990; 26:201–206.

10. Gilsbach JM, Reulen HJ, Ljunggren B, et al.: Early aneurysm surgery and preventive therapy with intravenously administered nimodipine: A multicenter, double-blind, dose-comparison study. *Neurosurgery* 1990; 26:458–464.

11. Goslinga H, Eijzenbach V, Heuvelmans BS, et al.: Custom-tailored hemodilution with albumin and crystalloids in acute ischemic stroke. *Stroke* 1992; 23:181–188.

12. Handa Y, Weir BKA, Nosko M, et al.: The effect of timing of clot removal on chronic vasospasm in a primate model. *J Neurosurg* 1987; 67:558–564.

13. Hasan D, Vermeulen M, Wijdicks EFM, et al.: Effect of fluid intake and antihypertensive treatment on cerebral ischemia after subarachnoid hemorrhage. *Stroke* 1989; 20:1511–1515.

14. Heros RC, Korosue K: Hemodilution for cerebral ischemia. *Stroke* 1989; 20:423–427.

15. Higashida RT, Halbach VV, Cahan LD, et al.: Transluminal angioplasty for treatment of intracranial arterial vasospasm. *J Neurosurg* 1989; 71:648–653.

16. Hino A, Mizukawa N, Tenjin H, et al.: Postoperative hemodynamic and metabolic changes in patients with subarachnoid hemorrhage. *Stroke* 1989; 20:1504–1510.

17. Jones TH, Morawetz RB, Crowell RM, et al.: Thresholds of focal cerebral ischemia in awake monkeys. *J Neurosurg* 1981; 54:773–782.

18. Kassel NF, Haley EC, Torner JC, et al.: Nicardipine and angiographic vasospasm. *J Neurosurg* 1991; 74:341A.

19. Kassell NF, Peerless SJ, Durward QJ, et al.: Treatment of ischematic deficits from vasospasm with intravascular volume expansion and induced arterial hypertension. *Neurosurgery* 1982; 11:337–343.

20. Keller T, McGillicuddy J, LaBond V, et al.: Volume expansion in focal cerebral ischemia: The effect of cardiac output on local cerebral blood flow. *Clin Neurosurg* 1982; 29:40–50.

21. Kosnik EJ, Hunt WE: Postoperative hypertension in the management of patients with intracranial arterial aneurysms. *J Neurosurg* 1976; 45:148–154.

22. Kudo T, Suzuki S, Iwabuchi T: Importance of monitoring the circulating blood volume in patients with cerebral vasospasm after subarachnoid hemorrhage. *Neurosurgery* 1981; 9:514–520.

23. Levy ML, Giannotta SL: Induced hypertension and hypervolemia for treatment of cerebral vasospasm. *Neurosurg Clin North Am* 1990; 1:357–365.

24. Linskey ME, Horton JA, Rao GR, et al.: Fatal rupture of the intracranial carotid artery during transluminal angioplasty for vasospasm induced by subarachnoid hemorrhage. *J Neurosurg* 1991; 74:985–990.

25. Maroon J, Nelson P: Hypovolemia in patients with subarachnoid hemorrhage: Therapeutic implications. *Neurosurgery* 1979; 4:223–226.

26. McGillicudy JE, Kindt GW, Keller TS: Effects of intravascular volume expansion on blood flow in ischemic brain: A clinical and laboratory study, in Cervos-Navarro J, Fritschka E (eds): *Cerebral Microcirculation and Metabolism*. New York, Raven Press, 1981, pp 415–419.

27. Medlock MD, Dulebohn SC, Elwood PW: Prophylactic hypervolemia without calcium channel blockers in early aneurysm surgery. *Neurosurgery* 1992; 30:12–16.

28. Nakagomi T, Kassell NF, Hongo K, et al.: Pharmacological reversibility of experimental cerebral vasospasm. *Neurosurgery* 1990; 27:582–586.

29. Neil-Dwyer G, Mee E, Dorrence D, et al.: Early intervention with nimodipine in subarachnoid hemorrhage. *Eur Heart J* 1987; 8 (Suppl K):41–47.

30. Newell DW, Eskridge JM, Mayberg MR, et al.: Angioplasty for the treatment of symptomatic vasospasm following subarachnoid hemorrhage. *J Neurosurg* 1989; 71:654–660.

31. Ohman J, Heiskanen O: Effect of nimodipine on the outcome of patients after aneurysmal subarachnoid hemorrhage and surgery. *J Neurosurg* 1988; 69:683–686.

32. Origitano TC, Wascher TM, Reichman OH, et al.: Sustained increased cerebral blood flow with prophylactic hypertensive hypervolemic hemodilution ("Triple-H" therapy) after subarachnoid hemorrhage. *Neurosurgery* 1990; 27:729–740.

33. Pare L, Delfino R, Leblanc R: The relationship of ventricular-drainage to aneurysmal rebleeding. *J Neurosurg* 1992; 76:422–427.

34. Petruk KC, West M, Mohr G, et al.: Nimodipine treatment in poorgrade aneurysm patients. Results of a multicenter double-blind placebo-controlled trial. *J Neurosurg* 1988; 68:505–517.

35. Phillippon J, Grob R, Dagreou F, et al.: Prevention of vasospasm in subarachnoid hemorrhage, a controlled study with nimopidine. *Acta Neurochir (Wien)* 1986; 82:110–114.

36. Pickard JD, Murray GD, Illingworth R, et al.: Effect of oral nimodipine on cerebral infarction and outcome after subarachnoid hemorrhage. British aneurysm nimodipine trial. *Br Med J* 1989; 298:636–642.

37. Pritz MB: Treatment of cerebral vasospasm: Usefulness of Swan-Ganz Catheter monitoring of volume expansion. *Surg Neurol* 1984; 21:239–244.

38. Pritz MB, Giannotta SL, Kindt GW, et al.: Treatment of patients with neurological deficits associated with cerebral vasospasm by intravascular volume expansion. *Neurosurgery* 1978; 3:364–368.

39. Rosenstein J, Suzuki M, Symon L, et al.: Clinical use of a portable bedside cerebral blood flow machine in the management of aneurysmal subarachnoid hemorrhage. *Neurosurgery* 1984; 15:519–525.

40. Seifert V, Eisert WG, Stolke D, et al.: Efficacy of single intracisternal bolus injection of recombinant tissue plasminogen activator to prevent delayed cerebral vasospasm after experimental subarachnoid hemorrhage. *Neurosurgery* 1989; 25:590–598.

41. Shah KB, Rao TLK, Laughlin S, et al.: A review of pulmonary artery catheterization in 624 patients. *Anesthesiology* 1985; 61:271–275.

42. Shibuya M, Suzuki Y, Sugita K, et al.: Effect of AT 877 on cerebral vasospasm after aneurysmal subarachnoid hemorrhage. *J Neurosurg* 1992; 76:571–577.

43. Solomon RA, Fink ME, Lennihan L: Early aneurysm surgery and prophylactic hypervolemic hypertensive therapy for the treatment of aneurysmal subarachnoid hemorrhage. *Neurosurgery* 1988; 23:699–704.

44. Solomon RA, Post KD, McMurtry JG: Depression of circulating blood volume in patients after subarachnoid hemorrhage: Implications for the management of symptomatic vasospasm. *Neurosurgery* 1984; 15:354–361.

45. Thomas DJ, Marshall J, Ross Russell R, et al.: Effect of hematocrit on cerebral blood-flow in man. *Lancet* 1977; 2:941–945.

46. Tohgi H, Yamanouchi H, Murakami M, et al.: Importance of the hematocrit as a risk factor in cerebral infarction. *Stroke* 1978; 9:369–374.

47. Tranmer BI, Keller TS, Kindt GW, et al.: Loss of cerebral regulation during cardiac output variation in focal cerebral ischemia. *J Neurosurg* 1992; 77:253–259.

48. Vander Ark G, Pomerantz M: Reversal of ischemic neurological signs by increasing the cardiac output. *Surg Neurol* 1973; 1:257–258.

49. Wilkins RH: Attempts at prevention or treatment of intracranial arterial spasm: An update. *Neurosurgery* 1986; 18:808–825.

50. Wood JH, Simeone FA, Kron RE, et al.: Experimental hypervolemic hemodilution: Physiological correlations of cortical blood flow, cardiac output, and intracranial pressure with fresh blood viscosity and plasma volume. *Neurosurgery* 1984; 14:709–723.

51. Wood JH, Simeone FA, Kron RE, et al.: Rheological aspects of experimental hypervolemic hemodilution with low molecular weight dextran: Relationships of cortical blood flow, cardiac output, and intracranial pressure to fresh blood viscosity and plasma volume. *Neurosurgery* 1982; 11:739–753.

52. Zubkov YN, Nikiforov BM, Shustin VA: Balloon catheter technique for dilatation of constricted cerebral arteries after aneurysmal SAH. *Acta Neurochir (Wien)* 1984; 70:65–79.

21

Treatment of Giant Cavernous Aneurysms: Endovascular vs. Reconstruction

CASE

A 53-year-old man complained of intermittent diplopia for the past 3 years. The diplopia worsened on right lateral gaze and, about 4 weeks before his admission to the hospital, it became continuous. He has had a persistent headache behind his right eye and a tingling sensation on the right side of his face. His examination is remarkable for a right sixth-nerve palsy, decreased sensation in the V1 distribution on the right, and a diminished corneal reflex. His right pupil is slightly larger than the left, but remains reactive. Computed tomography shows a right cavernous sinus mass; an angiogram shows a large right cavernous sinus aneurysm. On the left carotid injection, flow is seen through the right A1 segment with right carotid compression.

PARTICIPANTS

Endovascular Treatment of Giant Cavernous Aneurysms—Kimberly Livingston, M.D., Arvind Ahuja, M.D., Leo N. Hopkins, M.D.

Reconstruction to Treat Giant Cavernous Aneurysms—Takanori Fukushima, M.D., D.M.Sc., John D. Day, M.D.

Moderator—Vinko V. Dolenc, M.D., Ph.D.

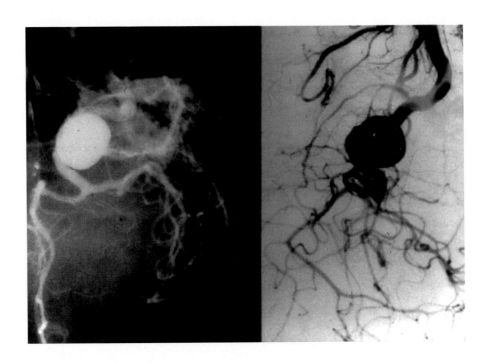

Endovascular Treatment of Giant Cavernous Aneurysms

Kimberly Livingston, M.D., Arvind Ahuja, M.D., Leo N. Hopkins, M.D.

Untreated cavernous carotid aneurysms are associated with a lower mortality compared with their supraclinoid counterparts, most likely because these lesions are confined by dura and bone, making rupture of an intracavernous aneurysm more likely to lead to carotid-cavernous fistula than to subarachnoid hemorrhage. For subarachnoid hemorrhage to occur, a portion of the ruptured cavernous aneurysm must extend through the dura of the cavernous sinus. Therefore, aneurysms of the anterior genu of the carotid siphon, giant intracavernous aneurysms, or aneurysms eroding into the sella turcica are more likely to cause dire consequences if they rupture.[5] Careful analysis of computed tomograms (CT), magnetic resonance images, and angiograms helps determine whether the subarachnoid space is preserved, but rarely with absolute certainty.

A review of the natural history of these lesions, based on a series of 44 aneurysms in 37 patients, suggests that the prognosis for cranial neuropathies or ipsilateral facial or orbital pain is quite variable.[5] Despite clinical progression, the cranial nerve symptoms from cavernous carotid aneurysms improved with time alone in some patients. The pathogenic mechanism for the cranial neuropathies associated with these lesions has not yet been proven. Cranial nerve compression certainly plays a role in many cases, but another possible mechanism is acute ischemia of the cranial nerve from thrombosis or compression of the branches of intracavernous arteries that supply the cranial nerves during their intracavernous course.

Radiographic indications for treating asymptomatic cavernous carotid aneurysms include an origin at the anterior genu of the siphon and extension of the aneurysm into the subarachnoid space. Indications for treating symptomatic lesions include subarachnoid hemorrhage, epistaxis, severe ipsilateral facial or orbital pain, radiographic evidence of aneurysm enlargement, progressive ophthalmoplegia, progressive visual loss,[5] and cerebral ischemic events secondary to emboli from giant aneurysms.

CASE ANALYSIS

Applying these criteria, the patient in question should be treated because of progressive visual deficit and a presumed increase in mass effect. Multiple angiographic views are required to establish the nature of the neck of this aneurysm, the turbulent flow within it, and the presence of mirror or multiple aneurysms. Magnetic resonance imaging is recommended to establish the true size of the lesion and the amount, if any, of partial thrombosis within the lumen. In cases of wide-neck lesions, endosaccular filling of the aneurysm with balloons, coils, or other embolic materials, while preserving normal flow through the parent vessel, is not possible with the technology presently available; these large lesions are dynamic entities with changes in turbulent flow and thrombus formation.[3] Therefore, even if embolic materials could be optimally positioned through endosaccular methods, they have a significant risk of migrating out of the aneurysm. The partial protrusion of a coil or balloon into the parent vessel can lead to embolic events and thrombosis of the parent vessel. For these reasons, endosaccular treatment of giant cavernous carotid aneurysms with a large neck is currently not recommended. Although not yet available for clinical use, intravascular stents placed across the orifice of the aneurysm, preserving flow through the parent vessel, may be the best treatment for this disease in the future.

OCCLUSION OF THE PARENT VESSEL

Can this patient tolerate sacrifice of the parent vessel, in this case, the right internal carotid artery? Angiographic demonstration of cross-flow with manual compression of the contralateral vessel is insufficient to answer this question; a balloon test occlusion should be done. This involves inflating a balloon in the parent vessel with fluoroscopic demonstration of stasis in the distal vessel and monitoring the patient's neurological status for at least 30 minutes to detect changes in vision, memory, speech, and motor function.

Erba and colleagues[1] categorized patients who could tolerate test occlusion with corroborative xenon/CT cerebral blood flow studies into 3 groups: Patients in group I had no significant change in cerebral blood flow with internal carotid artery occlusion; those in group II showed a symmetric decrease in cerebral blood flow; and those in group III had an asymmetric decrease in cerebral blood flow, always greater on the occluded side. A fourth group could not tolerate even brief carotid occlusion. Because disturbance of neuronal function may not occur until flow values reach 20 ml/100 g/min or lower, a patient may have compromised blood flow reserves with a clinically normal test occlusion, creating a susceptibility to a delayed deficit after occlusion. Patients in the group with asymmetric blood flow below 30 ml/100 g/min (group III) were considered at moderate to high risk for delayed deficit after carotid sacrifice.

An unequivocal intolerance of balloon test occlusion, that is, neurological deficit or evidence of hypoperfusion on transcranial Doppler or xenon/CT, suggests that strong consideration be given to an intracranial bypass before definitive surgical or endovascular treatment.

WHAT IS THE BEST TREATMENT?

Assuming the patient has evidence of good collateral flow, what is the best treatment? The best treatment is one that obliterates the lesion with minimal morbidity and mortality. In reasonably healthy individuals, if the size of the aneurysm and the configuration of its neck appear favorable on the angiogram and magnetic resonance images, the lesion should be surgically explored and clipped. In medically high-risk patients, those who have unclippable giant aneurysms or fusiform or wide-neck lesions, or those whose lesions can be surgically explored but are unclippable, endovascular balloon occlusion of the carotid artery proximal to the aneurysm can effectively treat the aneurysm, with protection from hemorrhage and clinical improvement.[4] Balloons can now be placed in the artery with maximum control and safety. Although the endovascular trapping of large, partially thrombosed aneurysms is technically possible, the thrombotic area may be disrupted by the distal balloon catheter, causing embolic infarction. If distal occlusion is necessary, surgery may be the treatment of choice.

RESULTS OF ENDOVASCULAR TREATMENT

How reliable is endovascular treatment? The largest series reported is from Fox and Higashida. In 1987, Fox and colleagues[2] reported on 68 patients with unclippable aneurysms (of which 37 were infraclinoid in origin) treated through proximal arterial occlusion with detachable balloons. They reported 9 cases (13%) of delayed cerebral ischemia, with 1 instance of permanent stroke. In 1990, Higashida and associates[4] reported a series of 87 patients with cavernous carotid aneurysms treated using endovascular detachable balloon techniques. Therapeutic occlusion of the internal carotid artery across, or just proximal to, the aneurysmal neck was done in 68 patients (78%). Endosaccular treatment was done in 19 patients (22%). Follow-up angiograms showed complete thrombosis with partial or total alleviation of symptoms in all patients with therapeutic occlusion of the parent vessel. Of the 19 patients undergoing endosaccular treatment, 12 (63%) had total exclusion and 7 (37%) had subtotal occlusion (85% or greater), with clinical improvement in all patients (no deaths). The morbidity rate for transient ischemia was 10.34% and the permanent morbidity rate was 4.6%.

In most patients, endovascular detachable balloon occlusion for carotid cavernous aneurysms is preferred to traditional Hunterian ligation. With a local anesthetic and the transfemoral approach, an awake patient can undergo continuous neurological monitoring during positioning of the balloon before detachment. Because the balloon is placed at or near the neck of the aneurysm, there may be less risk of filling from collateral branches of the internal carotid artery and a presumably lower chance of delayed washout of emboli during thrombosis of the aneurysm and carotid artery.[4]

OTHER CONSIDERATIONS

Bilateral cavernous carotid aneurysms present special challenges to an already difficult problem, yet the decision-making algorithms are similar to those for the solitary lesion. Subarachnoid hemorrhage, epistaxis, progressive ophthalmoplegia, progressive visual loss, ischemic episodes, or intractable facial pain are considerations for treatment. If a patient has a congenital condition that lends itself to multiple aneurysm formation, complete cure is unlikely. If the carotid artery is occluded to treat a mirror aneurysm, the contralateral lesion is more likely to grow. Nonetheless, if treatment of any kind is entertained, a balloon test occlusion is recommended. If the patient tolerates trial occlusion on both sides, the more accessible lesion may be surgically treated, followed by elective treatment of the inaccessible contralateral lesion through carotid balloon occlusion. If the patient does not tolerate occlusion on one or both sides, a bypass should be done before definitive treatment.

The optimum goals for treating patients with cavernous carotid aneurysms are eliminating mass effect, obliterating the aneurysm and risk of future rupture, and preserving the parent vessel or, at least, restoring normal territorial flow. These goals must be balanced with a reasonable knowledge of the nature of the disease and the limitations of the technology and technicians involved.

Reconstruction to Treat Giant Cavernous Aneurysms

Takanori Fukushima, M.D., D.M.Sc., John D. Day, M.D.

This patient shows the typical signs of an intracavernous giant aneurysm in a relatively young man. This patient has a slowly progressive disturbance of ocular motility, retro-orbital pain, and a trigeminal neuropathy. Studies of patients with intracavernous aneurysms have documented the low rate of symptoms resulting from aneurysmal rupture and the fairly high percentage of patients who are asymptomatic at presentation. In one study[13] of 37 patients with intracavernous aneurysms, 34% of patients had symptoms at presentation. Seven of these patients had giant aneurysms and, although it was not specifically stated, we suspect that the occurrence of symptoms was much higher in that subgroup. Of these 37 patients, 57% had symptoms of mass effect (43% with sixth-nerve paresis, 32% with trigeminal involvement, 20% with third-nerve paresis, and 16% with fourth-nerve paresis). About one third (36%) of the patients had headache. These numbers appear to be consistent with the senior author's personal experience with intracavernous aneurysms.[8]

This patient's angiogram clearly depicts the aneurysm, which probably originates from the C4 portion of the intracavernous carotid artery (Fischer nomenclature[5]). Unfortunately, however, the neck of the aneurysm is not well visualized. This aneurysm may be of the fusiform type, having no distinct neck, or it may have a wide, broad neck. The anatomy of the aneurysmal neck has a heavy impact upon the surgeon's decision regarding the approach to treatment. Considering the patient's age and the progressive nature of his symptoms, we favor aggressive treatment to prevent further compromise of the involved cranial nerves. Without therapy, this patient could have further dysfunction of ocular motility and increased pain in the trigeminal distribution or hypesthesia.

ENDOVASCULAR THERAPY

Several series report the results of patients with intracavernous aneurysms who have undergone endovascular occlusion of the intracavernous carotid artery. In 1974, Serbinenko[18] reported on 12 patients with intracavernous aneurysms treated through occlusion of the intracavernous segment. Since that time, several other authors have reported mostly favorable results in similar patients, from the standpoint of successful occlusion of the parent artery and relief of symptoms.[1,6,11,12,14,16,21] The major drawback of these methods has been the incidence of ischemic complications from propagation of thrombus and embolic phenomena. In the series of Fox and colleagues[6] describing 37 patients with cavernous aneurysms, 3 patients suffered ischemic complications, 1 permanent. The largest series reported to date describes 87 such patients with intracavernous aneurysms.[11] Of these, 39 patients had giant aneurysms. Temporary ischemic complications occurred in 10.3% of patients; and permanent ischemic complications were seen in 4.6%. In series reported in the medical literature, ischemic complications range from 4.6 to 50%.[11,21] Some surgeons have employed concomitant extracranial-intracranial bypass procedures, which have not met expectations in significantly reducing complications.[1,6]

A second issue involves the ability of these procedures to maintain the patency of the parent vessel. In several series,[1,6,18,21] all patients experienced complete occlusion of the intracavernous carotid artery (a total of 77 patients combined). Linskey and colleagues[14] reported that patency of the vessel was achieved in 5 of 11 patients undergoing endovascular treatment for large or giant intracavernous aneurysms. The highest percentage of parent vessel patency to date was reported in 1982 by Romodanov and Shcheglov,[16] who achieved a 73% patency rate in 67 patients with aneurysms of the internal carotid artery. Their series, however, showed a 9% mortality rate with 4.5% morbidity. In the series reported by Higashida and associates,[11] only 22% of patients had their aneurysms selectively occluded by detachable balloons; the rest had occlusion of the parent vessel. Of those patients with selective aneurysmal occlusion, all but 7 had complete occlusion of the aneurysm at 1-year follow-up. Four of these 22% underwent a second procedure to correct a defect in the aneurysm left by a shifting balloon. This seems to be a particular problem in the case of a giant aneurysm, which may require more than balloon for obliteration. A number of patients reported to have patency have not had complete embolization of the aneurysm, which maintains the risk of subsequent rerupture. On the basis of the information reported in these series, these balloon techniques are successful in occluding only the aneurysm in a limited number of cases, and obliteration is especially difficult in patients with giant intracavernous aneurysms.

In view of the angiographic features of the lesion in this patient, embolizing this aneurysm would be difficult with either detachable balloons or coils and preservation of the carotid artery. The treatment of giant aneurysms using such methods carries not only the risk of ischemic complications, but also the possibility of a fatal rupture during the procedure.[21] The inability to control an intraprocedural hemorrhage is a major disadvantage of these methods.

CAROTID LIGATION

Clearly, ligation of the cervical common or internal carotid artery has been the predominant form of surgical therapy for patients with intracavernous giant aneurysms in the past 30 years. As this technique has developed, it has been combined with extracranial-intracranial bypass procedures. The experience with these techniques is significant, and various authors have extensively documented the associated risks and resultant morbidity and mortality.[10,17] The cooperative study[15] published in 1966 cited an ischemic complication rate of 30% in all patients undergoing ligation of either the common or the internal carotid artery, for both ruptured and unruptured aneurysms. Of these complications, 89% occurred within the first 4 days after occlusion. Of patients with ruptured aneurysms, 8% suffered a delayed subarachnoid hemorrhage after occlusion, with 3.5% of unruptured aneurysms bleeding after ligation. In series published between 1960 and 1981, the ischemic complication rate varied between 0 and 32%, with mortality ranging from 0 to 29%. The late rebleed rate varied from 3.4 to 20%, and all repeated bleeding caused death.[17] Several other series of small numbers of patients published in the 1980s reported a high rate of ischemic morbidity.[2,3,9,19]

EC-IC Bypass

Extracranial-intracranial (EC-IC) bypass has been combined with carotid ligation with the goal of improving the high rate of ischemic complications. The neurosurgical literature reports a range from 0 to 60% of ischemia after EC-IC bypass done either concomitantly or before ligation.[9,17] The ischemic complications have varied, being both permanent and temporary. In the Japanese cooperative study of 137 patients,[15] all underwent EC-IC bypass either before ligation (63 patients) or at the same time (73 patients). Of these, 25% suffered ischemic complications, with 61% of these complications resulting in permanent deficits. Six of these 34 patients died as a result of the procedure. The ischemic complication rate of 25% should be considered high because these patients all had an EC-IC bypass to compensate for decreased distal flow.

The efficacy of the EC-IC bypass has been studied in experiments[9] which showed that a bypass can increase distal flow by only about 10 ml per 100 grams of tissue. Experimental studies have provided data about the minimum amount of cerebral blood flow necessary before changes are seen on an electroencephalogram. The values reported have been around 40 ml per 100 grams of tissue. In about 20% of patients undergoing carotid ligation, the distal flow is only about 20 ml per 100 grams. An EC-IC bypass provides only about 30 ml per 100 grams, which is not adequate. In Gelber and Sundt's clinical series of 10 patients undergoing ligation coupled with EC-IC bypass,[9] 7 patients had intracavernous aneurysms. None of these patients suffered permanent deficits from ischemia, but the authors estimated that the complication rate would have approached 60% without the bypass. This estimation was based on the fact that a number of these patients had a flow of under 20 ml per 100 grams with occlusion alone.

We conclude from this data that carotid ligation harbors many risks to the patient in terms of potential morbidity from ischemia, and a significant risk of mortality. In many patients, flow is not sufficient, even with an EC-IC bypass, to maintain adequate distal blood flow. The procedure also has caused a significant rate of late, fatal rebleeding. We believe that this method should, therefore, be reserved for a select subgroup of patients who cannot tolerate a direct approach.

DIRECT APPROACHES

The pioneering work of Dolenc[4] in the development of a combined epi- and subdural approach to the cavernous sinus has provided a method for safe access with acceptable morbidity. In addition to allowing a better understanding of the microsurgical anatomy involved, modern microsurgical techniques and refinements have made direct obliteration possible with a high success rate.[4,7,8,14,20] Our experience shows that most intracavernous aneurysms can be clipped safely. In patients with giant intracavernous aneurysms, however, significant technical difficulty and the risk of cranial nerve complications remain.[8] In the senior author's series of 37 patients with intracavernous giant aneurysms, 7 have been directly obliterated, 5 through direct clip ligation, and 2 through trapping after unsuccessful clip ligation. The remaining 30 aneurysms were treated with an interpositioned saphenous vein bypass that excludes the aneurysm from the circulation (Table 1).

Interpositioned Saphenous Bypass

Attempts to directly obliterate intracavernous giant aneurysms carry a significant risk of failure because of the difficulties encountered in dissecting the aneurysm neck and freeing the often-adherent cranial nerves. Determining the anatomy of the aneurysm's neck also can be difficult in these cases. Because of

Table 1. Direct Surgical Approach to Intracavernous Giant Aneurysms (n = 37)

Methods	No. of patients
Saphenous vein bypass	30
Clip ligation	5
Trapping	2
Complications	
Hemiparesis	2
Deafness	2
Blindness	1

these inherent difficulties, the senior author first carried out an interpositioned saphenous vein bypass of the intracavernous carotid artery to exclude a giant aneurysm from the circulation.[20] In this procedure, the anterior and posterolateral cavernous triangles are opened to expose the carotid siphon and intrapetrous carotid, respectively. The aneurysm is trapped and this segment is then replaced with a 6 to 7 cm saphenous vein interpositioned graft (Fig. 1). Either an end-to-end or end-to-side anastomosis is done, and occlusion time in this procedure has ranged from 1 to 2 hours. Patients undergoing this procedure are monitored by EEG and are administered various pharmacological agents to protect against ischemia. This procedure has been well-described in the literature.[8,20]

Results of the Series A 45-year-old woman came to medical attention with symptoms similar to those in the patient described in this case (Fig. 2). She had a giant aneurysm of the left C4 segment that was successfully treated with an interpositioned saphenous vein bypass (Fig. 3).

Two patients in this series had an ischemic complication from the bypass that resulted in permanent hemiparesis. One patient suffered an acute occlusion of the graft with temporary ischemia, which was corrected after a second surgery to open the graft. One patient had a late, asymptomatic occlusion of the graft discovered on routine postoperative angiography.[8] This series, therefore, has a 94% graft patency rate, and a 6.7% rate of permanent ischemic complications. In addition, 2 patients suffered ipsilateral deafness from cochlear damage during unroofing of the intrapetrous carotid artery in the middle fossa. Both of these patients were among the first to undergo this procedure. With refinements in technique regarding exposure of the intrapetrous carotid artery, no other patients suffered cochlear damage. One patient lost vision postoperatively secondary to an unknown cause. These figures yield a 16.7% complication rate. No mortality occurred. We expect the complication rate to fall as our experience increases with this procedure.

CONCLUSION

There are several advantageous features of the bypass procedure. The saphenous vein has about the same luminal size as the intracavernous carotid artery, preventing any significant reduction in flow. The graft is short and direct, and provides high flow in a physiological direction, and the anastomosis has a large diameter. In experienced hands, this procedure has a high rate of success. We, therefore, recommend that this procedure be used in this patient as it is most likely to allow obliteration of the aneurysm, with no chance of late rebleeding and minimal risk of ischemic complications.

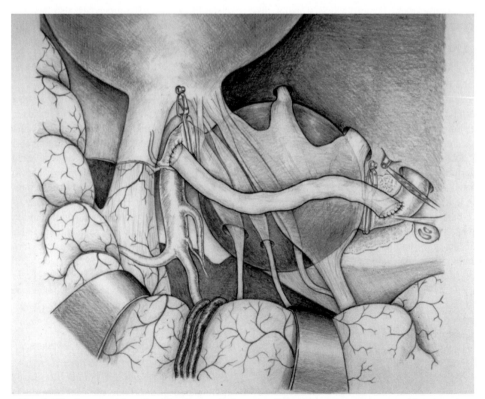

Fig. 1 The interpositioned saphenous vein bypass of the intracavernous carotid artery to treat a giant aneurysm.

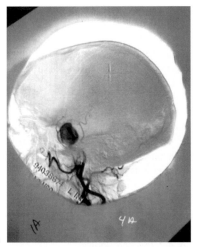

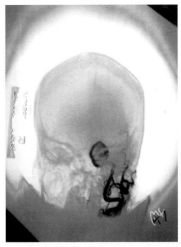

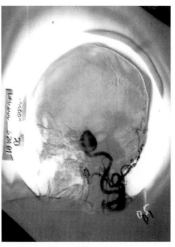

A B C

Fig. 2 (*A*) **Preoperative lateral angiogram of a giant intracavernous aneurysm of the C4 segment in a 45-year-old woman who presented with diplopia, headache, and hypesthesia of the left face.** (*B*) **Preoperative anteroposterior projection of the aneurysm.** (*C*) **Preoperative left anterior oblique view of the aneurysm.**

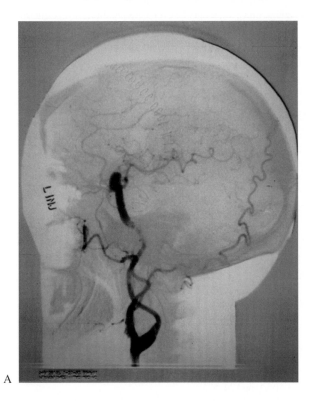

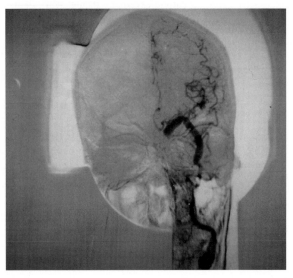

A B

Fig. 3 (*A*) **Postoperative lateral angiogram showing the bypassed intracavernous carotid artery excluding the giant aneurysm from the circulation.** (*B*) **Anterolateral projection of the postoperative angiogram.**

Treatment of Giant Cavernous Aneurysms: Endovascular vs. Reconstruction

Vinko V. Dolenc, M.D., Ph.D.

These 2 groups of authors describe the contemporary principle of treating large and giant intracavernous carotid aneurysms in a sound fashion. Both groups clearly emphasize that the site, size, and shape of the intracavernous aneurysm dictate the modality of treatment. For giant intracavernous aneurysms of the internal carotid artery, especially those that are partially thrombosed and have a broad neck, exclusion of the aneurysm is strongly indicated to prevent stroke. The indication for treatment is even

greater in patients with neurological deficits caused by stretching and compression of cranial nerves II–VI on the side of the lesion.

Both groups of authors agree that lesions with broad necks cannot be satisfactorily treated through endovascular techniques for various reasons: more than 1 balloon may be needed and coils could be brought further to the periphery, causing stroke. An incompletely occluded, partially thrombosed, large or giant aneurysm remains a permanent origin of emboli. Both groups of authors fully describe the necessary preoperative studies to determine brain perfusion. Carotid ligation is discredited because it does not solve the problem and risks postoperative complications.

ENDOVASCULAR TREATMENT

The authors advocating endovascular treatment of giant intracavernous aneurysms should clarify that aneurysms at the anterior genu are intracavernous when they originate from the proximal part of the anterior genu; they are carotid-ophthalmic when they originate from the distal segment of the anterior genu. The only exception is a traumatic aneurysm, which can be responsible for epistaxis, while other intracavernous aneurysms only occasionally, if ever, cause a nosebleed.

RECONSTRUCTION OF THE ARTERY WALL

The authors who advocate reconstruction to treat a giant aneurysm state that the rupture of such an aneurysm does not cause many symptoms. I cannot concur with this statement because the rupture of an intracavernous aneurysm of the internal carotid artery usually causes a carotid-cavernous fistula, with all its accompanying symptoms and signs. When the rupture of a small

intracavernous aneurysm does not cause a fistula but, instead, a large or giant aneurysm, the patient usually has a sudden onset of severe retrobulbar pain and ophthalmoplegia.

These authors recommend the use of a short venous bypass before dissecting the aneurysm. Although this is a good solution, it is not the only one.[1] Large or giant aneurysms with a neck should not be dissected circumferentially, but entered and then dealt with from inside. This approach allows the surgeon a good orientation of the neck, which can then be transected circumferentially from inside. This approach enables the surgeon to work far from the nerves on the surface of the aneurysm and occlude the neck with either a clip or a suture.

CONCLUSION

The patient described in this case has an intracavernous aneurysm of the internal carotid artery, for which endovascular treatment most probably is not the first choice. A direct surgical approach is indicated, and should be carried out by someone who has accumulated sufficient experience with this kind of lesion. The aneurysm could be trapped and the artery reconstructed through interpositioning of a venous graft.[2] In this patient, however, it may be even better to directly reconstruct the wall of the internal carotid artery.

REFERENCES

Kimberly Livingston, M.D., Arvind Ahuja, M.D., Leo N. Hopkins, M.D.

1. Erba SM, Horton JA, Latchaw RE, et al.: Balloon test occlusion of the internal carotid artery with stable xenon/CT cerebral blood flow imaging. *AJNR* 1988; 9:533–538.
2. Fox AJ, Viñuela F, Pelz DM, et al.: Use of detachable balloons for proximal artery occlusion in the treatment of unclippable cerebral aneurysms. *J Neurosurg* 1987; 66:40–46.
3. Graves VB, Strother CM, Partington CR, et al.: Flow dynamics of lateral carotid artery aneurysms and their effects on coils and balloons: An experimental study in dogs. *AJNR* 1992; 13:189–196.
4. Higashida RT, Halbach VV, Dowd C, et al.: Endovascular detachable balloon embolization therapy of cavernous carotid artery aneurysms: Results in 87 cases. *J Neurosurg* 1990; 72:857–863.
5. Linskey ME, Sekhar LN, Hirsch W Jr, et al.: Aneurysms of the intracavernous carotid artery: Natural history and indications for treatment. *Neurosurgery* 1990; 26:933–938.

Takanori Fukushima, M.D., D.M.Sc., John D. Day, M.D.

1. Berenstein A, Ransohoff J, Kupersmith M, et al.: Transvascular treatment of giant aneurysms of the cavernous carotid and vertebral arteries. *Surg Neurol* 1984; 21:3–12.
2. Diaz FG, Ohaegbulam S, Dujovny M, et al.: Surgical management of aneurysms in the cavernous sinus. *Acta Neurochir (Wien)* 1988; 91:25–28.
3. Diaz FG, Ohaegbulam S, Dujovny M, et al.: Surgical alternatives in the treatment of cavernous sinus aneurysms. *J Neurosurg* 1989; 71:846–853.
4. Dolenc VV: Direct microsurgical repair of intracavernous vascular lesions. *J Neurosurg* 1983; 58:824–831.
5. Fischer E: Die lagabweichrugan der vorderen hirnarterie in gefassbild. *Zentralb Neurochir* 1938; 3:300–312.
6. Fox AJ, Viñuela F, Pelz DM, et al.: Use of detachable balloons for proximal artery occlusion in the treatment of unclippable cerebral aneurysms. *J Neurosurg* 1987; 66:40–46.
7. Fukushima T: Direct operative approach to the vascular lesions in the cavernous sinus: Summary of 27 cases. *Mt Fuji Workshop Cerbrovas Dis* 1988; 6:169–189.
8. Fukushima T, Day JD, Tung H: Intracavernous carotid artery aneurysms, in Apuzzo MLJ (ed): *Brain Surgery: Complication Avoidance and Management*, vol. 1. New York, Churchill Livingstone, 1992, pp 925–944.
9. Gelber BR, Sundt TM: Treatment of intracavernous and giant carotid aneurysms by combined internal carotid ligation and extra- to intracranial bypass. *J Neurosurg* 1980; 52:1–10.
10. Hashi K, Nin K: Incidence of ischemic complications after carotid ligation combined with EC-IC bypass, in Spetzler RF (ed): *Cerebral Revascularization for Stroke*. New York, Thieme-Stratton, 1985, pp 570–577.
11. Higashida RT, Halbach VV, Dowd C, et al.: Endovascular detachable balloon embolization therapy of cavernous carotid artery aneurysms: Results in 87 cases. *J Neurosurg* 1990; 72:857–863.
12. Knuckey NW, Haas R, Jenkins R, et al.: Thrombosis of difficult intracranial aneurysms by the endovascular placement of platinum-Dacron microcoils. *J Neurosurg* 1992; 77:43–50.
13. Linskey ME, Sekhar LN, Hirsch W Jr, et al.: Aneurysms of the intracavernous carotid artery: Natural history and indications for treatment. *Neurosurgery* 1990; 26:933–938.
14. Linskey ME, Sekhar LN, Horton JA, et al.: Aneurysms of the intracavernous carotid artery: A multidisciplinary approach to treatment. *J Neurosurg* 1991; 75:525–534.
15. Nishioka H: Report on the cooperative study of intracranial aneurysms and subarachnoid hemorrhage: Section VIII, Part 1. Results of the treatment of intracranial aneurysms by occlusion of the carotid artery in the neck. *J Neurosurg* 1966; 25:660–682.

16. Romodanov AP, Shcheglov VI: Intravascular occlusion of saccular aneurysms of the cerebral arteries by means of a detachable balloon catheter. *Adv Tech Stand Neurosurg* 1982; 9:25–49.

17. Roski RA, Spetzler RF: Carotid ligation, in Wilkins RH, Rengachary SS (eds): *Neurosurgery*. New York: McGraw-Hill, 1985, pp 1414–1422.

18. Serbinenko FA: Balloon catheterization and occlusion of major cerebral vessels. *J Neurosurg* 1974; 41:125–145.

19. Silvani V, Rainoldi F, Gaetani P, et al.: Combined STA/MCA arterial bypass and gradual internal carotid artery occlusion for treatment of intracavernous and giant carotid artery aneurysms. *Acta Neurochir* 1985; 78:142–147.

20. Spetzler RF, Fukushima T, Martin N, et al.: Petrous carotid-to-intradural carotid saphenous vein graft for intracavernous giant aneurysm, tumor, and occlusive cerebrovascular disease. *J Neurosurg* 1990; 73:496–501.

21. Taki W, Nishi S, Yamashita K, et al.: Selection and combination of various endovascular techniques in the treatment of giant aneurysms. *J Neurosurg* 1992; 77:37–42.

Vinko V. Dolenc, M.D., Ph.D.

1. Dolenc VV: The necessity for intracavernous ICA reconstruction, in Sato K (ed): *Neurosurgeons. Proceedings of the Japanese Congress of Neurological Surgeons, Tokyo APPO*. Tokyo: Sci Med Publ, 1991, pp 299–307.

2. Spetzler RF, Fukushima T, Martui N, et al.: Petrous carotid to intradural carotid sphenous vein graft for intracavernous giant aneurysm, tumor, and occlusive cerebrovascular disease. *J Neurosurg* 1990; 73:496–501.

22

Conservative vs. Surgical Treatment of Unruptured Arteriovenous Malformations

CASE

A 24-year-old, right-handed man had intermittent episodes in which he lost his right visual field. This was not associated with any other neurological symptoms, and the field returned in 10 to 15 minutes with no residual deficit. Four years later, these episodes began to be associated with headaches, which were believed to be migraines with a visual aura. A magnetic resonance image showed a left posterior temporal arteriovenous malformation. The patient's neurological exam was normal.

PARTICIPANTS

Conservative Treatment of Unruptured Arteriovenous Malformations–Philip Azordegan, M.D.

Surgical Treatment of Unruptured Arteriovenous Malformations–Roberto C. Heros, M.D.

Moderator–Eugene George, M.D.

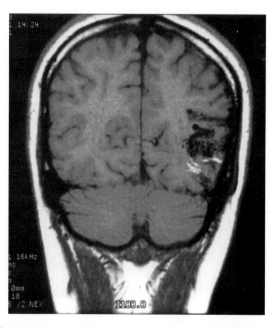 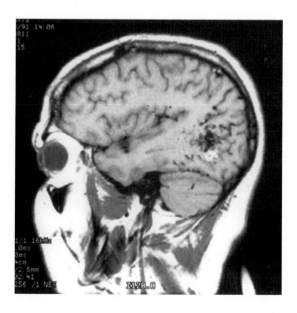

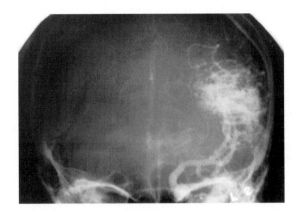
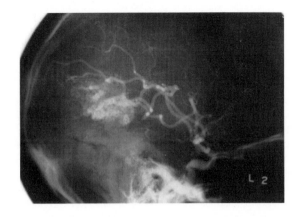

Conservative Treatment of Unruptured Arteriovenous Malformations

Philip Azordegan, M.D.

Before embarking on any treatment modality, a neurosurgeon must thoroughly define the problem at hand, delineate the goal of the treatment plan, review the various options in his or her therapeutic armamentarium, and carefully select the treatment that will best serve that particular patient. In doing so, a thorough knowledge of the natural history of the disease process, the patient's unique mental, physical, and emotional milieu, the potential complications (be they major or minor) of each therapeutic intervention, and the surgeon's own expertise must be considered. Only then may one recommend the "best" particular mode of treatment to preserve the patient's neurological function and quality of life.

This thorough, deliberate, and seemingly subliminal agenda grows even more imperative when a neurosurgeon deals with an arteriovenous malformation located within eloquent cortex—when the potential for a sudden, possibly catastrophic or fatal event entices the surgeon to "do something *now*." Notwithstanding the advances in microsurgical techniques, the modern neurosurgeon is no longer limited to the options of surgery and observation. Conservative nonoperative treatment of arteriovenous malformations no longer means that both the patient and the surgeon must passively wait for that patient's own unaltered natural history to unfold. There are still times, however, when our pledge first to do no harm should supersede our well-meaning desires to intervene.

CASE ANALYSIS

This case, in particular, underlines the sense of urgency one often feels when treating an arteriovenous malformation in a young person. Given an annual risk of hemorrhage estimated to be from 2.2 to 4% and about the same percentages for the combined annual mortality and morbidity,[4,6,10,17,18,20,21,23,25,26,28] the future for this 24-year-old man is unclear, if not precarious, and the urge to intervene is compelling. Notwithstanding this somber outlook, the physical characteristics of this patient's arteriovenous malformation, and symptoms unique to this particular lesion must temper the surgeon's zeal to "take it out" immediately.

This patient presents with headaches and intermittent symptoms consistent with a steal phenomenon affecting the visual cortex. Neither symptom has been associated with a statistically significant mortality rate versus other presenting symptoms of arteriovenous malformations.[5,11,16] In fact, the expected long-term morbidity rate would be lower in this patient as compared to a patient with a hemorrhage.[18] Yet, from an operative standpoint, Batjer and colleagues[2] have shown that evidence of a preoperative steal phenomenon is associated with higher incidences of postoperative morbidity and mortality.

Similarly, the most common error causing surgical morbidity is misjudging the topographical extent of the arteriovenous malformation.[19] The visual cortex is not the only eloquent area threatened by this malformation or its well-intentioned operative cure. In closely comparing this patient's magnetic resonance images and angiograms to previous radioisotope scans of lesions causing a Wernicke's aphasia[23] (Fig. 1), one would anticipate a significant operative risk to at least the posterior aspect of Wernicke's region. Although some might consider the loss of a visual field alone to be an acceptable outcome of a potentially life-preserving operation, few would argue that the quality of life for a patient with a life-expectancy approaching 50 years but with a debilitating postoperative Wernicke's aphasia justifies more than a minimal operative risk. This concern also extends

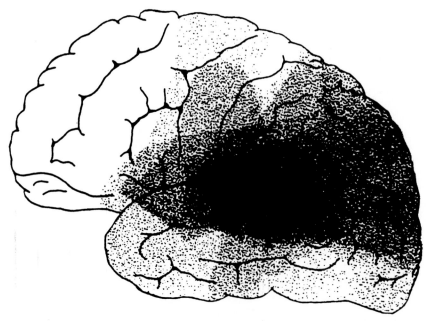

Fig. 1 Damaged areas resulting in Wernicke's aphasia. Infarcts in 13 patients, all causing Wernicke's aphasia, were superimposed after being determined by a technetium ⁹⁹ᵐTc scan.

to the quality of life of the family members entrusted with caring for this patient. Yet, as Heros and Korosue[19] have stated, a postoperative deficit is expected when an eloquent area is involved by an arteriovenous malformation.

GRADING AND RISKS

The risks for postoperative deficits depend greatly on the complexity of the malformation operated upon.[21,29] Thus, when estimating the size and drainage of this lesion to classify it according to the Spetzler-Martin system,[30,31] this arteriovenous malformation appears to be consistent with a grade IV or V. Unfortunately, even at centers of excellence, resecting malformations of grades IV or V (or those with similar physical characteristics) carries reports of major complications of surgery (defined as hemiparesis, aphasia, hemianopsia, or severe neurological deficit), poor outcomes (hemiplegia, severe speech deficits, akinetic mutism), and postoperative death or late serious morbidity (the patient was independent but unable to work, or incapacitated and incapable of independent living). Mortality ranged from about 2 to 35%, respectively.[11–14,22,23] Combined with the possible increased risk[2,19] from vessels of passage or perforating vessels from the middle cerebral artery and the lack of a significant, resolving hematoma to ease dissection,[29] the minimal risk of causing a permanent, debilitating postoperative deficit looms far more significant than the lifelong potential for a hemorrhage and its morbidity.

CONSERVATIVE TREATMENT

As stated earlier, nonoperative treatment of arteriovenous malformations is no longer confined to anxious observation of the patient. Recent studies involving embolization or radiosurgery for these lesions have shown some promising results. Multiple large series reporting embolization of arteriovenous malformations have shown angiographic cure rates between 5 and 17%, and partial reduction was seen in up to 95% of the malformations treated.[2,3,8–10,32,33] Embolization, however, is not immune to its own major complications. Reported stroke rates after embolization vary from 1.6 to 20%, and the overall risk of hemorrhage as a result of embolization in several large series was 4.3%,[1,2,4,7,8,10,11,16,19,24,26,32–34] almost one third of which were fatal.[1,4,7–9,26,33,34,36]

Treatment with radiosurgery alone has also demonstrated enticing results, with an overall 80% rate of angiographic obliteration within 2 to 3 years of treatment.[5,7,15,22,23,25,27,35] Regardless of whether the radiosurgery system is charged particle, gamma knife, or linac, the size of the lesion is a significant factor in the rates of both obliteration[22,23,25,28] and complication.[22,25] Using charged particles, Steinberg and colleagues[34] showed one of the best obliteration results of arteriovenous malformations greater than 25 cm³ (39% at 2 years and 70% at 3 years post-treatment). They also noted, however, a 12% incidence at follow-up of severe neurological complications, most being permanent neurological deficits (defined as gait ataxia, cranial nerve palsies, partial aphasia, hemiparesis, and hypothalamic syndrome). Steiner and colleagues[35,36] and other authors[13,23] have even suggested that most arteriovenous malformations are too large to be treated radiosurgically.

Combining embolization and radiosurgery as a nonoperative alternative shows promise in treating malformations such as the one in the patient presented here. By reducing the size of the arteriovenous malformation before radiosurgery, one conceivably could not only decrease the potential complications of an aggressive attempt to embolize 100% of a complicated malformation, but also reduce its volume. This should increase the chances of postradiation obliteration and reduce the volume-related complication rate of radiosurgery. Dawson and co-workers[9] showed a 2-year postradiation cure in 2 of 7 patients with large arteriovenous malformations reduced to 36 mm in greatest diameter before radiosurgery with only 1 transient complication. Similarly, Fournier and colleagues[13] showed a cure in 3 of 10 patients treated first through embolization and then with radiosurgery. Obviously, before this combined effort could be considered, the feasibility of partial embolization in the patient in this case would have to be ascertained during arteriography.

OTHER CONSIDERATIONS

Finally, and just as importantly as all of our systems and techniques, we must carefully consider the psychological effects on our patients produced by the various treatment options. Some patients deem living with a "time bomb" in their heads intolerable, irrespective of whether the lesion is untreated or within its postradiation, preobliteration latency period, and regardless of the potential risks of surgical intervention. Most patients, however, rely heavily or entirely upon the recommendations of their neurosurgeon.

For this 24-year-old, surgical eradication of this lesion, with its significant risk of postoperative hemianopsia and fluent aphasia, could submit him and his loved ones to decades of debilitation and adversity. It is incumbent upon us as neurosurgeons to show that our surgical results are clearly superior to the outcomes produced by nature. The fear of the potential future morbidity of this arteriovenous malformation must not hurry us towards surgical intervention and its potential for immediate and lifelong debilitation, unless we are certain of minimal risks.

Surgical Treatment of Unruptured Arteriovenous Malformations

Roberto C. Heros, M.D.

This patient has a cerebral arteriovenous malformation that has come to neurosurgical attention. The questions facing the neurosurgeon are:

- Should this lesion be treated at all?
- If treatment is to be recommended, what is the best form?
- How is that treatment best planned (i.e., if surgery is chosen,

which is the best approach and should preoperative embolization be considered; if radiosurgery is chosen, which modality would be best)?

Salient parts of the history that the neurosurgeon must factor in are the patient's age, the fact that the patient has no neurological deficit, the patient's right-handedness, indicating almost certainly that the lesion is located in the dominant hemisphere for speech, and the patient's presenting symptoms. In this case, the symptoms may all be related to migraine, which may or may not be relieved by excising the malformation. An important piece of history not given is the patient's occupation; it may make a difference as to whether the patient depends on the intactness of his speech for his livelihood or whether his job is more physical in nature.

ETHICAL ISSUES

I will begin by digressing into a question of ethics that is highly controversial. I firmly believe that a neurosurgeon has the responsibility to try to decide what is best for the patient, carefully considering all important factors such as age, medical and neurological condition, occupation and hobbies, family responsibilities and support systems, psychological make-up, and psychological reaction to the knowledge of having an arteriovenous malformation. To these patient-related factors must be added factors related to the lesion itself, including size, location, configuration, and pattern of arterial and venous supply. Finally, and very importantly, the surgeon must honestly consider his or her own experience with such lesions. In the end, the surgeon may believe that he or she has not had enough experience to expertly analyze these factors. If this should happen, referral to a neurosurgeon with more experience is indicated. If, however, the neurosurgeon believes he or she is capable of reaching an intelligent decision (whether the decision involves offering to excise the lesion himself or herself or to refer the patient to a more experienced surgeon or to a radiosurgeon), then he or she must forcefully convey this opinion to the patient. Only if the neurosurgeon truly believes that equally satisfactory options exist should these options be fairly presented as valid alternatives. Clearly, the surgeon must present alternatives that are, in the surgeon's opinion, less satisfactory, but they should be honestly presented as such. The "gold standard" should be "what I would chose for myself or my dear ones under your exact circumstances."

It is unfair to simply present a number of statistics to a patient and "wash our hands," thereby placing on the patient the entire burden of the decision. In most instances, the neurosurgeon is in a better position than the patient to know what is best for the patient. Although what to do is ultimately the patient's decision, the physician owes the patient unambiguous advice or referral to an expert who may be in a better position to give such advice.

Having been presented with the alternatives, the patient may still choose what the neurosurgeon considers a less satisfactory alternative, but we must then support that patient fully. He may choose to have no treatment, even though our unequivocal recommendation has been that he should have surgery. It is unkind at this point to emphasize that he has "a time bomb" in his head. The proper thing to do in this case is to be reassuring and emphasize that, in fact, the risk of a hemorrhage is "only" 3 to 4% per year and, of those malformations that do rupture, only about a third are of major clinical consequence.[8] I recommend to these patients a normal lifestyle without restrictions except for contact sports, competitive weight-lifting, sprinting, etc.

If surgical excision has been recommended, the patient may still opt for radiosurgery, in which case the neurosurgeon should facilitate referral to a reliable radiosurgical center. The problem is more difficult when the lesion is of borderline operability, the surgeon has recommended radiosurgery, and the patient responds, "I don't want any radiation to my body. I'd rather have it

taken out." There can be no rules about this. At this point, my approach—and I recall only a couple of instances of this situation—has been to refer the patient to a colleague for a second opinion and for my colleague to proceed with the surgery if he or she believes it should be done. I am reluctant to operate when I believe that another option is best.

If this is a valid ethical position for a surgeon when considering open surgery, should radiosurgery be subjected to the same standard? I believe that it should; that is, the radiosurgeon should not offer this modality of treatment unless he or she truly believes that it is, in fact, the best option, or at least an equally good option for the patient. Unfortunately, this standard is not held in several of the radiosurgical centers in which close to 50% of the lesions irradiated have been operable, generally meaning that surgical excision is the preferred modality for that lesion. The indications for radiosurgery in these cases has been given as "the patient's choice" or, worse, "preference of the referring physician."

CASE ANALYSIS

Let's go back now to the patient at hand. The lesion is moderate in size and superficial. The venous phase is not shown, but I assume that the venous drainage is primarily to the vein of Labbé. Is the lesion in an eloquent area? It certainly is at least adjacent to the angular gyrus of the dominant hemisphere. My sense, however, is that it is a bit below and posterior to it and, therefore, provided the surgeon stays right at the margin of the lesion, it can be excised without causing a significant speech deficit. I have found the Spetzler-Martin classification[11] both easy to use and reliable in predicting operative morbidity.

In this patient, however, the lesion may be borderline in 2 respects. For example, there may be a small deep vein even though, undoubtedly, the dominant venous drainage is superficial. Because the lesion is generally superficial to the plane of the posterior aspect of the insula, I would consider it superficial and not give it an extra point for deep venous drainage. Secondly, should the lesion be given an extra point for being in eloquent brain? With these lesions immediately adjacent to eloquent brain, where there is no margin of error, I have tended to classify them as eloquent; therefore, I would consider this a Spetzler-Martin Grade III (2 points for moderate size, 1 point for eloquence). In my reported series of 153 patients,[7] there was about 10% early surgical morbidity but no long-term serious disability or death with grade III lesions. Similar results are common in modern microsurgical series.[2,11,13] To the factors intrinsic to the lesion, we must add patient-related factors, such as age and general health, to estimate surgical morbidity. I will assume that, in fact, this young man is healthy and unlikely to suffer a major anesthetic or postoperative medical complication.

NATURAL HISTORY

Given the above analysis of the surgical risk, one must, of course, consider the natural history of this lesion. The fact that there is no history of hemorrhage has little bearing in overall yearly risk of hemorrhage, which has fairly consistently been established as 3 to 4% per year.[3,5,10,14] About a third of these hemorrhages lead to serious morbidity, and about 10% are fatal.[6] The patient's age is of paramount importance in the analysis of the natural history. The situation would be different if, instead of being 24 years of age with about another 50 years at risk from an actuarial point of view, the patient were 72 years with perhaps only about 8 more years at risk. General health, which I will assume here to be good, has a similar effect; I would not offer surgery to this patient if he had a malignancy that limits his life expectancy to a few years.

OTHER CONSIDERATIONS

In addition to surgical risk and natural history, other factors mentioned earlier are of importance. A knowledge of the patient's occupation and hobbies would allow us to predict the impact of a possible moderate speech deficit in his ability to earn a livelihood and on his quality of life. I assume that he is not incapacitated by his migraine spells, but what is his psychological reaction to his lesion? I have seen a number of patients who are devastated because they have been told of "the bomb in the head," and go from surgeon to surgeon begging to have their inoperable lesion removed, even if they are left paralyzed.

There is no formula, or decision-making statistical analysis that would allow us to weigh mathematically all of the above factors and arrive at a decision. Although based on some solid statistical information, such as the knowledge of the natural history and personal surgical results, the process of individual decision-making in these cases is highly subjective. It appears that this arteriovenous malformation can be removed with some risk, perhaps a 10 to 20% chance of a mild to moderate temporary speech deficit which, almost certainly, would improve to the point of being hardly noticeable in 3 to 6 months. In addition, I would tell the patient that there is a substantial risk of a permanent visual field deficit, but the risk of a complete hemianopsia is small. I would consider the risk of another major neurological deficit, such as hemiplegia or death, to be minimal and would quote it as less than 1%. Given the patient's young age and assumed good general condition, chances are high (at least 30%) that, if left untreated, this lesion eventually will bleed and lead to disability or death.

RECOMMENDATIONS

Considering all of the above, I would recommend surgical excision to this patient. If he told me that under no circumstance would he accept even a moderate speech deficit as a result of surgery and would rather have radiosurgery, I would gladly refer him, with my encouragement, for that procedure. Had the lesion been located 3 cm anterior and 3 cm superior to its real location, I would have recommended radiosurgery as the treatment of choice with conservative therapy (which, in the case of an arteriovenous malformation is essentially no therapy) as a reasonable option. I would not operate even if the patient said, "I can't stand the idea of having my head irradiated." If the lesion were located 3 cm inferiorly along the inferior temporal gyrus, I would be even more emphatic about recommending surgical excision. I would not present radiosurgery as a reasonable option, and would be disappointed to learn that one of my colleagues irradiated such a lesion.

There is no controversy here about the surgical approach, which must be through a standard temporal craniotomy and skin flap. Preoperative embolization is not necessary in this case. I use this modality for 2 reasons:

- To prevent normal perfusion breakthrough,[1,12] a complication that is extremely unlikely with this relatively small lesion with only moderate-size feeding arteries and no angiographic evidence of steal from the surrounding brain.
- To occlude major arterial pedicles that are difficult to reach through the surgical exposure.

Even though the vertebral injection was not shown, this lesion appears to be too high to have major posterior cerebral feeders. If it did, they would come around the convexity, where they could be readily controlled at surgery. Embolizing the middle cerebral supply to decrease flow and facilitate surgical dissection is reasonable, and I would not condemn it. These are long, tortuous feeders, however, some of which could be vessels in passage, and embolization has the risk of occluding some important branches. Overall, I would judge the risk of embolization and surgery as being greater than the risk of surgery alone; therefore, I would not recommend preoperative embolization.

Is embolization alone a reasonable option? I do not think so. First, embolization alone has practically no chance of eliminating this lesion completely.[4,15] Second, I know of no definite proof that partial reduction of flow through embolization (or any other means) has any beneficial effect on the natural history of these lesions. Finally, even when relatively permanent embolic agents are used, abundant evidence shows that recanalization occurs in time unless the lesion is excised.[4,9] The only instances in which I have recommended embolization without surgery is in cases of large, inoperable lesions to palliate symptoms referable to steal or increase intracranial pressure, or to relieve severe headaches, which are sometimes related to enlarged meningeal feeders that can be embolized. There is no question that embolization alone can cure simple, small arteriovenous malformations and fistulae with a limited number of feeders. I believe, however, that most lesions that can be cured through embolization alone can also be cured, with less risk, through surgical excision.

Conservative vs. Surgical Treatment of Unruptured Arteriovenous Malformations

Eugene George, M.D.

This patient certainly represents one of the most difficult therapeutic decisions facing neurosurgeons having the privilege to treat a significant number of intracranial arteriovenous malformations. This 24-year-old, right-handed man has a left post-temporal arteriovenous malformation presenting only with transient episodes of right visual field. There is no history of hemorrhage or seizures. The lesion appears to be about 4 cm in size, is likely located just adjacent to the angular gyrus, and is presumably draining only superficially. It should probably be classified as a Spetzler-Martin grade III.[1] Although we can presume left cerebral dominance, we cannot be sure about the speech location because it is often displaced in such patients. We do not know his occupation.

CONSERVATIVE TREATMENT

Azordegan has done an excellent job of presenting an extremely rational approach for carefully assessing the risk of intervening with current risk, in an attempt to prevent the possibility of an event with greater risk occurring in the future. He addresses the quality of years concept by discussing the effect on a young person with a fluent aphasia and right visual field loss to prevent a life-threatening or severely disabling deficit from potentially occurring. He rather deftly refers to a superb chapter by Heros and Korosue[1] that includes much discussion, referring to significant surgical morbidity incurred from lesions unexpectedly found to invade eloquent areas. Indeed, Heros lists this as one of the most common causes of significant surgical morbidity. Although the possible risk of a partial homonymous hemianopsia might be acceptable to most patients and neurosurgeons in return for removing this lesion, the more than remote possibility of a permanent dysphasia is the most troublesome aspect. One probably should disagree with Azordegan's seeming to include embolization and radiosurgery under conservative, nonoperative treatment because both of these modalities are therapeutic undertakings with significant risks. To embolize this lesion without some subservient therapeutic plan to obliterate it runs an excessively high therapeutic risk, for a rather low likelihood of really effecting the lesion's natural history. Certainly, there is as of yet no definite evidence that anything short of total obliteration really improves the long-term natural history of an arteriovenous malformation. And it is certainly doubtful that this is the type of malformation treatable with a combination of embolization and radiosurgery.

SURGICAL EXCISION

Heros likewise has done an excellent job in weighing out the salient features a surgeon should consider in assessing this problem. I strongly agree and recommend reading his discussions of surgical ethics regarding the responsibility of the surgeon to first thoroughly assess the problem, then clearly and fairly present the various therapeutic approaches to the patient and then to take a definite position, not merely assume the role of passive conveyor of statistics. With respect to this specific patient, he describes the lesion as "at least adjacent to the angular gyrus of the dominant hemisphere." Heros presents an adequate discussion of the pros and cons of radiosurgery and embolization. Because he believes there is no definite evidence that the absence of hemorrhage has any affect on the natural history of the lesion, and that the yearly risk of hemorrhage for this patient would be 3 to 4%, he recommends proceeding with an attempted surgical resection of this lesion. He also gives an overview of the operative considerations.

Both Azordegan and Heros correctly point out that we are progressively getting good data regarding the risk of hemorrhage for symptomatic patients with arteriovenous malformations, regardless of whether they have seizures or bleeding. However, I disagree slightly with Heros' effort to take current data about the natural history that was obtained almost entirely from symptomatic patients having either seizures or bleeding, and applying this data to patients who are either totally asymptomatic or who have only easily classifiable symptoms, such as cerebral steal or migraine-like vascular headaches.

NATURAL HISTORY

Data is still extremely sparse regarding the natural history of arteriovenous malformations in patients who are asymptomatic or, at least, who have not had hemorrhage or a definite seizure. Even in Troop's series of 168 patients followed postoperatively for more than 24 years,[1] a series which Steve Ondra and I had the privilege to review and carefully follow-up, there was not a sufficient number of patients with signs other than seizures and

hemorrhages for us to comment upon. Certainly, there was no difference between patients with hemorrhage versus those with only seizure. Furthermore, although the average bleed rate was at least 4% per year, and actually probably greater, with a mortality rate of 1% per year and a combined significant morbidity and mortality rate of 2.7% per year, the rebleed data naturally includes progressively a number of patients with serial rebleeding. Indeed, even at 24 years follow-up of these symptomatic patients, more than 50% of the individual patients have not re-bled. Hence, one can make the case that patients with lesions in extremely eloquent regions might reasonably be followed until they develop hemorrhage or seizures before recommending high-risk intervention. I am not saying that this lesion is precisely in that category but, on the other hand, it would certainly follow that a more conservative approach is increasingly justified for relatively asymptomatic patients with increasingly high-risk lesions.

OTHER CONSIDERATIONS

As Heros noted, this patient's occupation is also important; that is, if the patient is a linguist, translator, or in some language-related field, additional weight would be added to choosing a more conservative approach. Such patients are understandably more likely to have major problems in this area, even with a good resection in an area where primary speech should not be permanently affected. This risk may be more acceptable in a patient who has already had a bleed or seizures, but it becomes more of a concern for patients in whom the natural history is less clear.

I believe the risk of significant but temporary speech deficit after resection of the lesion in this patient is higher than 10 to 20%, and probably approaches 50%. Certainly, most of these patients would have their speech clear over the next 6 to 10 months. Unquestionably, however, some patients will have a permanent disabling deficit. All of us who have had the privilege of treating significant numbers of patients with intracranial arteriovenous malformations have individual recollections of such patients. If this lesion in this almost asymptomatic patient were further away from eloquent areas, such as at the anterior frontal pole or anterior-inferior temporal lobe, one could easily make an excellent case for surgical resection. If the lesion were smaller, a radiosurgical approach would also be a reasonable option and should at least be offered to the patient. For this patient, however, l would not recommend radiosurgery because this lesion is almost definitely at least 4 cm or greater in size, thus decreasing the likelihood of achieving a cure and increasing the likelihood of other untoward complications, such as radiation necrosis.

RECOMMENDATIONS

I would not recommend any therapeutic intervention at this time for this patient. If this young man had had a hemorrhage or seizures, or does so, I would recommend an attempted microsurgical resection. The approach to this lesion appears to be amenable to incorporating awake, open cortical mapping to carefully delineate speech areas before resection. One might possibly obtain this information sufficiently with miniballoon catheterization and barbiturate infusions, but this approach is much less reliable. This is a relatively small lesion; thus, one could easily map the lesion with the patient awake and then anesthetize the patient and proceed with a resection. Similarly, if this is one of those rare patients who has significant speech within the malformation, I would not recommend resection. Furthermore, one might consider preoperative embolization.

This lesion has fairly good flow in an eloquent area; embolization might well decrease the lesion to a minimal vascular malformation, allowing a more precise resection and decreasing the chance of potential trauma in at least closely adjacent eloquent areas. This approach is debatable, however, and I would be far more convinced of the value of cortical speech mapping.[1,3]

REFERENCES

Philip Azordegan, M.D.

1. Bank WO, Kerber CW, Cromwell LD: Treatment of intracranial arteriovenous malformations with isobutyl 2-cyanoacrylate: Initial clinical experience. *Radiology* 1981; 139:609–616.
2. Batjer HH, Devous MD, Seibert GB, et al.: Intracranial arteriovenous malformations: Relationship between clinical factors and surgical complications. *Neurosurgery* 1989; 24:75–79.
3. Barrow DL, Reisner A: Natural history of intracranial aneurysms and vascular malformations. *Clin Neurosurg* 1993: 40:3–39.
4. Berthelsen B, Lofgren J, Svendson P: Embolization of cerebral arteriovenous malformations with bucrylate: Experience in a first series of 29 patients. *Acta Radiol* 1990; 31:13–21.
5. Betti OO, Munari C, Rosler R: Serotactic radiosurgery with the linear accelerator: Treatment of arteriovenous malformations. *Neurosurgery* 1989; 24:311–321.
6. Brown RD Jr, Wiebers DO, Forbes C, et al.: The natural history of unruptured intracranial arteriovenous malformations. *J Neurosurg* 1988; 68:352–357.
7. Columbo F, Benedetti A, Pozza F, et al.: Linear accelerator radiosurgery of cerebral arteriovenous malformations. *Neurosurgery* 1989; 24:833–840.
8. Cromwell LD, Harris AB: Treatment of cerebral arteriovenous rnalformations: Combined neurosurgical and neuroradiologic approach. *AJNR* 1983; 4:366–368.
9. Dawson RC III, Tarr RW, Hecht ST, et al.: Treatment of arteriovenous malformations of the brain with combined embolization and stereotactic radiosurgery: Results after 1 and 2 years. *AJNR* 1990; 11:857–864.
10. Debrun G, Vinuela FV, Fox AJ, et al.: Embolization of cerebral arteriovenous malformations with bucrylate: Experience in 46 cases. *J Neurosurg* 1982; 56:615–627.
11. Deruty R, Lapras C, Patet JD, et al.: Intra-operative embolization of cerebral arteriovenous malformations by means of isobutylcyanoacrylate (experience in 20 cases). *Neurol Res* 1986; 8:109–113.
12. Fabrikant JI, Levy RP, Steinbert GK, et al.: Heavy charged-particle radiosurgery for intracranial arteriovenous malformations. *Stereotact Funct Neurosurg* 1991; 57:50–63.
13. Fournier D, TerBrugge KG, Willinsky R, et al.: Endovascular treatment of intracerebral arteriovenous malformations: Experience in 49 cases. *J Neurosurg* 1991; 75:228–233.
14. Fox AJ, Pelz DM, Lee DH, et al.: Arteriovenous malformations of the brain: Recent results of endovascular therapy. *Radiology* 1990; 177:51–57.
15. Friedman WA, Bova FJ: Linear accelerator radiosurgery for arteriovenous malformations. *J Neurosurg* 1992; 77:832–841.
16. Fults D, Kelly DL Jr: Natural history of arteriovenous malformations of the brain: A clinical study. *Neurosurgery* 1984; 15:658–662.
17. Graf CJ, Perret GE, Torner JC: Bleeding from cerebral arteriovenous malformations as part of their natural history. *J Neurosurg* 1983; 58:331–337.
18. Heros RC, Korosue K: Radiation treatment of cerebral arteriovenous malformations. *N Engl J Med* 1990; 323:127–129.
19. Heros RC, Korosue K: Parenchymal cerebral arteriovenous malformations, in Apuzzo MLJ (ed): *Brain Surgery: Complication Avoidance and Management.* New York, Churchill Livingstone, 1993, pp 1175–1192.
20. Heros RC, Morcos J, Korosue K: Arteriovenous malformations of the brain: Surgical management. *Clin Neurosurg* 1993; 40:139–173.
21. Heros RC, Tu Y-K. Unruptured arteriovenous malformations: A dilemma in surgical decision making. *Clin Neurosurg* 1985; 33: 187–236.
22. Jane J, Kassell N, Torner J, et al.: The natural history of aneurysms and arteriovenous malformations. *J Neurosurg* 1985; 62:321–323.
23. Kertesz A, Lesk D, McCabe P: Isotope localization of infarcts in aphasia. *Arch Neurol* 1977; 34:590–601.
24. Lunsford LD, Kondziolka D, Flickinger JC, et al.: Stereotactic radiosurgery for arteriovenous malformations of the brain. *J Neurosurg* 1991; 75:512–524.
25. Ondra SL, Troupp H, George ED, et al.: The natural history of symptomatic arteriovenous malformations of the brain: A 24 year follow-up assessment. *J Neurosurg* 1990; 73:387–391.
26. Pelz DM, Fox AJ, Viñuela F, et al.: Preoperative embolization of brain AVMs with isobutyl-2 cyanoacrylate. *AJNR* 1988; 9:757–764.
27. Pelz DM, Nishioka H: Report on the cooperative study of intracranial aneurysms and subarachnoid hemorrhage. Section VI. Arteriovenous malformations: An analysis of 545 cases of craniocerebral arteriovenous malformations and fistulae reported to the cooperative study. *J Neurosurg* 1966; 25:467–490.
28. Purdy PD, Samson D, Batjer HH, et al.: Preoperative embolization of cerebral arteriovenous malformations with polyvinyl alcohol particles: Experience in 51 adults. *AJNR* 1990; 11:501–510.
29. Samson DS, Batjer HH: Preoperative evolution of the risk/benefit ratio for arteriovenous malformations of the brain, in Wilkins RH, Rengachary SS (eds): *Neurosurgery Update II.* New York, McGraw-Hill, 1991, pp 129–133.
30. Spetzler RF, Hargraves RW, McCormick PW, et al.: Relationship of perfusion pressure and size to risk of hemorrhage from arteriovenous malformations. *J Neurosurg* 1992; 76:918–923.
31. Spetzler RF, Martin NA: A proposed grading system for arteriovenous malformations. *J Neurosurg* 1986; 65:476–483.
32. Stein BM, Wolpert SM: Arteriovenous malformations of the brain. I. Current concepts and treatment. *Arch Neurol* 1980; 37:353–371.
33. Stein RM, Wolpert SM: Arteriovenous malformations of the brain. II. Current concepts and treatment. *Arch Neurol* 1980; 37:1–5.
34. Steinberg GK, Fabrikant Jl, Marks MP, et al.: Stereotactic heavy-charged-particle Bragg-Peak radiation for intracranial arteriovenous malformations. *N Engl J Med* 1990; 323:96–101.
35. Steiner L, Lindquist C, Adler JR, et al.: Clinical outcome of radiosurgery for cerebral arteriovenous malformations. *J Neurosurg* 1992; 77:1–8.
36. Steiner L, Lindquist C, Cail W, et al.: Microsurgery and radiosurgery in brain arteriovenous malformations. *J Neurosurg* 1993; 79:647–652.

Roberto C. Heros, M.D.

1. Batjer HH, Devous MD, Meyer YJ, et al.: Cerebrovascular hemodynamics in arteriovenous malformation complicated by normal perfusion pressure breakthrough. *Neurosurgery* 1988; 22:503–509.
2. Batjer HH, Devous MD, Seibert GB, et al.: Intracranial arteriovenous malformation: Relationship between clinical factors and surgical complications. *Neurosurgery* 1989; 24:75–79.

3. Crawford PM, West CR, Chadwick DW, et al.: Arteriovenous malformations of the brain: Natural history in unoperated patients. *J Neurol Neurosurg Psychiat* 1986; 49:1–10.

4. Debrun G, Vinuela FV, Fox AJ, et al.: Embolization of cerebral arteriovenous malformations with bubrylate: Experience in 46 cases. *J Neurosurg* 1982; 56:615–627.

5. Graf CJ, Perrett GE, Torner JC: Bleeding from cerebral arteriovenous malformations as part of their natural history. *J Neurosurg* 1983; 58:331–337.

6. Heros RC: Arteriovenous malformations of the brain, in Ojemann RG, Heros RC, Crowell RM (eds): *Surgical Management of Cerebrovascular Disease*, ed 2. Baltimore, Williams and Wilkins, 1988, pp 347–413.

7. Heros RC, Korosue K, Diebold PM: Surgical excision of cerebral arteriovenous malformations: Late results. *Neurosurgery* 1990; 26: 570–578.

8. Heros RC, Tu Y-K: Unruptured arteriovenous malformations: A dilemma in surgical decision making. *Clin Neurosurg* 1985; 33: 187–236.

9. Luessenhop AJ, Rosa L: Cerebral arteriovenous malformations: Indications for and results of surgery, and the role of intravascular techniques. *J Neurosurg* 1984; 60:14–22.

10. Ondra SL, Troupp H, George ED, et al.: The natural history of symptomatic arteriovenous malformations of the brain: A 24 year follow-up assessment. *J Neurosurg* 1990; 73:387–391.

11. Spetzler RF, Martin NA: A proposed grading system for arteriovenous malformations. *J Neurosurg* 1986; 65:476–483.

12. Spetzler RF, Wilson CB, Weinstein P, et al.: Normal perfusion pressure breakthrough theory. *Clin Neurosurg* 1978; 25:651–672.

13. Steinmeier R, Schramm J, Muller H-G, et al.: Evaluation of prognostic factors in cerebral arteriovenous malformations. *Neurosurgery* 1989; 24:193–200.

14. Torner JC: *Natural history of AVMs*. Presented at the 53rd Annual Meeting of the American Association of Neurological Surgeons; April 12, 1984; San Francisco, California.

15. Viñuela F, Dion JE, Duckwiler G, et al.: Combined endovascular embolization and surgery in the management of cerebral arteriovenous malformations: Experience with 101 cases. *J Neurosurg* 1991; 75:856–864.

Eugene George, M.D.

1. Heros RC, Korosue K: Parenchymal cerebral arteriovenous malformations, in Apuzzo MLJ (ed): *Brain Surgery: Complication Avoidance and Management.* New York, Churchill Livingstone, 1993, pp 1175–1192.

2. Ondra SL, Troupp H, George ED, et al.: The natural history of symptomatic arteriovenous malformations of the brain: A 24 year follow-up assessment. *J Neurosurg* 1990; 73:387–391.

3. Samson DS, Batjer HH: Surface lesions: Lobar arteriovenous malformations, in Apuzzo MLJ (ed): *Brain Surgery: Complication Avoidance and Management.* New York, Churchill LIvingstone, 1993, pp 1142–1174.

4. Spetzler RF, Martin NA: A proposed grading system for arteriovenous malformations. *J Neurosurg* 1986; 65:476–483.

23

Surgical vs. Radiation Treatment of Small Arteriovenous Malformations

CASE

A 12-year-old boy had a tonic-clonic seizure at age 5. He had a second seizure at age 7 and was placed on phenobarbital. He had no other seizures until 2 recent ones, both of which were generalized and had no localizing features. His neurological exam was normal. A computed tomogram (CT) showed a contrast-enhancing lesion in the left rolandic area, and an angiogram confirmed that this lesion was an arteriovenous malformation. During surgical exploration with cortical stimulation, the malformation was found to lie in the central sulcus. Stimulating H produced flexion of the middle finger and G produced flexion of the hand.

PARTICIPANTS

Surgical Treatment of Small Arteriovenous Malformations–Bennett M. Stein, M.D., Michael B. Sisti, M.D.

Radiation Treatment of Small Arteriovenous Malformations–Tomasz K. Helenowski, M.D.

Moderators–M. Gazi Yasargil, M.D., Ali F. Krisht, M.D., Gerard Debrun, M.D., James I. Ausman, M.D., Ph.D.

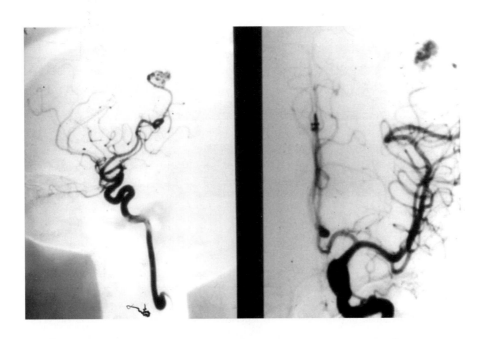

Surgical Treatment of Small Arteriovenous Malformations

Bennett M. Stein, M.D., Michael B. Sisti, M.D.

When reviewing the case of this 12-year-old boy, we must underscore certain points that help us decide how this particular patient should be treated. First, and most important, is the age of the patient, in this instance 12 years old and, therefore, young in the spectrum of patients having an arteriovenous malformation (AVM). Seizures that have been well-controlled since their onset at an early age are now manifest as a breakthrough seizure, which raises the issue of hemorrhage. The CT scan, presumably done at the time of this seizure, gives no indication of a hemorrhage. Whether or not previous seizures were associated with hemorrhage cannot be determined from the information provided. The anatomic aspects of the AVM indicate that it is located in an eloquent area of the brain, most likely in the arm or leg sensory area of the dominant cortex. Information regarding cortical stimulation is sketchy. Presumably, areas adjacent to the AVM were stimulated and the AVM "was found to lie in the central sulcus." In reviewing the angiogram, we would have thought that, even in a child, the AVM was situated behind the central sulcus in the sensory cortex.

We would categorize this AVM as small (under 3 cm in maximum diameter).[14] It appears to have a well-circumscribed border with minimal deep extension, a well-defined primary feeding artery (a terminal branch of the middle cerebral), and presumably, venous drainage that is not complex.

PRIORITIZING FACTORS WHEN CHOOSING A TREATMENT

The history and angiographic findings must be put into the context of a decision-making process leading to the best possible treatment for this particular patient.[14,17] Having operated on more than 400 AVMs of all sizes, we have developed a scheme to prioritize factors involved in this treatment program.[14]

There are two reasons for considering the patient's age of highest priority:

- A young patient is at greater risk of subsequent side effects of an AVM.
- The younger the brain, the better it adapts to treatment, regardless of the treatment chosen.

The response or "compliance" of the brain in a 12-year-old is far superior to that of the brain in a 55- or 60-year-old patient.

The second priority is the anatomy and size of the lesion. Anatomic features to be considered are:

- The margin of the AVM, whether diffuse or well circumscribed.
- The number and size of artery-to-vein shunts.
- Deep extension and presumably deep venous drainage, with maximum consideration given to deep arterial feeders such as the choroidal or lenticulostriate arteries.

Size is also a major factor. We consider AVMs under 3 cm in diameter to be small. In our series, these comprise about 20% of the lesions we have seen[14] (Fig. 1). Spetzler and colleagues[13] have recently theorized, based on intraoperative pressure studies, that smaller AVMs are at greater risk of hemorrhagic episodes.

The location of the lesion is of lesser importance. Most AVMs smaller than 3 cm in diameter can be removed safely, without permanent neurological deficits, regardless of whether their location is in eloquent or noneloquent portions of the brain. The only small AVMs that are inoperable because of location are those buried within the brain stem, diencephalon, or basal ganglion[9–12,14,16,17] (Fig. 2).

History is the least important of the criteria. Some have suggested that AVMs that have previously hemorrhaged are

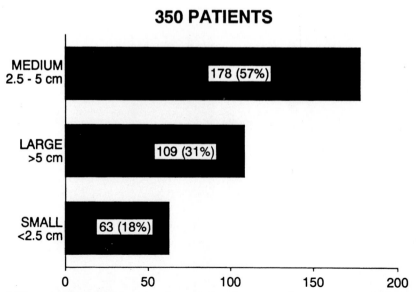

350 PATIENTS

MEDIUM 2.5 - 5 cm — 178 (57%)
LARGE >5 cm — 109 (31%)
SMALL <2.5 cm — 63 (18%)

0   50   100   150   200

Fig. 1 The categories of patients we have operated on according to the size of the AVM.

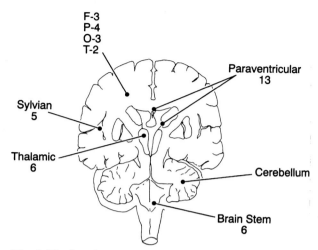

Fig. 2 The locations of small, deep AVMs we have resected.

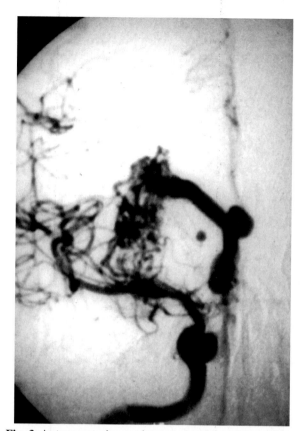

Fig. 3 Anteroposterior angiogram showing a deep AVM of the internal capsule and basal ganglia; this is one of the few small AVMs we consider inaccessible and, thus, a candidate for radiosurgery.

dangerous. When one considers that there must be a first hemorrhage, however, this theory is not logical. We do not believe that one hemorrhage predisposes to another hemorrhage. We consider the treatment of AVMs not as reconstructive, but as prophylactic. Accordingly, the ideal time to treat an AVM is when it is asymptomatic.

TREATMENT OPTIONS

For treatment, we have 4 options: observation, embolization, microsurgery, and radiation therapy.

The AVM can be observed when the risk of any curative treatment far outweighs what is presumed to be the natural history of the lesion. Quite frankly, no one knows for certain the natural history of AVMs in general, much less in any particular patient. Certain assumptions have been made, however, on the basis of retrospective studies.[8] These assumptions generally involve AVMs that have been excluded from treatment because of their size or location or the patient's age, or those that have been partially treated. There is not, and probably never will be, any large matched series of patients with AVMs who are followed prospectively for 2 or 3 decades without any treatment. Instead, we use an accumulative assumption that the catastrophic risk per year is in the range of 2%. Therefore, the older the patient, the less the overall cumulative risk. In a young patient, the risk could approach 100% during the patient's anticipated life span.

An insignificant number of AVMs have been cured through embolization. We consider embolization to be a preoperative adjuvant therapy and reserve it for patients with large AVMs of complex anatomy and those located in eloquent areas of the brain.

We have turned to surgery, with and without preoperative embolization, in the vast majority of cases and recommend it for patients with small AVMs.[14]

Focused radiation is a relatively new technique that is being adopted with increasing frequency. We do use the linear accelerator, but reserve it for very specific indications (Fig. 3).

RECOMMENDATIONS FOR THIS PATIENT

This patient's age is ideal, and the fact that the patient has no neurological deficits is extremely important. The malformation is small and, although located in a strategic area, is on the surface and, therefore, easily accessible. Because the lesion is congenital, it has displaced brain function to the periphery of the malformation. We would not consider simply observing this patient. Embolization might appear attractive because of the large, albeit distal feeding vessel, which may be the single or the only important artery feeding it. However, embolization of this vessel through its tortuous course to the distal area entails a risk and provides little, if any, benefit for subsequent surgery. We do not believe this lesion could be cured through embolization, even if there were a single arteriographically apparent artery supplying it. We would strongly advise microsurgical removal of this AVM.

There are good reasons for omitting corticography. First, adequate corticography must be done with the patient under local anesthesia. Because we use hypotension and controlled anesthetic techniques, local anesthesia cannot be used in this young patient. Second, whether done under general or local anesthesia, cortical mapping adds time to what are often already long operative procedures. Finally, we find no value in cortical mapping because we rely entirely on what is seen through the operating microscope and subscribe wholeheartedly to the theory that, if the AVM is accessible and small, it can be removed from any portion of the brain without causing neurological deficits. This assumes, and rightly so, that the congenital lesion displaces functional brain to the margin and that there is no functional brain within the malformation. Furthermore, the arteries that feed the malformation terminate at the malformation and do not supply important areas of the brain.

This patient would undergo surgery under general anesthesia, and a craniotomy would be done with a moderately wide margin around the malformation. The anatomy of the lesion is delineated on a preoperative magnetic resonance imaging (MRI) and preoperative lateral stereoscopic arteriography, which gives us a good clue as to the surface anatomy, most often the surface veins. In this patient, the feeding arteries appear to enter superficially into the malformation, a situation that could be identified early in the operation. AVMs are known to be much like icebergs—what is present on the cortical surface does not represent the extent of the AVM (Fig. 4). Therefore, the cortical incision must be small and the lips of this incision retracted to expose the main body of the AVM (Fig. 5). One draining vein must be left until the end, and hypotension is used liberally for AVMs having deep feeders (although probably not in this case).

DISCUSSION

The alternative to microsurgical removal is a radiosurgical approach with focused radiation through a variety of means: gamma knife, linear accelerator, proton beam, or helium ion. These techniques are only now being analyzed and follow-up information gathered. We prefer to cite what has been published rather than what has been presented at various meetings regarding this topic.[1-3,5,18,19] Anecdotal statistical presentations have been confusing and are impossible to analyze. For AVMs such as this one, many physicians consider radiosurgery to be the primary and appropriate treatment (Fig. 6). We disagree, based on our experience and the published experience of those using radiosurgery.[4,7,15]

In a worst-case scenario of microsurgery for this patient, we would not anticipate incomplete removal of the AVM and would expect a risk of serious permanent neurological deficit of less than 1%. For patients with small AVMs (3 cm or less in diameter) located in all areas of the brain, except the central brain stem, diencephalon, or basal ganglion (but including deep subcortical, periventricular, and surface or periventricular regions

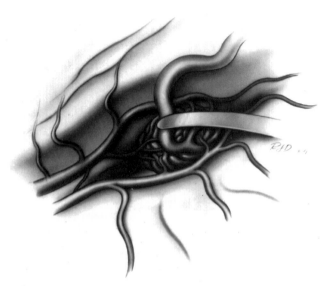

Fig. 5 The careful microdissection of a deep AVM at the sylvian fissure as a prelude to removal.

of the brain stem) we have had a 94% cure rate (without residual after appropriate surgery) and a 1.5% rate of serious neurological deficit.[14] Of all such small AVMs we see, fewer than 5% are located in areas we would consider inaccessible and, thus, candidates for radiotherapy. The other 95% of these lesions, regardless of their location and the patient's previous symptoms or age, have been microsurgically resected and form the basis of our statistics for small AVMs.

In comparing the best published data from radiosurgical treatment, it would appear that the overall cure rate of radiosurgery for AVMs under 3 cm ranges from 80 to 85%. Complications include a 4% rebleed rate occurring during the 2- to 3-year interval that it takes for radiosurgery to be maximally effective, and an additional 4 to 6% morbidity from radiation damage. This implies overall untoward results of 30%. The question that must be asked is: "What happens when the 2- to 3-year period passes and the AVM is still present?" One could not seriously recommend additional radiosurgery because the initial dose is believed to be the maximal tolerable dose. At the end of the 2- to 3-year interval, therefore, the neurological community is left with 15 to 20% of patients with small AVMs that are untreated and exposed to the future risks of hemorrhage, neurological deficit, or seizures. Furthermore, operating on AVMs that have been treated radiosurgically exposes the patient to increased postoperative risk from brain swelling and other unique neurological problems. The follow-up periods of patients undergoing radiosurgery for AVMs is limited and may overly discount the late effects of radiation.[3-5,7,15] We have seen patients who have had an excellent "cure" of the AVM through radiosurgery, but who then develop severe radiation necrosis in the area of the target and edema and histologic changes some distance from the focus (Fig. 7). These events may be irreversible and subject the patient to progressive, uncontrollable neurological deficits. When postoperative neurological deficits occur in patients undergoing microsurgery, however, most progressively improve and, to our knowledge, no late complications have occurred when the AVM is completely obliterated.

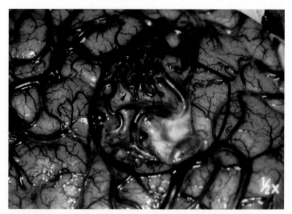

Fig. 4 Operative appearance of a small AVM. Note the small surface presentation (outlined by arrows) in comparison to the true subcortical extent of the AVM (outlined by the suture).

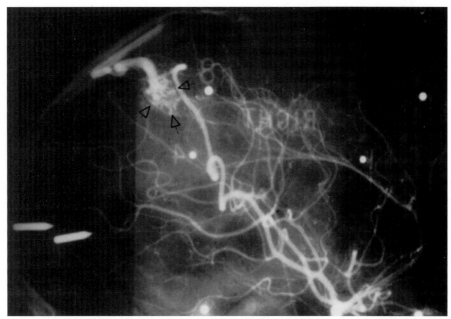

Fig. 6 Lateral angiogram showing a small AVM (arrows) in a 12-year-old patient who had a parietal hemorrhage and recovered without neurological deficit. Radiosurgery at a major gamma knife center was recommended; the patient's family opted for surgery, however, and we removed this lesion without incident.

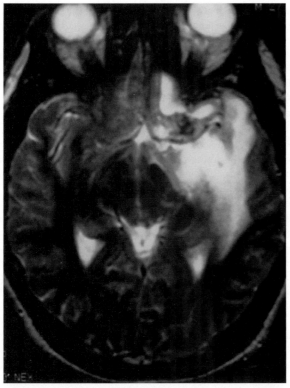

Fig. 7 A magnetic resonance image taken 3 years after successful gamma knife treatment of a deep AVM; the patient had developed a neurological deficit, and the scan shows extensive edema and radionecrosis.

CONCLUSION

Microsurgery is the ideal treatment for the patient described in this case, first because of the patient's age, second because of the anatomy and size of the lesion, third because of the lesion's location, and fourth, because the patient has no neurological deficits. Microsurgical removal can ensure a cure with minimal morbidity and without the fear of long-term neurological deficits. Based on published information, the acceptable results of radiosurgery for this particular patient would be far short of the microsurgical rate (Fig. 8). In those few cases in which radiosurgery is indicated, our experience shows that the linear accelerator is superior to the gamma knife because its installation is less expensive and no recharging is necessary. Thus, the cost of the procedure is less than that of the gamma knife.[6] However, microsurgical treatment of most small AVMs must still be considered unrivaled in terms of effectiveness and low morbidity.

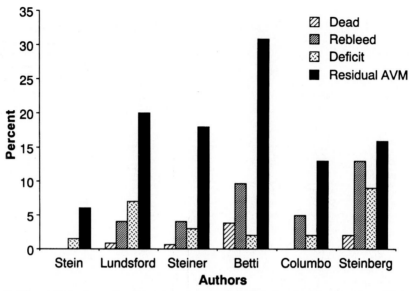

Fig. 8 The published results of treatment of small AVMs from various centers; Stein et al. represents the microsurgical series and the rest are radiosurgical series.

Radiation Treatment of Small Arteriovenous Malformations

Tomasz K. Helenowski, M.D.

Radiosurgery has become a useful and increasingly important neurosurgical technique for treating arteriovenous malformations and tumors. The term *radiosurgery* was defined by Leksell to describe a technique of delivering a focused, single high dose of radiation to obtain a specific biologic effect. Initially, he experimented with the linear accelerator but found it too cumbersome. He then developed the gamma knife to overcome the technical problems associated with focusing the radiation on a specific target.

THE GAMMA KNIFE

The present day gamma knife uses 201 ^{60}Co sources to produce gamma rays. The radiation is then collimated into 201 pencil beams that converge at the isocenter or focal point of the treatment. The radiation dose delivered to the isocenter is high and is distributed roughly spherically because of the additive effect of the numerous beams. Only a few beams traverse the tissues a few millimeters from the isocenter, delivering a significantly smaller dose to those tissues. Four different collimator helmets produce 4, 8, 14, and 18 millimeter isocenters at the focal point. Gamma knife radiosurgery has been used to treat 143 patients with AVMs at my institution.

Preoperative Evaluation

Patients referred for gamma knife radiosurgery are chosen by the Radiosurgery Patient Selection Committee, which consists of neurosurgeons, radiation oncologists, neuroradiologists, a medical oncologist, otolaryngologists, and nursing staff involved in the care of these patients. The relative risks of different treatment options are considered before patients are accepted for radiosurgery. Patients chosen for radiosurgery undergo tests the day before the procedure, including evaluation for general anesthesia in case it is needed during the procedure. Physical ther-

apy, occupational therapy, and speech therapy services evaluate the patients to determine their baseline function and to make sure that needed therapies are initiated. Depending on the location of the lesion being treated, the patient undergoes neurophysiological testing, including automated visual field testing, electroencephalography, evoked potentials, and audiograms, to obtain baseline values. Magnetic resonance images (MRI) of the brain are obtained in 3-mm or thinner axial sections with no gaps between the cuts. These images serve both as a baseline for future comparison studies and to help localize the boundaries of the lesion during the radiosurgical procedure.

Surgical Procedure

Gamma knife radiosurgery is usually carried out with the patient under local anesthesia. Patients younger than 5 years are typically treated under a general anesthetic. Patients from ages 5 and 17 years, and those who are claustrophobic, are treated under heavy sedation. Some patients with lesions in critical regions, who also have chronic obstructive pulmonary disease and use the accessory muscles of respiration, have been given general anesthesia for controlled ventilation during localization of the lesion. In these patients, controlled ventilation decreases head movements during imaging, allowing more accurate localization of these lesions.

After local anesthesia is administered, the Leksell G® stereotactic frame is attached to the patient's head with quick fixation screws. A cut-sheet selective or subselective angiogram is done with biplane angiography for all vessels feeding the malformation. The patient's head is then rotated 5 degrees and the angiogram is repeated to obtain stereoscopic views. Localizing the nidus of the AVM is critical, and the high-resolution stereoscopic angiogram is useful for discriminating the nidus from early draining veins and feeding vessels. A high-resolution contrast-enhanced computed tomograph (CT) of the brain is obtained in 1.5-mm thick contiguous axial sections to further define the lesion. During the CT scan, we use a gravity-activated electronic clinometer to monitor the position of the patient's head, which reduces the chance of localization errors from the patient's movement during the scan.

The nidus of the AVM is outlined on the angiogram and CT scan by the neuroradiologist and neurosurgeon involved in the procedure (Fig. 1). The coordinates of the center of the nidus are computed from the anteroposterior and lateral angiograms with an electronic digitizer and computer program from DosePlan®, Inc., and are verified by graphical calculations. A digitizer is then used to enter the contours of the nidus from the anteroposterior and lateral angiogram images into the DosePlan® treatment planning system. The CT images are transferred to the Helenowski-DosePlan® treatment-planning computer system over an Ethernet® network, and contours of the lesion are digitized on each image, using the radiologist's outline as a guide (Figs. 2, 3). If necessary, the MRIs may also be used in the planning process. Magnetic field inhomogeneity, however, makes localization on these images less accurate.

The contours derived from angiographic and CT images are integrated into a display file. This step is important because the angiographic images are two-dimensional but are being used to determine the treatment of a three-dimensional structure (Fig. 4). The CT and MRI images are not adequate alone because they may show draining veins, feeding arteries, and hematoma cavities that may not be discriminated from the nidus on these studies. In some patients with arteriovenous malformations, the CT and MRI images may not show the nidus at all, and a resolving hematoma cavity may be mistaken for the nidus of the AVM. The Helenowski-DosePlan® virtual reality treatment planning system (international patents pending) allows for dynamic, interactive, three-dimensional viewing of the lesion and surrounding critical structures, as well as shot placement. Multiple isocenter plans can be accurately and quickly calculated with the aid of virtual reality visualization to allow conformal treatment planning (Fig. 5). This type of planning allows maximal delivery of radiation to the nidus with minimal radiation to the surrounding tissues (Fig. 6). The average number of isocenters used for treatment of arteriovenous malformations has been 5.6 per case (range 1 to 12 shots per case) for the first 136 arteriovenous malformations treated.

After the plan is determined, the patient is treated in the Leksell® Gamma Knife Unit. Patients may be treated in the supine or prone position depending on the location of the lesion. Coordinates for an isocenter are set and verified on the stereotactic frame, and the patient's head is mounted in the collimator helmet. The operating team then moves to the control area and delivers the dose of radiation for the isocenter. This is repeated

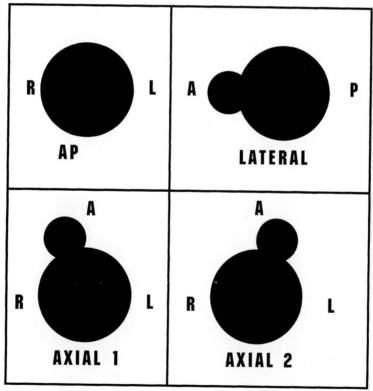

Fig. 1 This figure shows why serial axial CT images are integrated into the treatment planning for AVMs. The image may appear to be spherical on the anteroposterior view of the angiogram, but a portion of the nidus protrudes on the lateral view. On the CT images, the protrusion may be to the right (AXIAL 1 view), to the left (AXIAL 2 view), or a combination of locations anywhere between the 2 extremes. With only anteroposterior and lateral views on the angiogram (if no three-dimensional imaging is provided by CT or MRI), the proper location of a second isocenter to allow full treatment cannot be determined.

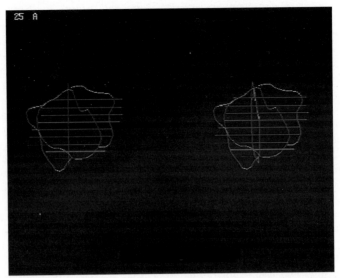

Fig. 2 A virtual reality image from the Helenowski-DosePlan® treatment planning system. The left and right images are a stereoscopic pair that allows three-dimensional viewing of the AVM. This is a view of the contour derived from the anteroposterior angiographic projection of the AVM. The horizontal lines are contours derived from axial CT images cutting through the AVM. The correlation of contours between the angiographic and CT images is excellent.

for all of the isocenters calculated to be necessary to treat the AVM. Once the radiation is delivered, the stereotactic frame is removed and the patient is monitored overnight in the hospital. Patients are discharged from the hospital the next day and allowed to return to their preoperative activities.

Follow-up

Follow-up MRIs of the brain are obtained 1 year after treatment. If the lesion appears to have been obliterated on MRIs, cerebral angiography is done to verify that the lesion has been oblite-

rated. Patients whose AVMs have been obliterated have had no further hemorrhage or recanalization of the lesion. If the lesion still shows flow at follow-up, cerebral angiography is done 2 years after the radiosurgical procedure. As long as the nidus appears to be decreasing on follow-up angiography, the angiograms are repeated on a yearly basis until the lesion disappears or stops shrinking. If the lesion stops shrinking, it is evaluated for further treatment, including possible further radiosurgery. Because of the improved dose-planning capabilities, a significant number of patients with lesions larger than 3.5 cm have

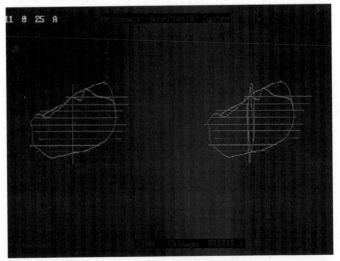

Fig. 3 A view of the contour derived from the lateral angiographic projection of the AVM. The horizontal lines are contours derived from axial CT images cutting through the AVM. The correlation of contours between the angiographic and CT images is excellent.

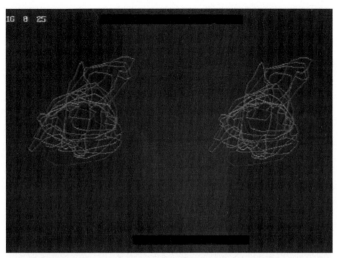

Fig. 4 When the contours are rotated to an oblique viewing angle, the irregular shape and three-dimensional configuration of the lesion is better appreciated.

been treated. A lower peripheral dose of radiation has been used in these patients, causing slower obliteration of the lesions as compared to other published results.

Results

Overall, in the first year, 25% of the lesions we treat appear to be obliterated. By the second year, 67% of the follow-up studies show that the lesions have been obliterated. At the end of the third year, the cumulative available follow-up angiograms show a 92% obliteration rate (Fig. 7). Most small lesions, however, which are covered by a single isocenter, are obliterated in 1 year, particularly in young patients. Permanent neurological deficits appear in less than 3% of patients; however, transient cerebral edema with increased symptoms may occur in as many as 30% of patients. These patients may experience headaches, weakness, numbness, and other symptoms, depending on the location of the AVM. Permanent deficits appear to be increased in patients with deeper lesions. The possibility of these symptoms increases with the size of lesion treated and usually lasts about 4

months. Some patients, however, may improve even 2 years after the onset of symptoms.

CASE DISCUSSION

The possibilities for this patient's AVM include no treatment, embolization of the lesion, surgical resection, and radiosurgery. Because the patient is young and the AVM has a 2 to 4% chance of hemorrhage per year, possibly causing severe neurological deficits or death, I recommend treating the lesion.

This lesion could be embolized because it has one main feeding vessel. The vessel is distal in the vascular tree, however, and takes a tortuous route to the AVM. Although embolization may be possible, the chances of getting a catheter distal enough in the vessel to safely occlude the AVM are poor. The patient may suffer permanent neurological deficits with this approach.

Because the AVM is in the left central sulcus, with hand and finger movement demonstrated by stimulating directly over the lesion, right hand dysfunction and speech problems would be likely after surgical excision.

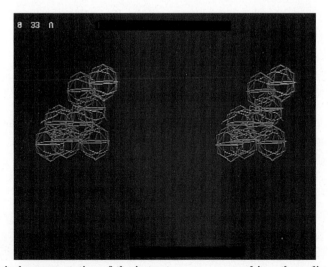

Fig. 5 Spherical representation of the isocenters are arranged in a three-dimensional configuration approximating the shape of the lesion as closely as possible. It is only possible to use multiple isocenters in this fashion if the three-dimensional configuration of the lesion is known.

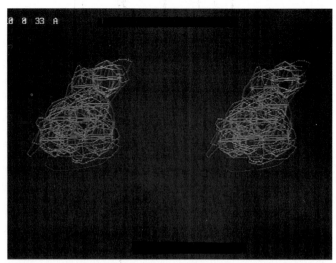

Fig. 6 The contours of the AVM derived from the anteroposterior and lateral angiograms and the CT images are displayed with the isocenters used to treat this lesion. The conformal planning derived from this technique allows the field of radiation to more closely approximate the size, shape, and position of the lesion and spare surrounding structures from excessive radiation.

The patient is an ideal candidate for gamma knife radiosurgery of the AVM. The lesion is small and could probably be treated with a single isocenter. A young patient with such a small lesion has a high probability (about 90%) of having the AVM obliterated in 1 year. Although we have seen a transient increase in seizures or the appearance of neurological deficits in 20 to 30% of patients such as this one, the symptoms tend to resolve within a few months. Permanent neurological deficits have been reported in only 3% of patients. In about two thirds of patients, seizure disorders are better controlled after the AVM is obliterated with the gamma knife. For these reasons, I would strongly recommend gamma knife radiosurgery for this patient.

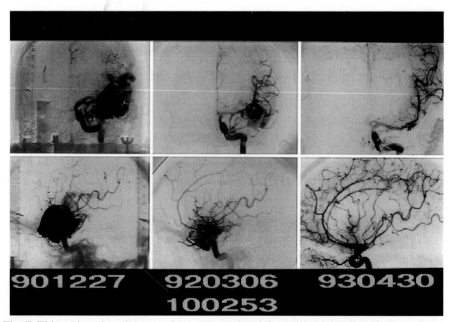

Fig. 7 This series of angiograms demonstrate the obliteration of a relatively large AVM after gamma knife radiosurgery. The left anteroposterior and lateral views show the lesion at treatment. The lesion is partially occluded 2 years later (middle images). Follow-up 3 years after treatment showed that the AVM was obliterated (right images).

Surgical vs. Radiation Treatment of Small Arteriovenous Malformations

M. Gazi Yasargil, M.D., Ali F. Krisht, M.D.

With great interest, we reviewed this controversial case of a 12-year-old boy who has a small (<3 cm) arteriovenous malformation (AVM) located in an eloquent brain area of the left dominant hemisphere. The information regarding the number, origin, and direction of the feeders of this malformation is, in our opinion, incomplete. The lateral view of the left internal carotid angiogram shows a small AVM probably localized in the posterior part of the middle frontal gyrus or within the precentral sulcus. No draining veins are evident, which may be a sign that the flow through the AVM is slow. The anteroposterior view shows 2 leptomeningeal branches in the direction of the AVM. Questionable evidence suggests slightly dilated veins within and around the malformation, but the direction of their drainage (superficial or deep) is not well visualized. In this particular situation, serial angiograms or multiplanar magnetic resonance images (MRI) would be helpful. The angiogram helps assess the hemodynamic aspect of the lesion and whether it is a slow- or high-flow malformation. The MRI can help localize the exact anatomic site of this lesion, its relationship to a sulcus or a gyrus, and whether the malformation has already bled. Nevertheless, we will pursue the discussion for its benefits as an academic exercise and try to find a balance between the opinions of Stein and Sisti, and Helenowski.

TREATMENT MODALITIES

In the past 3 decades, we have seen significant improvement in our microsurgical technical abilities, as well as important technological advancements that have helped establish a multimodality treatment for patients with AVMs of the brain. These modalities include microsurgery, radiosurgery, and endovascular techniques. The number of patients treated through any of these modalities lies between 2000 and 5000, great enough to support any one of these as a major player in the treatment of AVMs. In addition, each of these subspecialties is capable of presenting, in a sound way, arguments that support its effectiveness, success rate, and low morbidity and mortality rates. The arguments vary from the passionate and noncompromising ones to the more tolerant and flexible ones, which admit to benefits provided by other modalities. We believe that any of the 3 modalities in use has an important role, either separately or in combination. Our present ability to noninvasively follow the morphological features and behavior of lesions treated through any one or a combination of these modalities will provide us in the near future more reliable answers concerning the best treatment option to be recommended for a specific AVM.

Statistics vs. Reality

The discussions presented by both sides are well supported but, as we mentioned above, the information provided for this patient is incomplete. Therefore, the proponents' ability to prematurely formulate an opinion may reflect their bias towards the therapies they recommend. This brings us to an important issue. The best treatment for the patient should not be chosen solely on a biased opinion of the treating physician. It is important to take into account whether this is a symptomatic or an asymptomatic lesion, the exact location of the lesion, its hemodynamic proper-

ties, and the natural history of the disease because some low-flow AVMs occasionally thrombose spontaneously. In addition, we must address the potential role of other treatment modalities and, of utmost importance, the patient's and his family's wishes and their attitude toward the problem.

When we discuss the advantages and disadvantages of a particular treatment, we cannot generalize according to the best statistics reported for that modality. The best outcome scenario reflects the results obtained by the experts in a specific field and does not necessarily reflect the results achieved by the average specialist in the field. We stress this point because, although low mortality (0 to 0.8%) and morbidity (2 to 3%) have been reported for the treatment of AVM, this information should honestly be relayed to the patient by the treating physician as the results achieved by the experts in this field. Our opinion in this matter is driven by the fact that, when a complication occurs in a particular patient, it usually affects the patient 100%. Therefore, the patient and his family have the right to be fully informed about the results and experience of the treating physician, and they should actively participate in the decision-making process as to what they think is best in their specific situation.

SURGICAL EXCISION

In terms of deciding what is the potential role of any of the treatment modalities available, each one has its significant advantages and disadvantages. Microsurgical excision of the malformation promises to eliminate the lesion immediately, completely, and permanently in 85% of patients (diffuse hemispheric and large brain stem AVMs comprise the 15% of inoperable lesions). Surgical excision also has the advantage of removing any associated hematomas. On the other hand, the complications of surgery, including hemorrhage, infection, cerebral infarction, seizures, or even postsurgical hydrocephalus, are still potential problems that must be accounted for, no matter how low the risk.

EMBOLIZATION

Endovascular embolization of AVMs is an evolving modality that shows a lot of promise. Embolization can immediately obliterate AVMs in 40 to 50% of patients. This technique, no doubt, saves the patient from a craniotomy procedure and its potential risks, but whether embolization permanently obliterates the lesion has yet to be verified. On the positive side, embolization procedures are occasionally used to partially or totally occlude inoperable lesions, such as diffuse hemispheric and brain stem malformations. In these situations, embolization may be superior to both surgery and radiosurgery. On the other hand, embolization techniques cannot be used to evacuate adjacent intracerebral hematomas and they risk cerebral infarction. The ideal embolization material has not yet been determined and the equipment and techniques have yet to be standardized.

RADIOSURGERY

Radiosurgery of small AVMs is effective in up to 90% of patients. It involves no craniotomy, a short hospital stay, and immediate return of the patient to his or her usual daily activities. Similar to endovascular treatment, however, long-term follow-up is not established and we do not yet know whether these lesions recur. In addition, although radiosurgery may seem to be a benign treatment, it has its own risks. Helenowski admits that radiosurgery carries a risk of permanent neurological deficit in up to 3% of patients. Transient cerebral edema with a possibility of an increase in a patient's symptoms occurs in as many as 30% of patients. In addition, we have to keep in mind that, in 10% of patients, the lesion may still be present after 1 year and continue to have the potential of hemorrhage and severe neurological deficits or death. Radiosurgery is limited for lesions adjacent to eloquent parts of the brain. It is not recommended, for example, for lesions located in the brain stem. Like embolization, it is also an evolving treatment modality for AVMs that has yet to be standardized.

Discussion

We understand the opinions of both sides regarding the indications to treat this lesion. We see how they concur that this is a treatable lesion and, in a patient as young as this boy, some form of intervention is needed. The information provided in this case is not complete, however, and we have seen spontaneous and permanent obliteration of small AVMs that have no venous drainage and with features consistent with a low-flow lesion. This possibility is an important piece of information that must be relayed to the patient and the family during the decision-making process. We agree with Stein and Sisti that the microsurgical excision of this small AVM carries a low risk that would make this option, in the appropriate experienced hands, superior to

radiosurgery. This choice is supported by the lower risks of permanent neurological deficit and an immediate complete removal of the AVM, with no further risks of hemorrhage or other problems. On the other hand, we disagree with their opinion about embolization. In the same way that neurosurgeons improved on their microsurgical techniques and decreased the surgical mortality and morbidity of AVM surgery, the neuroradiologists are achieving significant advances in their field and are becoming more and more able to safely embolize distant AVMs that are supplied by long and tortuous blood vessels. Embolization is a less invasive option, and a relatively safe one in experienced hands. It may very well be the best option for patients with medical problems that put them in a high surgical risk category.

CONCLUSION

In conclusion, the information included in this case did not provide all the data necessary to decide in favor of any of the available treatment modalities. The 3 available modalities have excellent potentials for treating a small lesion, but only when the treatment is delivered by the experts. For this reason, the average specialist with not enough experience cannot generalize and use the data of the best results. He or she must be honest with his or her patients and provide them the results of his or her own experience. It is important to educate the patient and his family and to take into consideration their wishes and attitudes toward the problem.

Surgical vs. Radiation Treatment of Small Arteriovenous Malformations

Gerard Debrun, M.D.

I strongly disagree with Stein and Sisti's statement that embolization would have been risky and could not cure this AVM. The chances of anatomic cure are high. The tortuous course to this distal area is not a contraindication, and interventionists with good experience using the "magic" microcatheter routinely reach vessels more tortuous and distal than this one. This is a small nidus, of less than 2 cm, with a single arterial feeder and one single cortical vein of drainage. The risks associated with selective catheterization of this feeder are low, close to 0. The nidus can be completely filled with acrylic glue in one sitting with a high chance of success, I would say 90%. The risks of stroke or hemorrhage from the AVM after embolization are low, close to 3%. Therefore, I believe that the risks associated with embolization and the chances of cure are similar to those of

surgical resection.

I agree that radiosurgery is less attractive because it takes 2 years for the AVM to be cured with a 10 to 15% chance of incomplete cure and a 4% risk of radionecrosis. Considering that a small AVM may have a greater chance of bleeding than a large one and also the young age of the patient, radiosurgery should not be the first and best choice.

It is worth noting that the neurosurgeon recommends neurosurgery, the oncologist recommends radiation, and the interventionist recommends endovascular embolization. Each one believes the risks of his treatment to be extremely low and the chance of cure high. Could it be that any of these 3 alternatives is equally good?

Surgical vs. Radiation Treatment of Small Arteriovenous Malformations

James I. Ausman, M.D., Ph.D.

The basic principle of any therapy is to provide the best possible treatment with the lowest possible risks. For this patient, we have 3 choices: embolization, surgery, or radiosurgery. If embolization were not to succeed, one of the other 2 alternatives could then be used. I do not believe that observation only would be an adequate therapeutic choice for this patient.

The next principle is, if the lesion were in my brain, what would I want done? Having worked with endovascular therapists who use both principles of feeder embolization and nidus embolization, I am convinced that the few interventional radiologists who use the nidus embolization technique have the method that will prevail. Embolization of the feeders only leads to further recanalization and recruitment of vessels for the AVM and necessitates surgery. This is the background from which most neurosurgeons in the United States and other countries argue, because their experience is with feeder-embolizing interventionists. Debrun has made a strong case for nidus embolization, and I have seen malformations larger than this patient's obliterated with this technique. I have also seen Debrun navigate catheters through vessels as tortuous as the one in this patient precisely to the nidus, for the administration of glue. I believe this is the method of embolization of the future.

If the malformation were not eliminated through embolization, either surgery or radiosurgery could be used. Obviously, if the lesion were smaller, radiosurgery could be used, avoiding a craniotomy and the complications of surgery. However, this would expose the patient to the risks of the long-term results of radiosurgery, which at this point are not fully known. On the other hand, if a highly skilled surgeon could remove this lesion

with little or no deficit, that would certainly be a consideration. Most people would not like to have a craniotomy. At my institution, we remove malformations like this while the patient is awake. Cortical stimulation helps identify the lesion and carry out a resection during which a neurological exam is continuously done. I have used this approach in 3 patients with lesions in the middle of the motor sensory cortex and have had excellent results in 2 and a minor deficit in one.

Thus, I believe that, after a nidus embolization, either surgical resection or radiosurgery can be used. The choice would depend upon the skills of the people available in the unit and the patient's decision. Radiosurgery would be attractive because the lesion is small, the chance of success should be high, and there would be no intervention. The advantage to surgery is that the lesion could be confirmed as being totally removed. Given these choices, I believe most people would choose radiosurgery if embolization should fail.

REFERENCES

Bennett M. Stein, M.D., Michael B. Sisti, M.D.

1. Betti OO, Munari C, Rosler R: Stereotactic radiosurgery with the linear accelerator: Treatment of arteriovenous malformations. *Neurosurgery* 1989; 24:311–321.
2. Colombo F, Benedetti A, Pozza F, et al.: Linear accelerator radiosurgery of cerebral arteriovenous malformations. *Neurosurgery* 1989; 24:833–840.
3. Friedman WA, Bova FJ: Linear accelerator radiosurgery for arteriovenous malformations. *J Neurosurg* 1992; 77:832–841.
4. Heros RC, Korosue K: Radiation treatment of cerebral arteriovenous malformations. *N Engl J Med* 1990; 323:127–129.
5. Lunsford LD, Kondziolka D, Flickinger JC, et al.: Stereotactic radiosurgery for arteriovenous malformations of the brain. *J Neurosurg* 1991; 75:512–524.
6. Luxton G, Petrovich Z, Jozsef G, et al.: Stereotactic radiosurgery: Principles and comparison of treatment methods. *Neurosurgery* 1993; 32:241–259.
7. Ogilvy CS: Radiation therapy for arteriovenous malformations: A review. *Neurosurgery* 1990; 26:725–735.
8. Ondra SL, Troupp H, George ED, et al.: The natural history of symptomatic arteriovenous malformations of the brain: A 24-year follow-up assessment. *J Neurosurg* 1990; 73:387–391.
9. Sisti MB, Solomon RA, Stein BM: Stereotactic craniotomy in the resection of small arteriovenous malformations. *J Neurosurg* 1991; 75:40–44.
10. Solomon RA, Stein BM: Interhemispheric approach for the surgical removal of thalamocaudate arteriovenous malformations. *J Neurosurg* 1987; 66:345–351.
11. Solomon RA, Stein BM: Management of arteriovenous malformations of the brain stem. *J Neurosurg* 1986; 64:857–864.
12. Solomon RA, Stein BM: Surgical management of arteriovenous malformations that follow the tentorial ring. *Neurosurgery* 1986; 18:708–715.
13. Spetzler RF, Hargraves RW, McCormick PW, et al.: Relationship of perfusion pressure and size to risk of hemorrhage from arteriovenous malformations. *J Neurosurg* 1992; 76:918–923.
14. Stein BM, Kader A: Intracranial arteriovenous malformations. *Clin Neurosurg* 1992; 39:76–113.
15. Stein BM, Mohr JP, Sisti MB: Is radiosurgery all that it appears to be? (letter). *Arch Neurol* 1991; 48:19–20.
16. Stein BM: Arteriovenous malformations of the medial cerebral hemisphere and the limbic system. *J Neurosurg* 1984; 60:23–31.
17. Stein BM: General techniques for surgical removal of arteriovenous malformations, in Wilson CB, Stein BM (eds): *Current Neurosurgical Practice: Intracranial Arteriovenous Malformations.* Baltimore, Williams & Wilkins, 1984, pp 143–155.
18. Steinberg GK, Fabrikant Jl, Marks MP, et al.: Stereotactic heavy-charged-particle Bragg-peak radiation for intracranial arteriovenous malformations. *N Engl J Med* 1990; 323:96–101.
19. Steiner L, Lindquist C, Adler JR, et al.: Clinical outcome of radiosurgery for cerebral arteriovenous malformations. *J Neurosurg* 1992; 77:1–8.

24

Treatment of Soft Cervical Disc Herniation

CASE

A 41-year-old woman developed pain in her neck and right arm. Upon examination, her deltoid and bicep muscles on the right were weak. Her right thumb was numb, and her right biceps reflex was diminished. Despite 4 weeks of conservative treatment, her symptoms persisted. A magnetic resonance image (MRI) at this time showed a lateral soft-disc herniation at the C5-C6 level compressing the right C6 nerve root.

PARTICIPANTS

Posterior Discectomy for Soft Cervical Disc Herniation–Frederick A. Simeone, M.D.

Anterior Discectomy without Fusion for Soft Cervical Disc Herniation–W. Michael Vise, M.D.

Anterior Discectomy with Interbody Fusion for Soft Cervical Disc Herniation–
    Deiter Grob, M.D.

Moderator–Fraser Henderson, M.D.

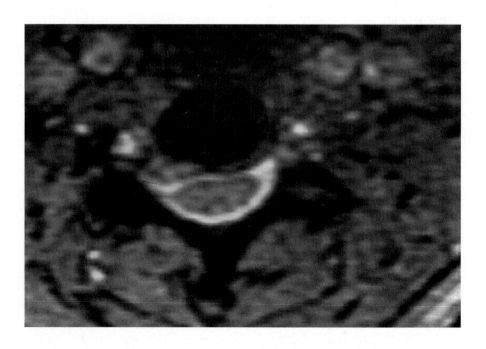

Posterior Discectomy for Soft Cervical Disc Herniation

Frederick A. Simeone, M.D.

This patient has a history compatible with acute cervical radiculopathy and neurological findings that confirm compression of the right C6 nerve root. The magnetic resonance image (MRI) clearly shows a soft lateral disc herniation as the cause of these symptoms, and a reasonable period of nonoperative therapy has been ineffective. Both from the point of view of pain relief and protection from permanent nerve root damage, surgical decompression of this nerve root is indicated.

PREOPERATIVE IMAGES

Computed tomography (CT) and MRI do not always clearly delineate the source of nerve root compression as nicely as they do in the patient in this case. In patients with chronic disc degeneration and foraminal narrowing, the exact mechanism of compression or the specific nerve root involved may be even less obvious on scans. Therefore, we have a low threshold for the performance of cervical myelography in such patients. A C1-C2 puncture myelogram is a safe, well-tolerated study, and it can avoid some of the pitfalls associated with relying entirely on scanning. Although improvements in the quality of CT and MRI scans have reduced the necessity for myelography, greater experience in the performance of myelograms has made the test safer, and there should be little hesitancy in ordering the study.

SURGICAL TECHNIQUE

The surgical approach is through a posterior partial foraminotomy and laminotomy, the so-called *keyhole* technique, with the patient in the face-down, kneeling, and sleep reverse Trendelenberg position.

With the aid of the operating microscope, the dorsal portion of the intervertebral foramen is drilled at C5-C6, thereby decompressing the nerve. The bony removal proceeds until an instrument can be passed cleanly through the intervertebral foramen along any part of the circumference of the nerve root. This ordinarily involves removal of a portion of the medial half of the facet joint, but a significant articular surface remains even after an aggressive foraminotomy. When the nerve is fully decompressed, the procedure can be considered complete. In his series of 846 cases reported in 1988, Henderson and colleagues[1] achieved excellent results (96% relief) without any attempt to remove disc material. I have found that, since the advent of MRI and the improved resolution of the CT scan, it is possible to predict with reasonable accuracy whether a soft disc herniation is present. This information is not available on the basis of myelography alone. Consequently, with the operating microscope, it is possible to pass a microsurgical instrument, such as a Rosen® knife, under the nerve root and retrieve fragments of soft herniated disc. This is a technically satisfying maneuver, and immediately and visibly relieves nerve root compression. Whether it affects the overall outcome of the surgical procedure is unclear because Henderson achieved such excellent results without removal.

In a large series in which I was an investigator, there were 2 recurrences in the early postoperative period (3 days in 1 patient and 4 months in another) despite decompressive foraminotomy. In neither of these patients was a soft-disc fragment removed at the time of the first operation. I believe that these recurrences could have been avoided through removal of the disc fragments, which were found during subsequent surgery. Therefore, I now attempt to retrieve disc fragments whenever they are suspected from a review of the scan. There have been no instances of nerve root injury as a result of this maneuver, which is done under the operating microscope. Care must be taken, however, to avoid the ventral root, which may leave the dural canal in its separate sleeve and may be attenuated over a tight disc herniation. Under the operating microscope, the ventral root sleeve can be gently retracted and a flat instrument passed beneath it to remove soft disc material.

Postoperative Results

Because the surgical approach can be done with an incision as small as 3 cm, the patient can be mobilized promptly and discharged on the first or second postoperative day. Collars are not required, except empirically for patient comfort, particularly while riding in a car. Postoperative radiographs are not necessary, and the recurrence rate is negligible. Significant complications are rare. With the use of the operating microscope, injury to the nerve root has been avoided. Temporary motor deficit has been seen on a few occasions, always involving the C5 root, but these have been transient. Preoperative fingertip numbness can be aggravated and is sometimes persistent, although rarely troublesome. Almost all instances of persistent fingertip numbness occur in patients with a long history of preoperative numbness that simply never cleared. The infection rate is low and infection is easily treated when it occurs. Cerebrospinal fluid leaks have not been seen in our series of microsurgical cervical discectomies, and no instances of cervical instability or subluxation could be attributed to the operation.

ANTERIOR DISCECTOMY

Equally good results for pain relief and control of neurological deficit can be obtained through an anterior cervical discectomy. Although complications are rare with that operation as well, aggregately, the anterior procedure exposes the patient to a broad variety of risks that are unnecessary when one considers that equally good results can be obtained through the posterior approach.

The complications of anterior cervical discectomy include hoarseness, tongue paralysis, difficulty swallowing, Horner's syndrome, esophago-cutaneous fistula, spinal cord injury, vertebral artery injury, failure of fusion without angulation deformity, and donor site problems, among others. Fortunately, all of these complications are rare. A more common complication, but one not seen until years after the operation, results from the added stress to adjacent spinal levels as a result of a solid fusion. There is no doubt that anterior fusion predisposes a patient to disc degeneration and instability at adjacent levels, which can lead to more disc surgery in the future. It is far preferable to decompress a nerve root without altering the dynamic function of the cervical spine. With posterior microsurgical discectomy, only a small portion of the disc material, if any at all, is removed. Although some of the facet joint is channeled over the nerve root, the joint and the disc space both function normally in flexion and extension of the spine.

CONCLUSION

If this patient had a large midline soft-disc herniation with cord compression, the operation of choice would be an anterior dis-

cectomy. For laterally placed discs, however, more than 98% of patients can have satisfactory results with a posterior foraminotomy, with fewer complications, freedom from the use of a collar, and better long-term spinal function.

Anterior Discectomy without Fusion for Soft Cervical Disc Herniation

W. Michael Vise, M.D.

Patients with soft disc herniation respond well to either anterior or posterior cervical discectomy. I prefer the anterior approach and nongrafting techniques. For more than 10 years, I used the Cloward method of bone grafting with good results and few complications. I now exclusively use a microsurgical technique called *radical* cervical discectomy without bone grafting for both hard and soft disc herniations, and in the resection of ventral osteophytic lesions that produce myelopathy.

CHOOSING THE ANTERIOR APPROACH

In choosing to use this method, I have followed a simple line of reasoning: A more thorough resection of the offending pathologic process is required than with traditional methods because immediate segmental stabilization and interspace expansion with a bone graft are not done. Otherwise, postoperative settling of the interspace may lead to neural compromise with recurrence of symptoms if a complete neural decompression has not been achieved.

The reasons I would choose this particular operation for this patient are:

1. It is a gentle technique for the patient;
2. One can completely excise the segmental pathologic process with radical excision of the disc, which obviates the need for a graft;
3. The patient has no hip pain because a bone graft is not taken;
4. Delayed fusion always occurs, although total radiographic fusion may be incomplete in some patients;
5. The patient's hospital stay is brief and, with refinement of surgical technique, many of these patients can be treated on an outpatient basis;
6. I have achieved good or excellent results in 93% of my patients according to the criteria of either Odom[16] or Rosenørn and colleagues[19] (Table 1).

Contraindications

Reasons for not selecting this procedure are:

1. The surgical technique is more demanding than that of traditional methods if a radical rather than a simple discectomy is done;
2. Neurological risk is increased because of wide exposure of the neural elements through an anterior approach. This increase can be offset, however, with the use of the operating microscope and meticulous hemostasis;
3. Although most patients do not experience immediate postoperative pain, 25% develop settling pain, primarily limited to the neck and shoulders, within a few days of surgery, as there is axial loading of the spine. When it occurs, it is

Table 1. Results of Operations with Radical Microsurgical Anterior Cervical Discectomy

Outcome	Number of Procedures	Percentage of Patients
Excellent	122	65
Good (mild pain)	53	28
Fair (moderate pain)	7	4
Poor (unimproved)	5	3
TOTAL	187	
Overall good to excellent outcome		93

relatively brief. In a few patients, however, the pain is severe and may last for several weeks. This pain always resolves and does not require reoperation if the surgeon has carried out a truly radical excision and is certain that there is no remaining compression of the nerve root.

SIMPLE ANTERIOR DISCECTOMY

Anterior cervical discectomy without bone grafting has been practiced for 35 years, with results comparable to the more widely accepted methods of discectomy with fusion.[11,13,18] Table 2 summarizes a literature review of more than 1600 cases of anterior cervical discectomy without bone grafting. Fewer than half of the authors of these studies opened the posterior longitudinal ligament and excised the pathologic process behind it. Many described a simple discectomy alone, and a few made reference to a more radical resection of the posterior wall of the interspace with exposure of neural elements. Several authors discouraged venturing beyond this boundary.[1,8,15,23] Benini and colleagues[1] only tried to "fish out" free fragments if a tear was seen in the posterior annulus, and stated that exploration of the spinal canal, visualization of the nerve roots, and removal of osteophytes are useless and dangerous surgical acrobatics.

I disagree with this point of view and have found that, with the use of the operating microscope and wide exposure of the neural elements, one can further improve the patient's outcome and shorten hospital stays. In my experience, a visible tear in the annulus occurred in no more than 1 in 5 cases with associated free fragments. Furthermore, it seldom coincided with the location of the fragment, that is, a tear may be central yet the fragment may be laterally placed. Therefore, when the surgeon tries to read the posterior longitudinal ligament and fish out hidden fragments, he or she is unaware of the pathologic process left behind, and may be unable to adequately retrieve fragments.

Table 2. Anterior Cervical Discectomy Without Bone Grafting*

Authors	No. of Cases	Opened Posterior Ligament	Results or Major Complications	Levels Re-op	Fusion	Instability	Hospital Stay (days)
†Benini, et al.[1]	25	no	88% good/improved		–	none	5
Bertalanffy, Eggert[2]	164	yes	82% good/excellent		75%	1%	6
Bertalanffy, Eggert[3]	286	yes	17 worsened myelopathy, 5 epidural hematomas	5	–	1%	6
Cuatico[4]	81	no	95% good/excellent		–	none	
DeTribolet, Zander[5]	17	yes	76% good/excellent		–	–	–
Dunsker[6]	11	yes	100% good/excellent		–	–	–
Giombini, Solero[7]	100	sometimes	80% good/excellent; 3 deaths, 3 quadraparesis	3	45%	none	5
Granata, et al.[8]	24	no	88% good/excellent		63%	–	7
†Grisoli, et al.[9]	120	yes	87% good/improved		70%	none	3
Hankinson, Wilson[10]	52	sometimes	89% good/excellent		–	2%	8
†Hirsch, et al.[11]	45	no	83% good/improved		–	none	4
Husag, Probst[12]	60	yes	82% good/excellent		70%	none	7
Lunsford, et al.[13]	135	–	69% good/excellent	4	–	–	7
Martin[14]	26	yes	65% good/excellent		–	4%	–
†Murphy[15]	26	no	92% good/improved	1	72%	none	–
O'Laoire, Thomas[17]	25	sometimes	96% recovery from myelopathies		–	–	–
Robertson, Johnson[18]	135	sometimes	52% good/excellent—hard discs; 85% good/excellent—soft discs		88%	–	–
Rosenørn, et al.[19]	32	–	87% good/excellent		–	–	6
Smith[20]	50	no	90% good/excellent		90%	–	–
Tew, Mayfield[21]	50	–	–	–	100%	–	–
U, Wilson[22]	100	sometimes	3 epidural hematomas	3	–	–	–
†Wilson, Campbell[23]	71	no	78–95% good/improved		28%	none	5
Vise	187	always	93% good/excellent		66%	none	1.9 (34 outpatients)
Total series: 23	Total patients: 1822	< half opened the posterior longitudinal ligament	52–100% good/excellent results	16 reoperations	about 70% fusion	excellent stability	Average about 6 days

*Table 2 reviews publications in the English medical literature and the 187 cases of the author not previously published. These used different methods of reporting outcome and types of cases selected for treatment; most were soft or soft/hard disc herniation. Most authors reverted to bone grafting for spondylosis. In some instances, outcome or fusion percentages had to be derived from the information available. Authors who did not use the outcome classification proposed by Rosenørn and colleagues[19] or Odom[16] (excellent, good, fair, poor) are indicated by †. The series reported by O'Laoire and Thomas[17] represented a group of patients treated for myelopathy. There were differences among authors in reporting fusion; most listed the incidence of complete radiographic fusion; this had no bearing upon outcome. Several authors opened the posterior longitudinal ligament, but few resected most of it and included foraminotomies. Martin[14] defined a radical discectomy, but he did not mention foraminotomies. Bertalanffy and Eggert[2] radically excised the posterior longitudinal ligament in many patients and described an anterior foraminotomy; their most recent report of 450 cases is an addition of 286 to their earlier series of 164. Information not commented upon or that could not be derived from reported data is indicated by a dash.

Nor can one rely upon the concept of "the tail" leading to a lesion behind the posterior longitudinal ligament because, in my experience, this is only an occasionally reliable finding.[4,23]

SIMPLE VS. RADICAL DISCECTOMY

How one deals with the posterior boundary of the interspace differentiates a *simple* from a *radical* discectomy and determines whether one can consistently achieve good or excellent results with nongrafting techniques and avoid the need for a second operation. A simple discectomy alone may suffice for epiligamentous herniations, that is, those that have stretched the posterior longitudinal ligament and remain anterior to it. But a simple discectomy does not remove subligamentous herniations that penetrate the posterior longitudinal ligament and constitute the majority of soft-disc ruptures. Furthermore, excising the posterior longitudinal ligament greatly facilitates removal of an osteophyte by allowing excellent purchase of bone punches upon vertebral margins, rather than attempting to undermine osteophytes when this barrier remains.

Although several authors have used the term *radical* to describe cervical discectomy,[12,14,18] it has not been properly defined. Thus, I offer the following definition. A radical cervical discectomy is that which includes:

- Complete excision of the disc,
- Wide resection of the anterior and posterior longitudinal ligaments,
- Removal of pathologic bone and disc posterior to the posterior longitudinal ligament,
- Foraminal resection of the uncovertebral joints.

Surgical Technique

After induction of anesthesia, the interspace is marked percutaneously with indigo carmine with a 20-gauge spinal needle. This mark locates the skin incision for precise alignment of the operating microscope with the interspace, and stains the disc and posterior wall of the interspace to help differentiate the interspace from the dura.

After discectomy and with the interspace expanded, a portion of the posterior vertebral margins is removed with curettes or bone punches to expose the posterior longitudinal ligament, which is fused with the posterior annulus. The posterior annulus is incised with a number 15 blade, and the posterior longitudinal ligament is separated from the dura with a microdissector. In a few instances, the dura adheres to the posterior longitudinal ligament and may be inadvertently nicked or opened. If this happens, a piece of Gelfoam® can be left over the site at the time of closure. (Other authors have used muscle and fibrin glue.[9]) The epidural venous plexus is usually laterally placed; therefore, bleeding that interferes with visualization seldom occurs at this point. Initial resection of the posterior longitudinal ligament begins with a thin-tipped ½-mm bone punch and continues with 1- and 2-mm rongeurs. Free disc fragments can then be retrieved.

Then, a much wider resection of the posterior longitudinal ligament can be done, making it flush with the resection of the posterior vertebral margins and osteophytes (Figs. 1, 2). This maneuver prevents postoperative buckling of the ligament. Bleeding is controlled with packing. Occasionally, application of bone wax to a few sites is necessary.

Bilateral foraminotomies are then done with bone punches (Fig. 2). The uncovertebral joint should be resected as much as possible. With this instrumentation, the vertebral artery is beyond reach. The anterior canal branch of the vertebral artery, however, can be opened or avulsed; bleeding from this artery can be stopped with temporary packing. Vigorous venous bleeding always occurs from resection of the epidural venous plexus at the root axillae. This bleeding, however, is readily controlled with packing.

Postoperative narrowing of the interspace primarily occurs anteriorly, rather than at the foramen. Nevertheless, bilateral foraminotomies should be carried out to assure that neural compromise does not occur with settling. The opposite foramen is

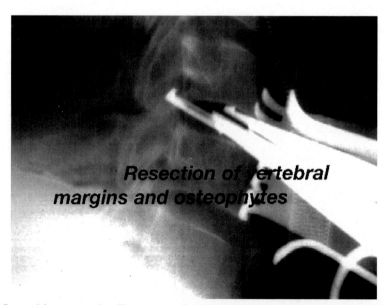

Fig. 1 Lateral intraoperative X-ray taken for demonstration purposes only during excision of the posterior vertebral margins and the posterior longitudinal ligament. This maneuver removes osteophytes and makes the resection of the posterior longitudinal ligament flush with the bone margins to prevent postoperative buckling of the ligament.

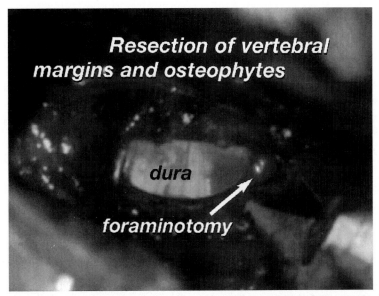

Fig. 2 Intraoperative photomicrograph of the completed resection of the vertebral margins and posterior longitudinal ligament. The left foraminotomy and root axilla are seen from this view (arrow); the dura is widely exposed.

within the curative field and can be opened without much additional time. This should not be compared to operating on an asymptomatic side from a posterior approach, which is quite another matter and is generally contraindicated. Furthermore, contralateral settling pain may occur in some instances, and one must be certain that it does not stem from neural compromise.

One can often retrieve additional free disc fragments well out into a foramen; these fragments can be easily missed if the foraminotomies are incomplete and not thoroughly cleared with a right-angled probe. If the operative approach is from the patient's right side, resection of the left foramen is always easier than the right. This approach is not improved by the surgeon simply moving to the opposite side of the table. The converse is true for an opposite, left-sided incision.

Sometimes, part or all of the posterior longitudinal ligament is ossified, which may not be discovered until resection of the ligament is initiated. Resection of an ossified ligament and the occasional ossified disc may be required to gain access to the osteophytes producing neural compression. In this event, the procedure becomes a tedious excavation and reconstitution of the interspace, but can be accomplished with patience.

With a calcified posterior longitudinal ligament, slow, controlled picking-away with a small curette at a portion of the ligament and adjacent bone margins eventually exposes a membrane over the cord, which is then opened. Once a foothold is established, resection of the calcified ligament is not much harder than in the routine resection of the posterior longitudinal ligament except for greater bleeding at the bone margins.

Decortication of the vertebral surfaces need not be excessive. All that is required is thorough excision and curettage of cartilaginous plates. This step is done with the initial disc excision, but is rechecked for completeness at the time of closure. Only curettes are used; high-speed drills are not needed and may cause unnecessary bleeding, which may explain the series of epidural hematomas reported by U and Wilson[22] (Table 2).

Hemostasis must be almost perfect and is achieved through the measures noted above, in addition to repeated gentle packing of the interspace. Irrigation with hydrogen peroxide is useful.

The interspace is repeatedly inspected until all bleeding is stopped. In some instances, an additional 15 to 25 minutes may be required to complete this step. Gelfoam® is removed from the interspace, or a small pledget may be left posteriorly on either side. The wound is then closed.

RESULTS

In my series of 187 operations, the average hospitalization time was 1.9 days. Thirty-four patients were treated as outpatients, and I am now doing about half of these operations on an outpatient basis. Postoperatively, patients are instructed to continue bed rest for a week at home and to wear a soft collar when up. Most patients return to work within 3 to 6 weeks.

Good or excellent results were achieved in 93% of these patients and no levels required reoperation (Tables 1, 3). This is several percentage points better than the results generally reported for either graft or nongraft techniques.[13,18] Complications have been minimal and include: seroma (2.7%), transient hoarseness (3.2%), and Horner's syndrome (0.6%). There were no neurological deficits.

Table 3. Total Levels Operated on Through Radical Microsurgical Anterior Cervical Discectomy

Total levels operated on	225
Total operations	187
Number of patients	182
with radiculopathy	172 (92%)
with myelopathy	15 (8%)
reoperated at another level	5 (3%)
undergoing multilevel operations	37 (20%)
2 levels	36
3 levels	1
with adjacent fusion before surgery	18 (10%)
Levels reoperated	0

CONCLUSION

This surgical experience has taught me three important lessons:

1. Often, there is more pathology behind the posterior longitudinal ligament than suspected. In my patients, free disc fragments were found behind the ligament in two thirds of those with soft-disc herniations and in one third of other patients;
2. Although it is sometimes brisk, bleeding associated with

resection of the posterior wall of the interspace and uncovertebral joints is mostly venous and quite manageable;
3. Although the neurological risk is increased during the procedure, radical disc resections can be done safely with the aid of the operating microscope. Whereas the goals of traditional procedures are decompression, immediate stabilization, and delayed resorption of osteophytes, the goals of radical discectomy are complete neural decompression and delayed fusion.

Anterior Discectomy with Interbody Fusion for Soft Cervical Disc Herniation

Deiter Grob, M.D.

For the patient described in this case, the indications for surgery can be justified because of the triad of:

- Pain,
- Neurological deficit (the symptoms of numbness in the right thumb, a diminished biceps reflex and weakness in the deltoid indicate malfunction of the C6 nerve root),
- The radiologic finding of a lateral soft herniated disc at the C5-C6 level, which localizes the origin of compression; in addition, the MRI shows no obvious degenerative signs of the facets nor are severe uncarthrosis or other possible sources of pain identifiable.

The patient has a monosegmental pathologic process and the site of compression can be identified. Therefore, mechanical removal of the compressive agent is justified. If the patient has no contraindications, surgery is recommended.

RATIONALE FOR SURGERY

Once the decision to do surgery is made, the aim of the intervention should be clearly defined. Because every surgical intervention has certain risks, the risk:benefit ratio should be influenced as much as possible in favor of the benefit. Therefore, surgery should fulfill a maximum of advantages rather than aim at a minimal advantage at a given risk rate. At a minimum, surgery must relieve pain and decompress the nerve root. The best surgical outcome is a patient with a cervical spine free of pain, a normal range of spinal motion, and an anatomy restored as much as possible to normal.

Choice of Procedure

Removing the disc and herniated material decompresses the nerve root. Therefore, pain relief and, to a certain extent, neurological recovery are to be expected. If a nucleotomy is done through a posterior approach, stability might be a concern because of a partial facetectomy. With the anterior approach, a major part of the disc must be removed for the surgeon to reach and extract the herniated disc material. In patients with dislocated disc material in the spinal canal, it may even be necessary to do a partial vertebrectomy to safely remove the herniated material.

Surgical intervention with a nucleotomy is impossible without altering the mechanical properties of the segment. Removing the intervertebral disc produces a certain instability. Nature may compensate for this instability by narrowing the disc space and producing a kyphotic deformity.[5] Eventually, spontaneous fusion occurs in this position. The timing of fusion and the degree

of deformity remains unpredictable. To avoid this uncertain situation, an anterior interbody fusion can be done. With appropriate technique, a predictable fusion in a defined position is possible; additional decompression through the application of distraction might be of value.

Operative Technique

The technique of anterior fusion through removal of the intervertebral disc and insertion of a bone graft is a well-known and established technique.[1,7] Through an anterolateral approach, the C5-C6 level is exposed. The correct level is identified intraoperatively with lateral X-rays and a C-arm. Incising the ante-

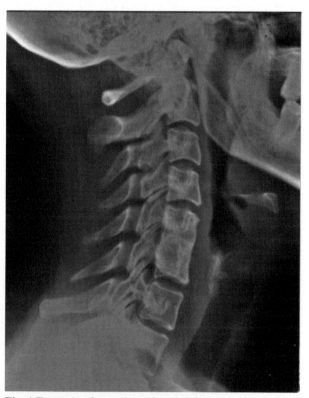

Fig. 1 Example of a patient 12 months after nucleotomy and simultaneous fusion. Note the correct alignment, with physiological lordosis and equal distances between the spinous processes; physiological load distribution of the cervical spine is assured.

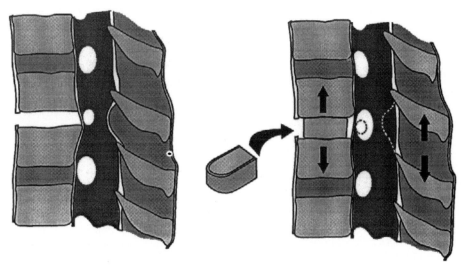

Fig. 2 The principle of anterior interbody fusion with distraction. The intervertebral foramen is opened and the spinal canal decompressed through segmental distraction. Moving the vertebral bodies into the original position allows the foramen to return to its original size. Through the same maneuver, the bulging ligaments are stretched and the spinal cord enlarged. (Modified from: White AA, Panjabi MM: *Clinical Biomechanics of the Spine,* **ed. 2. Philadelphia, JB Lippincott, 1990.[8])**

rior longitudinal ligament and the annulus fibrosus of the disc opens the access to the disc. With the magnification and illumination of the microscope, the nucleus pulposus and parts of the disc material are removed and the posterior annulus fibrosus is exposed. With a dissector, the defect in the posterior wall is identified and enlarged, if necessary, to remove the herniated material. Removing bone might be necessary to identify a dislocated hernia.

After the herniated disc material is extracted, the bed for the bone graft is prepared. The cartilaginous tissue of the disc is carefully removed to expose the bony surface of the endplate. In addition, a thin layer of bone is removed down to 3 to 4 mm of the posterior annulus fibrosus, thus preventing the graft from protruding into the spinal canal.

A bone graft is taken from the anterior iliac wing. The cut surfaces of the graft converge slightly to obtain a physiological lordosis after insertion. The graft is placed under distraction. Removing the distraction creates tension in the tissue that locks the graft firmly in place.

DISCUSSION

To treat the patient described in this case, I prefer an anterior discectomy and interbody fusion. The advantage of the addi-

tional fusion is the predictability of the final position of the cervical spine and preservation of the physiological lordosis[2] (Fig. 1). Procedures that do not employ fusion rely on nature to compensate for the defect. The inevitable narrowing of the disc space means that the patient must accept a posterior narrowing of the intervertebral foramen. Through distraction with an appropriately-shaped bone graft, the foramen gets wider and additional decompression can be achieved through the reduction of posterior ligaments (Fig. 2). The immediate segmental stability reduces the period of postoperative pain.[6]

Arguments against fusion include the possibility of complications with bone graft (extrusion, resorption) and at the donor site.[4] These problems exist, but they occur relatively infrequently. With fusion, the risk of complications might be slightly increased, but the advantages outweigh these risks. Reports in the medical literature of fusion techniques using allografts are promising.[3] With this option, complications at the donor site are eliminated.

With newer techniques, such as percutaneous nucleotomy, fusion can possibly be avoided. At present, however, I believe that simultaneous anterior interbody fusion with a cervical discectomy is the most reliable technique.

Treatment of Soft Cervical Disc Herniation

Fraser Henderson, M.D.

Presented is the case of a young woman with neck and right arm pain, weakness, and sensory deficits referable to the C6 dermatome. Conservative therapy has not been successful. The MRI confirms a lateral soft-disc herniation at the appropriate level. No myelopathy is suggested, and the MRI shows no spinal cord compression, stenosis, or spondylitic hard disc. Based on

these facts, I favor the posterior "keyhole" foraminotomy for this patient for 3 reasons:

- There is less potential for complications,
- There are fewer long-term adverse biomechanical consequences,

- The simplicity of the procedure.

The arguments raised by the previous authors provide an excellent basis for discussion.

THE ANTERIOR APPROACH

The author who argues for anterior discectomy with interbody fusion emphasizes that the risk:benefit ratio should be favorable. What are the risks of the anterior approach? In good hands, serious complications are uncommon.

Common Complications

Flynn[6] compiled the complications reported on questionnaires sent to those surgeons who use the anterior approach. Of those surgeons responding to the questionnaire, 71% claimed to have had no complications in their patients. The remaining 29% reported 311 serious complications from a total of 36,657 cases. These included 78 cases of transient or permanent myelopathy, and 22 cases of significant permanent radiculomyelopathy. There were 128 cases of radiculopathy of "intraoperative etiology," and 52 cases of laryngeal nerve palsy. These rates of peripheral nerve injury are most certainly low. Cloward[4] reported that hoarseness complicated 8% of all of his cases; in 2% the hoarseness was permanent. This rate is more in line with that of Heeneman[9] who noted voice changes in 11% of his patients, all of whom were found to have impaired or unilateral mobility of the vocal cord on indirect laryngoscopy.

A more recent retrospective study[2] elicited histories of hoarseness in 22% and dysphagia in 17% of patients. These symptoms lasted only 2 days to 3 months. Permanent recurrent nerve palsy and superior nerve palsy occurred in only 2% of these patients. The authors cautioned that 1% of laryngeal nerves do not recur, arise from the vagus nerve and pass to the posterior aspect of the cricoarytenoid joint. Thus, they are subject to injury during dissection. More commonly experienced are traction injuries to the superior laryngeal nerve in the upper cervical levels. While unilateral palsy is usually associated with mild hoarseness from paralysis of the cricothyroid muscle, it can also cause aspiration because the patient loses sensation in the larynx above the glottis. (I always reoperate on the cervical spine on the same side as the previous surgical approach, so as not to risk creating a bilateral nerve palsy.)

Other Complications

The sympathetic plexus may also be injured, causing Horner's syndrome. The cervical portion of the sympathetic trunk lies within the carotid sheath. When joined with the first thoracic ganglion, the inferior cervical ganglion, or stellate ganglion, it lies on the ventral aspect of the head of the first rib, and then ascends within the sheath posteromedial to the carotid artery over the lateral border of the vertebrae. Approaching the vertebra too laterally may cause Horner's syndrome; this complication sometimes occurs because of scarring. The surgeon is often unable to identify the longus colli muscles and the midline space between them.

Infections may occur from injury to the viscera. Laceration of the viscera is not rare, and unrecognized contamination of the wound by esophageal organisms can cause a life-threatening infection. Flynn[6] reported 3 deaths from esophageal perforation. Fortunately, esophageal lacerations are easily closed in a single layer. In fact, most wound infections are superficial and easily treated.

Vascular complications are uncommon in anterior approaches. The most life-threatening of these is delayed retropharyngeal bleeding, which is caused by pressure on the trachea that compromises the airway.[20] Other complications, such as stroke, may stem from carotid compression, and a few rare cases of cerebral infarction have been reported. Injury to the vertebral artery may result from overly ambitious rongeuring of the uncus in an effort to decompress the root. The vertebral artery lies 2 mm from the tip of the uncal process in the undistracted spine and 1.6 mm from the tip of the uncal process in the distracted spine.[14] Thus, there is clearly a greater risk to the vertebral artery when the vertebrae are distracted. On occasion, one may inadvertently tear a branch of the vertebral artery. While most of these bleeds respond to packing, many surgeons prefer to dissect and clip the vertebral artery to prevent a delayed hemorrhage.

Dural laceration is infrequent. Grisoli and colleagues[8] reported 2 cases in their series of 120 patients. In these patients, scarring between the posterior longitudinal ligament and the dura caused shearing of the dura. In each case, the tear was repaired with muscle and glue. Others have reported series of corpectomies to treat ossification of the posterior longitudinal ligament and commented that even large tears in the dura heal without problems.

Complications Related to the Graft

Complications related to removing the graft usually stem from the surgeon's inexperience and include osteomyelitis, fracture of the iliac crest, and injury to the superficial femoral, iliohypogastric, or ilioinguinal nerves. Great blood loss may result from inadequate hemostasis, and may even lead to breakdown or infection of the wound. The most enduring of problems relating to graft removal, however, is that of pain at the graft site. When reviewing all types of grafts, Prolo reported a 25% incidence of unacceptable pain at graft sites. Others report 0% morbidity at the graft site and attributed their success to removing the graft well lateral to the anterior superior iliac crest,[3] away from the superficial femoral nerve, which lies within 2 cm of the anterior superior iliac spine. Patients seem to do better when the graft is taken more laterally, hemostasis is complete, the bone is thoroughly waxed, and the wound thoroughly lavaged and closed in several watertight layers.

Complications of the graft itself include delayed graft extrusion (2 to 27%), graft fracture and recurrent radiculopathy, and mild transient myelopathy from fracture of the bone graft.[19] Collapse of the posterior disc space may cause interscapular pain or recurrent radiculopathy from narrowing of the neural foramen. Although no evidence has been shown for this, entrapment of the posterior longitudinal ligament after graft collapse has been suggested to provoke neck pain.[8]

Pseudoarthrosis

Pseudoarthrosis remains a potential problem with the anterior approach. Robinson reported a 12% nonfusion rate per level.[17] Other authors have reported rates of pseudoarthrosis of 12%.[5] A subsequent study using a modified technique, in which the vertebral end plates were burred down to bleeding subchondral bone, resulted in a 4% nonunion rate and, significantly, a correspondingly improved outcome in terms of pain. Others have reported a nonunion rate of 4%[3] and 2%.[7] However, whether pseudoarthrosis causes pain is uncertain. One series reported nonunion in 4 patients, of which 2 had incomplete relief of pain, and 1 developed early recurrence of neck and arm pain.[7] Another author[3] reported that 50% of pseudoarthroses were symptomatic. Yet, others have reported that pseudoarthrosis does not cause pain. Grisoli and colleagues[8] reported on 120 patients who underwent discectomy without fusion; there was a fusion rate of 70%, but pain recurred in only 10%. Thus, only 1 in 3 patients with failed fusions had recurrent pain. This statistic seems more in line with my experience and that of others with whom I have spoken.

Is Fusion Necessary?

It is also uncertain whether or not patients undergoing anterior cervical discectomy without interbody fusion eventually require fusion for a good result. In their series of anterior cervical discectomies without interbody grafting, Benini and colleagues[1] found no instability on dynamic radiographs and no correlation between the quality of clinical results and the radiographic appearance. Perhaps the importance (or lack of it) of fusion in anterior procedures without interbody fusion is underscored by the absence of any statistic of fusion rate in the series of 187 patients described by Vise.

ANTERIOR DISCECTOMY WITH FUSION

The author advocating anterior discectomy with interbody fusion stated that decompression of the nerve root, a pain-free cervical spine, and restoration of normal anatomy and range of motion are the goals of treatment. However, restoration of normal anatomy is not achieved with the anterior approach; instead, the biomechanics and long-term functioning of the cervical spine are significantly altered.

An anterior discectomy with fusion is a destructive and reconstructive process. Clearly, major elements of the anterior and middle columns—the anterior longitudinal ligament, the intervertebral disc, and sometimes the posterior longitudinal ligament—are removed. This does not have a big effect on short-term stability.[1,8] Restoration of the disc height with a graft does seem to restore adequate stability to the motion segment; however, questions about long-term biomechanical consequences remain unanswered. For instance, the torque generated by a fused segment in the sagittal and coronal planes exerts a fulcrum effect proportional to the length of the fused segment. The potential consequences of this fulcrum effect are empirically obvious.

Adjoining Degeneration

Long-term radiographic follow-up studies have suggested that patients undergoing anterior cervical fusions develop adjoining degenerative disease. In a retrospective review of 49 cervical fusions for degenerative disc disease,[13] the authors were able to obtain follow-up X-rays in only 9 patients 7 to 15 years after the initial surgery. Of these 9 patients, 8 were found to have increased degenerative changes above and below the level of fusion. In their series, Williams and colleagues[20] reported the rate of disc extrusion at levels adjacent to the fusion to be 16.6%.

Not only does interbody fusion increase degenerative disease at adjacent levels, but the presence of spondylosis at adjacent levels appears to affect the patient's outcome after interbody fusion. A retrospective study of 94 patients[3] showed that the efficacy of anterior cervical discectomy and fusion significantly decreased in the presence of adjacent asymptomatic spondylosis. When no additional levels of spondylosis were present, 88% of patients had a good or excellent outcome. When additional levels of spondylosis were present above or below the

level of discectomy and fusion, however, only 60% of patients had a good or excellent outcome. The presence of cervical spondylosis at adjoining levels should promote the consideration of a posterior approach.

Other Complications

There are other biomechanical consequences of interbody fusion. First, if one considers that all motions of one segment of the cervical spine are coupled with the motions of contiguous segments, and that each vertebra relates with the one above and below, then the abnormal movement of 2 fused vertebrae directly involves the motions of 4 vertebrae, or 3 motion segments. Second is the obvious decrease in range of motion. At the C5-C6 level, fusion creates a loss of 3 to 5 degrees of rotation, 6 degrees of flexion, and 4 degrees of lateral bending. Although the loss is trivial if only 1 segment is fused, the restriction may become important if subsequent fusions are necessary at adjacent levels.

WITH OR WITHOUT FUSION?

There is no doubt that the anterior discectomy and interbody fusion removes the source of compression and immediately relieves pain in most patients. I do not advocate this procedure for the patient described in the case presented, but it is the procedure with which I am most comfortable and which has been without serious complication. It is rapid, bloodless and, from a surgical perspective, a satisfying operation.

Some surgeons leave the posterior longitudinal ligament intact and probe for herniated fragments. For patients in whom disc fragments cannot be retrieved through a tear in the annulus— the majority in the opinion of one of the foregoing authors—the technique relies on the indirect decompression of the nerve root through interbody distraction with a bone graft. When taking the anterior approach, I prefer to remove the posterior longitudinal ligament on the side of the disc to ensure the removal of disc fragments and to more completely remove bars or hard discs that often compromise the spinal canal. With the posterior ligament removed, the nerve root can be directly palpated and the spinal canal probed. I stand on the side opposite the site of the disc herniation; this gives the maximum visualization of the lateral recess. As Raynor[15] points out, however, the lateral extent of resection of the uncus can be easily overestimated because there are no good landmarks. With the anterior approach, under direct vision, only the first 1 to 2 mm of the nerve root are exposed. Therefore, the last few millimeters of uncal resection must be carried out without direct observation to fully decompress the root. Unfortunately, the root may actually exit the spinal canal above the level of the disc; thus, the root impingement may be inaccessible through the anterior approach.[15] Superb instrumentation has greatly enhanced the exposure and safety of the operation.

Are there fewer potential complications in performing the anterior cervical discectomy without fusion? Certainly there is a big advantage; there is no need for grafting and, hence, graft harvesting. There are, however, 2 major disadvantages:

- The radical discectomy necessary to decompress the nerve roots involves a more extensive removal of both uncovertebral joints and longitudinal ligaments, and there is increased risk associated with radical discectomy;
- Postoperative pain complicates 25% of cases because of settling, which usually resolves within several weeks.

In my lesser experience, however, the pain occasionally lingers for longer periods, and the patient may have some loss of lordosis and even slight kyphosis. Wide resection of the uncal joints is necessary to allow the disc space to collapse and, yet, preserve the foraminal space; this carries the small, but real, risk of injury to the vertebral artery. In the near future, new bone substitutes may obviate the need for obtaining autologous bone grafts. The excellent results achieved by the proponent of this procedure are a tribute to his surgical skill; I remain unconvinced as to the superiority of the concept.

THE POSTERIOR APPROACH

For the patient described in this case, I favor a posterior "keyhole" foraminotomy. The advantages of this approach include its safety, simplicity, and speed. The only complications are an occasional wound hematoma, infection, and neck pain that is related to the incision and resolves in several days or a week. Good exposure of the nerve root can be obtained by removing the medial 30 to 50% of the facet joint.[16] On average, 4 mm of the nerve root can be exposed through removal of the medial one third of the facet.[16] This is probably adequate to decompress most nerve roots, although occasionally more of the facet must be removed. Removing more than 50% of the facet compromises the strength of the remaining facet. An overly aggressive resection of the facet theoretically predisposes the contralateral facet to fracture under loads within the physiological range.[16] However, this complication is exceptionally rare. Nerve-root injury is also rare because the nerve root is clearly visualized. The nerve root may leave the dural tube horizontally directly overlying the disc, or may exit at oblique angles well above the disc space, in which case it lies above the uncovertebral joint.[15]

From a biomechanical perspective, the posterior approach is more sound. The keyhole foramen does not interfere with the disc space or the anterior or posterior longitudinal ligaments. There is no alteration in the vertebral height, no significant loss of motion, and no interference with movements of vertebrae. When subsequent discectomies are anticipated or required on the initial approach, two-level foraminotomies can be executed without significantly altering the biomechanics of the cervical spine. Because of its economy of time and materials, the keyhole foraminotomy is attractive. In the prone position, a unilateral approach can be performed through a small midline incision or a paramedian oblique incision that centers over the facet joint.[12] In his series of 846 patients who underwent posterolateral foraminotomy, Henderson and colleagues[10] showed that removing the disc is not usually necessary because the foraminotomy is adequate to decompress the nerve root in most instances. Scoville and colleagues[18] concurred that simple decompression of the nerve root sleeve overlying a lateral osteophyte has given good results although, in cases of lateral soft disc, they generally incised the posterior longitudinal ligament and milked out the extruded fragment. Henderson and colleagues[10] and Scoville and associates[18] reported good or excellent results in 98% and 95% of their cases, respectively. One of the authors discussing the patient presented here carefully notes that removing herniated disc fragments from the neural foramen might lessen the number of recidivus discs.

Only 2 long-term, prospective, randomized studies compare posterior cervical laminotomy-foraminotomy with anterior cervical discectomy. In 1 study, 44 patients with anterolateral disc herniations alternately underwent either the anterior or posterior procedure, and were followed for a mean of 4 years. No statistical significance was found as to the relative efficacy of the 2 procedures, but there was a tendency toward an improved outcome in those patients undergoing the anterior approach (100% improved) versus those undergoing the posterior approach (93% improved). Similarly, in the study by Herkowitz and colleagues,[11] 94% of patients undergoing anterior discectomy with fusion enjoyed good or excellent results while 75% of those undergoing a posterior laminectomy-foraminotomy had good or excellent results. The authors cite increased stability of the motion segment and distraction of the neural foramen as factors favoring successful outcome in the anterior approach. Unfortunately, the number of cases was too small to appreciate the complications possible, and no statistical significance of results was achieved in either study.

CONCLUSION

In general, I reserve the anterior approach for hard central discs, bilateral pathologic processes, and cervical myelopathy from stenosis and discs. I generally avoid the anterior approach in the presence of scarring in the anterior neck or known recurrent laryngeal or superior laryngeal palsy, and in the presence of spondylitic disease adjacent to the level of proposed discectomy. Most neurosurgeons agree, however reluctantly, that the posterior approach is underused. It is an adequate, safe, and simple procedure for soft lateral discs and for unilateral hard discs. The opinions of the foregoing authors are forged on an anvil of experience greater than mine. Therefore, I defer, with some reservations, to the assessment of de Tribolet, who stated that the choice between the 2 approaches mostly depends on the experience of the surgeon and one should not be too dogmatic on this issue.

REFERENCES

Frederick A. Simeone, M.D.

1. Henderson CM, Hennessy RG, Shuey HM, et al.: Posterolateral foraminotomy as an exclusive operative technique for cervical radiculopathy: A review of 846 consecutively operated cases. *Neurosurgery* 1983; 13:504–572.

W. Michael Vise, M.D.

1. Benini A, Krayenbühl H, Bruderl R: Anterior cervical discectomy without fusion: Microsurgical technique. *Acta Neurochir (Wien)* 1982; 61:105–110.
2. Bertalanffy H, Eggert HR: Clinical long term result of anterior discectomy without fusion for treatment of cervical radiculopathy and myelopathy, a follow-up of 164 cases. *Acta Neurochir (Wien)* 1988; 90:127–135.
3. Bertalanffy H, Eggert HR: Complications of anterior cervical disc-

ectomy without fusion in 450 consecutive patients. *Acta Neurochir (Wien)* 1989; 99:41–50.

4. Cuatico W: Anterior cervical discectomy without interbody fusion: An analysis of 81 cases. *Acta Neurochir (Wien)* 1981; 57:269–274.

5. De Tribolet N, Zander E: Anterior discectomy without fusion for the treatment of ruptured cervical discs. *J Neurosurg Sci* 25: 217–220.

6. Dunsker SB: Anterior cervical discectomy with and without fusion. *Clin Neurosurg* 1977; 24:516–521.

7. Giombini S, Solero CL: Considerations on 100 anterior cervical discectomies without fusion, in Grote W, Brock M, Clar HE (eds): *Advances in Neurosurgery*, vol 8. New York, Springer, 1980, pp 302–307.

8. Granata F, Taglialatela G, Graziussi F, et al.: Management of cervical disc protrusions by anterior discectomy without fusion, personal contribution. *J Neurosurg Sci* 1981; 25:231–234.

9. Grisoli F, Graziani N, Fabrizi AP, et al.: Anterior discectomy without fusion for treatment of cervical lateral soft disc extrusion: A follow-up of 120 cases. *Neurosurgery* 1989; 24:853–859.

10. Hankinson HL, Wilson CB: Use of the operating microscope in anterior cervical discectomy without fusion. *J Neurosurg* 1975; 43:452–456.

11. Hirsch C, Wickbom II, Lindstrom A, et al.: Cervical-disc resection: A follow-up of myelographic and surgical procedure. *J Bone Joint Surg* 1964; 46A:1811–1821.

12. Husag L, Probst C: Microsurgical anterior approach to cervical discs: Review of 60 consecutive cases of discectomy without fusion. *Acta Neurochir (Wien)* 1984; 73:229–242.

13. Lunsford LD, Bissonette DJ, Janetta PJ, et al.: Anterior surgery for cervical disc disease. Part 1: Treatment of lateral disc herniation in 253 cases. *J Neurosurg* 1980; 53:1–11.

14. Martin AN: Anterior cervical discectomy with and without interbody bone graft. *J Neurosurg* 1976; 44:290–295.

15. Murphy MG, Gado M: Anterior cervical discectomy without interbody bone graft. *J Neurosurg* 1972; 37:71–74.

16. Odom GL, Finney W, Woodhall B: Cervical disc lesions. *JAMA* 1958; 166:23–28.

17. O'Laoire SA, Thomas DG: Spinal cord compression due to prolapse of cervical intervertebral disc (herniation of nucleus pulposus). Treatment in 26 cases by discectomy without interbody bone graft. *J Neurosurg* 1983; 59:847–853.

18. Robertson JT, Johnson SD: Anterior cervical discectomy without fusion: Long term results. *Clin Neurosurg* 1980; 27:440–449.

19. Rosenørn J, Hansen EB, Rosenorn MA: Anterior cervical discectomy with and without fusion. A prospective study. *J Neurosurg* 1983; 59:252–255.

20. Smith RA: Anterior cervical discectomy without grafting. *J Med Assoc Ga* 1985; 74:642–647.

21. Tew JM, Mayfield FH: Anterior cervical discectomy: A microsurgical approach (abstract). *J Neurol Neurosurg Psychiatry* 1975; 38:413.

22. U HS, Wilson CB: Postoperative epidural hematoma as a complication of anterior cervical discectomy. Report of three cases. *J Neurosurg* 1978; 49:288–291.

23. Wilson DH, Campbell DD: Anterior cervical discectomy without bone graft. *J Neurosurg* 1977; 47:551–555.

Deiter Grob, M.D.

1. Bailey RW, Badgley CE: Stabilization of the cervical spine by anterior fusion. *J Bone Joint Surg* 1960; 42A:565–594.

2. Chesnut RM, Abitbol JJ, Garfin SR: Surgical management of cervical radiculopathy: Indication, techniques and results. *Orthop Clin North Am* 1992; 23:461–474.

3. Ferneyhouyn JC, Whit JI, LaRocca SH: Fusion rates in multilevel spondylosis comparing allograft fibula with autograft fibula. Paper presented at Cervical Spine Research Society Annual Meeting, San Antonio, Texas, 1990.

4. Hankinson HL, Wilson CB: Use of the operating microscope in anterior cervical discectomy without fusion. *J Neurosurg* 1975; 43:452–456.

5. Husag L, Probst CH: Microsurgical anterior approach to cervical discs: Review of 60 consecutive cases of discectomy without fusion. *Acta Neurochir (Wien)* 1984; 73:229–242.

6. Kadoya A, Nakamura T, Kwak R: A microsurgical anterior osteophytectomy of cervical spondylotic myelopathy. *Spine* 1984; 9: 437–441.

7. Smith GW, Robinson RA: The treatment of certain cervical spine disorders by the anterior removal of the intervertebral disc and interbody fusion. *J Bone Joint Surg* 1958; 40A:607–613.

8. White AA, Panjabi MM: *Clinical Biomechanics of the Spine*, ed. 2. Philadelphia, JB Lippincott, 1990.

Fraser Henderson, M.D.

1. Benini A, Krayenbühl H, Bruderl R: Anterior cervical discectomy without fusion: Microsurgical technique. *Acta Neurochir (Wien)* 1982; 61:105–110.

2. Bulger RF, Rejowski JE, Beatty RA: Vocal cord paralysis associated with anterior cervical fusion: Considerations for prevention and treatment. *J Neurosurg* 1985; 62:657–661.

3. Clements DH, O'Leary PF: Anterior cervical discectomy and fusion. *Spine* 1990; 15:1023–1025.

4. Cloward RB: New method of diagnosis and treatment of cervical disc disease. *Clin Neurosurg* 1962; 8:93–132.

5. Emery SE, Bohlman HH, Goodfellow DB: Robinson anterior cervical discectomy and fusion for cervical radiculopathy: Long-term follow-up on 122 patients. *Orthop Trans* 1991; 15:678.

6. Flynn TB: Neurologic complications of anterior cervical interbody fusion. *Spine* 1982; 61:537–539.

7. Gore DR, Sepic SB: Anterior cervical fusion for degenerated or protruded discs: A review of 146 patients. *Spine* 1984; 9: 667–671.

8. Grisoli F, Graziani M, Fabrizi AP, et al.: Anterior discectomy without fusion for treatment of cervical lateral soft disc extrusion: A follow-up of 120 cases. *Neurosurgery* 1989; 24:853–859.

9. Heeneman H: Vocal cord approaches to the anterior cervical spine. *Laryngoscope* 1973; 83:17–21.

10. Henderson CM, Hennesy RQ, Sherry HM, et al.: Posterolateral foraminotomy as an exclusive operative technique for cervical radiculopathy: A review of 846 consecutively operated cases. *J Neurosurg* 1983; 13:504–512.

11. Herkowitz HN, Kurz LT, Overholt DP: Surgical management of cervical soft disc herniation: A comparison between anterior and posterior approach. *Spine* 1990; 15:1026–1030.

12. Hunt WE, Miller CA: Management of cervical radiculopathy. *Clin Neurosurg* 1985; 33:485–502.

13. Hunter LY, Brauenstein EM, Bailey RW: Radiographic changes following anterior cervical fusion. *Spine* 1980; 5:399–401.

14. Pait TG, Killefer JA, Kaufman HH: *Surgical anatomy of the anterior cervical spine*. Paper presented at the Tenth Annual Meeting for the Spine and Peripheral Nerves, Ft Lauderdale, Florida, 1994.

15. Raynor RB: Anterior and posterior approach to the cervical spine: An anatomical and radiographic evaluation and comparison. *Neurosurgery* 1983; 12:7–13.

16. Raynor RB, Pugh J, Shapiro I: Cervical facetectomy and its effect on spine strength. *J Neurosurg* 1985; 63:278–282.

17. Robinson RA, Smith GW: Anterolateral cervical disc removal and interbody fusion of the cervical spine. *J Bone Joint Surg* 1962; 44A:1569–1587.

18. Scoville WB, Dohrmann GJ, Corkill G: Late results of cervical disc surgery. *J Neurosurg* 1976; 45:203–210.

19. Shapiro SA, Scully T, Campbell R, et al.: *Cervical spondylosis with radiculopathy and no myleopathy*. Paper presented at the Ninth Annual Meeting of the Joint Section on Disorders of the Spine and Peripheral Nerves, Tuscon, Arizona, 1983.

20. Williams JL, Allen MB, Harkess JW: Late results of cervical discectomy and interbody fusion: Some factors influencing the results. *J Bone Joint Surg* 1968; 50A:277–286.

25

Treatment of Thoracic Disc Herniation with Myelopathy: Thoracotomy vs. Costotransversectomy vs. the Lateral Extracavitary Approach

CASE

A 39-year-old man came to medical attention with a 3-month history of progressive weakness of his legs. Upon examination, he had a relative sensory level just below the nipple line that was more pronounced in the right leg. He had profound weakness of the left leg and moderate weakness in the right leg. His leg reflexes were abnormally brisk and he had a Babinski reflex on the left. Magnetic resonance images demonstrated disc herniation at T4-T5.

PARTICIPANTS

Thoracotomy and Discectomy for Thoracic Disc Herniation with Myelopathy–
Noel Perin, M.D.

*Costotransversectomy for Thoracic Disc Herniation with Myelopathy–*Sean O'Laoire, M.D.

The Lateral Extracavitary Approach for Thoracic Disc Herniation with Myelopathy–
Edward C. Benzel, M.D.

*Moderator–*Edward S. Connolly, M.D.

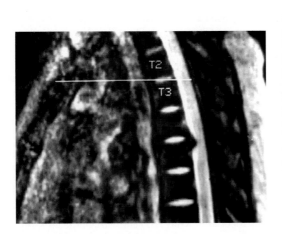
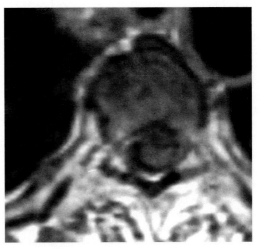

Thoracotomy and Discectomy for Thoracic Disc Herniation with Myelopathy

Noel Perin, M.D.

Thoracic disc herniation is a relatively uncommon condition, accounting for less than 2% of all disc operations.[1,3] More recent imaging modalities, especially magnetic resonance imaging (MRI), have shown a greater prevalence of thoracic disc herniation than previously suspected.[4] The upper thoracic spine is the least common site for disc herniation; however, the lower 4 thoracic levels account for one half to two thirds of all cases of symptomatic thoracic disc herniation. The increased occurrence of disc herniation in the lower thoracic spine might result from the greater mobility at the thoracolumbar junction, compared with other levels in the thoracic spine.[5]

CASE ANALYSIS

In this case, a 39-year-old man presented with a 3-month history of progressive weakness in his legs. Examination showed a partial Brown-Séquard syndrome with weakness predominantly on the left side, and a sensory level just below the nipple line. Deep tendon reflexes were brisk with a positive Babinski on the left side.

CHOOSING A SURGICAL APPROACH

Because of this patient's progressive neurological deterioration, early surgical intervention is indicated to arrest the progression and reverse the deficits. The decision to operate and the approach adopted depends upon the surgeon's training and experience, as well as the patient's overall medical condition. Patients in poor general condition may not tolerate a transthoracic, transpleural approach or an extensive extracavitary approach. These patients may be best treated through a posterior laminectomy and a transpedicular or a limited costotransversectomy approach.

Other factors to consider in choosing the optimal approach to this disc herniation include the location of the disc herniation in relation to the spinal canal (i.e., lateral, central, or centrolateral). Lateral herniations are best treated through a transpedicular-transfacetal approach. Large central disc herniations are more appropriately treated through a transthoracic-transpleural approach. Centrolateral herniations can be treated through either a transthoracic or a posterolateral approach. A third consideration in choosing the approach is the level of the herniation in the thoracic spine. From T2 to T4, a traditional costotransversectomy or a transthoracic approach may be difficult because of the presence of the scapula. A transmanubrial-transsternal approach or a third rib approach may be required to reach this area of the spine. An extended costotransversectomy or extracavitary approach can be done in the upper thoracic spine through the parascapular approach.[2] Migration of a disc fragment upward or downward at any level can necessitate a more anterior approach to retrieve the free fragment.

Other conditions that present with thoracic disc herniations, and are usually treated through an anterior approach, include juvenile kyphosis dorsalis (Scheuermann's disease) with disc herniations occurring at the apex of the kyphotic deformity. The kyphotic deformity may be corrected at the same time as the discectomy tthrough a transthoracic-transpleural approach. The consistency of the disc, especially the presence of calcification, is another indication for the use of the anterolateral approach.

This is especially true in a large, calcified herniation of the central disc. The patient in this case has a left centrolateral disc herniation at T4-T5 with significant cord compression and draping of the cord around the herniated disc. The anterior and anterolateral regions of the spinal cord are seen more effectively through the transthoracic approach to the T4-T5 interspace than with the posterolateral approaches. Therefore, I recommend approaching this disc herniation through a right T5 thoracotomy (transpleural).

OPERATIVE TECHNIQUE

Positioning, Intubation, and Monitoring

In the operating room, the patient undergoes electrode placement for monitoring of somatosensory evoked potentials. A baseline study is obtained before the induction of anesthesia. The patient is intubated with a double-lumen endotracheal tube to enable the collapse of the right lung during the procedure. The anesthesiologist administers low concentrations of halogenated inhalation agents, as well as muscle relaxants and narcotics, to prevent interference with evoked potential monitoring. The patient is placed in the lateral decubitus position with the right side up. An axillary roll is placed below the left axilla and an abdominal roll is placed in front of the left chest and abdomen. All pressure points are padded and a pillow is placed between the patient's knees. The right arm is pulled forward and supported on a padded stand. The patient is adequately taped to the operating table to enable lateral tilting during the operation.

Exposure

An oblique incision is made over the fifth rib starting from the lateral margin of the paraspinal muscles posteriorly to the anterior axillary line (Fig. 1). The incision is carried down to the trapezius and rhomboid muscles posteriorly and the serrati anteriorly. The muscles are divided with a coagulating current. The intercostal muscles are encountered between the ribs and are divided at the superior margin of the fifth rib to avoid injuring the neurovascular bundle. The parietal pleura is visualized and opened along the length of the exposure.

A self-retaining retractor is used to open the intercostal space, and the ribs are counted subcutaneously to verify the level. The anesthesiologist deflates the right lung at this point. The fifth rib is followed down to the spine to locate the T4-T5 disc space. Spinal needles are inserted into 2 adjacent disc spaces, and an anteroposterior X-ray is obtained to confirm the level. The parietal pleura and endothoracic fascia are reflected as a flap poste-

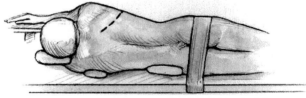

Fig. 1 The lateral decubitus position with the incision outlined.

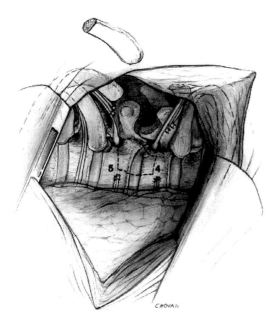

Fig. 2 After the head and neck of the fifth rib are removed to expose the pedicle of T5, the area outlined is drilled.

riorly and sutured to the adjacent chest wall. The intercostal artery and vein course over the vertebral bodies in the anterior-posterior direction midway between 2 adjacent disc spaces. They can be dissected free and retracted rostrally and caudally or divided between ligatures.

Discectomy

The head and neck of the fifth rib are removed with a rongeur to expose the pedicle of T5. The vertebral bodies adjacent to the

T4-T5 disc space and the pedicle of T5 are outlined (Fig. 2). The disc is entered in its anterior two thirds, and the posterior third and the herniated fragment are spared until later in the procedure. Disc material is removed piecemeal anteriorly. A high-speed air drill is used to drill the bodies of T4 and T5 adjacent to the T4-T5 disc space in its posterior third together with the pedicle of T5. Drilling continues until a thin shell of cortical bone is left covering the anterior aspect of the spinal cord from pedicle to pedicle. This shell is next opened rostrally and caudally with a nerve hook and on the right side at the thinned out pedicle. This enables the surgeon to free the shell of bone with the attached herniated disc from the adjacent dura and to pull this segment anteriorly into the cavity created by the drilling of the bodies of T4 and T5 (Fig. 3). An assistant holds the shell of cortical bone and the attached disc with a clamp while the surgeon, under direct vision using the microscope, frees the disc from the underlying spinal dura, where it might be stuck.

When the dura has been decompressed from root to root, the segment of the fifth rib previously removed is used as a bone graft. Two pieces of rib are placed in the trough anterior to the cord and wedged into position (Fig. 4). The flap of parietal pleura is sutured back with chromic catgut, and the wound is closed with an apical chest drain in place.

CONCLUSION

Once a decision has been made to treat a patient surgically, determining which approach is most appropriate for that patient is key to a successful outcome. This decision is based on the anatomy of the disc herniation as determined by MRI findings, the general medical status of the patient, the presence of coexisting conditions in the spine (for example, thoracic canal stenosis or Scheuermann's disease), and the surgeon's expertise with different approaches.

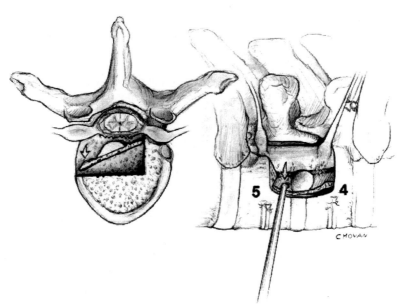

Fig. 3 The shell of cortical bone with the herniated disc attached posteriorly is pulled away from the cord into the area of decompression anteriorly.

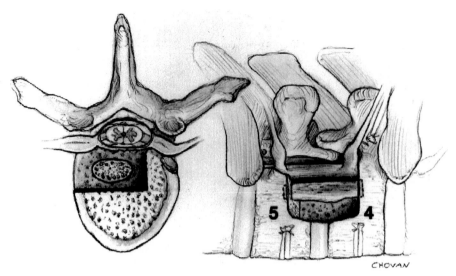

Fig. 4 The decompressed cord with the rib graft in place.

Costotransversectomy for Thoracic Disc Herniation with Myelopathy

Sean O'Laoire, M.D.

The case presented is one of a thoracic disc prolapse causing compression of the spinal cord, the compressive lesion being off-center. The surgical requirements include excision of an anteriorly placed intraspinal mass that compresses the spinal cord without undue manipulation of the cord, thereby avoiding trauma. The nerve root and the vascular supply thereto must be preserved, and spinal stability should be maintained to allow for early mobilization. Adequate surgical access to the anterior aspect of the spinal canal with minimal interference of spinal integrity is, therefore, required.

COSTOTRANSVERSECTOMY

The features described above are provided through a modification of the traditional costotransversectomy approach using microsurgical principles. For this approach, the patient is placed face down after transfixion under radiological guidance of the head of the rib or the tip of the transverse process, immediately above or below the diseased disc on the side for which the approach is planned. The approach should be from the side of maximum protrusion if the disc is not central. In the case of a truly central disc, the approach may be from either side, depending on the surgeon's preference.

Surgical Technique

An incision 7 to 10 cm long is made about 5 cm from the midline. A muscle-splitting incision is then made obliquely in the direction of the costal transverse junction. The muscle origins are detached from the transverse processes and the medial 2 to 3 cm of rib above and below. After subperiosteal dissection, the medial 2 to 3 cm of the upper rib and the head of the inferior rib are excised. The transverse processes are trimmed back to the junction of the lamina and pedicle. The intercostal nerve and vessels are then identified and traced proximally to the intervertebral foramen. The radicular artery is identified, and the vessels and nerve are mobilized in the intervertebral foramen by dividing the

tissue bands lying between them and the disc with microscissors. The pleura is then separated from the posterior centimeter or 2 of the vertebral body and pedicle. The pedicles above and below the intervertebral foramen are then thinned down to the inner cortex using the high-speed drill. Removal of the inferior third of the upper pedicle and the superior two thirds of the lower pedicle is usually sufficient.

A trench is then cut using the high-speed drill in the posterior aspect of the vertebral bodies above and below the disc. This maneuver preserves the posterior cortex about half a centimeter in the anteroposterior direction. The trench is carried towards the opposite side to a depth of about 1.5 cm, which is usually enough to reach the opposite pedicle. The cephalad and caudal limits should be beyond any osteophytes, that is, at the level of the normal anterior wall of the spinal canal. Small Kerrison® punches are then used to remove the inner cortex of the pedicles to expose the dura. It is then possible to inspect the anterior aspect of the dura and the disc protrusion.

The posterior vertebral body cortex is then cut using the high-speed drill above and below the disc. Inspection and palpation with microinstruments reveals whether or not the disc protrusion adheres to the dura. If not, the disc material between the vertebral body trenches can be transected. Then, it is often possible to lever the entire protrusion and attached osteophytes and endplates forward, away from the dura, and to displace the disc and bone complex forward into the vertebral trench and remove it in one piece by fracturing its opposite base. This maneuver should be done under direct vision and only when the bone on the opposite side has been undermined so that it will crack forward. If undermining is insufficient, the bone may snap backwards and traumatize the spinal cord.

If the disc adheres to the dura or is likely to have eroded, a lateral dural opening should be made. The intradural mass is then treated as an anterior tumor. Its base is cut through and, if the disc protrusion is heavily calcified, the use of a high-speed

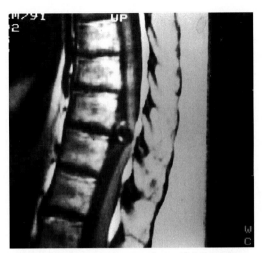

Fig. 1 Sagittal MRI showing a substantial, largely intradural, calcified disc protrusion at T9-T10. This patient had a 2-year history of painful dysesthesia in the lower limbs, mild difficulty in walking, and extensor plantar responses. She underwent a costotransversectomy to repair the herniation.

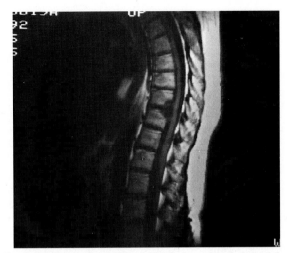

Fig. 2 Postoperative MRI, sagittal view, showing that the normal position and contour of the spinal cord was restored after surgery; note the extent of limited resection of the vertebral body.

drill may be necessary. The intradural mass is then debulked slice-by-slice on its most anterior aspect with the drill, rongeurs, or an ultrasonic aspirator, and the dome of the disc is moved forward. The spinal cord itself commonly is not visualized until the dome of the disc has collapsed forward. This dome is then dissected through the arachnoid layers, allowing the spinal cord to fall forward; this often being no more than a thin ribbon of tissue, sometimes transparent, in the midline. The spinal cord should not be manipulated in any way.

After the intradural disc is excised, the anterior dural defect is readily repaired with a patch of dural substitute (lyophilized dura) and sealed with fibrin glue. The lateral dural incision is closed using absorbent suture material, and the wound is closed over a vacuum drain.

Postoperative Course and Surgical Considerations

After surgery, the wound tends not to be very painful. Patients do not complain of unpleasant dysesthesia, and they usually walk within 24 hours. There is some risk of injuring the spinal cord (one out of 25 patients). Once mastered, the procedure is not difficult and is very safe, but familiarity with the use of the high-speed drill in confined spaces and in conjunction with the operating microscope is necessary, particularly in terms of changing the angle of approach by altering the microscope and the operating table. Even the largest of calcified intradural discs can be safely and effectively excised through a costotransver-sectomy (Figs. 1 to 3).

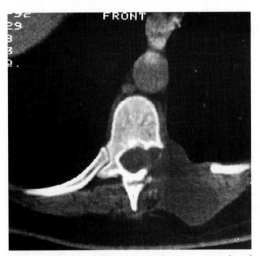

Fig. 3 Postoperative axial computed tomogram showing the extent of resection of the rib, the transverse process and the pedicle; the patient walked without deficit the day after surgery.

The Lateral Extracavitary Approach
for Thoracic Disc Herniation with Myelopathy

Edward C. Benzel, M.D.

The patient is a 39-year-old man with a 3-month history of progressive weakness and an MRI scan showing a T4-T5 central disc.

PREOPERATIVE STUDIES

I would begin my clinical treatment of this patient with a computed tomography (CT) myelogram. Although an MRI can define pathologic spinal anatomy, particularly in the sagittal plane, axial views can be difficult to interpret. A CT myelogram with intrathecal contrast clearly delineates the location of the disc herniation, particularly in the coronal plane.[1] In addition, the myelogram confirms the precise location of the herniated disc in relation to surgically definable anatomy (for example, ribs). This confirmation is critical because intraoperative definition of the pathologic anatomy is not always accurate.

After the precise location of the pathologic level is confirmed with MRI and CT myelogram, I order a spinal angiogram to confirm the absence of the radicular artery in the region of the herniation. If the artery is not present on the left, I would perform a lateral extracavitary surgical approach on the left. If, however, a radiculomedullary artery appears on the left in the region of the planned surgery, I would use a right-sided lateral extracavitary approach. A radiculomedullary branch rarely occurs in the upper thoracic region of the spine. Nevertheless, the risk of angiography must be weighed against the advantage of the procedure.

SURGICAL TECHNIQUE

A paramedian vertical incision is made about 3 cm from and parallel to the midline (Fig. 1). This incision is about 10 to 14 cm long and is centered on the T5 rib. Intraoperative radiography is used to locate this rib. The erector spinae muscles are freed from the ribs, transverse processes, lateral facet joints, and laminae in the region of exposure and retracted medially with self-retaining retractors, Figure 2 (**A**). Subperiosteal dissection is performed circumferentially around the T5 rib with periosteal and rib dissectors. The rib is transected 8 to 10 cm from the costotransverse junction. To minimize the chance of pleural penetration by a bony spicule, the remaining portion of the rib is rongeured to provide a blunt bony margin. Extrapleural and subperiosteal dissection is performed underneath the rib to its terminus at the costovertebral joint, thus freeing the pleura from extrapleural attachments. The rib is freed of soft tissue confines and removed after its disarticulation from the costotransverse and costovertebral joints, Figure 2 (**B**), allowing excellent lateral exposure of the region of concern. Any intercostal muscle obscuring the view is removed.

The T4 nerve underlying the rib and superior to the resected rib is dissected free of its associated soft tissues, including the pleura, intercostal muscles, and intercostal artery and vein. A tie is placed about the T4 intercostal nerve, which is transected lateral to this tie. The proximal nerve is followed to its exit point from the spinal canal at the T4-T5 neural foramina. After bipolar coagulation of the vascular component of the nonneural tissue of the foraminal region, the extraneous nonneural foraminal tissue

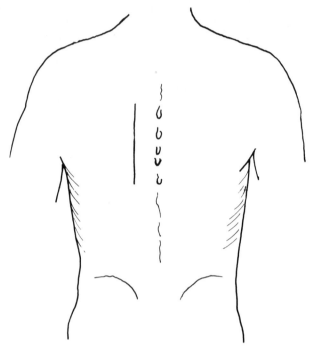

Fig. 1 For the lateral extracavitary approach, a paramedian incision is made about 3 cm from and parallel to the midline.

is removed, Figure 2 (**C**). The operating table may be rotated away from the surgeon to facilitate visualization.

A curved instrument, such as a nerve hook, is passed into the spinal canal to document the location of the margins and size of the neural foramina. A small amount of the superior margin of the dorsal aspect of the foramina (facets) and the superior and inferior aspects of the foramina (pedicles), are resected with a thin, plated, 45-degree Kerrison® rongeur, thus exposing the lateral aspect of the dura and the exit point of the T4 nerve root. Under the lateral aspect of the dura at the level of the neuroforamina lies the pathologic T4-T5 disc, Figure 2 (**C**).

The lateral aspect of the disc annulus is then incised with a 15 blade, and the disc is removed with small pituitary biopsy forceps, Figure 2 (**D**). A downward-facing 3-0 curette can be used to push the bulging disc into the cavity left by this maneuver, Figure 2 (**E**). Great care is taken to avoid plunging into the spinal canal at this point. After the dural sac is completely decompressed and the remainder of the offending disc material removed, a high-speed burr is used to create a trough about 1 to 1.5 cm deep in the vertebral body above and below the T4-T5 disc interspace. This trough is taken about three quarters across the diameter of the vertebral body.

The resected rib is then cut into 2 segments that fit snugly into the trough. These segments are placed into the trough sequentially, Figure 2 (**F**). The first rib graft is secured with a suture placed around it, so that the second rib graft can be secured to the first with a circumferential suture around both bone grafts. The

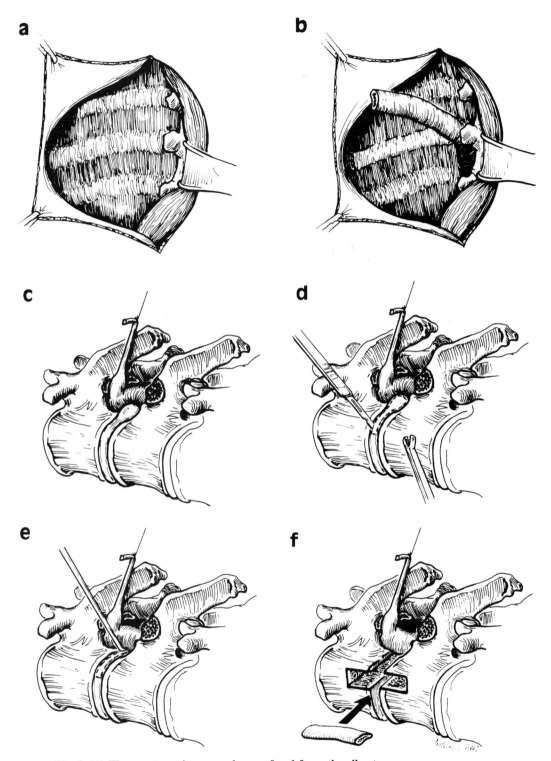

Fig. 2 (*A*) The erector spinae muscles are freed from the ribs, transverse processes, lateral facet joints, and laminae, and retracted medially with self-retaining retractors. (*B*) The rib is freed of soft tissue and removed after it is disarticulated from the costotransverse and costovertebral joints. (*C*) The vascular component of the nonneural tissue of the foramen is coagulated and extraneous nonneural tissue is removed. The damaged disc lies under the lateral aspect of the dura at the level of the neuroforamina. (*D*) The lateral aspect of the disc annulus is incised with a 15 blade and the disc is removed with small biopsy forceps. (*E*) A 3-0 curette is used to push the bulging disc into the cavity left after the disc is removed. (*F*) The resected rib is cut in two; each piece of this rib is placed into the trough.

wound is closed in multiple layers. A pleural tear can be sutured while the lung is inflated by the anesthesiologist, or a tube thoracostomy can be done. For 3 months after surgery, the patient must wear a cervicothoracic brace with a long thoracic extension whenever he or she is out of bed.

DISCUSSION

A variety of surgical approaches for thoracic disc resection have been used, including a laminectomy, a transpedicular approach, a costotransversectomy, the lateral extracavitary approach, and anterior or anterolateral (transthoracic) approaches.[3] The laminectomy and posterolateral approaches (costotransversectomy and transpedicular) carry, to varying degrees, a risk of neural injury during disc resection, particularly with discs extending to the midline, as is the case here. These discs require dural retraction if a posterior angle of approach is used, which is exceptionally dangerous in the region of the spinal cord.[2,5–13] These approaches do not allow for the placement of an interbody bone graft, which may be important to prevent further disc herniation. In a relatively immobile joint (e.g., mid- and upper thoracic intervertebral joints), a loss of mobility in a single motion segment is inconsequential.

The best angle to view the dural sac in each of the posterior and lateral approaches is illustrated in Figure 3. The direction in which the erector spinae muscle is retracted (medial vs. lateral) has significant implications regarding the best angle of view, because both the mass of the muscle itself and the self-retaining retractors partially obstruct the view if the muscle is retracted laterally with a midline exposure. Garrido[4] eliminated this problem by transsecting this muscle. The morbidity of transsecting the erector spinae and trapezius muscles, however, is not insignificant. The lateral extracavitary approach eliminates this problem by allowing a view under the erector spinae muscle, thus gaining at least 20 degrees of anterior view (regarding both decompression of the dural sac and placement of interbody fusion), and an excellent view of the lateral aspect of the vertebral body and disc.

The anterolateral or anterior approaches[9,12] require a thoracotomy and do not permit visualization of the dura until after substantial disc tissue has been removed, thus increasing the risk of the procedure. In the low thoracic region, incision of the diaphragm and retroperitoneal dissection is necessary, further augmenting the risk of these procedures.

The lateral extracavitary approach is simple and straightforward, facilitates X-ray localization of the level of the pathologic anatomy, provides direct visualization of the disc, and allows safe anterior resection of the disc and placement of an interbody fusion with an already accessible bone graft. Although this approach allows for anterior decompression and fusion, its extrapleural nature causes less respiratory embarrassment and allows simple and safe postoperative care, when compared with transthoracic approaches.

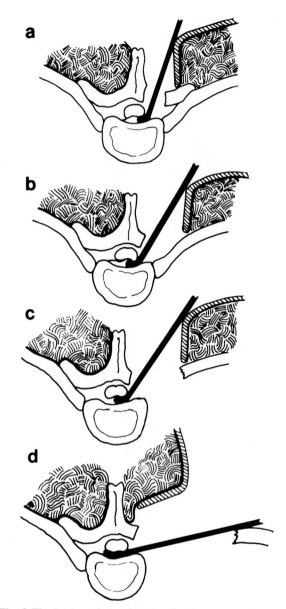

Fig. 3 The best angle to view the dural sac according to several approaches: (*A*) The best angle in the laminotomy. (*B*) The best angle in the transpedicular approach. (*C*) The best angle in the costotranversectomy. (*D*) The best angle in the lateral extracavitary approach.

Treatment of Thoracic Disc Herniation with Myelopathy: Thoracotomy vs. Costotransversectomy vs. the Lateral Extracavitary Approach

Edward S. Connolly, M.D.

All authors agree that thoracic disc herniation causing myelopathy should be treated surgically. The treatment of thoracic disc herniation producing pain alone is more controversial, but is not the subject of this chapter. Controversies in the treatment of myelopathy producing thoracic discs are related to preoperative diagnostic studies and operative approaches to thoracic discs.

CONTROVERSIES REGARDING IMAGING

The Use of Angiography

The first controversy is the necessity of spinal angiography in the evaluation of thoracic disc herniation from T8 to T12. The great radicular artery of Adamkiewicz usually enters the spinal canal from T8 to L1 and is located on the left side 60% of the time. Injury to this vessel may produce transverse myelitis; therefore, theoretically, in surgical approaches to thoracic discs from T7 to T12, it is important to know the exact location of this vessel.

Several groups of authors[5,9,13] are strong proponents of preoperative spinal angiography. Stillerman and Weiss[13] used it in 22 of 42 patients with thoracic disc herniation between T7 and T12, and changed their surgical approach in 1 patient because of the angiographic findings. Maiman and colleagues[5] used spinal angiography in all 25 patients with herniation from T7 to T12, and changed the side of approach in 6 patients based on the angiograms. Ransohoff and associates[9] concluded that, if the lesion is above T9, preoperative intercostal angiography should be done to determine the side and level of the artery of Adamkiewicz.

On the other hand, Sekhar and Jannetta[11] used angiography in 1 of 12 cases they presented, but considered it unnecessary. In their review of 280 cases of thoracic disc herniation, Arce and Dohrmann[1] made no mention of spinal angiography. Perot and Munro[8] reported 2 cases at T6 and T7 that were successfully treated without angiography. El-Kalliny and colleagues[4] did not mention the use of angiography in their report of 21 patients (17 between T7 and T12), but suggested that the approach to these levels be made on the right side to avoid injury to the artery of Adamkiewicz. Otani and colleagues[7] also made no mention of the use of spinal angiography in 23 cases of successfully-treated thoracic disc herniation. Bohlman and Zdeblick[3] reviewed 22 herniated thoracic discs in 19 patients, 18 of which were between T8 and T12, without the use of angiography. Blumenkopf[2] reported 9 patients successfully treated without angiography. Rosenbloom[10] did not mention spinal angiography in his article on the use of imaging in patients with thoracic disc disease. Singounas and colleagues[12] also did not use angiography in their 14 cases. In his chapter on thoracic disc herniation, Ogilvie[6] states that, if the segmental vertebral artery is ligated anterior to the neural foramen, preoperative arteriography is not necessary.

Although radiographic identification of the artery of Adamkiewicz in patients with thoracic disc herniation from T7 to T12 is appealing, no scientific evidence supports the routine use of spinal angiography, even though digital techniques are less dangerous than direct arterial injections. If the surgical approach to be used requires resection of the radicular artery, angiographic identification of the artery of Adamkiewicz seems prudent. If high-quality spinal magnetic resonance arteriography becomes available, this problem will be moot.

Alternative Modalities

Since the advent of high-resolution magnetic resonance imaging (MRI), most patients with thoracic myelopathy have been screened with this form of imaging. Those unable to tolerate MRI because of claustrophobia or the presence of a pacemaker or other magnetic metallic foreign body are usually screened with water-soluble contrast myelography followed by computed tomography (CT) with high-contrast resolution. The controversy revolves around who needs only 1 form of imaging. If 1 imaging modality shows a disc herniation that correlates with the physical findings, another type of imaging is not necessary. If the lesion appears to be calcified, however, a CT scan at that level helps delineate the extent of bone removal not easily seen or appreciated on MRI.

CHOOSING THE SURGICAL APPROACH

The second controversy is surgical approach to thoracic disc herniation. Because of the poor results of thoracic laminectomy with extradural removal of thoracic disc herniation (28% of 119 cases made worse[1]), a number of operative approaches previously described to treat Pott's disease were developed to treat patients with thoracic disc herniation.

The surgical approaches used to treat thoracic disc herniation are best described as anterior, anterolateral, lateral, posterolateral, and posterior. Except for the posterior approach alone, each of these approaches has its proponents. There are also proponents of approaching the thoracic spine on one side or the other, depending on the level, and various approaches advocated according to the location of the disc herniation (central, paracentral, and lateral). Other approaches are based on whether the disc is hard or soft and whether or not there is an intradural component or multiple herniations.

A review of 363 reported operative cases of thoracic disc herniation (Table 1) suggests that there is no significant difference in outcome among patients undergoing the posterolateral (transpedicular-transfacet) approach, the lateral (costotransversectomy or lateral extracavitary) approach, and the anterolateral (transthoracic) approach, but each approach has its advantages and disadvantages (Table 1).

The Direct Anterior Approach

The direct anterior approach to herniation (Fig. 1) is applicable only to the first 3 thoracic discs; at lower levels, the aortic arch, the heart, and the great vessels interfere. This approach requires a sternal splitting incision or partial resection of the manubrium and proximal clavicle, which puts at risk the recurrent laryngeal

Table 1. Outcome Analysis of Various Surgical Approaches to Thoracic Disc Herniation*

Approach	Total	Asymptomatic	Improved	Unchanged	Worse	Died
Laminectomy	129	19 (15%)	55 (43%)	14 (11%)	36 (28%)	5 (4%)
Posterolateral	38	16 (42%)	17 (45%)	5 (13%)	0	0
Lateral	120	44 (37%)	66 (55%)	8 (5%)	2 (2%)	–
Anterolateral	76	15 (20%)	59 (78%)	1 (1%)	1 (1%)	–
TOTAL	363	94 (26%)	197 (54%)	28 (8%)	39 (11%)	5 (1%)

*Composite of seven clinical reports; totals from each are as follows: 211,[1] 51,[13] 23,[5] 23,[7] 19,[3] 21,[4] and 15 (present study).

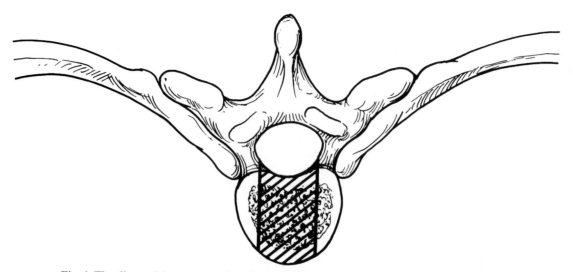

Fig. 1 The disc and bone removal in the anterior approach to the upper thoracic disc.

nerves, the thoracic duct, and the subclavian vessels, but provides an excellent direct view of the disc with the operative microscope. Either soft or calcified discs may be removed, with or without interbody fusion.

The Anterolateral (Transthoracic) Approach

The anterolateral, or transthoracic, approach (Fig. 2) is ideal for herniations at T4 or below, but is associated with the morbidity of thoracotomy: atelectasis, pneumonia, pneumothorax, and injury to the great vessels, as well as the necessity to take down the diaphragm at the thoracolumbar level and the possibility of a cerebrospinal fluid-pleural fistula and the post-thoracotomy pain syndrome. The anterolateral approach allows access to adjoining levels in cases of multiple disc herniation. It also allows access to central, paracentral, and lateral lesions and allows one to look across the entire anterior surface of the dural sac. Both soft and hard discs may be removed, and the body of the vertebrae may be drilled out and interbody fusion carried out with rib grafts from the thoracotomy incision. Perot and Munro[8] advised using a right-sided approach to midthoracic discs because the heart and great vessels do not impair exposure and the chance of injuring a significant radicular artery is less; however,

they recommended the left-sided approach for the lower thoracic discs because the vena cava obscures the vertebrae and disc on the right side and is more difficult to mobilize than the aorta on the left side. This direction, however, may create a greater risk of injury to the radicular artery of Adamkiewicz. Ransohoff and colleagues[9] suggested using the left side at all levels because it is easier to work with the aorta than the vena cava. Most of the reported series of transthoracic disc removals are from the left side, regardless of the level.

The Lateral Approach

The lateral approach to thoracic discs appears to be the most popular alternative among neurosurgeons because it provides visualization almost equal to that of the transthoracic approach, without the potential pulmonary complications and possible injury to the great vessels. This approach may be either a standard costotransversectomy (Fig. 3) for a lateral soft disc herniation or a more extensive, extrapleural lateral extracavitary approach (Fig. 4) to midline and calcified lesions. The advantage is that the dural sac and pathologic process can be visualized during removal of the disc, potentially minimizing cord injury. Extensive removal of the vertebral body, interbody fusion with a

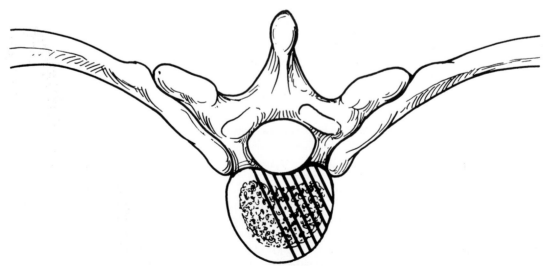

Fig. 2 The disc and bone removal in the transthoracic anterolateral approach to the upper thoracic disc.

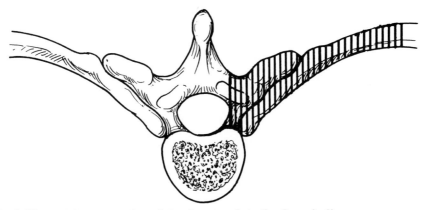

Fig. 3 The costotransversectomy lateral approach to the thoracic disc.

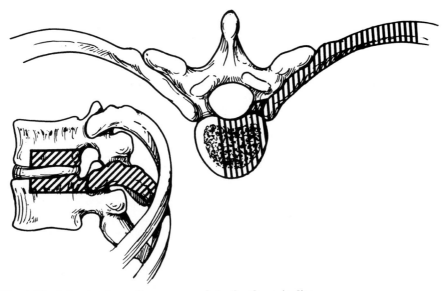

Fig. 4 The lateral extracavitary approach to the thoracic disc.

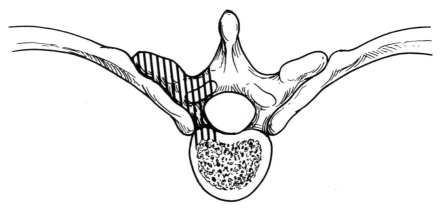

Fig. 5 The posterolateral or transpedicular approach to the thoracic disc.

rib graft, and posterior stabilization can also be done if necessary. This approach may also be advantageous if the disc herniation has an intradural component.

The Posterolateral (Transpedicular) Approach

The posterolateral or transpedicular approach (Fig. 5) provides the technically easiest approach to the thoracic disc, but offers the poorest visualization of the anterior aspect of the dural sac. It is, therefore, limited to lateral soft disc herniation.

Complications

Although, in a few reported series, cases of transverse myelopathy have occurred after the previously described approaches, many anecdotal cases are seen, usually in reviews of malpractice litigation. These cases appear at random, even in the hands of technically adept surgeons and have no obvious cause recognized by the surgeon or case reviewer. They resemble similar cases of transverse myelitis that occur after anterior cervical discectomies in which no obvious technical difficulties were encountered. Are these caused by mechanical compression unrecognized by the surgeon, vascular insufficiency secondary to spasm, or poor perfusion pressure in a vascular watershed area? The answer has yet to be determined and may be multifactoral. It is difficult to find the rate of complications associated with these procedures or the occurrence of transverse myelopathy, which is well-known if one reviews many malpractice cases. The rate is probably similar to that of transverse myelopathy occurring in patients after anterior cervical discectomy, and its cause is just as obtuse.

REFERENCES AND SUGGESTED READING

Noel Perin, M.D.

1. Arseni C, Nash F: Thoracic intervertebral disc protrusions: A clinical study. *J Neurosurg* 1960; 17:418–430.
2. Fessler RG, Dietze DD, MacMillan MM, et al.: Lateral parascapular extrapleural approach to the upper thoracic spine. *J Neurosurg* 1991; 75:349–355.
3. Gowers WR: *Diseases of the Nervous System*, ed. 2, vol. 1. London, Churchill, 1892, p 260.
4. Sekhar LN, Janetta PJ: Thoracic disc herniation: Operative approaches and results. *J Neurosurg* 1983; 12:303–305.
5. William MP, Cherryman GR, Husband JE: Significance of thoracic disc herniation demonstrated by MR imaging. *J Comput Assist Tomogr* 1989; 13:211–214.

Sean O'Laoire, M.D.

1. Young S, Karr G, O'Laoire SA: Spinal cord compression due to thoracic disc herniation: Results of microsurgical posterolateral costotransversectomy. *Br J Neurosurg* 1989; 3:31–38.

Edward C. Benzel, M.D.

1. Arce CA, Dohrmann G: Thoracic disc herniation: Improved diagnosis with computed tomographic scanning and a review of the literature. *Surg Neurol* 1985; 23:356–361.
2. Arseni C, Nash F: Thoracic intervertebral disc protusion: A clinical study. *J Neurosurg* 1960; 17:418–430.
3. Cybulski GR: Thoracic disc herniation: Surgical technique. *Contemp Neurosurg* 1992; 14:1–6.
4. Garrido E: Modified costotransversectomy: A surgical approach to ventrally placed lesions in the thoracic spinal canal. *Surg Neurol* 1980; 13:109–114.
5. Love JG, Keifer EJ: Root pain and paraplegia due to protrusions of thoracic intervertebral discs. *J Neurosurg* 1950; 7:62–69.
6. Love JG, Schorn VG: Thoracic-disc protrusions. *JAMA* 1965; 91:91–95.
7. Maiman DJ, Larson SJ, Luck E, et al.: Lateral extracavitary approach to the spine for herniation: Report of 23 cases. *Neurosurgery* 1984; 14:178–182.
8. Otani K, Nakai S, Fujimura Y, et al.: Surgical treatment of thoracic disc herniation using the anterior approach. *J Bone Joint Surg* 1982; 64B:340–343.
9. Perot PL, Munro DD: Transthoracic removal of midline thoracic disc protrusions causing spinal cord compression. *J Neurosurg* 1969; 31:452–458.
10. Ransohoff J, Spencer F, Siew F, et al.: Trans-Thoracic removal of thoracic disc: Report of three cases. *J Neurosurg* 1969; 31:459–461.
11. Ravichandran G, Frankel HL: Paraplegia due to intervertebral disc lesions: A review of 57 operated cases. *Paraplegia* 1981; 19:133–139.
12. Sekhar LN, Janetta PJ: Thoracic disc herniation: Operative approaches and results. *Neurosurgery* 1983; 12:303–305.
13. Terry AF, McSweeney T, Jones HWF: Paraplegia as a sequela to dorsal disc prolapse. *Paraplegia* 1981; 19:111–117.

Edward S. Connolly, M.D.

1. Arce CA, Dohrmann G: Thoracic disc herniation: Improved diagnosis with computed tomographic scanning and a review of the literature. *Surg Nevrol* 1985; 23:356–361.
2. Blumenkopf B: Thoracic intervertebral disc herniations: Diagnostic value of magnetic resonance imaging. *Neurosurgery* 1988; 23:36–40.
3. Bohlman HH, Zdeblick TA: Anterior excision of herniated thoracic discs. *J Bone Joint Surg* 1988; 70A:1038–1047.
4. El-Kalliny M, Tew JM Jr, Van Loveren H, et al.: Surgical approaches to thoracic disc herniations. *Acta Neurochir* 1991; 111:22–32.
5. Maiman DJ, Larson SJ, Luck E, et al.: Lateral extracavitary approach to the spine for thoracic disc herniation: Report of 23 cases. *Neurosurgery* 1984; 14:178–182.
6. Ogilvie JW: Thoracic disc herniation, in Bridwell KH, DeWald RL (eds): *The Textbook of Spinal Surgery*, vol. 2. Philadelphia, JB Lippincott, 1991, pp 711–718.
7. Otani K, Yoshida M, Fujii E, et al.: Thoracic disc herniation: Surgical treatment in 23 patients. *Spine* 1988; 13:1262–1267.
8. Perot PL Jr, Munro DD: Transthoracic removal of midline thoracic disc protrusions causing spinal cord compression. *J Neurosurg* 1969; 31:452–458.
9. Ransohoff J, Spencer F, Siew F, et al.: Transthoracic removal of thoracic disc: Report of three cases. *J Neurosurg* 1969; 31:459–461.
10. Rosenbloom SA: Thoracic disc disease and stenosis. *Radiol Clin North Am* 1991; 29:765–775.
11. Sekhar L, Jannetta PJ: Thoracic disc herniation: Operative approaches and results. *Neurosurgery* 1983; 12:303–305.
12. Singounas EG, Kypriades EM, Kellerman AJ, et al.: Thoracic disc herniation: Analysis of 14 cases and review of the literature. *Acta Neurochir (Wien)* 1992; 116:49–52.
13. Stillerman CB, Weiss MH: Management of thoracic disc disease. *Clin Neurosurg* 1992; 38:325–352.

26

Treatment of Lumbar Disc Protrusion with Unilateral Radiculopathy: Percutaneous Aspiration Discectomy vs. Microdiscectomy vs. Conservative Treatment

CASE

After a brief period of lower back pain, a 35-year-old woman developed pain radiating into the posterior lateral thigh and, subsequently, the anterior lateral calf. She had no previous history of lumbar disc surgery or rheumatologic disorder. On examination, she had numbness to pinprick in the left great toe and weakness of the left extensor hallucis longus muscle. Her deep tendon reflexes were normal and her toes flexed to plantar stroke. Left straight-leg raising reproduced the radiating pain into the leg. Plain lumbosacral spine X-rays were normal. Her symptoms and signs persisted despite 6 weeks of conservative treatment. Axial magnetic resonance images demonstrated herniated disk at the L4-L5 level.

PARTICIPANTS

Percutaneous Aspiration of Lumbar Disc Protrusion with Unilateral Radiculopathy–
Joseph C. Maroon, M.D., Gary Onik, M.D.

Microdiscectomy for Lumbar Disc Protrusion with Unilateral Radiculopathy–Paul Young, M.D.

Prolonged Conservative Therapy for Lumbar Disc Protrusion with Unilateral Radiculopathy–
Edward Tarlov, M.D.

Moderator–Stephen J. Haines, M.D.

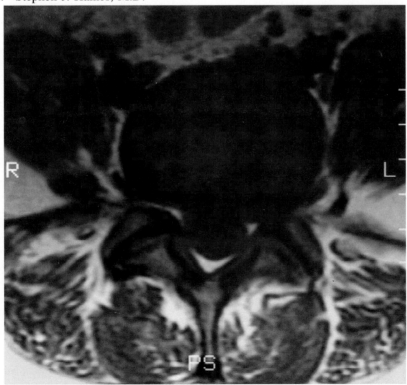

Percutaneous Aspiration of Lumbar Disc Protrusion with Unilateral Radiculopathy

Joseph C. Maroon, M.D., Gary Onik, M.D.

Safety and efficacy are the primary reasons to consider automated percutaneous lumbar discectomy in this patient. The growth of percutaneous intradiscal therapy, as an alternative to traditional open laminectomy and microdiscectomy, occurred because of the perception by both patients and some in the medical profession that the risks of laminotomy and laminectomy were significant and an alternative was needed.

THE RISKS OF OPEN SURGERY

Recent reports confirm this perception of open discectomy as a potentially high-morbidity procedure. A recent prospective study gathered the experience of neurosurgeons who have performed more than 100 surgical discectomies.[29] Data were collected on the open discectomies these neurosurgeons performed over a 1-year period to assess the incidence and type of complications. In this study, 481 operations were carried out using microsurgical and macrosurgical techniques. Intraoperative complications included perforation of the dura, significant hemorrhage, nerve root damage, and exposure of the wrong interspace. Overall, significant intraoperative complications occurred in 7.8% of the microdiscectomies, 13.7% of the macrodiscectomies, and in 27.5% of patients who underwent repeated operations. Postoperative complications included delayed wound healing, discitis, early recurrence of herniated discs, and worsened paresis. Postoperative complications ranged from 1.4% in the repeated operations to 4% in both micro- and macrodiscectomies.

Complications associated with open discectomy were reconfirmed by a report reviewing 28,000 patients who underwent lumbar discectomy at community hospitals.[25] This study showed that the incidence of death was 6 per 10,000, or 1 in 1700. The incidence of at least 1 major complication was 157 per 10,000. Although neurosurgeons carried out 60% of the operations and orthopedic surgeons 40%, no difference was found between the risk of surgery based on the surgeon's specialty.

A more recent report studied 654 patients, all of whom had procedures carried out under the operating microscope.[23] This study revealed that 11% of these patients had complications, with 1 death caused by abdominal arterial bleeding. After surgery, 3 patients had discitis, 3 had postoperative pseudomeningoceles requiring further surgery, 1 had an arterial injury, and 1 had a small-bowel injury.

PERCUTANEOUS LUMBAR DISCECTOMY

Automated percutaneous lumbar discectomy is a low-risk alternative to the high morbidity associated with open discectomy, as well as other intradiscal therapies including chemonucleolysis and the rongeur method of percutaneous discectomy. It has now been used for almost 10 years in more than 50 separate surgical series (many of them prospective multi-institutional studies) reported in the literature.[1–5,7,8,10–13,15,20,24,26–28,30–34] These studies, comprising more than 5000 patients, reported no major complications. Specifically, no permanent nerve injury, great vessel damage, or deaths were reported. The complication of discitis was reported at a rate of 0.2%, 3 to 5 times lower than that reported for open discectomy. At this point, the mortality

rate of this procedure is 0%. Two major complications of cauda equina injury mar an otherwise excellent safety record in our 70,000 patients. These complications were associated with major breaks in the recommended surgical protocol and were errors in radiographic localization.[9,21] The procedure has now been reviewed by the Technology Assessment Committee of the American Medical Association and has been given a CPT code. The National Blue Cross/Blue Shield Technology Assessment Committee no longer considers the technique experimental. The success rate of automated percutaneous lumbar discectomy has been consistently reported to be between 70 and 90%, with the range related to patient selection. A number of reports in the literature have compared open discectomy to percutaneous lumbar discectomy, with the slightly higher success rate of open discectomy balanced by the lower morbidity of percutaneous discectomy. A recent, prospective, randomized study presented at a meeting of the European Spine Society showed a difference in success rate between open discectomy and percutaneous lumbar discectomy of only 8%.[34] This study concluded that, based on its low morbidity rates, percutaneous lumbar discectomy was the procedure of first choice in properly selected patients.

CASE PRESENTATION

Based on these facts, we believe we are justified in offering this patient a percutaneous discectomy. She fits the criteria for this procedure, with a typical history of a herniated L4-L5 disc with compression of the L5 nerve root. The patient's leg pain is greater than her back pain and she has associated physical findings including numbness, weakness, and a positive straight-leg raising sign.

While this patient clinically fits the criteria of a candidate for percutaneous lumbar discectomy, the justifiable question can be raised as to whether 6 weeks of conservative therapy is sufficient. The answer to this question is determined by the patient and the treating physician. If all conservative treatment has failed and the patient continues to have intractable pain as a neurological defect, surgical treatment should be considered.

At this stage, the radiographic appearance of the herniation determines the type of operative treatment appropriate for the patient (that is, either an open microdiscectomy or a percutaneous discectomy). In this patient, the herniation is focal, with smooth margins consistent with the patient's symptoms. This herniation is most likely contained by the patient's annulus and posterior longitudinal ligament. For this patient, we would need more information to absolutely rule out a migrated fragment (that is, other axial magnetic imaging slices above and below to look for fragment migration into the lateral recess, and sagittal slices to look for migration and determine whether the annular fibers are intact). If there is any doubt as to whether the herniation is contained, computed tomography discography should be done to look for gross free-flow of contrast into the epidural space; this would indicate a complete tear of the annulus and posterior longitudinal ligament.

The communication between the center of the disc and the herniation can also be an important criteria indicating whether or not a percutaneous lumbar discectomy will be successful. A

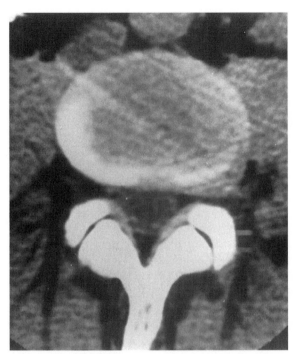

Fig. 1 Axial computed tomogram shows a far-lateral herniation at the L4-L5 disc level on the left. Note that no space exists between the disc and the L4 nerve root (compared with the right). The margins of the herniation are smooth, and there is no migration superiorly or inferiorly, indicating a contained herniation. This patient was successfully treated by automated percutaneous lumbar discectomy.

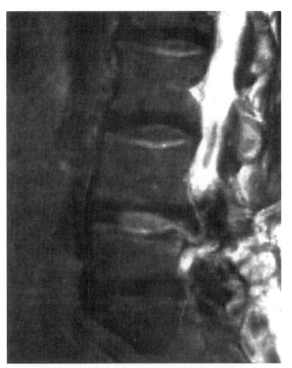

Fig. 2 Magnetic resonance image showing a herniated nucleus pulposus in the L4-L5 position in a 64-year-old woman. The patient had a microdiscectomy at this level 2 years before this scan, which shows herniated nuclear material and scar. The patient's symptoms resolved completely after automated percutaneous lumbar discectomy.

wide communication indicates that the patient would have a good result. A narrow communication that creates a mushroom effect indicates that a patient is less likely to be helped by this procedure.[6]

Having decided that this patient has a contained herniation consistent with the clinical picture, opponents of the lumbar discectomy might say that nothing needs to be done because patients with contained herniation eventually get better, regardless of the treatment used. This position is unsupported by the literature. In a multi-institutional study carried out on 500 patients undergoing conservative treatment, the mean duration of symptoms was 11.5 months.[22] This rather prolonged period of conservative therapy has been confirmed by other studies, clearly indicating that these patients do not necessarily improve spontaneously. In another report, 20% of operated herniated discs were contained at the time of operation.[14]

In this patient, the herniated disc is in a foraminal, almost far lateral, position. The location of the disc, however, is not of value in determining the eventual success of the procedure; even

far lateral herniated discs can be successfully treated through a percutaneous lumbar discectomy (Fig. 1). Although this patient did not undergo previous surgery, patients who have previous surgery at the same level of a reherniation do well with percutaneous lumbar discectomy (Fig. 2). These patients may be successfully treated with exposure to minimal morbidity.[3,8,10]

ADVANTAGES OF PERCUTANEOUS DISCECTOMY

The advantages of automated percutaneous lumbar discectomy include: (1) lower morbidity when compared to open discectomy; (2) the performance of the procedure under local anesthesia on an outpatient basis with early return to function (about 70% of patients can return to work within 2 weeks of the procedure); (3) the procedure avoids the epidural space; therefore, it does not cause epidural fibrosis and has no subsequent effect on the success of an open procedure; and (4) this procedure costs about half that of a microdiscectomy. Even when the 15% of patients who need an open operation are factored in, marked financial savings can result.

Microdiscectomy for Lumbar Disc Protrusion with Unilateral Radiculopathy

Paul Young, M.D.

The representative axial image from the magnetic resonance image (MRI) of this patient reveals primarily a paracentral and subarticular disc herniation. I would describe this abnormality

as a contained (within a thinned annulus) disc protrusion. With only 1 axial image supplied, I cannot be certain of the rostral-caudal extent of this disc abnormality, but I will assume that the only significant radicular compression occurs adjacent to the disc space. This certainly fits the patient's clinical signs and symptoms, which are referable to an L5 radiculopathy (and not L4). In addition, there is evidence of facet hypertrophy, which supports the likely pathophysiological basis of this disc abnormality, that is, motion segment instability. The patient's plain spine films are normal, so, clearly, the instability is physiological and not (as yet) anatomic.

CASE ANALYSIS

It is surprising that the patient did not respond to an adequate conservative treatment program. I will assume that this program included rest at home, physiotherapy, anti-inflammatory medicines, and mild exercise (extension-type). In my experience, most patients with this particular anatomic disc abnormality, indeed, respond to conservative treatment modalities over the short term. Unfortunately, many of these "responders" will, over months to years, develop recurrent sciatica of a more chronic nature, often eventually requiring surgical intervention. The fact that this patient did not respond to initial conservative treatment implies that the radiculopathy may be related to factors other than just the disc herniation. These possible associated etiologies include: a conjoint root abnormality at this level, subarticular or foraminal narrowing of the lateral recess secondary to facet joint arthrosis, or a missed, extruded, or sequestered fragment on imaging studies. In other words, my index of suspicion is high that the actual degree of radicular compression is greater than the imaging studies suggest.

SURGICAL TECHNIQUE

I would treat the patient with a lumbar microdiscectomy. Briefly, my operative procedure is as follows.

With the patient prone, a 2-cm midline incision and a curvilinear fascial incision are made off the midline to spare the supra-interspinous ligamentous complex. The epidural space is entered through the left lateral L4-L5 interlaminar space (Fig. 1). After adequate lateral exposure of the exiting nerve root and retraction of the root medially, the disc space can be identified (Fig. 2). With the patient in this position, one may be surprised to find less disc protrusion than anticipated. After confirming the

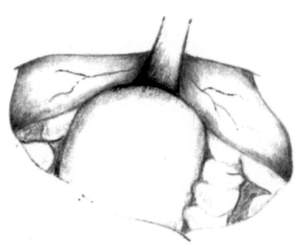

Fig. 2 The disc protrusion after the root is retracted; note that the degree of disc herniation observed in the prone position may be less than anticipated.

disc space radiographically, the disc nucleus is injected with 0.5% bupivacaine (Marcaine®) (1 or 2 cc) to confirm and better visualize the pathologic reaction of the annulus to increased intradiscal pressure. This maneuver may show leakage through an unsuspected tear in the annulus (and help identify a sequestered fragment) or, more commonly, better identify functional annular alterations.

The annulus is incised as far laterally as possible in a thin and incompetent area (Fig. 3). The thicker, more resilient portions of the annulus are preserved, particularly those segments intimately related to the exiting nerve root. All underlying herniated soft-disc fragments are removed after gentle dissection from the surrounding annulus (Fig. 4). Other fragments located centrally, laterally, and deeper in the interspace are gently loosened or teased from the surrounding annulus and cartilaginous endplates and removed (Fig. 5). The intradiscal decompression is completed only when firm, attached nuclear or nuclear-annular material is identified (Fig. 6). No rough curettage or massive avulsion of tissue is necessary. Upon completion of the discectomy,

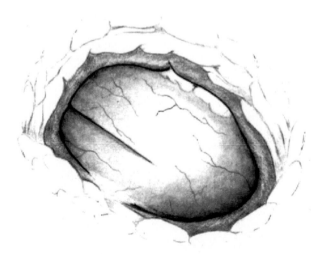

Fig. 1 The L4-L5 left interlaminar space is opened through a 2-cm skin incision; notice the discal pressure underlying the proximal portion of the root.

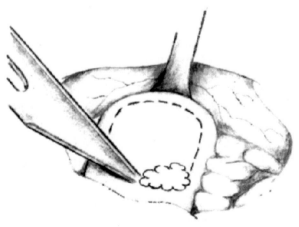

Fig. 3 Incision of the disc space in the area of incompetent annulus.

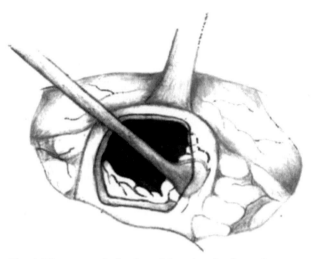

Fig. 4 The removal of soft and herniated subannular nuclear material.

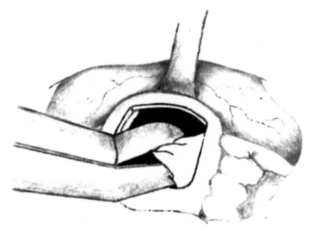

Fig. 6 The removal of disc material is completed when firm, attached nuclear material is identified.

the disc space is irrigated with antibiotic solution through a small catheter to flush out any other hidden fragments.

Before closure, the epidural space surrounding the disc space (medial, lateral, cranial, and caudal) is explored for unrecognized disc fragments. In turn, the epidural space surrounding the nerve root (laterally and axillary) is explored for further sources of compression. Finally, the subarticular and foraminal zones are inspected for evidence of stenosis, which is corrected if found. Upon satisfactory completion of the procedure, the previous protruded annulus should be retracted into the plane of the disc space and nerve root mobility should be restored (Fig. 7).

Closure includes absolute hemostasis, the placement of Gelfoam® over the annular and ligamentous defects, and the injection of the paraspinous muscles with 0.5% bupivacaine (Marcaine®). Postoperatively, the patient should be walking within a few hours and discharged that evening or the next morning. The patient is encouraged to return to a normal home activity program over the next 3 weeks, at which point a progressive exercise and rehabilitation program is prescribed.

SURGICAL RESULTS

The overall results of microdiscectomy for lumbar disc disorders and for this type of disc protrusion are summarized in Table 1.[2] The reason for the slightly higher rate of recurrence in young patients with this type of disc protrusion relates to the presence of motion segment instability. These patients have a higher postoperative recurrence of ongoing back pain related to this abnormality. They do, however, have complete relief of sciatica, which allows most of them to resume full, normal activity (even strenuous job-related activities).

ADVANTAGES OF MICRODISCECTOMY

In experienced hands, microdiscectomy for this group of patients is a safe and effective treatment that results in minimal morbidity and no mortality. Microdiscectomy has significant advantages over blind procedures (enzyme nucleolysis, percutaneous discectomies, etc.),[1] because it permits an accurate assessment of the topography of the disc herniation, the etiology of the radicular compression, and associated anomalies (conjoint roots, missed sequestration, and associated stenosis). This pro-

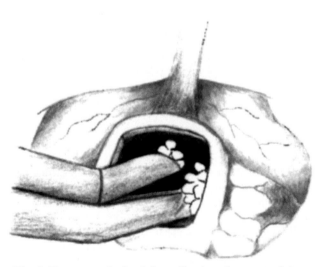

Fig. 5 The removal of soft intradiscal nuclear material.

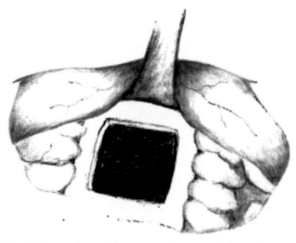

Fig. 7 Retraction of the previously protruded annulus into the plane of the disc space.

Table 1. Results of Lumbar Microdiscectomy

	Number of patients	Recurrent or persistent back pain	Recurrent sciatica	Additional surgery
Total	481	62 (12.9%)	42 (9.5%)	24 (5%)
Young patients (<40 years) with contained disc herniation	66	21 (32%)	6 (9.5%)	5 (8%)

cedure avoids the morbidity of a classic laminectomy and, yet, affords an improved opportunity for precisely identifying both normal and pathologic tissue. Although our follow-up is rela-tively short (up to 9 years), there is no support for the suggestion that these patients should undergo a stabilization procedure at the time of discectomy.

Prolonged Conservative Therapy for Lumbar Disc Protrusion with Unilateral Radiculopathy

Edward Tarlov, M.D.

A protruded intervertebral disc is a ubiquitous phenomenon in the adult population. I see no justification for surgical interven-tion in patients such as the one described. The long-term natural history of this problem is far less disabling than the effects of intervention. This is a nondisease. It is a sad commentary on the commercial aspects of modern medicine that the application of operative therapy to this problem may be increasing, fueled by the burgeoning of gimmicks.

Imaging techniques now available, including computed to-mography and MRI, allow for the accurate diagnosis of disc herniation and the gradations of disc protrusion, including the mildest forms such as this. No surgery whatsoever is advisable for this patient's disorder. It is not clear that so-called conserva-tive therapy is any better than the natural history of a protruded disc with reassurance and no treatment at all. It is hazardous for patients with mild disc protrusions such as this to make repeated follow-up visits to surgical offices, because this may increase the likelihood of ill-advised surgical treatment.

Treatment of Lumbar Disc Protrusion with Unilateral Radiculopathy: Percutaneous Lumbar Discectomy vs. Microdiscectomy vs. Conservative Treatment

Stephen J. Haines, M.D.

The authors evaluating this patient have nicely outlined the controversy surrounding the choice of initial surgical treatment for single-level, first-time, contained lumbar disc herniation pre-senting with unilateral radiculopathy. Each is confident that his (or their) recommendation represents the best initial treatment for the patient. They have all based their opinions on individual and collective experience with the recommended procedures. The experience with both procedures is extensive, although microsurgical discectomy clearly has a longer collective experi-ence than automated percutaneous discectomy.

CONSERVATIVE TREATMENT

The recommendation to avoid any form of surgical treatment at this time is an interesting one. It represents a very conservative view that is outside the mainstream of neurosurgical practice in the United States. This is not to say that it is wrong, for a substantial proportion of patients in this setting gradually im-prove over a prolonged period of benign neglect. The temporary disability that this theory imposes exceeds that tolerated by most North American patients and, for many, creates a significant financial hardship. Therefore, most neurosurgeons would con-sider a 6-week trial of nonsurgical treatment in a patient with radicular pain and an appropriate motor deficit to be more than sufficient to justify surgical intervention. A better answer to the question of when to intervene surgically requires more detailed research than is currently available.

SURGICAL INTERVENTION

The argument in favor of automated percutaneous discectomy relies essentially on 2 points: (1) that it is a less morbid proce-dure than microsurgical discectomy; (2) that its efficacy is close enough to that of microsurgical discectomy that the percentage of patients who do not respond to the percutaneous procedure, and require a microsurgical procedure, is small enough to justify the addition of percutaneous discectomy to the current standard of treatment with microsurgical discectomy. The morbidity and mortality figures given to justify the first contention are bother-some, in that there is a wide variation in the incidence of complications among the studies cited. Mortality ranges from 0 to 0.15% and complications from 1.6 to 11%. I suspect that such wide variations do exist in practice; that was certainly the case when carotid endarterectomy was examined. Nonetheless, death, paralysis, and disabling nerve injury remain extremely uncommon events in the practice of microdiscectomy as carried out by well-trained, experienced surgeons, and it has already been shown that serious complications can occur with automated percutaneous discectomy. The typical surgeon will never experience mortality with either procedure and is unlikely to encounter more than a handful of serious complications in the same period of time. Therefore, the choice between these procedures must be based more on questions of efficacy than on safety.

DETERMINING EFFICACY

Assessing the efficacy of surgical treatment is difficult. The outcome of importance in the treatment of this disease is primarily a subjective one. Physician and patient evaluations of such outcomes obtained by the operating surgeon are notoriously overly optimistic and subject to the effects of expectation before the procedure. The enthusiasm with which a new, apparently less invasive, procedure is received is known to have a substantial impact on the way patients are treated postoperatively. In addition, the selection of patients for procedures that appear to have different levels of risk contributes to subtle selection bias that can alter outcome. Despite the optimistic figures cited for success rates in automated percutaneous discectomy and the reported results of an unpublished controlled trial showing only an 8% difference in outcome between the automated and microsurgical procedures, the bulk of the literature (based on uncontrolled trials) suggests that the response rate to this procedure approximates 75%, and the rates reported for microdiscectomy from similar series are in the 85 to 90% range. No one has seriously proposed that automated percutaneous discectomy is superior to microdiscectomy in terms of success in relieving symptoms.

COST EFFECTIVENESS

The issue of cost savings with percutaneous lumbar discectomy is a very complex one. One cannot simply compare the cost of the procedures and hospitalization, but must include the cost for those patients who do not respond to the first procedure and require repeated surgery. To control for the effects of expectation in determining postoperative treatment, a controlled trial must remove the decision from the operating surgeon. Such a trial has not been done, and cost estimates taking into account all of these factors have not been made in truly comparable groups of patients.

CONCLUSION

With all of these caveats, I can only conclude at this time that the role of automated percutaneous lumbar discectomy in the treatment of first-time contained lumbar disc herniation presenting with radiculopathy remains unclear. There is certainly a solid rationale for considering the possibility that its use as the first procedure for such patients may lower the overall use of resources, and might produce fewer long-term complications. The case remains unproved, however, and no surgeon with a good track record in microdiscectomy should be criticized for continuing to recommend this as the procedure of choice. In these days of outcome scrutiny and cost containment, one would hope that surgeons treating such patients could come together to carry out a well-designed comparative trial of the two procedures, so that the role of percutaneous lumbar discectomy can be clearly and unequivocally defined. This would be in the best long-term interests of our patients and our profession.

REFERENCES AND SUGGESTED READING

Joseph C. Maroon, M.D., Gary Onik, M.D.

1. Benoist M, Bonneville JF, Lassale B, et al.: A randomised, double-blind study to compare low-dose with standard-dose chymopapain in the treatment of herniated lumbar intervertebral discs. *Spine* 1993; 18:28–34.
2. Blanc C, Meyer A, Tang YS, et al.: Treatment of herniated lumbar disc by percutaneous nucleotomy with aspiration: Preliminary results in 70 cases. *J Neuroradiol* 1990; 17:182–189.
3. Bocchi L, Ferrata P, Passarello F, et al.: La nucleoaspirazione secondo Onik nel trattamento dell'ernia discale lombare analisi multicentrica dei primi risultati su oltre 650 trattamenti. *Riv Neuroradiol* 1989; 2(Suppl 1):119–122.
4. Bonneville JF, Runge M, Paris D, et al.: CT of the lumbar intervertebral disc space after automated percutaneous nucleotomy. Comparison with chemonucleolysis. *Rachis* 1989; 1:113–121.
5. Cartolari R, Davidovits P, Gagliardelli M: Automated percutaneous lumbar discectomy (APLD), in Mayer HM, Brock M (eds): *Percutaneous Lumbar Discectomy.* Berlin, Springer, 1989, pp 157–162.
6. Castro WH, Jerosch J, Halm H: *Do we really remove as much nuclear material with percutaneous or conventional nucleotomy as we think?* Toft/Hoogland Course, November 1991, Munich, Germany.
7. Cooney FD: Comparison of chemonucleolysis with chymopapain to percutaneous automated discectomy: A surgeon's first 50 cases of each, in Mayer HM, Brock M (eds): *Percutaneous Lumbar Discectomy.* Berlin, Springer, 1989, pp 163–168.
8. Davis GW, Onik GM, Helms CA: Automated percutaneous discectomy. *Spine* 1991; 16:359–363.
9. Epstein NE: Surgically confirmed cauda equina and nerve root following percutaneous discectomy at an outside institution: A case report. *J Spinal Disord* 1990; 3:380–383.
10. Gill K, Blumenthal SL: Clinical experience with automated percutaneous discectomy—the Nucleotome system. *Orthopedics* 1991; 14:757–760.
11. Gobin P, Theron J, Courtheoux F, et al.: Percutaneous automated lumbar nucleotomy. *J Radiol* 1990; 71:401–406.
12. Hammon W: Percutaneous lumbar nucleotomy. *Neurosurgery* 1989; 24:635.
13. Hidalgo Ovejero AM, Garcia Mata S, Antunano Zarraga P, et al.: Resultados iniciales de la nucleotomia percutanea automatizada en el tratamiento de las hernias discales. *Rev Ortop Traum* 1991; 35:428–433.
14. Jackson RP, Cain JE Jr, Jacobs RR, et al.: The neuroradiographic diagnosis of lumbar herniated nucleus pulposus: I. A comparison of computed tomography (CT), myelography, CT myelography, discography, and CT-discography. *Spine* 1989; 14:1356–1361.
15. Kahanovitz N, Viola K, Goldstein T, et al.: A multicenter analysis of percutaneous discectomy. *Spine* 1990; 15:713–715.
16. Kaps HP, Cotta H: The value of automated percutaneous lumbar discotomy in the herniated lumbar disc. *Med Orthop Tech* 1989; 109:147–150.
17. Lisai P, Gasparini G, Laneri P, et al.: Percutaneous nucleotomy: The indications and limits. *Arch Putti Chir Organi Mov* 1990; 38:311–319.
18. Luft C, Weber J, Horvath W, et al.: Automated percutaneous lumbar discectomy (APLD)—Method and 1-year follow-up. *Europ Radiol* 1992; 2:292–298.

19. Magalhaes ACA, Weigand H, Barros Filho TE: Lumbar disc hernia: Indications for percutaneous discectomy. *Rev Hosp Clin Fac Med Sao Paulo* 1989; 44:285–287.

20. Maroon JC, Allen RC: A retrospective study of 1,054 APLD cases: A twenty-month clinical follow-up at 35 US centers. *J Neurol Orthop Med Surg* 1989; 10:L335–L337.

21. Onik G, Maroon JC, Jackson R: Cauda equina syndrome secondary to an improperly placed nucleotome probe. *Neurosurgery* 1992; 30:412–415.

22. Onik G, Mooney V, Maroon JC, et al.: Automated percutaneous discectomy: A prospective multi-institutional study. *Neurosurgery* 1990; 26:228–233.

23. Pappas CTE, Harrington T, Sonntag VKH: Outcome analysis in 654 surgically treated lumbar disc herniations. *Neurosurgery* 1992; 30:862–866.

24. Pitto E, Fabbri D, Pitto RP: Clinical experience with automated percutaneous discectomy. *Arch Putti Chir Organi Mov* 1990; 38:321–326.

25. Ramirez LR, Thisted R: Complications and demographic characteristics of patients undergoing lumbar discectomy in community hospitals. *Neurosurgery* 1989; 25:226–231.

26. Rezaian SM, Silver ML: Percutaneous discectomy—personal observations of 27 cases, in Mayer HM, Brock M (eds): *Percutaneous Lumbar Discectomy*. Berlin, Springer, 1989, pp 173–176.

27. Seibel RMM, Gronemeyer DHW, Sorensen RAL: Percutaneous nucleotomy with CT and fluoroscopic guidance. *JVIR* 1992; 3: 571–576.

28. Solini A, Paschero B, Ruggieri N: Automated percutaneous discectomy according to the Onik method: Conclusive considerations. *Ital J Orthop Traumatol* 1991; 17:225–236.

29. Stolke D, Sollmann WP, Seifert V: Intra- and postoperative complications in lumbar disc surgery. *Spine* 1989; 14:56–58.

30. Swiecicki M: Results of percutaneous lumbar discectomy compared to laminectomy and chemonucleolysis, in Mayer HM, Brock M (eds): *Percutaneous Lumbar Discectomy*. Berlin, Springer, 1989, pp 133–137.

31. Vanneroy F, Courtheoux F, Huet H, et al.: Percutaneous automated nucleotomy in the treatment of foraminal and extra-foraminal lumbar disc herniation: Review of 18 cases. *Rachis* 1991; 3:323–333.

32. Vogl G, Pallua A, Mohsenipour I, et al.: Neuroradiologic treatment possibilities of intervertebral disc displacement. *Wien Klin Wochenschr (Austria)* 1992; 104:243–247.

33. Weigand H, Weissner B: Percutaneous nucleotomy: A new interventional radiological technique for lumbar disc removal. *Ann Radiol* 1989; 32:34–37.

34. Wilson LF, Mulholland RC: *Automated percutaneous discectomy versus surgery: A prospective randomised study of treatment for lumbar disc protrusions*. Paper presented at the Third Annual Meeting of the European Spine Society, Cambridge, England, September 1992.

Paul Young, M.D.

1. Herkowitz HN: Current states of percutaneous discectomy and chemonucleolysis. *Orthop Clin North Am* 1991; 22:327–332.

2. Young PH: Microsurgery of the lumbar spine: A 4-year experience, in Williams RE, McCulloch JA, Young PH (eds): *Microsurgery of the Lumbar Spine*. Rockville, Aspen, 1990, pp 215–222.

Edward Tarlov, M.D.

1. Tarlov E (ed): *Complications of Spine Surgery*. Park Ridge, American Association of Neurological Surgeons, 1991.

2. Tarlov E, D'Costa D: *Back Attack*. Little, Brown, and Company, Boston, 1985.

27

Approaches to Multilevel Cervical Spondylotic Myelopathy

CASE

A 65-year-old man sought medical attention for long-standing neck pain, a recent onset of numbness in his hands, and progressive difficulty walking. Upon examination, he had mild muscle wasting in his hands, a slightly diminished grip strength, and clumsiness of fine finger function. He walked with a scissors gait and had abnormally brisk reflexes. His sensation was diminished to pinprick in the hands, bilaterally.

PARTICIPANTS

Anterior Corpectomy vs. Laminectomy for Cervical Spondylotic Myelopathy–
   Paul C. McCormick, M.D.

Posterior Cervical Decompression for Cervical Spondylotic Myelopathy–
   Peter M. Klara, M.D., Ph.D., Kevin T. Foley, M.D.

Moderator–H. Louis Harkey, M.D.

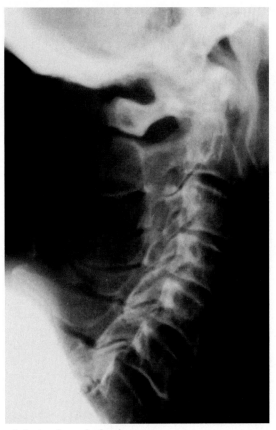

Fig. 1 Lateral cervical spine x-ray.

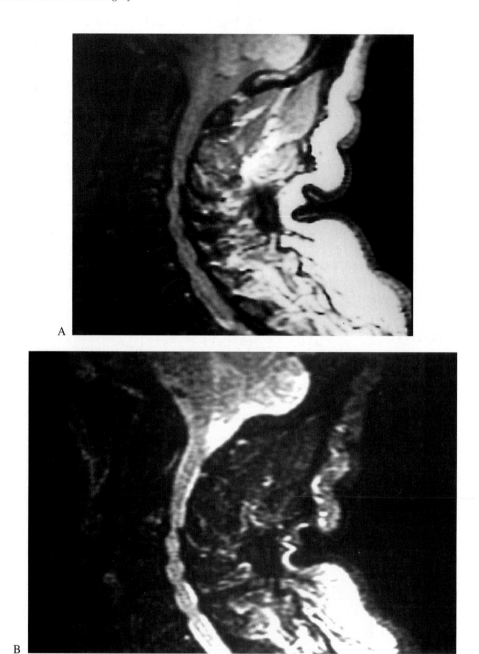

Fig. 2 Sagittal magnetic resonance images: (*A*) T-1 weighted. (*B*) T-2 weighted.

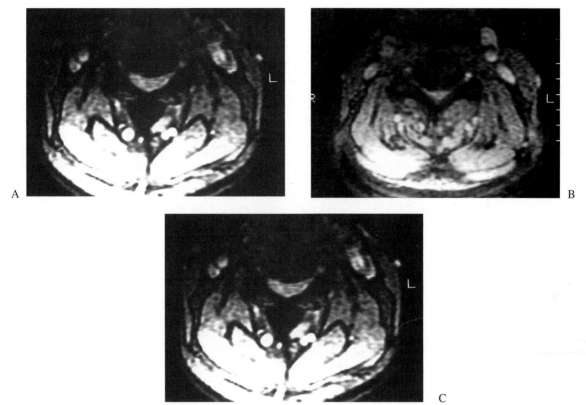

Fig. 3 Axial magnetic resonance images: (*A*) **C3-C4.** (*B*) **C4-C5.** (*C*) **C5-C6.**

Anterior Corpectomy vs. Laminectomy for Cervical Spondylotic Myelopathy

Paul C. McCormick, M.D.

This patient has the classic syndrome of cervical spondylotic myelopathy (CSM). Although the natural history of this disorder varies and is individually enigmatic, few would argue with the appropriateness of surgical intervention in a patient with a well-established clinical syndrome and significant multilevel compression of the spinal cord. Nevertheless, the surgical treatment of CSM, until recently consisting primarily of laminectomy, is associated with a relatively high failure rate. Although most series report a 70 to 80% improvement rate after laminectomy, only about one half of patients show significant improvement or resolution that is maintained long-term.[3,10] These inconsistent results have led some investigators to question whether or not there is any advantage of surgery over the natural history of this disorder.[9]

WHEN SURGICAL TREATMENT FAILS

The inability to reverse a neurological deficit or halt a progressive myelopathy defines the failure of surgical treatment. Recurrence of myelopathy after an initially successful operative result may also occur. The causes of failure vary and have not been entirely elucidated, which reflects an incomplete understanding of the pathophysiology of CSM. One cause is inaccurate diagnosis. Although cervical spondylosis is the most common cause of myelopathy in adults over 50 years of age, degenerative or inflammatory diseases, such as amyotrophic lateral sclerosis, primary lateral sclerosis, and multiple sclerosis, can produce myelopathy in this age group. Some of these patients may have significant radiographic spondylosis, which complicates the differential diagnosis. About 5% of patients with amyotrophic lateral sclerosis have had, or will, undergo surgical decompression.[10]

Another cause of surgical failure assumes that the spinal cord has sustained permanent damage at the time of treatment. It is difficult to identify preoperatively to what degree an established neurological deficit is reversible. Advanced age, severe and long-standing deficit, multilevel involvement, and severe morphological alterations and signal abnormalities seen on a magnetic resonance image have all been cited as negative predictive factors, but are not absolute.[5,8,12]

Unfortunately, all too often the patient who does not improve after surgery is assumed to have irreversible injury of the spinal cord or an alternative diagnosis. Only recently has surgical failure been recognized as a significant cause of poor outcome. In these cases, surgery does not achieve the required objective. This failure can result from a technically inadequate operation or an inappropriately chosen procedure that does not address the factors responsible for the myelopathy. Because our understanding of the pathophysiology of CSM is incomplete, however, defining clear treatment objectives is difficult.

IS COMPRESSION A CAUSE?

Compression is believed to be the primary cause of CSM. Indeed, the diameter of the sagittal spinal canal correlates with the incidence of myelopathy.[7] Direct compression may impair spinal cord function by causing pathologic mechanical stress (force per unit area) within the spine, interfering with its vascular supply, or both. The deleterious effects of multilevel cord compression appear to be additive.[11] Pathologic forces may be further influenced by the motion of the spinal column, which may intermittently exacerbate spondylotic compression or generate pathologic axial tension (stretch) within the spinal cord. Several investigators have shown a correlation between the severity of myelopathy and the degree of cervical spine motion.[1,2] Thus, compression alone as the sole cause of CSM seems unlikely.

Many Factors

Some patients have relatively severe cervical spondylosis without significant signs or symptoms, or their symptoms may remit or stabilize despite ongoing severe compression of the spinal cord. Other patients may show significant neurological deficit with less severe compression. Although the pathologic changes that define cervical spondylosis are progressive, the natural history of this clinical disorder can vary. This suggests that the pathogenesis of CSM is probably multifactorial, with both static and dynamic elements. The relative contributions of these pathologic factors probably differs among patients, which may explain the variable natural history of this disorder. In attempting to achieve the appropriate anatomic objective during surgery, therefore, all factors that may have contributed to the myelopathy must be addressed.

CASE DISCUSSION

This patient presents with diffuse congenital spinal stenosis that has been exacerbated by anterior formation of spurs and infolding of the posterior ligamentum flavum. One cannot be too dogmatic about the operative treatment of this patient. Adequate decompression and comparable surgical results can probably be achieved with either an anterior or posterior approach.

The multilevel spinal stenosis, the posterior component of cord compression, the absence of a dominant ventral spur, and a retained cervical lordosis are favorable predictive factors for posterior cervical laminectomy. Nevertheless, medial corpectomy and reconstruction is the preferred treatment in most patients with multilevel stenosis producing myelopathy. Only in unusual cases of a hyperlordotic cervical spine or dominant posterior compression of the spinal cord does laminectomy remain the treatment of choice. A trilevel (C4-C6) medial corpectomy with fibular reconstruction using an allograft would be recommended in this patient. Multiple discectomies do not produce comparable clinical results because pre-existing spinal stenosis is not adequately decompressed. Aggressive long-segment decompression, to include all levels of stenosis, prevents clinical recurrence as a result of deterioration of the marginally stenotic areas. Further, pathologic tension within the spinal cord may develop at these marginal levels through tethering or exacerbation of compression, as the spinal cord migrates into the defect left by the corpectomy. This is more likely to occur in patients who have retained some degree of spinal curvature, as is seen in this patient.

ANTERIOR DECOMPRESSION VS. LAMINECTOMY

Anterior cervical decompression has several advantages over laminectomy. Anterior decompression eliminates the main source of compression in most patients with CSM, the anterior osteophyte. Pre-existing spinal stenosis is also corrected with a multilevel corpectomy. Excessive motion is eliminated and iatrogenic spinal instability is avoided.

Cervical laminectomy enlarges the spinal canal and eliminates posterior compression, when present. Decompression from anterior osteophytes can only be achieved indirectly by disengaging the posterior spinal cord. Excessive cervical motion, if clinically relevant, is not addressed and there is a risk of delayed instability. This procedure may also be associated with debilitating postoperative pain syndromes, with significant impairment of the biomechanics of the cervical spine that results from removal of the posterior element and extensive disruption of muscular attachments.

The unacceptably high failure rate of laminectomy cannot simply be ascribed to incorrect diagnosis or irreversible spinal cord injury, particularly if the surgical objective has not been identified and critically evaluated. In one recent study, for example, Batzdorf and Flannigan[3] noted that 8 of 16 patients had persistent impingement of the spinal cord on magnetic resonance images after cervical laminectomy for spondylotic myelopathy. Further, long-term structural instability of the cervical spine, such as loss of lordosis, an S-shaped deformity, or kyphosis, has been reported in up to 25% of patients after laminectomy for CSM and is obviously a cause of late neurological deterioration.[6] Dense posterior scarring that does not allow the posterior spinal cord to disengage and exacerbation of excessive motion probably also compromise the surgical objective of laminectomy. Indeed, in light of the clearly superior results of medial corpectomy for patients with multilevel CSM in the hands of an increasing number of neurosurgeons having experience with anterior and posterior approaches, a significant number of treatment failures after laminectomy probably stem from a failure to adequately decompress the cord, eliminate excessive motion, or prevent future instability.[4]

CORPECTOMY

Complications

Limited exposure and poor bone graft technique are the main sources of complications in patients undergoing multilevel corpectomies. Small incisions and inadequate fascial release cause 2 problems. First, limited exposure compromises the surgeon's ability to adequately decompress the spinal cord. Second, excessive retraction of soft tissue increases the risk of postoperative swallowing and voice complications.

To prevent these complications, I prefer to use a generous skin incision that parallels the anterior border of the sternocleidomastoid muscle. The platysma muscle is divided and undermined in line with this skin incision. The fascia investing the anterior border of the sternocleidomastoid muscle is widely released, as far as possible. This maneuver is key. Each fascial layer is similarly opened widely until the prevertebral space is reached. The omohyoid muscle crosses the field at about the C5-C6 level, and can be divided. Small crossing blood vessels, such as the thyroid arteries and facial vein, may be divided as necessary. The hypoglossal, superior laryngeal, and recurrent laryngeal nerves are identified and preserved. Intraoperative fluoroscopy confirms the vertebral levels. The longus colli muscles are elevated with electrocautery. Identifying the uncovertebral joints helps determine the extent of the corpectomy. Table-mounted retractors are particularly useful, but must be periodically released to reduce the incidence of postoperative pharyngeal complications.

Surgical Technique

The technique of corpectomy begins with a multilevel discectomy. A high-speed drill is used to drill the endplates back to the posterior longitudinal ligament at each disc level. This drilling minimizes blood loss, which occurs primarily from the basovertebral vein in the center of the vertebral body. Once the discectomies have been done, a rongeur is used to carry out the anterior corpectomy, which is accomplished quickly with minimal blood loss. The bone is saved to later augment the allograft fusion. The high-speed drill is then used to widen the troughs and remove the rest of the vertebral body back to the posterior longitudinal ligament. The drilling is done early and completed before the dura is exposed. The decompression should be about 15 to 16 mm wide. This distance assures adequate decompression of the spinal cord, which is about 13 to 14 mm at its widest transverse diameter. Wider decompressions (for example, 18 to 20 mm) might be associated with a higher risk of postoperative radiculopathy, especially of the C5 root. (A satisfactory explanation of this phenomenon has yet to be made.) Wider decompressions may also increase the risk of complications after a bone graft.

Removing the Posterior Ligament

Removal of the posterior longitudinal ligament is controversial. Ossification of the ligament obligates its removal, but adequate decompression can often be achieved without its excision. In most patients, it is simply easier to incise the posterior longitudinal ligament and remove it along with the posterior osteophytes. Once the central dura has been decompressed, small angled curettes and microkerasins are used to widen the corpectomy, particularly at the level of the disc space. The table can be angled toward the surgeon so that the ipsilateral foramina are better seen and decompressed.

Complications of the Bone Graft

Bone graft complications add significantly to the morbidity of this procedure. The longer the graft, the more likely extrusion or collapse will occur. A good-quality fibular allograft, however, rarely collapses. Graft extrusion is a complication of technique; most occur in the first few postoperative days, and adequate attention to fashioning a mortise virtually eliminates this complication. Mortises are recessed about 3 to 4 mm under the anterior cortical surface of the adjacent vertebral bodies, and there must be maximum surface contact between the bone graft and mortise. This contact reduces the risk of graft extrusion and minimizes the piston effect of the allograft into the cancellous mortise bone. The mortises may not be parallel because of the spinal curvature; therefore, the fibular ends should be sculpted accordingly. Distraction is achieved manually with tongs or vertebral screw retractors. (I prefer the retractors.) The bone is placed into the mortises and the distraction is released. A stable construct is usually achieved. An anterior cervical plate or postoperative halo immobilization is, rarely, required to secure the bone graft, but the long-term effectiveness of these adjuncts in maintaining sagittal alignment or increasing fusion rates has not been prospectively evaluated. The autograft that was harvested during the corpectomy is morcellized and placed in the lateral gutters and over the surface of the ventral allograft. The wound is closed in standard fashion. The patient should begin walking the day after surgery and wear a Philadelphia® collar for 6 to 8 weeks.

CONCLUSION

The reluctance to embrace multilevel corpectomy as the preferred treatment for most patients with CSM stems from the unfamiliar and technically demanding nature of the procedure. Nevertheless, as the surgeon gains ability and experience with this approach, this treatment "controversy" will likely resolve. Only the surgeon who is comfortable with both corpectomy and laminectomy will be able to compare treatment strategies objectively. Most will find that anterior corpectomy and reconstruction is superior to laminectomy, from both a conceptual and clinical perspective.

Posterior Cervical Decompression for Cervical Spondylotic Myelopathy

Peter M. Klara, M.D., Ph.D., Kevin T. Foley, M.D.

The combination of lower motor neuron findings in the arms with upper motor neuron findings in the legs is a common pattern of presentation of cervical spondylotic myelopathy (CSM).

CASE ANALYSIS

The magnetic resonance images of the patient described in this case show multilevel spondylosis with significant cord compression at C3-4, C4-5, C5-6, and C6-7. This compression arises, not only ventrally from spondylotic bars and degenerated cervical discs, but also dorsally from infolding and hypertrophy of the ligamenta flava. The axial images show evidence of a small cervical canal, with relatively symmetrical encroachment ventrally and dorsally. The patient's lateral plain film shows that the lordotic curvature is preserved. In particular, a cord constructed from the posterior inferior "corner point" of the C7 vertebral body runs directly through the spinal canal without intersecting any portion of the intervening cervical vertebral bodies. One needs to keep in mind, however, that other entities can produce similar clinical findings in the presence of incidental radiographic changes. These include primary motor system disease such as amyotrophic lateral sclerosis, and demyelinating diseases, such as multiple sclerosis and subacute combined degeneration.

CHOOSING AN APPROPRIATE SURGICAL APPROACH

Once the diagnosis of CSM had been confirmed, treatment considerations can be entertained. Although the natural history of CSM can vary considerably, the patient's history of progressive difficulty with gait argues for surgical intervention.[8] Although several surgical options exist to treat patients with CSM, we advocate a posterior approach for this patient.

With regard to the best surgical approach for an individual with CSM, several factors enter into our decision:

- Is the curvature of the cervical spine lordotic, neutral, or kyphotic?
- Is the predominant compression of the cervical cord from a ventral or dorsal pathologic process or is the compression relatively symmetric?
- How many levels require decompression?

A kyphotic cervical spine, in which the spinal cord drapes over the kyphotic deformity, is a contraindication to a primary posterior surgical approach. In these circumstances, the spine should be decompressed anteriorly. A lordotic cervical spine lends itself to posterior decompression, with good results.[3] A neutral cervical curvature (or "gray zone" configuration[4]) can be approached either anteriorly or posteriorly.

Significant ventral cord compression should be approached anteriorly. On the other hand, many cases of cervical spondylosis result from a "washboard" configuration of the cervical canal, with relatively small ventral osteophytic bars and degenerated discs found in association with hypertrophic, infolded ligamenta flava. Additionally, congenital stenosis of the cervical canal is frequently superimposed. We believe it is critical to obtain axial images of the cervical canal, not only at the level of the interspace, but also at the level of the midcervical bodies to assess the degree of cervical canal stenosis. In particular, we prefer to obtain a computed tomogram to assess the diameter of the canal. Certainly, when the cervical cord is compressed symmetrically or no focal ventral compressive lesion of significant size exists, the cervical spinal cord can be nicely decompressed through a posterior approach.

When several levels (more than 2 to 3) require decompression, we favor a posterior approach. We can carry out a multilevel laminectomy faster and with less *potential* morbidity than a multilevel anterior cervical corpectomy or multilevel discectomies. Data collected by the Cervical Spine Research Society underscores the difference in morbidity between anterior and posterior approaches to the cervical spine.[10]

CONSIDERING FUSION

Once a decision has been made to decompress the cervical spine posteriorly, cervical fusion must be considered. This, in itself, is a controversial topic. Cervical laminectomy can be associated with instability.[11] Careful attention to surgical detail, especially to ensuring that a laminectomy is extended no farther into the facet joints than one quarter to one third of their width can minimize the incidence of kyphosis after a laminectomy.

True instability may coexist with cervical spondylosis and should be looked for before surgery. Cusick and associates[5] reported on 3 patients with CSM and coexistent instability in the upper vertebral column who were treated with posterior fusion and wiring without decompression. All 3 patients had severe and progressive myelopathy preoperatively and all showed significant clinical improvement postoperatively.

Even in the absence of gross instability, however, an argument can be made for fusion. Evidence indicates that normal motion of the cervical spine is a significant factor in the genesis and progression of cervical spondylosis. In particular, Barnes and Saunders[2] found that a flexion-extension arc of more than 60 degrees correlated with clinical deterioration in a group of patients with CSM who were treated without surgery. Adams and Logue[1] correlated deterioration after laminectomy with a flexion-extension arc of 40 degrees or more. Conversely, those patients with less than 40 degrees of motion on flexion-extension (using a line drawn from the posterior aspect of the odontoid to the posterior inferior corner of the C7 vertebral body) did well after laminectomy. Maurer and associates[9] reported on 10 patients with advanced CSM who underwent combined posterior decompression and fusion in conjunction with internal fixation with a Luque rectangle. Nine of the 10 patients experienced significant neurological improvement, while the tenth patient, who had progressive myelopathy preoperatively, showed no evidence of clinical progression postoperatively.

Alternative Surgical Approaches

Cervical laminectomy alone is associated with variable results in patients with CSM. The reported rate of improvement after laminectomy alone ranges from 25[1] to 70%.[6] Several studies have documented late deterioration after posterior decompressive operations.[3] For these reasons, we obtain preoperative flexion-extension radiographs for every patient with CSM who is being considered for posterior decompression. If there is a significant flexion-extension arc (40 degrees or more), we combine the posterior decompression with a posterior (facet) fusion. Although we have used facet wiring and Luque rectangles in the past, our current preference is to supplement the posterior fusion

with the placement of titanium lateral mass plates. These can be applied quickly, are compatible with magnetic resonance images, and provide excellent fixation.

Laminoplasty is an alternative to posterior decompression and fusion. Proponents of laminoplasty maintain that it is superior to cervical laminectomy alone. The efficacy of laminoplasty has been shown in cervical spondylosis.[7] We have limited experience with this technique.

CONCLUSION

Our current approach to patients with CSM is outlined in Figure 1. We believe that applying a single surgical technique to this complex clinical phenomenon is shortsighted. Rather, we advocate a broader approach and attempt to tailor the specific surgical procedure to each patient. Clearly, controversy will continue regarding the proper treatment of patients with cervical spondylotic myelopathy, until prospective randomized trials comparing these various approaches have been conducted.

With this in mind, and knowing that one man's dogma is another man's anathema, we would recommend a cervical laminectomy from C3 through C7 for this 65-year-old man. We would combine the laminectomy with a bilateral facet fusion from C3 through C7, using portions of the removed posterior elements as autogenous graft material. In addition, we would supplement this fusion with titanium lateral mass plates (Figs. 2, 3). This approach presupposes, of course, that this patient's flexion-extension radiographs show a significant arc of motion. Surely, we would have our patient in and out of the operating room in a shorter time and put him at less risk than the advocate of a multilevel anterior cervical decompression.

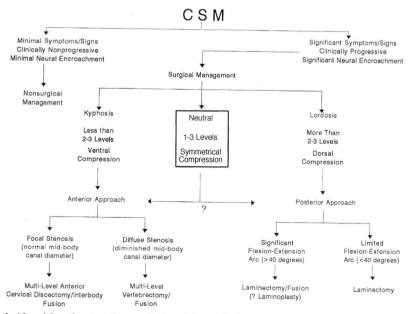

Fig. 1 Algorithm for treating patients with cervical spondylotic myelopathy.

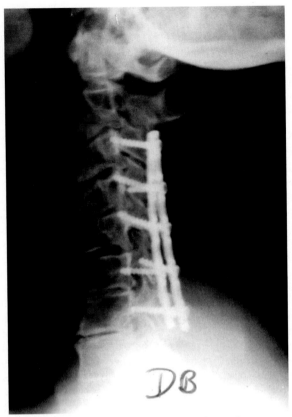

Fig. 2 Plain lateral X-ray of a patient who underwent decompressive laminectomy (C3-C7) with the placement of lateral mass plates.

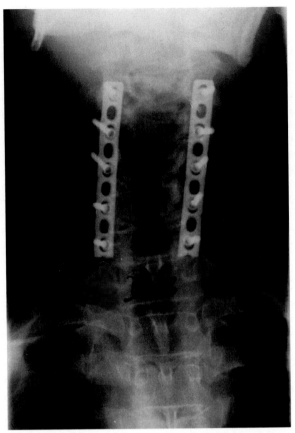

Fig. 3 Plain X-ray of the same patient (anteroposterior view).

Approaches to Multilevel Cervical Spondylotic Myelopathy

H. Louis Harkey, M.D.

The case presented is one with typical signs and symptoms of cervical spondylotic myelopathy (CSM).

CASE REVIEW

Based on the described numbness, spastic gait, and brisk reflexes, this patient has clear evidence of long-tract dysfunction. The muscle wasting in the hands may be evidence of bilateral root compression at C8 and T1 or, alternatively, of more proximal cord compression in the midcervical spine. The numbclumsy hand has been recognized as a manifestation of CSM, even in the absence of compression of lower cervical roots.[8,12,25]

The lateral X-ray of the spine shows congenital stenosis with superimposed degenerative changes. The disc spaces are narrow, and osteophytes have formed both anteriorly and posteriorly. Although the magnetic resonance image may misrepresent the actual degree of canal stenosis, comparing the T1- and T2-weighted images, one can clearly appreciate the compromise of the spinal cord. Disc herniations are evident at several levels, compressing the anterior cord. The posterior compression results from redundant ligamentum flavum at several levels and a prominent C4 lamina. These degenerative changes combine to obliterate the cerebrospinal fluid signal around the cord, partic-

ularly at the level of the disc spaces. The cervical spine has maintained the normal lordotic curvature, despite significant degenerative changes. The axial views show foraminal stenosis at multiple levels, as well. The constellation changes seen on the diagnostic images are consistent with the diagnosis of CSM.

Although CSM is a common disease of the cervical cord in middle-aged patients, one must consider other causes, such as amyotrophic lateral sclerosis and multiple sclerosis. A complete evaluation of this patient should include a careful review of his history and a complete physical and neurological examination. If any doubt exists regarding the diagnosis, the work-up should also include an evaluation of the cerebrospinal fluid, magnetic resonance images of the brain, and an electrodiagnostic examination. The failure to recognize other causes of myelopathy in middle-aged patients may explain some of the poor results of surgery in patients with CSM.

THE PATHOPHYSIOLOGY OF CSM

Before choosing a treatment, one must consider the pathophysiology of CSM and the goals of therapy. Although the pathophysiology is not fully understood, it seems to relate to a reduction in the volume of the spinal canal, either anatomically or mechanically or as a combination of the two. The effect of stenosis upon the spinal cord is a source of some controversy. I currently subscribe to a theory that explains the neurological and anatomic manifestations of CSM based upon intermittent, but chronic, microvascular insufficiency within the spinal cord.[1]

When the cervical spine is extended, the ligamentum flavum infolds[17] and the cervical cord fattens.[26] In the normal spinal canal, ample reserve space surrounds the spinal cord to accommodate the changes associated with motion of the cervical spine. In spondylosis, however, this reserve space is gradually consumed by bulging discs, redundant or hypertrophied ligaments, and enlarging osteophytes. Ultimately, the spine reaches a point at which it no longer has sufficient room to accommodate the changes in the spinal canal associated with motion. At this point, the spinal cord is intermittently compressed between the anterior osteophyte and infolding posterior ligamentum flavum each time the neck is extended.

Intermittent compression of the spinal cord, in turn, interferes with microvascular blood flow, producing periods of relative ischemia within the watershed zone of the spinal cord. Repeated episodes of ischemia eventually injure the most vulnerable cells, the large motor neurons. Over time, as the compression becomes more severe and the effects of repeated episodes of ischemia accumulate, more severe pathologic changes occur. These changes include edema, cell loss, necrosis, and cavitation, and are manifested clinically as the myriad of findings associated with CSM. Based on this theory, the correct approach to treating this patient must take into account both the anatomic compression and the mechanical effects of motion on the cervical cord.

SURGICAL APPROACHES

Historically, patients with CSM were treated conservatively because the disorder was benign. Because the disease is prolonged and rarely progressive, and because early surgical reports were discouraging, certain authors recommended that surgery be avoided.[5,18,21] As surgical experience improved, however, posterior decompression became popular and reports indicated that 60 to 70% of patients improved after a laminectomy for CSM.[2,10,11]

As it came into widespread use, the anterior cervical approach was applied to CSM with good results.[4] Anterior cervical discectomy, with or without fusion, however, was generally limited to two-level disease. Even "anterior" surgeons relied on cervical laminectomy to treat cervical spondylotic compression involving more than 2 levels. In recent years, surgeons have become more aggressive in using anterior decompression, performing discectomies at 3 or more levels and even doing corpectomies at multiple levels.[24] The complications of pseudoarthrosis and graft dislodgement that accompany these more aggressive anterior decompressions have been reduced through the use of anterior plate fixation. Reported outcomes of anterior cervical decompression in patients with CSM are generally good and, in some reports, are superior to posterior decompression.[16,22]

The complications associated with multilevel anterior decompression and the concerns of kyphosis after laminectomy led to the development of a variety of laminoplasty techniques. Laminoplasty has been used most extensively to treat ossification of the posterior longitudinal ligament, but has also been used for more typical CSM.[15] The benefits of laminoplasty over a simple laminectomy are controversial, with any advantage afforded by laminoplasty probably resulting from the enhanced stability of the cervical spine after decompression.[9,20]

THE OPINIONS

Klara and Foley would treat this patient with posterior decompression, but argue that simultaneous stabilization of the segments may be critical for successful outcome if this patient has a flexion-extension arc of 40 degrees or more. This approach addresses both the static and the dynamic compression that contribute to the patient's myelopathy. Additionally, stabilization prevents the possibility of subluxation or kyphosis after the laminectomy. A similar technique has been reported with excellent results in a small number of patients.[19] In fact, posterior stabilization alone has been reported to reverse deficits in 3 patients with CSM.[7]

I tend to side with McCormick's recommendation of anterior decompression. I also agree with his statement that the results of medial corpectomy are superior to those of multilevel discectomy. In fact, I think that a more complete decompression can be achieved in less time if the intervening bodies are removed along with the disc. I should also emphasize that a corpectomy for CSM should extend to the lateral gutters of the canal, and that anterior foraminotomies should be done at each level. All too often, when performing a corpectomy, surgeons drill tangentially through the cervical vertebra because of the angle of exposure, producing a trough that fails to adequately decompress the spinal cord (Fig. 1). Special care must be taken to ensure that sufficient bone is removed from the vertebral body on the side of the exposure. The lateral osteophytes within the foramen can tether the cord and require resection, to allow the cord to prolapse into the defect left by the corpectomy. The posterior longitudinal ligament, which may be responsible for some of the cord compression, should be resected, as well, to ensure that the cord is thoroughly decompressed.[9]

I would, likewise, reconstruct the spine with a fibular allograft, as McCormick has described, but I would not bother with mortises to secure the graft. I create a flat plane on the vertebral endplates above and below the corpectomy defect by drilling away the anterior and posterior lips of the vertebral body.[14] Then, I cut the fibula so that it slides into the defect while the vertebral bodies are maximally distracted. The graft is then secured and the spine stabilized with an anterior cervical plate, preferably a Caspar® plate, using bicortical screw fixation into the bodies and the graft itself. After a single-level corpectomy, I frequently use a locking plate because it is easier to place and more rigid. For longer decompressions, however, I find the Caspar® plate to be more easily contoured and fixed to the bodies above and below the decompression. In addition, long plates are more prone to fail at the interface with the vertebral body because they have a long lever arm on a rigid construct.[13]

Both authors allude to a treatment algorithm for determining the appropriate way to treat patients with CSM. This algorithm must take into consideration the levels of cord compression, whether most of the compression is anterior or posterior, and the shape of the cervical spine. Batzdorf and Batzdorf[3] have shown that posterior migration of the spinal cord after a laminectomy may be inadequate to clear osteophytes in the kyphotic, or even straight, cervical spine. Clearly, it does no good to remove the lamina if the spinal cord remains draped over a kyphotic hump or large osteophytes. Therefore, posterior decompression is only appropriate in the presence of a normal lordotic curvature. Considering the complexity of CSM, the best overall surgical outcome should stem from the use of a variety of surgical procedures tailored to the individual patient.[6]

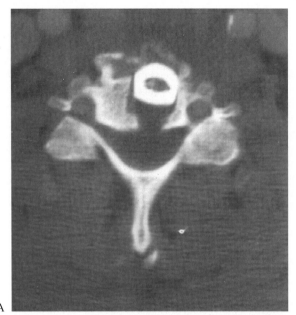

A

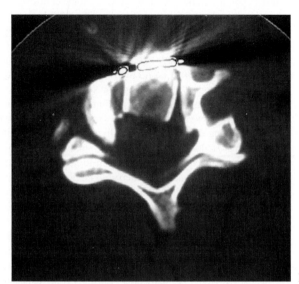

B

**Fig. 1 Computed tomograms after corpectomy for cervical spondylotic myelopathy:
(*A*) Inadequate decompression. (*B*) Adequate decompression.**

Recently, there has been a call for close scientific scrutiny of the treatment of patients with CSM. Citing the lack of sound data supporting the benefits of surgery, and the preponderance of data indicating that the natural history of CSM is at least as good as surgery, Rowland[23] has suggested a cooperative trial comparing conservative and surgical treatment of CSM. Although his argument that our current treatment lacks a solid scientific foundation is compelling, this view ignores the overwhelming weight of clinical experience and common sense. In some cases, it is neither necessary nor ethical to subject patients to scientific evaluation to "prove" that a certain therapy works. The failure of surgery to produce perfect outcomes does not mean that it is the wrong therapy but, in part, reflects the difficulty of diagnosis, the risk of surgical intervention, and other factors beyond control in a clinical setting. None of these issues would be resolved by a randomized prospective study.

REFERENCES

Paul C. McCormick, M.D.

1. Adams CBT, Logue V: Studies in cervical spondylotic myelopathy: II. The movement and contour of the spine in relation to the neural complications of cervical spondylosis. *Brain* 1971; 94:569–586.
2. Barnes MP, Saunders M: The effect of cervical mobility on the natural history of cervical spondylotic myelopathy. *J Neurol Neurosurg Psychiatry* 1984; 47:17–20.
3. Batzdorf U, Flannigan BD: Surgical decompressive procedures for cervical spondylotic myelopathy: A study using magnetic resonance imaging. *Spine* 1991; 16:123–127.
4. Ducker TB: Cervical stenosis: Myelopathy hand. *J Spin Disord* 1992; 5:374–380.
5. Epstein JA, Epstein NE: The surgical management of cervical spinal stenosis, spondylosis, and myeloradiculopathy by means of the posterior approach, in *The Cervical Spine*, ed. 2. Philadelphia, JB Lippincott, 1989, pp 625–643.
6. Fukuda S, Ogata M, Slitikawa K: Laminectomy versus laminoplasty for cervical myelopathy. *J Bone Joint Surg* 1988; 70B: 325–326.
7. Nagata K, Kiyonaga K, Ohashi T, et al.: Clinical value of magnetic resonance imaging for cervical myelopathy. *Spine* 1990; 16:1088–1093.
8. Okada Y, Ikata T, Yamada H, et al.: Magnetic resonance imaging study on the results of surgery for cervical compression myelopathy. *Spine* 1993; 18:2024–2029.
9. Rowland LP: Surgical treatment of cervical spondylotic myelopathy: Time for a controlled trial. *Neurology* 1992; 42:5–13.
10. Saunders RL, Bernin PM, Shirretts TG Jr, et al.: Central corpectomy for cervical spondylotic myelopathy: A consecutive series with long-term follow-up evaluation. *J Neurosurg* 1991; 74: 163–170.
11. Shinomiya K, Mutoh N, Furuya K: Study of experimental cervical spondylotic myelopathy. *Spine* 1992; 17:S383–S387.
12. Yone K, Sakou T, Yanase M, et al.: Pre-operative and postoperative magnetic resonance image evaluations of the spinal cord in cervical myelopathy. *Spine* 1992; 17:S388–S392.

Peter M. Klara, M.D., Ph.D., Kevin T. Foley, M.D.

1. Adams CBT, Logue V: Studies in cervical spondylotic myelopathy: III. Some functional effects of operations for cervical spondylotic myelopathy. *Brain* 1971; 94:587–594.
2. Barnes MP, Saunders M: The effect of cervical mobility on the natural history of cervical spondylotic myelopathy. *J Neurol Neurosurg Psychiatry* 1984; 47:17–20.
3. Batzdorf U, Batzdorf A: Analysis of cervical spine curvature in patients with cervical spondylosis. *Neurosurgery* 1988; 22:827–836.

4. Benzel EC: Cervical spondylotic myelopathy: Posterior surgical approaches, in Cooper PA (ed): *Degenerative Diseases of the Cervical Spine*, Park Ridge, AANS Publications, 1992, pp 91–103.
5. Cusick JF, Steiner RE, Berns T: Total stabilization of the cervical spine in patients with cervical spondylotic myelopathy. *Neurosurgery* 1986; 18:491–495.
6. Fager C: Results of adequate posterior decompression in the relief of spondylotic cervical myelopathy. *J Neurosurg* 1973; 38:684–692.
7. Herkowitz H: A comparison of anterior cervical fusion, cervical laminectomy, and cervical laminoplasty for the surgical management of multilevel spondylotic radiculopathy. *Spine* 1988; 13:774–780.
8. Klara PM, Foley K: Surgical treatment of osteophytes and calcified discs of the cervical spine. *Neurosurg Clin North Am* 1993; 4:53–60.
9. Maurer PK, Ellenbogen R, Ecklund J, et al.: Cervical spondylotic myelopathy: Treatment with posterior decompression and Luque rectangle bone fusion. *Neurosurgery* 1991; 28:680–685.
10. Raynor RB: Anterior and posterior approaches to the cervical spinal cord, discs and roots: A comparison of exposures and decompression, in The Cervical Spine Research Society, Editorial Committee (ed): *The Cervical Spine*, ed. 2. Philadelphia, JB Lippincott, 1989, pp 659–669.
11. Yasuoka S, Peterson HA, MacCarty CS: Incidence of spinal column deformity after multilevel laminectomy in children and adults. *J Neurosurg* 1982; 57:441–445.

H. Louis Harkey, M.D.

1. Al-Mefty O, Harkey HL, Marawi I, et al.: Experimental chronic compressive cervical myelopathy. *J Neurosurg* 1993; 79:550–561.
2. Bakay L: Postoperative myelography in spondylotic cervical myelopathy. *Acta Neurochir* 1973; 28:123–133.
3. Batzdorf U, Batzdorf A: Analysis of cervical spine curvature in patients with cervical spondylosis. *Neurosurgery* 1988; 22:827–836.
4. Bohlman HH: Cervical spondylosis with moderate to severe myelopathy: A report of seventeen cases treated by Robinson anterior cervical discectomy and fusion. *Spine* 1977; 2:151–162.
5. Campbell AMG, Phillips DG: Cervical disc lesions with neurological disorder: Differential diagnosis, treatment, and prognosis. *Br Med J* 1960; 2:481–485.
6. Carol MP, Ducker TB: Cervical spondylitic myelopathies: Surgical treatment. *J Spinal Disord* 1988; 1:59–65.
7. Cusick JF, Steiner RE, Berns T: Total stabilization of the cervical spine in patients with cervical spondylotic myelopathy. *Neurosurgery* 1986; 18:491–495.
8. Ebara S, Yonenobu K, Fujiwara K, et al.: Myelopathy hand characterized by muscle wasting: A different type of myelopathy hand in patients with cervical spondylosis. *Spine* 1988; 13:785–791.
9. Epstein N: The surgical management of ossification of the posterior longitudinal ligament in 51 patients. *J Spinal Disord* 1993; 6: 432–455.
10. Epstein JA, Janin Y, Carras R, et al.: A comparative study of the treatment of cervical spondylotic myeloradiculopathy: Experience with 50 cases treated by means of extensive laminectomy, foraminotomy, and excision of osteophytes during the past 10 years. *Acta Neurochir* 1982; 61:89–104.
11. Fager C: Results of adequate posterior decompression in the relief of spondylotic cervical myelopathy. *J Neurosurg* 1973; 38:684–692.
12. Good DC, Couch JR, Wacaser L: "Numb, clumsy hands" and high cervical spondylosis. *Surg Neurol* 1984; 22:285–291.
13. Harkey HL: Synthes cervical spine locking plate (Morscher plate). *Neurosurgery* 1993; 32:682–683.
14. Harkey HL, Caspar W, Tarassoli Y: Caspar plating of the cervical spine, in Wilkins RH, Rengachary SS (eds): *Neurosurgical Operative Atlas*. Baltimore, Williams and Wilkins, 1991, pp 261–271.
15. Herkowitz H: A comparison of anterior cervical fusion, cervical laminectomy, and cervical laminoplasty for the surgical management of multiple level spondylotic radiculopathy. *Spine* 1988; 13:774–780.
16. Jeffreys RV: The surgical treatment of cervical myelopathy due to spondylosis and disc degeneration. *J Neurol Neurosurg Psychiatry* 1986; 49:353–361.
17. Key CA: On paraplegia depending on disease of the ligaments of the spine. *Guys Hosp Rep* 1838; 3:17–34.
18. Lees F, Turner JWA: Natural history and prognosis of cervical spondylosis. *Br Med J* 1963; 2:1607–1610.
19. Maurer PK, Ellenbogen RG, Ecklund J, et al.: Cervical spondylotic myelopathy: Treatment with posterior decompression and Luque rectangle bone fusion. *Neurosurgery* 1991; 28:620–684.
20. Nakano N, Nakano T, Nakano K: Comparison of the results of laminectomy and open-door laminoplasty for cervical spondylotic myeloradiculopathy and ossification of the posterior longitudinal ligament. *Spine* 1988; 13:792–794.
21. Nurick S: Cervical spondylosis and the spinal cord. *Br J Hosp Med* 1975; 13:668–676.
22. Phillips DG: Surgical treatment of myelopathy with cervical spondylosis. *J Neurol Neurosurg Psychiatry* 1973; 36:879–884.
23. Rowland LP: Surgical treatment of cervical spondylotic myelopathy: Time for a controlled trial. *Neurology* 1992; 42:5–13.
24. Saunders RL, Bernini PM, Shirreffs TG Jr, et al.: Central corpectomy for cervical spondylotic myelopathy: A consecutive series with long-term follow-up evaluation. *J Neurosurg* 1991; 74:163–170.
25. Voskuhl RR, Hinton RC: Sensory impairment in the hands secondary to spondylotic compression of the cervical spinal cord. *Arch Neurol* 1990; 47:309–311.
26. Waltz TA: Physical factors in the production of the myelopathy of cervical spondylosis. *Brain* 1967; 90:395–404.

28

Treatment of Lumbosacral Spondylolisthesis with Radiculopathy

CASE

A 23-year-old laborer with a known history of spondylolisthesis injured his back, developing low back pain and numbness in both legs. Upon examination, he had exaggerated lumbar lordosis and back pain on extension. He had mildly diminished sensation in both the anterior lateral legs and great toes, and weakness of both extensor hallucis longus muscles. His deep tendon reflexes were normal. The symptoms persisted despite conservative treatment, including a complete course of physical therapy and bracing for 6 months.

PARTICIPANTS

Stabilizing Lumbar Spondylolisthesis with Decompression, Fusion, and Instrumentation– Charles L. Branch, Jr., M.D.

Treating Lumbar Spondylolisthesis with Decompression and Fusion Alone– Edward N. Hanley, Jr., M.D., Mark E. Coggins, M.D.

Moderator–Thomas Ducker, M.D.

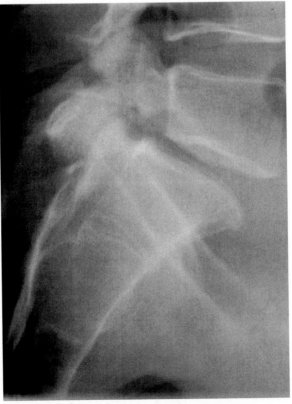

Fig. 1 Lumbar spine x-ray demonstrating pars interarticularis defects and grade I spondylolisthesis.

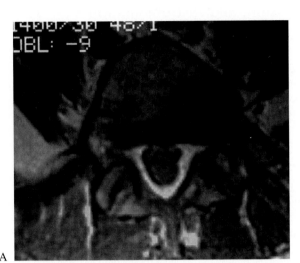

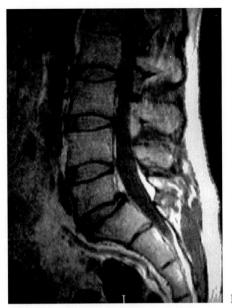

Fig. 2 Lumbar magnetic resonance images showing absence of disc herniation: (*A*) **Axial view of L5-S1.** (*B*) **Sagittal view.**

Stabilizing Lumbar Spondylolisthesis
with Decompression, Fusion, and Instrumentation

Charles L. Branch, Jr., M.D.

In the young patient with lytic spondylolisthesis who becomes symptomatic after a work-related injury, the ultimate outcome may be affected by a variety of factors, among them socio-economic factors. Disregarding these, however, the 2 issues that must be addressed are neural decompression and stabilization of the pathologic segment of the spine.

DECOMPRESSION ALONE

In the case presented, most of the initial symptomatic relief is related to decompression of the L5 nerve roots bilaterally. The classic operative technique for decompression removes the dorsal arch (the Gill procedure). Removing the arch alone, however, does not decompress the attenuated neural foramen. Therefore, I remove the dorsal arch to enhance exposure and adequately decompress the neural foramen, and to carry out a posterior interbody fusion. I morcellize the bone from the dorsal arch and reuse it as part of the fusion material. There is always thick, fibrous tissue at the pathologic pars interarticularis and over-lying the attenuated neural foramen. The sequential use of a 3-mm, 45-degree Kerrison® punch with 3 to 4 mm angled curettes and a diamond-tipped burr on a high-speed drill allows for safe, complete decompression of the nerve roots. In the patient without frank disc herniation at this level, removing the pannus or fibrous tissue with some of the pars or pedicle, without manipulating the nerve root, should relieve some, if not all, of the symptoms of radicular pain or motor dysfunction. From this perspective, one could limit the operation to decompression alone and have early, satisfactory results in a number of patients. This concept has been validated in the past.

THE NEED FOR FUSION

Despite the results achieved with decompression alone, I believe that lumbosacral fusion or immobilization of the pathologic segment is essential for symptomatic relief of the back pain and to prevent recurrence or progression of the listhesis. In the presence of a listhesis of less than one third of the vertebral body (grades 1 or 2) with adequate neural decompression, there is no advantage in reducing the listhesis, and an *in situ* fusion or stabilization eliminates a pathologic or dysfunctional motion segment.[7] Historically, a simple bilateral lateral fusion of the transverse process from L5 to S1 has a reasonable success rate, but this rate is far from 100%.[10] A successful lateral fusion without internal fixation requires meticulous dissection of soft tissue from the transverse process at L5 and creates bleeding cortical surfaces over the transverse processes, the superior facets of L5, and the inferior facets of S1.[4] Generous portions of cancellous autologous bone compacted laterally without compression of the L5 root are essential for a satisfactory fusion.

Factors Impairing Fusion

This joint can be temporarily immobilized only with a rigid lumbar orthosis with a hip spica cast. This orthotic device, however, is cumbersome and many patients find it unacceptable. The segments may fuse without this degree of external immobilization, but it is less likely. Probably most important is the presence of a competent annulus and longitudinal ligament both anteriorly and posteriorly. Excessive anteroposterior translational or angular motion secondary to an incompetent or severely degenerated disc may also impair fusion. Other factors impeding fusion in the young or middle-aged patient include smoking, nutritional deficiencies, a lack of compliance with external orthoses, and radicular symptoms.[3]

INTERBODY FUSION

Among other authors, Cloward[2] has popularized the use of the posterior lumbar interbody fusion to treat patients with spondylolisthesis. This technique uses the axial loading force on the disc space and its contents to compress the bone graft, thereby increasing the potential for fusion. The theoretical advantages of interbody fusion and descriptions of safe effective techniques appear elsewhere.[1] Decompression and interbody fusion historically have a success rate similar or superior to that of lateral fusion alone.

The concept of a 360-degree fusion has merit in that the posterior lateral fusion or stability is augmented by the graft in the interspace and vice versa, immobilizing the spine to a greater degree and creating the potential for fusion of the lumbosacral joint.[6] Increasing experience with posterior exposure and interbody fusion allows for both interbody and lateral fusion during the same procedure, without undue increases in operative time or morbidity. Although long-term studies indicating that this approach is substantially superior to a lateral fusion or interbody fusion alone currently do not exist, theoretically this technique appears to be superior if it can be done safely and expeditiously.[11]

INTERNAL FIXATION

Instrumentation or internal fixation to immobilize the pathologic segment while fusion occurs appears to have a theoretical advantage over fusion alone.[9] The benefits include immediate internal fixation, which should enhance the fusion rate and facilitate more rapid mobilization of the patient in a less cumbersome external orthosis.[5] In this patient, the pathologic segment is L5-S1; occasionally, however, L4 is incorporated in the internal fixation as well. This is accomplished with a variety of devices that may use the L4 lamina, pedicles, or spinous process for fixation with subsequent fixation to L5 and the sacrum. I generally include L4 in the fusion or fixation when the patient has a significant pathologic process at the disc or facet of L4-L5 or a high grade of listhesis at L5-S1. Again, long-term studies do not yet uniformly substantiate the benefits of internal fixation, in spite of its theoretical advantage. This variation in results may relate to factors ranging from the technical skills of the surgeon to the socioeconomic factors surrounding the patient.

SURGICAL TECHNIQUE FOR FIXATION

My approach to the patient in the case presented here would use all the techniques described to create the greatest potential for osteosynthesis and immobilization of the pathologic segment at the first operation. This approach requires the development of technical skills and a knowledge of exposure and anatomy that allow the surgeon to use this technique without an undue increase in operative time, blood loss, or morbidity.

Through a midline exposure, the neural arch can be removed as a single piece by abrading the L5-S1 joint with a small curette and removing sublaminar ligamentous structures often densely adherent to the facets. These structures are usually tough and require careful removal of the fibrous tissue using curettes and the 3-mm Kerrison® punch. I often use a 3-mm diamond-tipped burr to enlarge the bony foramen before removing the pannus or tough fibrous tissue. After satisfactory decompression of the nerve roots bilaterally, the soft tissue from the superior facet and transverse process at L5 and the residual S1 joint surface is thoroughly debrided using the drill or curette. At this point, the S1 nerve root is retracted medially and the epidural veins are coagulated bilaterally. This maneuver exposes the annulus at the L5-S1 disc space, which is generally associated with a step-off of 3 to 8 mm in the patients with grades 1 or 2 disease. The annulus is incised and various-sized curettes are sequentially inserted into the attenuated disc space, removing the annulus and disc material until clean cortical surfaces are felt above and below, and the surfaces bleed. This maneuver is done bilaterally, but most of the midline posterior longitudinal ligament and annulus are left intact.

At this point, the pedicle screws are inserted into the L5 and S1 pedicles, with the S1 screw just penetrating the ventral or anterior cortex of the sacrum. After the screws are in place, the interspace is again entered and multiple small fragments of morcellized bone from the arch are compacted anteriorly. For interbody fusion, I generally use cadaveric grafts of iliac crest that are 25 mm deep, 12 to 15 mm high, and about 10 mm wide. After some small morsels are compacted in place, these larger grafts are sequentially compacted into the disc space. Before the first graft is inserted, a spreader or osteotome is inserted into the disc space on the opposite side to open the space for the graft.

Three grafts are inserted, with one being manipulated under the midline using small osteotomes or chisels as pry bars.

After the interbody grafts are in place, the slotted plates are contoured to fit on the pedicle screws. I generally contour the plates to the lordosis at this level. Before seating the plate on the screws, autologous bone from the morcellated arch and facets is compacted laterally over the transverse processes, the facets, and the sacrum. Occasionally, bone from the iliac crest is harvested, but this is seldom necessary if a good supply of banked bone is available for interbody grafting. The plate is then tightened down onto the screws with no effort made to reduce the spondylolisthesis. This technique provides for a 360-degree fusion with internal fixation, in addition to satisfactory neural decompression.

Postoperative Course

On the second or third postoperative day, the patient is allowed to walk while wearing a canvas lumbosacral corset. Depending upon the symptoms and the radiographic appearance of the spine, the patient can return to work between 3 and 6 months after surgery.

Attempts to reduce the listhesis may place undue stress upon the hardware and cause the screws to break or fail, negating the potential benefit of this technique over *in situ* fusion techniques alone. *In situ* fusion also takes advantage of existing ligamentous support to further immobilize the pathologic segment. True reduction of the listhesis may require extensive disruption of ligamentous support, placing further stress on the instrumentation or interbody graft material.

Published reports of long-term outcomes with this technique are still sporadic or anecdotal.[8] However, this approach appears to be theoretically superior and, if it can be done expeditiously without dramatic increases in cost, operative time, or morbidity, I believe it has merit.

Treating Lumbar Spondylolisthesis with Decompression and Fusion Alone

Edward N. Hanley, Jr., M.D., Mark E. Coggins, M.D.

The young adult laborer presented here has persistent, functionally-incapacitating back pain, bilateral leg numbness, and motor weakness caused by isthmic lumbosacral spondylolisthesis. His symptoms persist despite appropriate conservative treatment. Radiographic studies show an L5-S1 olisthesis (slip) of about 25% with a nonpathologic slip angle. The magnetic resonance images show minimal evidence of disc degeneration above the slip level. The patient's disease probably developed in childhood or early adolescence, and has probably become symptomatic only recently.[3]

DECOMPRESSING THE NERVE ROOT

When a nonoperative course of treatment fails, surgery may be indicated in an attempt to improve the patient's functional capacity by lessening low back pain and neurological symptoms. Because this patient has radicular signs and symptoms consistent with typical compression of the L5 nerve root, neural decompression is appropriate.[14] Removing the loose posterior elements is done first, to gain access for formal decompression of the reactive fibrocartilaginous tissue that compresses the exit-

ing L5 nerve root near the site of the isthmic defects. The roots should be fully decompressed for their entire course in the lateral recesses, as they swing beneath the pedicle and out the complete length of the neural foramina. Both sides should be addressed. Although sublaminar decompression has been done in some instances without removing the loose element, this technique may not permit complete decompression of the nerve root throughout its course, and is not recommended.

FUSION

After the nerve has been decompressed, posterolateral fusion is performed from the L5 transverse process and lateral aspects of the facet joints at L5 and S1 to the sacral alae bilaterally. With a relatively horizontal slip angle and fairly normal L4-L5 disc (according to the magnetic resonance images), fusion in this patient need not extend above L5. An autologous bone graft should be used for the arthrodesis; allograft bone should be avoided.[5] Because of the young age of this patient, the chances of an excellent or good result are high (Table 1).[4]

Table 1. Success Rate by Age and Compensation Status*

Age (yrs)	Entire group	Compensation group	Noncompensation group
10–19	5/5 (100%)	0/0 (0%)	5/5 (100%)
20–29	8/11 (73%)	2/4 (50%)	6/7 (86%)
30–39	8/14 (54%)	3/9 (33%)	5/5 (100%)
40–49	3/11 (27%)	2/7 (28%)	1/4 (25%)
50–59	4/6 (67%)	2/4 (50%)	2/2 (100%)
60–69	2/3 (67%)	1/2 (50%)	1/1 (100%)
TOTAL	30/50 (60%)	10/26 (38%)	20/24 (83%)

*The success in 50 patients undergoing *in situ*, noninstrumented fusion for isthmic lumbosacral spondylolisthesis based on patient age and compensation status. Note the profound negative influence of a compensation predicament.[4]

WHEN TO REDUCE THE SLIP

In some patients with higher-grade slips (>50%), an argument can be made for reducing the slip. This approach has been proposed for patients with substantial kyphotic and cosmetic deformities, which are often associated with functional and neurological incapacity. Because of the high rate of complications (nerve root dysfunction, recurrent slip, pseudoarthrosis, instrument problems, etc.) with reduction of spondylolisthesis, reduction is never indicated for patients having lower-grade olisthetic deformities. In these situations, reduction adds only risks but no benefits.[2]

THE RISKS OF INSTRUMENTATION

In patients with lower-grade spondylolisthesis, as illustrated by the patient described here, some surgeons might supplement the posterolateral fusion with instrumentation to add stability and enhance the arthrodesis rate. We do not believe, however, that pedicle screw or other instrumentation devices are indicated for fusion of grade 1 or 2 spondylolisthesis; many reviews substantiate high rates of fusion (>80%) without its use,[4,8,13] even after formal decompression.

Instrumentation is not without risks, although, as the surgeon gains experience, these problems may decrease.[10] Potential complications of screw placement include malposition, pedicle fracture, foraminal encroachment, adjacent facet injury, instrument failure or dislodgement, and a prominence caused by the instrument. Although the operative time increases by a factor of two, the reported rate of infection in patients with posterior spine fusion appears to be similar with or without instrumentation.[1,11]

Malposition of the inserted pedicle screw relates somewhat to the variability in pedicle shape and angle. The most critical region for nerve root damage is where the root passes around the inferomedial aspect of the pedicle. The nerve may be damaged by the pedicle probe, tap, or the screw itself. Rates of neurological complication from screw-related injury range from 0.82 to 4.9%.[1,9,11] Most authors have noted that these complications are more likely to occur early in their experience with these devices.

Mechanical failure of the instrumentation is an additional potential problem. Screws may bend or break. When McAfee and colleagues[7] reviewed their 120 patients with pedicle instrumentation, they found that 22 of the 526 screws placed were "problem" screws (6 bent, 16 broken). In less than one half of the patients, however, there was a clinical problem with the breakage. In their series, West and associates[12] noted 12 of 124

patients with broken screws, while the series of Matsuzaki and co-workers showed screw breakage in 21% of patients.[6]

Despite the lack of radiographic evidence of pseudoarthrosis, posterolateral fusion can be associated with some loss of deformity correction over time. This problem may also occur despite the use of instrumentation. In fusions done without instrumentation, this problem is believed to be related to plastic deformation of the fusion over time, and may be associated with forces tangential to the weight-bearing plane (that is, kyphosis). This problem may also occur in patients with instrumented fusions and is likely related to the same factors. In the review of their patients with pedicle screw instrumentation, Matsuzaki and associates[6] noted an average deformity correction of 53% immediately after surgery, which decreased to 31% by 2 months after the procedure.

FUSION WITH VS. WITHOUT INSTRUMENTATION

When deciding whether to perform lumbosacral fusion with or without instrumentation, the surgeon must weigh the risks and benefits of these undertakings. There is no need for instrumentation in a procedure such as single-level decompression and fusion for low-grade spondylolisthesis, which has an approximate 80 to 90% fusion rate without instrumentation.[4,8,13]

By far, the more important issue is that of intrinsic patient variables. These patient characteristics include cigarette smoking, compensation-related work issues, age, and negative psychosocial factors (depression, family life situation, job dissatisfaction, etc.), and may well be the most important factors that determine how a patient will do postoperatively.[4] In our previously published series of 50 patients operated on for isthmic spondylolisthesis,[3] the fusion rates for patients without these negative factors was 83% versus 38% for patients with them (Table 1).

CONCLUSION

In summary, adolescent or young adult patients with functionally incapacitating pain in the back or legs from isthmic lumbosacral spondylolisthesis, who exhibit no or minimal inherent negative characteristics, are candidates for surgical treatment. If the disease is isolated to the lumbosacral articulation and is low-grade, a one-level posterolateral fusion without instrumentation is all that is necessary for stabilization (Fig. 1). If symptomatic irritation of the nerve root is present, formal decompression at the slip level should be done, ensuring that the irritated nerve roots remain free throughout their entire exit from

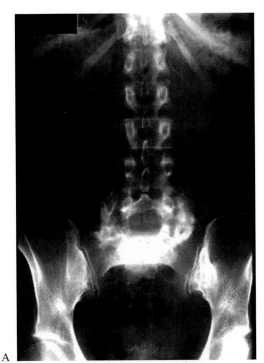
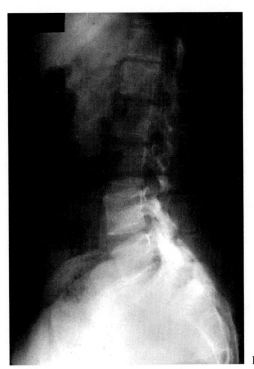

A   B

Fig. 1 Postoperative radiographs of a 30-year-old patient with symptomatic isthmic spondylolisthesis (back and leg pain) treated through decompression and posterolateral *in situ* arthrodesis. The patient's clinical outcome was satisfactory. (*A*) Anteroposterior view. (*B*) Lateral view.

the spinal canal. Because risks far outweigh any potential benefits of these minimally unstable situations, operative reduction and instrumentation is not appropriate. Further guidelines for what procedure to perform based on symptoms and degrees of olisthesis are presented in Table 2. Probably most important is the recognition of intrinsic patient variables that may drastically influence indications for surgery and functional outcomes, in patients with symptomatic isthmic lumbosacral spondylolisthesis.

Table 2. Guidelines for Treatment of Spondylolisthesis Based on Symptoms and Degree of Olisthesis

	Low back pain only	*Back and neural symptoms*
I (<25%)	One-level fusion or deficit repair	One-level fusion with or without neural decompression
II (25–50%)	One-level fusion	One-level fusion with neural decompression
III (50–75%)	Two-level fusion with or without instrumentation	Two-level fusion with or without instrumentation
IV (75–100%)	Two-level fusion (selective reduction) with or without instrumentation	Two-level fusion with neural decompression (selective reduction) with or without instrumentation)
Spondyloptosis	Two-level fusion (selective reduction) with or without instrumentation	Two-level fusion neural decompression (selective reduction) with or without instrumentation

Treatment of Lumbosacral Spondylolisthesis with Radiculopathy

Thomas Ducker, M.D.

Spondylolisthesis commonly occurs in the lumbar spine and at the lumbosacral junction. There are 5 types of this pathologic slippage, and each case must be properly classified. The dysphasic type occurs in children, the traumatic type occurs with severe lower hyperextension injuries, the pathologic type can cause slippage in patients with cancer, and degenerative spondylolisthesis occurs in elderly patients. The degenerative type produces neurogenic claudication, which is a type of bilateral radiculopathy; the other 3 types primarily cause problems with back pain. The fifth type of spondylolisthesis results from isthmic failure; this discussion deals only with that disease.

PREDISPOSING FACTORS

Isthmic spondylolisthesis with fracture or a defect in the pars interarticularis is common in older children and young adults. The isthmic abnormality precedes the slippage. Once spondylolisthesis occurs, the patients are more likely to be symptomatic. Whether some patients have a congenitally weakened pars interarticularis is not clear, but repeated stress fractures are considered the more common cause of this disorder. The prevalence is increased in patients active in certain sporting activities, including weight-lifting, gymnastics, and football. Forced hyperextension with rotary movements of the lumbar spine predispose the athlete to a pars stress fracture. At least half of patients relate their symptoms to competitive sports activities. This condition occurs more commonly in white men but, for some reason, certain populations, such as Eskimos, have an increased rate of occurrence.

SIGNS AND SYMPTOMS

Persistent significant symptoms from spondylolysis and early spondylolisthesis is the exception in patients with this disease. The bony defect occurs in 3% of the population; yet, less than 1% of the population has significant symptoms of the condition. In a review of patients who came to a low back pain clinic, Macnab[2] found the incidence of a pars defect to be slightly over 7%, which is not much higher than that in the general population. Once the spondylolysis is associated with a progressive spondylolisthesis, especially in patients in their 20s and 30s, associated disc degeneration often occurs at that level and the number of symptomatic patients increases.

CASE ANALYSIS

The case presented in this controversy is that of a 23-year-old laborer who already had significant symptoms for 6 months and who has definite signs and symptoms of L5 root dysfunction. When a patient has persistent symptoms, in spite of bracing, physical therapy, and anti-inflammatory medications, operative intervention is a serious consideration. The symptoms of L5 root dysfunction stem from far lateral entrapment of the L5 nerve root. As it passes beneath the pars defect, the root is subjected to repeated trauma from false overgrowth of the joint, a buildup of cartilage, and actual osteophytic bone encroachment. The L5 root symptoms can be relieved only through far lateral foraminotomies, which entail decompressing the fifth root from the medial aspects of the pedicle within the canal, and following the root clear out for nearly 2 cm. All the compressive material must be removed and the pars defect taken down completely. The symptoms do not stem from compression of the canal. The laminectomy per se does nothing to relieve the patient's symptoms. It is done, in part, to gain access to the canal. The importance of decompressing the root rather than the canal cannot be overemphasized.

Magnetic resonance images are of great importance in these patients. Many of the patients undergo successful fusion of the lumbosacral spine only to have continued symptoms because the next disc, L4-L5, has seriously degenerated. This disc can be the source of pain but, in this particular patient, the images show a healthy L4-L5 disc. Therefore, that level need not be treated surgically. Historically, some physicians have recommended discometric and discogram studies at L4-L5, but we recently have found this not to be necessary because magnetic resonance images appear to be adequate. In this patient, therefore, the fusion need only be carried from L5 to S1.

Decompression Alone

The first question placed before us in deciding the appropriate treatment for this patient is whether or not decompression alone would suffice to relieve the patient's symptoms. The answer to this question is yes; however, the good results would be short-lived. My experience shows that, within 5 years, 50% of the patients treated without fusion were again symptomatic, with increased spinal slippage. Instead of being simply a grade 1 slippage, as in this patient, the disorder would rapidly progress to a grade 2 or 3, making fusions even more difficult.

Fusion Alone

On the other hand, if the patient were considerably younger, with incapacitating back pain and minimal neurological signs and symptoms, I would recommend fusion alone without decompression of the nerve root. In those cases, parallel exposures in the back to carry out posterior lateral fusions or *in situ* fusions certainly work well in 80% of patients, but only 60% can then return to full sporting and other activities.

Instrumentation

If the patient truly has a grade 2 or 3 spinal slippage, I am inclined to use internal spinal fixation. It is only in that fashion that the spine can be held still enough to fuse. The pedicle screw devices are, by far, the most common screws used. To completely decompress the nerve root, the stubby end of the pedicle must be visualized clearly at the L5 vertebra. The landmarks of the sacrum are adequate in placing the pedicle screws of an internal fixation device, but the device will fail if bone grafting is not adequate. The fixation devices simply provide an internal brace while the fusion becomes solid. With spinal slippage greater than grade 3, I believe instrumentation is necessary.

Forcing a reduction in slippage with instrumentation carries a high rate of complications with increased symptoms stemming from the L5 root. The slippage can be partially reduced, but only if it can be done easily. Reduction is not a priority of treatment; fusion is the priority.

APPROPRIATE TREATMENT FOR THIS PATIENT

In this patient with a grade 1 spondylolisthesis and about 5 mm of slippage, a far lateral foraminotomy must be done through a fusion, but no clear evidence determines whether internal fixation is required. Fortunately, when fusing L5 to the sacrum, the sacroilia are large and vascular enough to be taken down and peeled back to provide a periosteal bed for the fusion to take. Many patients have a large L5 transverse process; therefore, any graft is likely to take if, indeed, there is not a great deal of slippage.

The X-rays of this patient's spine do not show a major vertebral dislocation. Therefore, to execute a lateral decompression and a standard posterolateral fusion, the bony elements must be completely exposed, the sacral prominence is turned down internally where it comes into contact with the L5 transverse process, and the L5 transverse process is properly denuded. In addition, strong grafts of both cancellous and cortical bone must be packed in tightly. The patient can then be placed in a body jacket that incorporates the most symptomatic leg. That brace must be used whenever the patient is upright; however, the patient can sleep in a canvas corset. After 2 months, the awkward brace can be replaced with a chair-back brace for 2 months, for a total bracing time of 4 months. Such standard techniques are the most accepted, but the patient must cooperate fully.

Instrumentation as an Alternative

Patients who believe they would not tolerate such bracing, and those who the physician believes would not comply with bracing, must undergo internal fixation with pedicle screws. Only through internal fixation will the fusion be solid. Several fixation devices are adequate.[3] My own experience has been with the VSP® plates or the TSRH® bar system. More recently, I have used the Universal AO® bar system as well. But, the U.S. Food and Drug Administration (FDA) has recently reviewed these devices and declared them to be investigational or Class 3. According to the FDA, pedicle screw fixation devices are neither safe nor effective; yet, we continue to use them. All the authors writing about the patient described here chose similar surgical procedures with internal fixation. These are reasonable ways to handle this patient. For properly trained and educated professionals, I recommend the same operation, but each surgeon must now obtain a separate consent form from the patient stating the position held by the FDA, followed by a reason for recommending the pedicle screw fixation.

Interbody Fusion

To make the fusion 360 degrees or circumferential, some surgeons have advocated using interbody fusion. On only 2 occasions have I found it necessary to do this. Both patients had a grade 2 slippage wherein the spine was extremely mobile. With the internal fixation device, the patients' slippages were easily corrected. Because of the stresses on these patients' spines, we believed the pedicle fixation device might fail; therefore, bone was placed in the interbody space. As a general rule, an interbody fusion is not part of the therapy for this condition.

Repairing the Pars Fracture

When patients have good spinal alignment, and when the back pain from the pars fracture exceeds the leg discomfort, the patients can be treated through direct repair of the pars fracture itself. This can be done after the far lateral foraminotomies. A screw is placed in the lateral aspect of the pedicle near the transverse process and angled in. The entire posterior element or Gill body is then replaced. The edges of the bone are roughened, and small cancellous grafts are placed in the area. The Gill body is replaced and brought down tightly with #18 wire onto the far lateral pedicle screw. (Other physicians advocate simply placing the wire around the transverse process to accomplish the same type of lateral fixation.) I have used this particular procedure on two athletes, one of whom later competed in the Olympics. Because the patient's anatomy had to be as normal as possible for competition, I believed this procedure was appropriate. For a 23-year-old laborer, however, this is probably not the treatment of choice.

SUMMARY

Considering the many options to treat the patient described here, decompression is essential and it must be far lateral. A fusion must be added. Admittedly, that doubles the operative and recovery time, but this is the only way to ensure long-term results. If the malalignment is minimal and if the L5 to S1 vertebrae are fairly fixed intraoperatively, a standard fusion will suffice. This fusion must be done well and the patient must be adequately braced postoperatively.

If, at the time of the operation, the area from L5 to S1 is greatly mobile and, if the physician believes the patient will not comply with the brace, pedicle screw fixation along with the fusion allows enough internal bracing for a solid fusion to occur in as many as 80 to 90% of patients. Internal fixation can be done safely. The pedicle screws must be placed high in the pedicle; the complications always occur when placement is too low. Less than 2% of patients have an increased neurological deficit after such procedures. The rate of infection rate is also about 2%. The operation can be carried out successfully in 95% of patients, with at least two thirds being quite well when fully evaluated a year later.

REFERENCES

Charles L. Branch, Jr., M.D.

1. Branch CL Jr: Posterior lumbar interbody fusion, in Hardy RW (ed): *Lumbar Disc Disease*, ed. 2. New York, Raven Press, 1993, pp 187–200.
2. Cloward RB: Spondylolisthesis: Treatment by laminectomy and interbody fusion. *Clin Orthop* 1981; 154:74–82.
3. Hanley EN Jr, Levy JA: Surgical treatment of isthmic lumbosacral spondylolisthesis: Analysis of variables influencing results. *Spine* 1989; 14:48–50.
4. Johnson LP, Nasca RJ, Dunham WK: Surgical management of isthmic spondylolisthesis. *Spine* 1988; 13:93–97.
5. Kaneda K, Satoh S, Nohara Y, et al.: Distraction rod instrumentation with posterolateral fusion in isthmic spondylolisthesis: 53 cases followed for 18-89 months. *Spine* 1985; 10:383–389.
6. Kim SS, Denis F, Lonstein JE, et al.: Factors affecting fusion rate in adult spondylolisthesis. *Spine* 1990; 15:979–984.
7. Saraste H: Spondylolysis and spondylolisthesis. *Acta Orthop Scand* (Suppl) 1993; 251:84–86.
8. Schlegel K, Pon A: The biomechanics of posterior lumbar interbody fusion in spondylolisthesis. *Clin Orthop Rel Res* 1985; 93:115–119.
9. Steffee AD, Brantigan JW: The variable screw placement spinal fixation system: Report of a prospective study of 250 patients enrolled in Food and Drug Administration clinical trials. *Spine* 1993; 18:1160–1172.
10. Suzuki I, Pearcy MJ, Tibrewal SB, et al.: Posterior intertransverse fusion assessed clinically with biplanar radiography. *Internat Orthop* 1985; 9:11–17.
11. Yashiro K, Homma T, Hokari Y, et al.: The Steffee variable screw plate system using different methods of bone grafting. *Spine* 1991; 16:1329–1334.

Edward N. Hanley, Jr., M.D., Mark E. Coggins, M.D.

1. Davne SH, Myers DL: Complications of lumbar spinal fusion with transpedicular instrumentation. *Spine* 1992; 17:S184–S189.
2. Garfin SR, Heller J: The operative reduction of spondylolisthesis: Indications, results, complications. *Semin Spine Surg* 1989; 1:125–132.

3. Hanley EN: Operative treatment: Children and adolescents, in Weinstein JN, Wiese SW (eds): *The Lumbar Spine*. Philadelphia, WB Saunders, 1990, pp 515–528.

4. Hanley EN Jr, Levy JA: Surgical treatment of isthmic lumbosacral spondylolisthesis: Analysis of variables influencing results. *Spine* 1989; 14:48–50.

5. Hanley EN, Phillips E, Harvell JC: Allograft, in Rothman RH, Simeone FA (eds): *The Spine*. Philadelphia, WB Saunders, 1992, pp 1766–1773.

6. Matsuzaki H, Tokuhashi Y, Matsumoto F, et al.: Problems and solutions of pedicle screw plate fixation of lumbar spine. *Spine* 1990; 15:1159–1165.

7. McAfee PC, Weiland DJ, Caralow JJ: Survivorship analysis of pedicle spinal instrumentation. *Spine* 1991; 16:S422–S427.

8. Savini R, Cervellati S, Draghetti M, et al.: The surgical treatment of spondylolisthesis in the adult, in *Progress in Spinal Pathology*, vol. II. Bologna, Italian Scoliosis Research Group.

9. Scoliosis Research Society Morbidity and Mortality Committee: *Member Survey*, 1987.

10. Weinstein JN, Spratt KF, Spengler D, et al.: Spinal pedicle fixation: Reliability and validity of roentgenogram based assessment and surgical factors on successful screw placement. *Spine* 1988; 13: 1012–1018.

11. West JL, Bradford DS, Ogilvie JW: Results of spinal arthrodesis with pedicle screw-plate fixation. *J Bone Joint Surg* 1991; 73A: 1179–1184.

12. West JL, Ogilvie JW, Bradford DS: Complications of the variable screw plate pedicle screw fixation. *Spine* 1991; 16:576–579.

13. Wiltse LL: Spondylolisthesis and its treatment: Conservative treatment; fusion with and without reduction, in Ruge D, Wiltse LL (eds): *Spinal Disorders: Diagnosis and Treatment*. Philadelphia, Lea and Febiger, 1977, pp 193–217.

14. Zendrick MR, Lorenz MA: The nonreductive treatment of spondylolisthesis. *Semin Spine Surg* 1989; 1:116–124.

Thomas Ducker, M.D.

1. Krag MH: Spinal Fusion: Overview of options and posterior internal fixation, in Frymoyer J (ed): *The Adult Spine*. New York, Raven Press, 1991, pp 1919–1945.

2. Macnab I: *Backache*, ed. 2. Baltimore, Williams and Wilkins, 1990, pp 84–103.

29

Treatment of Rheumatoid Arthritis with Atlantoaxial Subluxation

CASE

A 59-year-old woman with long-standing rheumatoid arthritis came to medical attention with right occipital headache and neck pain. She had a progressive loss of function in her arms and legs over a 6-month period. On examination, her sensation was normal, but she had generalized weakness throughout. Her deep tendon reflexes were hyperactive and she had bilateral Babinski reflexes.

PARTICIPANTS

Anterior Decompression and Posterior Arthrodesis for the Treatment of Rheumatoid Arthritis with Atlantoaxial Subluxation–H. Louis Harkey, M.D.

Posterior Arthrodesis for the Treatment of Rheumatoid Arthritis with Atlantoaxial Subluxation– H. Säveland, M.D., S. Zygmunt, M.D., Ph.D.

Moderator–Arnold H. Menezes, M.D.

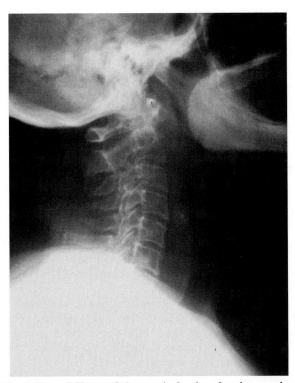

Fig. 1 Lateral X-ray of the cervical spine showing erosion of the odontoid and atlantoaxial subluxation.

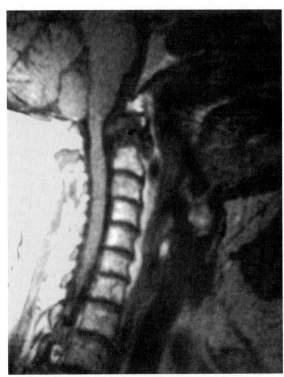

Fig. 2 Magnetic resonance image (MRI) of the craniovertebral junction in extension showing pannus formation.

279

Anterior Decompression and Posterior Arthrodesis for the Treatment of Rheumatoid Arthritis with Atlantoaxial Subluxation

H. Louis Harkey, M.D.

The case presented is typical of rheumatoid arthritis. Although some unfortunate individuals develop atlantoaxial instability within a few years of the initial diagnosis of rheumatoid arthritis, this woman has likely had long-standing disease, probably in excess of 20 years. The usual presenting complaints in the patient with rheumatoid atlantoaxial subluxation are pain and progressive loss of function. As primary care physicians have become more aware of this manifestation of rheumatoid arthritis, however, atlantoaxial instability is being recognized more frequently in asymptomatic patients.

The headaches this patient describes are probably occipital neuralgia from compression or stretching of the second cervical root.[15] Her neck pain may originate from C1-C2 instability and muscle spasm attempting to stabilize the joint, or it may originate from arthritis involving the subaxial cervical spine.

DIFFERENTIATION FROM MYELOPATHY

It is often difficult to differentiate loss of function due to myelopathy from that of progressive arthritis or other effects of the disease and its treatment.[2] The severe deformities in the hands commonly interfere with dexterity, while arthritis in the hip, knee, and ankle often make walking difficult, leaving a patient quite handicapped even in the absence of neurological deficits. Long-term steroid therapy and other immunosupressants can affect both peripheral nerves and muscles, with resulting numbness and weakness. However, a careful history often differentiates the onset of myelopathy from progression or flare-up of arthritis. Recognizing the onset of myelopathy in rheumatoid patients is critical; death rates are high in conservatively treated patients with rheumatoid arthritis after the onset of myelopathy.[10,12] Although little in the patient's examination except hyperactive and abnormal reflexes suggests progressive myelopathy, a detailed history from this patient would probably lead to the appropriate diagnosis.

Analysis of Images

The lateral X-ray of the cervical spine shows some erosion of the odontoid and suggests that the atlantoaxial subluxation is fully reducible. On MRI, however, pannus formation is seen compressing the cervicomedullary junction, even in the fully reduced position. Although subtle, some increased signal intensity appears within the spinal cord at the level of compression, suggesting the presence of edema or myelomalacia, or both. In addition to the diagnostic studies provided, a computed tomogram of the craniovertebral junction would be useful to evaluate the integrity of the lateral masses of the atlas. If the lateral masses of C1 are intact and the course of the vertebral artery through the transverse processes of C2 is normal, this patient might be a candidate for transarticular screw fixation. If the lateral masses of C1 are severely eroded, stabilization must incorporate the occiput, particularly if the anterior arch of C1 is removed during anterior decompression. In this patient, neither the plain X-ray nor the MRI suggest severe erosion of C1; there is no evidence of odontoid translocation.

GOALS OF SURGERY

The goals of surgery in this patient are twofold:[13]

- Decompress the cervicomedullary junction;
- Restore stability to the craniovertebral junction.

The cervicomedullary junction can often be decompressed through simple reduction of the atlantoaxial subluxation. If postural reduction alone is insufficient, a brief trial of cervical traction sometimes restores alignment. Some authors recommend prolonged traction in an attempt to achieve reduction, particularly when the odontoid has invaginated into the foramen magnum.[14] Experience indicates that skeletal traction beyond a few days rarely reduces rheumatoid atlantoaxial subluxation and odontoid translocation.[3] Because the risks of prolonged traction in a rheumatoid patient are not insignificant, I recommend surgical decompression if reduction is not achieved within a few days.

Reduction of atlantoaxial subluxation alone may not be sufficient to decompress the cervicomedullary junction, as is shown in this case.[8] Pannus may continue to compress the neural structures with resulting myelopathy, which may partially explain the lack of correlation between the degree of subluxation seen on X-ray and neurological function.[4] Some surgeons argue that simply immobilizing the atlantoaxial joint through posterior stabilization is sufficient treatment and that the pannus will eventually resolve.[11,20] Because pannus is reactive tissue caused by chronic instability, stabilization of the abnormally mobile joint should cause a regression of the reactive tissue. This argument is similar to that used in anterior cervical interbody arthrodesis, that is, fusion alone causes resorption of osteophytes.[17] However, it is not clear that the pannus completely resolves or at what rate it resolves. A period of persistent spinal cord compromise may follow surgical stabilization, during which the myelopathy may not improve and the spinal cord may suffer additional, possibly irreversible, damage. Additionally, the risk of spinal cord injury during posterior stabilization with anterior cord compression is significantly increased.[7]

Transoral Decompression

For this patient, I recommend an initial anterior decompression through the transoral approach. In experienced hands, this is a relatively quick procedure that is tolerated amazingly well. This is particularly true for irreducible atlantoaxial subluxation without associated basilar invagination, which can make the caudal exposure more difficult. In this patient, the anterior atlas and axis should be easily exposed by simply elevating the soft palate and depressing the tongue.

Depending on the type of transoral retractor used, nasal or oral intubation is generally satisfactory. A tracheostomy is rarely necessary, except in the few patients who require an extended transoral approach. I prefer the supine position because it is easier to maintain sagittal orientation and I do not typically rely on fluoroscopy for intraoperative guidance. The anterior tubercle of C1 is readily palpable and identifies the center of the pharyngeal incision. The muscle and mucosa are reflected together to expose the anterior arch of C1, the body of C2, and the base of the odontoid. Carrying the exposure out to the facet joints helps to maintain orientation and allows any residual subluxation to be appreciated. I typically enter the C1-C2 joint and remove cartilage or other soft tissue, making it easier to fully reduce the atlantoaxial subluxation and encouraging a bony union across the facet.

Usually, only the lower half of the anterior arch of C1 must be removed to complete the decompression. Working above and below the remaining bridge of the anterior arch of C1, the entire odontoid can typically be removed—unless the odontoid is severely translocated. In this case, I would remove pannus until the dura bulges into the defect and pulsations of cerebrospinal fluid can be seen. Removing all vestiges of pannus that adhere to the dural surface is unnecessary and can be risky. A leak of cerebrospinal fluid after transoral surgery can be extremely problematic. By removing the pannus, a complete decompression at the time of surgery is ensured.

The endotracheal tube can be removed once the patient is fully awake, if the tongue and soft palate are not excessively swollen from prolonged traction or surgical trauma. The patient should not take anything orally for 2 to 3 days after surgery to allow the mucosa time to heal.

Sakou and colleagues[18] have reported success with anterior arthrodesis after transoral surgery. Although concerns about placing a foreign body into an oral wound have not borne out, maintaining stability until the bony union occurs is a problem. Many surgeons avoid using the halo for rheumatoid patients because the device is so poorly tolerated.[5] Devices and procedures for anterior fixation of the craniovertebral junction have been devised, but experience with them is limited. Anterior plates designed to attach to the lateral masses of C1 and body of C2 are not biomechanically sound, and may fail to adequately restore stability. Unlike an anterior plate for the subaxial spine, no load-sharing graft is interposed between the atlas and axis. The forces in atlantoaxial subluxation are directed anteriorly and are magnified by the lever arm of the plate, generating tremendous stress upon the screws in the body of C2. Eventually, the screws will loosen and, ultimately, the device will fail. Anterior transarticular screw placement is extremely demanding and requires a separate incision in the neck. There is very little tolerance for proper screw placement. Even in the best situations, only a small portion of bone is present in the body of C2 for the screw to purchase. Again, the leverage applied by way of the screw may easily overwhelm its bony purchase in the body of C2. Therefore, anterior fusion and stabilization after transoral decompression is not a viable alternative.

POSTERIOR STABILIZATION

After decompression, the stability of the atlantoaxial joint must be restored, and the specific technique for stabilizing atlantoaxial subluxation in rheumatoid arthritis must be tailored to the patient. If the lateral masses of C1 are significantly eroded, the fixation must include the skull.[16] Fixing the posterior elements of C1 and C2 would do little to stabilize the craniovertebral junction in this patient. Disrupting the anterior arch of C1 during decompression produces a condition not unlike that of an un-

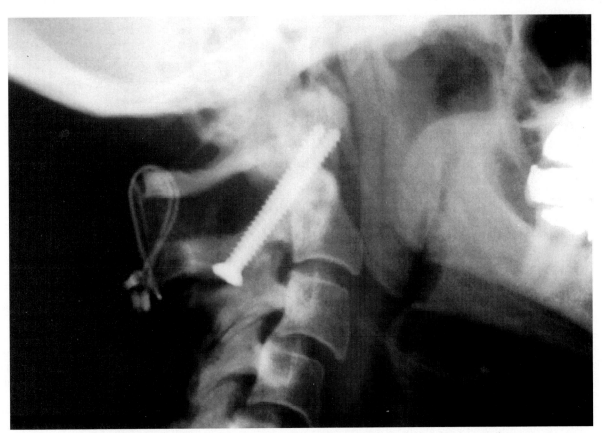

Fig. 1 Postoperative X-ray showing posterior transarticular C1-C2 fixation in a patient with rheumatoid arthritis and atlantoaxial subluxation.

stable Jefferson's fracture, and may require the skull to be incorporated in the fixation. Because the transverse ligament is typically incompetent, removing the anterior arch of C1 allows the lateral masses to migrate under the weight of the skull. If the anterior arch and the lateral masses of C1 remain intact, however, stability can be restored through C1-C2 arthrodesis alone.

Assuming that the lateral masses of C1 are intact, I recommend restoring stability with a modified transarticular C1-C2 screw fixation (Fig. 1). This technique requires significant skill and precise placement of the transarticular screws, but affords some advantages.[11] The primary advantage lies in the superior stability achieved when compared to traditional techniques for posterior C1-C2 arthrodesis. If adequate screw purchase is achieved, external immobilization with a halo is unnecessary. When the anterior arch of C1 is destroyed during transoral decompression, transarticular screws prevent lateral migration

and stability can be achieved without incorporating the skull. Another advantage of transarticular C1-C2 fusion is a higher fusion rate.[6] Posterior C1-C2 fusions, particularly in patients with rheumatoid arthritis, have a relatively high rate of pseudoarthrosis.[1,9,19]

CONCLUSION

There is no argument that surgical intervention is indicated for this patient, as she has evidence of myelopathy associated with an unstable atlantoaxial subluxation. A good clinical outcome may result from either a posterior stabilization alone or an anterior decompression followed by a posterior fixation. Surgical intervention, however, must ensure that the cervicomedullary junction is completely decompressed and that lasting stability is restored to the atlantoaxial junction.

Posterior Arthrodesis for the Treatment of Rheumatoid Arthritis with Atlantoaxial Subluxation

H. Säveland, M.D., S. Zygmunt, M.D., Ph.D.

This unfortunate woman with chronic rheumatoid arthritis is suffering from occipital headache, neck pain, and progressive myelopathy. In patients with cervical rheumatoid arthritis, the pain is often intractable, but the most hazardous clinical sign is progressive myelopathy. The radiographic investigation shows the most common type of rheumatoid cervical subluxation—atlantoaxial subluxation. Her myelopathy is most likely caused by cord compression by the subluxation in combination with periodontoid pannus. In view of the progressive neurological dysfunction, there is a strong indication for surgical treatment.

Before deciding on the surgical approach, and to verify the degree of atlantoaxial instability, the radiographic investigations must be supplemented with plain views in flexion and extension. If there is a significant instability, we recommend occipitocervical fusion alone. If the subluxation is irreducible, however, we recommend a posterior or transoral decompression.

SURGICAL APPROACH

The first fusion technique used for rheumatoid atlantoaxial dislocation was described by Hamblen in 1967.[5] Hamblen's method included wiring bone grafts to the occiput and the cervical spine. To provide immediate internal fixation, Brattström and Granholm[1] employed a fusion technique using wires, bone grafting, and methylmethacrylate cement (Figs. 1, 2). The first procedure was done in 1970 and the technique has been used in 180 patients with rheumatoid arthritis.

The Brattström-Granholm Technique

For this approach, the patient is placed on a Stryker® frame and intubated in the supine position. After this, the patient's skull is placed in traction, and the patient is turned prone. Through a midline incision, the muscles are stripped subperiosteally from the occiput and the laminae of C1 and C2. Four burr holes are drilled in the occiput, 2 on each side of the midline. The lower burr holes should be placed close to the posterior edge of the foramen magnum. A loop of wire is passed under the laminae of the atlas and then cut in two. The upper free ends are twisted together in the midline. A pin is then inserted through the

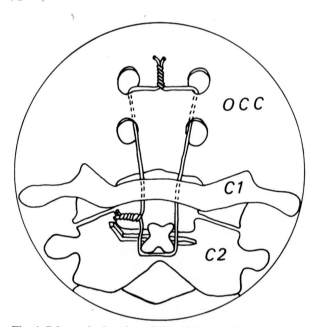

Fig. 1 Schematic drawing of the wiring used in Brattström-Granholm fusion. The pin in the spinous process of the axis is bent on the left side. The bent pin and the two twisted ends of the wires are encased in acrylic cement. The exposed occipital bone and the laminae opposite the cement are covered with bone chips. OCC: occipital bone.

spinous process of C2 and, to provide better anchorage in the cement, one end of the pin is bent slightly. The caudal ends of the wires are passed over the pin and twisted together, thus reducing the atlantoaxial subluxation.

If the arch of the atlas is thin or displaced rostrally and ventrally, a laminectomy of C1 is done. In such cases, the wire is placed under the pin. The burr holes, the twisted wire ends, and the bent end of the pin are encased in the methylmethacrylate cement on one side. The uncovered occipital bone and the

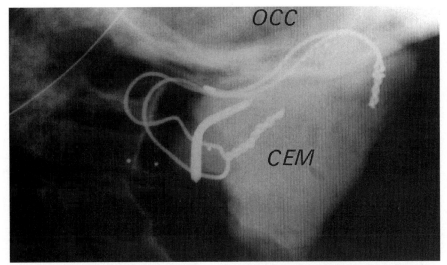

Fig. 2 Lateral radiograph of the Brattström-Granholm fusion. Tantalum markers for roentgen analysis have been implanted in the occipital bone and C2. OCC: occipital bone; CEM: acrylic cement.

laminae opposite the cement are partly decorticated and covered with bone chips. The wound is closed in layers and the patient's skull is removed from traction. The patient is mobilized on the first postoperative day. No external support other than a soft collar is used.

Clinical Results

The long-term results of the first 100 consecutive fusion procedures in patients with rheumatoid atlantoaxial subluxation were presented in 1988.[12] In our series, 81% of the patients improved. Seven patients underwent a second operation, 5 for infection and 2 for rupture of the wires. There was no operative mortality. A review of reported results after both occipitocervical and atlantoaxial fusion seems to favor the inclusion of the occiput in the fusion (Table 1).[11] Most authors used occipitocervical fusion for patients with more severe cases. In spite of this, bony union

was observed more frequently after occipitocervical fusion and nonunion was more common after atlantoaxial fusion.

REDUCING PERIODONTOID PANNUS

From a study of magnetic resonance images, we concluded that posterior occipitocervical fusion alone reduced or even eliminated periodontoid pannus.[13] The reduction was seen within 6 weeks of surgery (Fig. 3), and the neuraxis at the craniocervical junction expanded after the periodontoid pannus was reduced. In the study, all 6 patients with clinical signs of myelopathy improved after the fusion. Thus, transoral removal of the pannus in patients with rheumatoid arthritis and cord compression from soft-tissue periodontoid pannus appears to be redundant. We believe that transoral decompression should be restricted to patients with cord compression from irreducible lesions, cranial

Table 1. Reports Including Atlantoaxial and Occipitocervical Fusions

Authors	No. of patients*	Mean age	Bony union (%)	Fibrous union (%)	Nonunion	Success (%)**	Death (%)***
			Atlantoaxial fusion				
Ranawat, et al.[7]	13	63	67	–	33	31	31
Conaty, Mongan[3]	17	50	76	12	12	71	–
Larsson, Toolanen[6]	25 (2)	56	52	32	16	96	–
Clark, et al.[2]	20	57	75	10	15	65	–
Santavirta, et al.[8]	24	57	50	17	33	91	–
			Occipitocervical fusion				
Ranawat, et al.[7]	9	61	55	–	11	67	11
Conaty, Mongan[3]	10 (1)	54	80	–	10	60	10
Larsson, Toolanen[6]	4	60	100	–	–	75	–
Clark, et al.[2]	16	56	100	–	–	69	–
Santavirta, et al.[8]	5 (1)	47	100	–	–	100	–

* The number of patients without rheumatoid arthritis appears in parentheses.
** Success as defined by the authors.
***Death within 4 months.

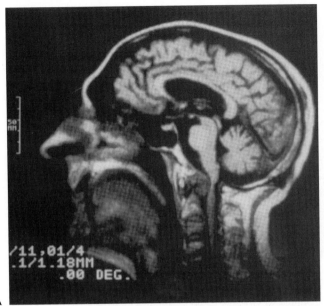
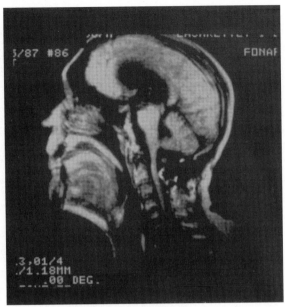

A   B

Fig. 3 (*A*) **Preoperative magnetic resonance image showing cord compression from periodontoid pannus.** (*B*) **Magnetic resonance image in the same patient 6 weeks after occipitocervical fusion alone; the pannus is drastically reduced.**

settling, or horizontal atlantoaxial subluxation caused by pannus anterior to the odontoid peg.

MICROMOTION AFTER FUSION

Some investigators have questioned the use of methylmethacrylate cement in spinal fusion because of a decrease in stability with time or potential resorption of bone.[4,9,10] Recently, we used roentgen stereophotogrammetric analysis to study the stability of the spine after Brattström-Granholm fusion.[14] This study included 10 patients with chronic rheumatoid arthritis and atlanto-axial instability who underwent occipitocervical fusion. Tantalum markers were implanted into the occipital bone and axis preoperatively to facilitate stereophotogrammetric analysis. Conventional radiography showed that all patients were stable after the fusion. The analysis showed small movements—micromotion—in all patients. In most patients, however, the motion was less than 0.5 mm and probably reflected the elasticity between the fused components. We, therefore, conclude that the Brattström-Granholm fusion technique creates stable fusions, even when measured with the highly sensitive stereophotogrammetric method.

Treatment of Rheumatoid Arthritis with Atlantoaxial Subluxation

Arnold H. Menezes, M.D.

The case presented is that of a 59-year-old woman with long-standing rheumatoid arthritis. This patient has right occipital headache, neck pain, and high cervical myelopathy. The lateral cervical radiograph shows erosion of the odontoid process without any subluxation. The T1-weighted magnetic resonance image (MRI) of the cranial cervical junction documents that a large mass has replaced the odontoid process, with ventral indentation of the cervicomedullary junction. The posterior arch of C1 is also displaced ventrally, such that there is a mild hour-glass constriction of the cervicomedullary junction.

This study is incomplete without axial images. In addition, the status of the lateral masses of the atlas and axis must be defined, and is best done with computed tomography and T1- and T2-weighted axial images of the MRI.

IDEAL TREATMENT

I believe that the odontoid process has been replaced by pannus. This replacement usually accompanies destruction of the synovial joints around the odontoid process and the atlantoaxial and occipital-atlantal lateral joints. The fact that the posterior arch of C1 has been displaced signifies that the lateral atlantal masses are involved. Thus, this patient has the potential for occipitocervical and atlantoaxial instability. I believe that the ideal treatment is ventral decompression of the mass, which requires removing the anterior arch of the atlas along with the offending pathologic process. The procedure is done with the patient in halo traction; the patient then should undergo a dorsal occipital cervical fixation.

Osseous fusion is mandatory in these patients, and can be supplemented with methylmethacrylate or a contoured metallic loop. My experience has been extremely satisfactory with bone grafts spanning the occiput and the posterior arch of C1 and C2, wired to all 3 structures. If methylmethacrylate is used, the patient does not require fixation in a halo brace postoperatively. In gross occipitocervical instability, a contoured loop fashioned out of a threaded Stinneman® pin provides the internal stability.

The stance supporting transoral decompression and anterior arthrodesis assumes that the lateral atlantal masses are normal.

This is not the case when rheumatoid granulation tissue appears at the craniovertebral junction. A donor bone graft (after transoral decompression) fixed in the ventral clivus and the axis vertebra is relatively unstable because of problems with graft fixation; hence, this approach must be supplemented with dorsal fixation. Thus, the anterior route for arthrodesis is not efficacious in this patient.

A simple posterior C1-C2 arthrodesis is unlikely to solve this patient's compressive myelopathy, nor will it take care of the potential instability between the occiput and the atlas. In such a situation, the patient's neurological condition progressively deteriorates, which, unfortunately, can be precipitous after the operation. This damage stems from the ventral compression and a progressive instability between the occiput and atlas, and because the dynamic load is transferred.

REFERENCES

H. Louis Harkey, M.D.

1. Clark CR, Goetz DD, Menezes AH: Arthrodesis of the cervical spine in rheumatoid arthritis. *J Bone Joint Surg* 1987; 71A:381–392.
2. Crellin RQ, Maccabe JJ, Hamilton EBD: Severe subluxation of the cervical spine in rheumatoid arthritis. *J Bone Joint Surg* 1970; 52B:244–251.
3. Crockard HA, Calder I, Ransford AO: One-stage transoral decompression and posterior fixation in rheumatoid atlanto-axial subluxation. *J Bone Joint Surg* 1990; 72B:682–685.
4. Crockard HA, Stevens JM, Kendall BE, et al.: Transoral decompression and posterior fusion for rheumatoid atlanto-axial subluxation. *J Bone Joint Surg* (Br) 1986; 68B:350–356.
5. Ferlic DC, Clayton ML, Leidholt JD, et al.: Surgical treatment of the symptomatic unstable cervical spine in rheumatoid arthritis. *J Bone Joint Surg* 1975; 57A:349–354.
6. Grob D, Jeanneret B, Aebi M, et al.: Atlanto-axial fusion with transarticular screw fixation. *J Bone Joint Surg* 1991; 73B:972–976.
7. Hamblen DL: Surgical management of rheumatoid arthritis: The cervical spine, in Harris NH (ed): *Postgraduate Textbook of Clinical Orthopaedics*. Bristol, Wright PGS, 1983, pp 487–497.
8. Kenez J, Turoozy L, Barsi P, et al.: Retro-odontoid "ghost" pseudotumours in atlantoaxial instability caused by rheumatoid arthritis. *Neuroradiology* 1991; 35:367–369.
9. Kourtopoulos H, von Essen C: Stabilization of the unstable upper cervical spine in rheumatoid arthritis. *Acta Neurochir* 1988; 91:113–115.
10. Marks JS, Sharp J: Rheumatoid cervical myelopathy. *Q J Med* 1981; 50:307–319.
11. McGuire RA, Harkey HL: Modification of technique and results of atlantoaxial transfacet stabilization. *Orthopedics* (in press 1995).
12. Meijers KAE, van Beusekom GT, Luyendijk W, et al.: Dislocation of the cervical spine with cord compression in rheumatoid arthritis. *J Bone Joint Surg* 1974; 56B:668–680.
13. Menezes AH, VanGilder JC: Transoral-transpharyngeal approach to the anterior craniocervical junction. *J Neurosurg* 1988; 69:895–903.
14. Menezes AH, VanGilder JC, Clark CR, et al.: Odontoid upward migration in rheumatoid arthritis. *J Neurosurg* 1985; 63:500–509.
15. Papadoupoulos SM, Dickman CA, Sonntag VKH: Atlantoaxial stabilization in rheumatoid arthritis. *J Neurosurg* 1991; 74:1–7.
16. Ransford AO: The cervical spine in rheumatoid arthritis. *Semin Orthopaed* 1987; 2:94–100.
17. Robinson RA, Walker AE, Ferlic DC, et al.: The results of anterior interbody fusion of the cervical spine. *J Bone Joint Surg* 1962; 44A:1569–1587.
18. Sakou T, Morizono Y, Morimoto N: Transoral atlantoaxial anterior decompression and fusion. *Clin Orthop* 1984; 187:134–138.
19. Santavirta S, Konttinen YT, Laasonen E, et al.: Ten-year results of operations for rheumatoid cervical spine disorders. *J Bone Joint Surg* 1991; 73B:116–120.
20. Zygmunt S, Säveland H, Brattstrom H, et al.: Reduction of rheumatoid periodontoid pannus following posterior occipito-cervical fusion visualised by magnetic resonance imaging. *Br J Neurosurg* 1988; 2:315–320.

H. Säveland, M.D., S. Zygmunt, M.D., Ph.D.

1. Brattström H, Granholm L: Atlanto-axial fusion in rheumatoid arthritis: A new method of fixation with wire and bone cement. *Acta Orthop Scand* 1976; 47:619–628.
2. Clark CR, Goetz DD, Menezes AH: Arthrodesis of the cervical spine in rheumatoid arthritis. *J Bone Joint Surg* 1989; 71A:381–392.
3. Conaty JP, Mongan ES: Cervical fusion in rheumatoid arthritis. *J Bone Joint Surg* 1981; 63A:1218–1227.
4. Crockard HA, Ransford AO: Stabilization of the spine, in Krayenbühl H (ed): *Advances and Technical Standards in Neurosurgery*. New York, Springer, 1990, pp 159–188.
5. Hamblen DL: Occipito-cervical fusio: Indications, technique, and results. *J Bone Joint Surg* 1967; 49B:33–45.
6. Larsson SE, Toolanen G: Posterior fusion for atlanto-axial subluxation in rheumatoid arthritis. *Spine* 1986; 11:525–530.
7. Ranawat CS, O'Leary P, Pellicci P, et al.: Cervical spine fusion in rheumatoid arthritis. *J Bone Joint Surg* 1979; 61A:1003–1010.
8. Santavirta S, Konttinen YT, Laasonen E, et al.: Ten-year results of operations for rheumatoid cervical spine disorders. *J Bone Joint Surg* 1991; 73B:116–120.
9. Whitehill R, Drucker S, McCoig JA, et al.: Induction and characterization of an interface tissue by implantation of methylmethacrylate cement into the posterior part of the cervical spine of a dog. *J Bone Joint Surg* 1988; 70A:51–59.
10. Whitehill R, Stowers SF, Fechner RE, et al.: Posterior cervical fusions using cerclage wires, methylmethacrylate cement, and autogenous bone graft: An experimental study of a canine model. *Spine* 1987; 12:12–22.
11. Zygmunt S: *Rheumatoid arthritis of the cervical spine: Aspects on the surgical treatment*. Thesis, Lund, University of Lund, 1992.
12. Zygmunt S, Ljunggren B, Alund M, et al.: Realignment and surgical fixation of atlanto-axial and subaxial dislocations in rheumatoid arthritis (RA) patients. *Acta Neurochir* 1988; 43:79–84.
13. Zygmunt S, Säveland H, Brattström H, et al.: Reduction of rheumatoid periodontoid pannus following posterior occipito-cervical fusion visualised by magnetic resonance imaging. *Br J Neurosurg* 1988; 2:315–320.
14. Zygmunt S, Säveland H, Selvik G, et al.: Micromotions in occipito-cervical fusion for rheumatoid atlanto-axial instability: A clinical and roentgen stereophotogrammetric study. *J Orthop Rheumatol* 1991; 4:213–222.

30

Treatment of Type II Odontoid Fractures

CASE

An otherwise healthy, 54-year-old woman suffered a fracture of the odontoid as a result of a motor vehicle accident. She was neurologically intact and the fracture was well aligned. Cervical tomograms of the AP and lateral views were taken.

PARTICIPANTS

Screw Fixation for Type II Odontoid Fractures–Ronald I. Apfelbaum, M.D.

The Halo Brace for Type II Odontoid Fractures–Stephen M. Papadopoulos, M.D., Michael Polinsky, M.D.

Moderator–Volker K.H. Sonntag, M.D.

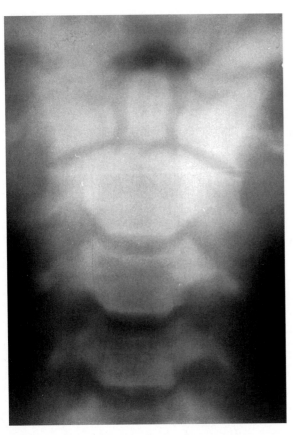 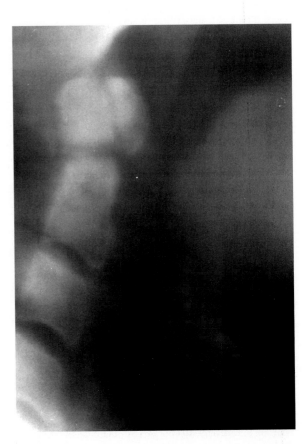

Screw Fixation for Type II Odontoid Fractures

Ronald I. Apfelbaum, M.D.

Type II odontoid fractures are best treated in most patients through direct screw fixation. Although this statement may seem controversial, it represents, I believe, a defensible position that is the best option for most patients with a Type II odontoid fracture. Consider the facts.

THE PROBLEM

Type II odontoid fractures (Anderson and D'Alonzo classification)[2] are the most frequent type of odontoid fracture. They occur at the junction of the odontoid process and the body of C2 and result in potentially disastrous cervical instability. The biomechanical design of the C1-C2 complex is such that more motion occurs here than at any other single level in the cervical spine. This motion is primarily rotation, accounting for one half of the axial rotation of the neck.[32] Translational motion is restricted by the strong transverse ligament containing the odontoid process in the anterior portion of the ring of C1. All other supporting ligaments are substantially weaker than in the subaxial spine, to facilitate the motion that occurs at this joint.

With a fracture of the odontoid, there is no longer significant restriction of translational movements. Anterolisthesis, retrolisthesis, or both, of the C1 odontoid complex may occur relative to the body of C2. If of a significant degree, it may jeopardize the function and integrity of the spinal cord. Indeed, this is one of the commonest sites of disruption in fatal cervical spine injuries.[1,13] Treatment, therefore, clearly is required.

SOLUTIONS

Conventional neurosurgical treatment has been to immobilize the patient in the minerva jacket[26] or halo brace orthosis,[10,12,16,25,27,31] or to carry out a C1-C2 posterior fusion as a primary treatment[22,25,28–30] or after a trial of immobilization fails. Few would argue against surgery in the latter circumstance, but the choice of initial treatment remains controversial. Let's examine each of these alternatives.

External Orthotic Immobilization

For simplicity, I will refer to all external immobilization as halo brace immobilization because that is the most common type of external orthosis in use. Halo brace immobilization has been reported as successful in promoting bone union and, therefore, stability in 0 to 100% of cases in various series. Despite these extremes, most series report success in the 35 to 80% range, with an average of about 50% success (my estimation of the reported

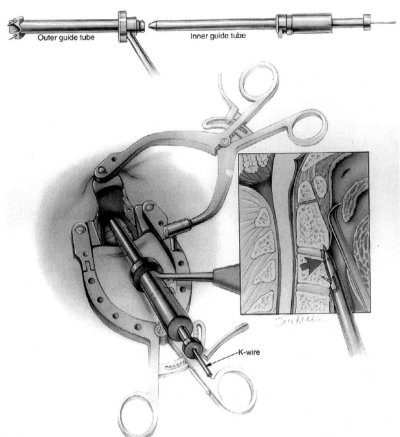

A

Fig. 1 (A) The guide tube system used to facilitate odontoid screw fixation. A low cervical approach is employed. The entire procedure is carried out under biplanar fluoroscopic control. (Figure continued on the next page.)

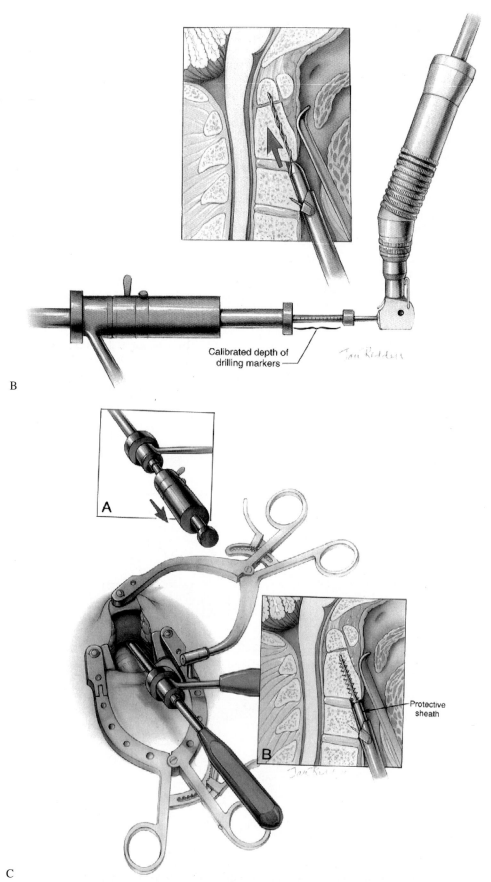

Fig. 1 (Continued). (*B*) A special retractor creates a tunnel for placement of the guide tube and through which drilling can be done. (*C*) Tapping of the hole. (Figure continued on the next page.)

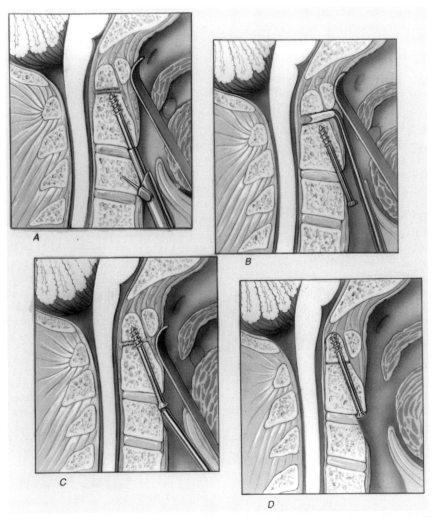

D

Fig. 1 (Continued). (*D*) Screw placement (letters show the sequence). (Reproduced with permission from Apfelbaum RI: Anterior screw fixation of odontoid fractures, in Wilkins RH, Rengachary SS (eds): *Neurosurgical Operative Atlas*. Baltimore, Williams and Wilkins, 1992, pp 189–199.)

series). Why there should be such variability is unclear and a number of authors have attempted to analyze their series, in an attempt to predict the success of immobilization or to define patients who should be offered early surgery.

In their series of 128 patients, Dunn and Seljeskog[15] found a nonunion rate with immobilization of 32%. They found that posterolisthesis greater than 2 mm and a patient age of more than 65 years were associated with the highest nonunion. In analyzing 45 patients in 1985, Apuzzo and colleagues[6] found a 33% instance of nonunion in patients treated conservatively. These authors suggested that displacement greater than 4 mm and a patient age of more than 40 years predicted a higher chance of nonunion. Clark and White[11] found that 5 mm or more of anterior or posterior displacement and angulation of 10 degrees or more significantly increased nonunion rates. Hadley, Browner, and Sonntag[21] could not correlate these findings in 40 patients. The only factor they identified as predisposing to failure to unite with immobilization was greater than 6 mm listhesis in any direction. No author recommended flexion/extension views; therefore, the degree of offset seen on radiographs is really in a random sample and not the extremes that may occur. This may explain some of the variability. If immobilization is successful, it results in an ideal resolution: healing of the fracture with

preservation of normal C1-C2 motion. The fact that it fails so often, perhaps in 50% of cases, limits its usefulness. Also to be considered are the medical *and social* morbidity of halo immobilization. Patients require daily care of the pin sites, may suffer complications, such as local infections and skull osteomyelitis, and require ongoing medical supervision. They usually cannot return to work in the halo and, thus, can suffer a loss of income as well as restriction in most of their activities.

If the outcome of immobilization with the halo brace were assured, this form of treatment might be acceptable. But with a 50% success rate, is it acceptable?

C1-C2 Posterior Fusion

Atlantoaxial posterior fusion can be accomplished through a number of techniques. The Gallie,[19] Brooks,[9] and Sonntag[14] constructs are the most commonly employed. These, too, are not universally successful, but nonunion rates are generally reported as less than 10%. A few, well-documented series, however, report less successful fusion rates, including the report by Fried[18] of 80% failed C1-C2 posterior fusions. The concomitant use of a halo is frequently recommended because most wire and bone graft constructs do not provide strong immobilization before bone union.

Most importantly, if successful, such surgery sacrifices 50% of the normal axial rotation of the neck to achieve stability. Such stability is so important to a patient's future well-being that it would be a reasonable exchange were it the only alternative, *but it is not.*

ODONTOID SCREW FIXATION

Odontoid screw fixation is not a new technique. In 1982, Böhler[7] described his experience with 11 patients dating back to 1968, and Lesoin and colleagues[24] reported on 5 patients in 1987. The technique these authors used involved extensive exposure to achieve odontoid screw placement; therefore, their procedure has not been widely accepted.

The Technique and Results

I have developed a set of instruments that greatly facilitate screw placement, Figure 1 (**A**) to (**D**). The entire operation is done through a small, unilateral, low-cervical linear incision, exactly as though one were doing an anterior cervical discectomy. Special retractors and guide tubes facilitate realigning the fractured odontoid, which then is fixed to the body of C2 with 1 or 2 lag screws placed from the anterior inferior lip of C2 to the tip of the odontoid under biplanar fluoroscopic control,[3–5] Figure 2 (**A**), (**B**).

Direct screw fixation provides immediate stability without an external orthosis. As such, it allows the patient to resume most normal activities of daily living and to promptly return to work, in most cases. By immobilizing the odontoid at the fracture site, rather than remotely, and by reapproximating the bone edges (in the case of acute fractures), optimal conditions for bony healing are achieved. This advantage is reflected in the excellent results of the procedure.

I have employed this technique in 33 patients since 1986. Nineteen procedures were for acute fractures defined as less than 6 months old. Solid bony union was achieved in 15 of the 17

available for evaluation. (One was lost to follow-up, and 1 expired several weeks after surgery of unrelated pulmonary problems.) One recent patient is doing well, but not yet showing solid bony union, and 1 patient's screw pulled out of C2 because of a concomitant (recognized, but underestimated) body fracture.

Of the 14 patients with chronic nonunited fractures (all over 6 months of age and most over 18 months), 4 achieved solid bony union and another 5 have a stable (fibrous) union. Two had fractured screws, one at 2 months and another at 2 years, and 1 screw pulled out of a small odontoid. In 2, the outcome is pending.

For patients with acute fractures, 15 of the 16 procedures were successful (94%), and for those with chronic nonunions apparent, success was achieved in 9 (75%) of 12 patients. Other series have also shown comparable results.[8,17,20]

The procedure is relatively easy and can be accomplished in about 1 hour of surgery time, with another hour required for patient positioning and setting up the fluoroscope. Patients can usually be discharged from the hospital in 1 to 2 days, and promptly resume most nontraumatic or strenuous activities. It is a safe procedure. The only complication in our series was a minor esophageal leak at the site of the retractor at C5-C6 (not at the upper pharyngeal area), which resolved with 2 days of nasogastric suction.

CONCLUSION

Direct screw fixation of odontoid fractures treats the problem at the site of the pathologic process—the fracture. It optimizes the chance of bony union by providing the 2 requisites needed for fracture healing: immobilization at the fracture site and reapproximation of the fragments under compression. It has an excellent success rate in regard to bony fusion, preserves normal C1-C2 motion,[23] and is a safe procedure requiring minimal hospital time. Patients can return immediately to most activities, reducing greatly the social morbidity of their injury. Therefore,

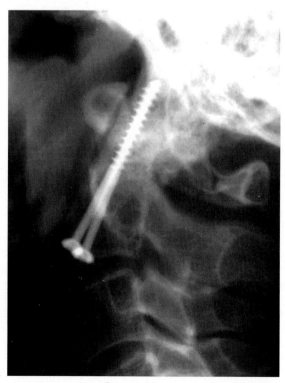

A

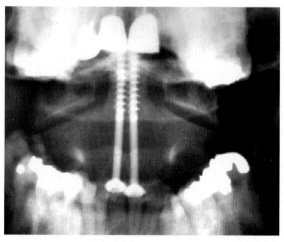

B

Fig. 2 (*A*), (*B*) **Postoperative images of a patient undergoing screw fixation. The spine has been realigned and the odontoid reattached to the body of C2 with 2 lag screws.**

why subject these patients to long periods of immobilization with only fair success, or more painful operative procedures that often also require immobilization and that, if successful, obviate

the superb bioengineering and design of the C1-C2 complex and eliminate up to 50% of the rotation of the neck? Clearly, Type II odontoid fractures are best treated through direct screw fixation.

The Halo Brace for Type II Odontoid Fractures

Stephen M. Papadopoulos, M.D., Michael Polinsky, M.D.

The initial treatment of Type II odontoid fractures remains controversial. Many investigators have directed attention at identifying factors that might predict which patients require surgical fusion and which patients are successfully treated nonoperatively.[2,3,5–7] The halo brace has been useful for immobilizing the cervical spine with few and minor associated complications.[4] In addition, use of the halo brace has the advantage of high success rates in treating most patients with Type II odontoid fractures, avoiding an operative procedure and substantial cost. The patient presented is a healthy 54-year-old woman with minimal displacement, a criterion for an anticipated good outcome if treated with a halo brace (Table 1).

DISCUSSION

Type II odontoid fractures comprise about 60% of all dens fractures and are associated with 6% mortality and morbidity rates.[1,6] Of the various dens fractures, Type II has the highest fusion failure rate when treated solely with external immobilization. The initial treatment of this fracture subtype has, therefore, been controversial. Halo brace immobilization and C1-C2 posterior intraspinous wiring are the most common treatments. Posterior transarticular and anterior transodontoid screws have recently gained popularity as alternative surgical techniques.

Several factors have been identified as predictors of whether stable fracture healing will occur with nonoperative treatment of Type II axis fractures. One of the most commonly cited predictors is the degree of fracture displacement, with a value of greater than 4 to 6 mm being associated with higher failure rates.[2,4–7] In patients treated with a halo brace, Hadley and colleagues[5,6] showed that nonunion occurred in only 5 of 50

Table 1. Factors Increasing the Incidence of Nonunion

Displacement	>6 mm
	Anterior > posterior
Age	>40–65 years
Delay of treatment	>1 week
Fracture type	Type IIA[6]

patients with less than 6 mm of displacement, but occurred in 14 of 18 patients with greater than 6 mm. An age exceeding 40 to 65 years has also been associated with higher rates of nonunion.[2–4] In a series of patients studied by Apuzzo and associates,[2] nonunion occurred in only 4 of 23 younger than 40 years old, but in 9 of 17 patients older than 40 years. Posterior displacement has been less consistently associated with a higher nonunion rate than anterior displacement.[3,4,7] Dunn and Seljeskog[3] noted that delay in treatment was associated with a higher nonunion rate and that those patients treated within a week of their injury were more likely to have fusion than those patients treated after 1 week. Hadley and colleagues[6] recently described a subtype of the Type II fracture (Type IIA), in which bone fragments were noted at the base of the dens at the fracture site. All 3 patients studied could not undergo adequate reduction in a halo brace.

The cost and convenience of treatment cannot be ignored. Others have estimated that the cost of treating a patient with a halo brace is about $3200, which is in accordance with our experience. This should be compared to an estimated total cost of about $20,000 to $25,000 for an operative fusion procedure, including surgeon's fees and hospital costs.

Treatment of Type II Odontoid Fractures

Volker K.H. Sonntag, M.D.

Fractures of the second vertebral body constitute 18% of all cervical spine fractures.[3] Of the various types of C2 fractures, odontoid Type II fractures are the most common (40%).[3] Treatment of this particular fracture is also the most controversial of all C2 fractures, especially when the odontoid fracture is not displaced. Displaced odontoid Type II fractures more than 6 mm anterior or posterior have a 78% chance of failure when treated with a halo brace and, therefore, should not be treated with this modality but, rather, with early surgical stabilization. Treatment of Type IIA fractures, an odontoid type II fracture with bone fragments at the base of the odontoid, in our experience has a 100% failure rate with the halo and should have early surgical stabilization as well.[2]

The case presented here is that of a woman who has a nondisplaced Type II odontoid fracture. The 2 arguments presented

provide valid reasons for both treatments; that is, with halo stabilization or with direct anterior odontoid screw fixation. Papadopoulos and Polinsky argue that, in most studies, the success rate of fusion in odontoid Type II fractures displaced less than 6 mm treated with a halo brace is about 80 to 90%. This treatment also avoids an operative procedure and is relatively inexpensive. Apfelbaum's success rate in patients with Type II odontoid fractures treated acutely with an anterior odontoid screw fixation is 94%. He emphasizes that this technique preserves the normal C1-C2 motion and provides immediate stability without an external orthosis.

I will not discuss chronic nonunited odontoid Type II fractures, except to agree that surgical stabilization needs to be done; however, I favor a procedure such as the posterior transfacet screw fixation because it has a success rate of greater than 75%.

CHOOSING BETWEEN TWO TREATMENTS

Table 1 lists the advantages and disadvantages of the two procedures favored by the different authors. Although the application of a halo is thought to be a nonoperative technique, it is nonetheless invasive (having at least 4 pin sites) and has complications much like that of an operative procedure, including infection, hematoma, and loosening of the construct. The screw fixation technique is an invasive procedure with its associated morbidity. Apfelbaum reports having 1 esophageal leak. The success rate appears to be equivocal: 90% vs. 94%. Apfelbaum cites a lower success rate with the halo brace, but several of the papers quoted include chronic fractures and dislocation of larger than 5 to 6 mm, which is not applicable in this case. If successful, both treatment modalities preserve the C1-C2 motion. The transverse ligament must be intact for odontoid screw fixation. The halo brace, however, could be successful in a patient who has a Type II odontoid fracture with a ruptured transverse ligament, if the rupture resulted from a fracture of the tubercle of C2.[1]

By definition, the halo brace is an external orthosis and may be uncomfortable for the patient. After a screw fixation of the odontoid, however, most surgeons place the patient in some sort of orthosis, such as a rigid or soft collar, for several weeks. Initially, the cost of applying the halo is cheaper than the operative procedure of an odontoid screw fixation. However, with the extended and more intensive follow-up needed for patients wearing the halo (e.g., repeated office visits, X-rays, a consequent convalescence period, and work disruption), the costs of the 2 treatment modalities are most likely similar.

A definite advantage of screw fixation is the immediate stability it provides the odontoid. The 2 forehead scars left by the halo pins sometimes indicate that the patient should undergo a cervical approach for screw fixation. Screw fixation leaves a scar in the mid- to lower anterior cervical area that is less conspicuous than those left by the halo brace and, therefore, more desirable to the patient. To carry out anterior screw fixation, special techniques and instrumentation are required and may not be available in every institution.

SUMMARY

To summarize, both techniques are viable options to treat the patient with a nondisplaced odontoid Type II fracture. My preference is to allow the patient to choose the treatment after presenting the advantages and disadvantages of each. Over the past few years, both patients and I have preferred screw fixation because it seems to mobilize the patient more rapidly, allowing him or her to return to work sooner with no disfiguring scars, and without the burden of the halo.

Table 1. Comparison of the Halo Brace and Screw Fixation for Treating Odontoid Type II Nondisplaced Fractures

	Halo	*Screw fixation*
Avoids operative technique	yes/no	no
Success rate	90%	94%
Preserves C1-C2 motion	yes	yes
External orthoses	yes	no/yes
Cost	?	?
Immediate stability	no	yes
Visible external scars	yes	no/yes
Special technique/instruments	no	yes

REFERENCES

Ronald I. Apfelbaum, M.D.

1. Alker GJ, Oh YS, Leslie EV, et al.: Postmortem radiology of head and neck injuries in fatal traffic accidents. *Radiology* 1975; 114: 617–661.
2. Anderson LD, D'Alonzo RT: Fractures of the odontoid process of the axis. *J Bone Joint Surg* 1974; 56A:1663–1674.
3. Apfelbaum RI: Anterior screw fixation of odontoid fractures, in Camins MD, O'Leary PF (eds): *Diseases of the Cervical Spine.* Baltimore, Williams and Wilkins, 1992, pp 603–608.
4. Apfelbaum RI: Anterior screw fixation of odontoid fractures, in Wilkins RH, Rengachary SS (eds): *Neurosurgical Operative Atlas.* Baltimore, Wiliams and Wilkins, 1992, pp 189–199.
5. Apfelbaum RI: Ventral cervical spine fixaton techniques, in Benzel EC (ed): *Spinal Instrumentation.* Park Ridge, American Association of Neurological Surgeons, 1994.
6. Apuzzo ML, Heiden JS, Weiss MH, et al.: Acute fractures of the odontoid process: An analysis of 45 cases. *J Neurosurg* 1978; 48:85–91.
7. Böhler J: Anterior stabilization for acute fractures and non-unions of the dens. *J Bone Joint Surg* 1982; 64A:18–27.
8. Borne GM, Bedou GL, Pinaudeau M, et al.: Odontoid process fracture osteosynthesis with a direct screw fixation technique in nine consecutive cases. *J Neurosurg* 1988; 68:223–226.
9. Brooks AL: Atlanto-axial arthrodesis by the wedge compression method. *J Bone Joint Surg* 1978; 60A:279–283.
10. Chan RC, Schweigel JF, Thompson GB: Halo-thoracic brace immobilization in 188 patients with acute cervical spine injuries. *J Neurosurg* 1983; 58:508–515.
11. Clark CR, White AA: Fractures of the dens: A multicenter study. *J Bone Joint Surg* 1985; 67A:1340–1347.
12. Cooper PR, Maravilla KR, Sklar FH, et al.: Halo immobilization of cervical spine fractures. *J Neurosurg* 1979; 50:603–610.
13. Davis D, Bohlman H, Walker AE, et al.: The pathological findings in fatal craniospinal injuries. *J Neurosurg* 1971; 34:603–613.
14. Dickman CA, Sonntag VKH, Papadopoulos SM, et al.: The interspinous method of posterior atlantoaxial arthrodesis. *J Neurosurg* 1991; 74:190–198.
15. Dunn ME, Seljeskog EL: Experience in the management of odontoid process injuries: An analysis of 128 cases. *Neurosurgery* 1986; 18:306–310.
16. Ekong CE, Schwartz ML, Tator CH, et al.: Odontoid fracture: Management with early mobilization using the halo device. *Neurosurgery* 1981; 9:631–637.
17. Etter C, Coscia M, Jaberg H, et al.: Direct anterior fixation of dens fractures with a cannulated screw system. *Spine* 1991; 16:S25–S32.
18. Fried LC: Atlanto-axial fracture-dislocation: Failure of posterior C1 to C2 fusion. *J Bone Joint Surg* 1973; 55B:490–496.
19. Gallie WE: Fractures and dislocations of the cervical spine. *Am J Surg* 1939; 46:495–499.

20. Geisler FH, Cheng C, Poka A, et al.: Anterior screw fixation of posteriorly displaced type II odontoid fractures. *Neurosurgery* 1989; 25:30–38.

21. Hadley MN, Browner C, Sonntag VK: Axis fractures: A comprehensive review of management and treatment in 107 cases. *Neurosurgery* 1985; 17:281–290.

22. Hentzer L, Schalimtzek M: Fractures and subluxations of the atlas and axis. A follow-up study of 20 patients. *Acta Orthop Scand* 1971; 42:251–258.

23. Jeanneret B, Magerl F, Ward EH, et al.: Posterior stabilization of the cervical spine with hook plates. *Spine* 1991; 16:S56–S63.

24. Lesoin F, Autricque A, Franz K, et al.: Transcervical approach and screw fixation for upper cervical spine pathology. *Surg Neurol* 1987; 27:459–465.

25. Lind B, Nordwall A, Sihlbom H: Odontoid fractures treated with halo-vest. *Spine* 1987; 12:173–177.

26. Maiman DJ, Larson SJ: Management of odontoid fractures. *Neurosurgery* 1982; 11:471–476.

27. Ryan MD, Taylor TKF: Odontoid fractures: A rational approach to treatment. *J Bone Joint Surg* 1982; 64B:416–421.

28. Schatzker J, Rorabeck CH, Waddell JP: Fracture of the dens (odontoid process): An analysis of thirty seven cases. *J Bone Joint Surg* 1971; 53B:392–405.

29. Schiess RJ, DeSaussure RL, Robertson JT: Choice of treatment of odontoid fractures. *J Neurosurg* 1982; 57:496–499.

30. Waddell JP, Reardon GP: Atlantoaxial arthrodesis to treat odontoid fractures. *Can J Surg* 1983; 26:255–258.

31. Wang GJ, Mabie KN, Whitehill R, et al.: The nonsurgical management of odontoid fractures in adults. *Spine* 1984; 9:229–230.

32. White AA, Panjabi MM: Kinematics of the spine, in White A, Panjabi M (eds): *Clinical Biomechanics of the Spine*. Philadelphia, JB Lippincott, 1990, pp 92–97.

Stephen M. Papadopoulos, M.D., Michael Polinsky, M.D.

1. Anderson LD, D'Alonzo RT: Fractures of the odontoid process of the axis. *J Bone Joint Surg* 1974; 56A:1663–1674.

2. Apuzzo ML, Heiden JS, Weiss MH, et al.: Acute fractures of the odontoid process: An analysis of 45 cases. *J Neurosurg* 1978; 48:85–91.

3. Dunn ME, Seljeskog EL: Experience in the management of odontoid process injuries: An analysis of 128 cases. *Neurosurgery* 1986; 18:306–310.

4. Ekong CE, Schwartz ML, Tator CH, et al.: Odontoid fracture: Management with early mobilization using the halo device. *Neurosurgery* 1981; 9:631–637.

5. Hadley MN, Browner C, Sonntag VK: Axis fractures: a comprehensive review of management and treatment in 107 cases. *Neurosurgery* 1985; 17:281–290.

6. Hadley MN, Dickman CA, Browner C, et al.: Acute axis fractures: A review of 229 cases. *J Neurosurg* 1989; 71:642–647.

7. Schatzker J, Rorabeck CH, Waddell JP: Fractures of the dens (odontoid process): An analysis of thirty seven cases. *J Bone Joint Surg* 1971; 53A:392–405.

Volker K.H. Sonntag, M.D.

1. Dickman CA, Mamourian A, Sonntag VK, et al.: Magnetic resonance imaging of the transverse atlantal ligament for the evaluation of atlantoaxial instability. *J Neurosurg* 1991; 75:221–227.

2. Hadley MN, Browner C, Liu SS, et al.: A new subtype of acute odontoid fractures (Type IIA). *Neurosurgery* 1988; 22:67–71.

3. Hadley MN, Dickman CA, Browner C, et al.: Acute axis fractures: A review of 229 cases. *J Neurosurg* 1989; 71:642–647

31

Treatment of Traumatic Instability of the Cervical Spine: The Halo Brace vs. Posterior Stabilization vs. Anterior Stabilization

CASE

A 17-year-old boy was rendered quadriplegic after diving into shallow water. Upon examination, he had posterior cervical tenderness and no other external signs of trauma. He had a complete cord injury with C5 sensory and motor levels. He was in spinal shock and had no rectal tone or perirectal sensation. An X-ray of the cervical spine showed a fracture subluxation of C4 on C5. After the fracture was reduced (Fig. 1), a magnetic resonance image (MRI) showed no significant cord compression by disc, bone, or blood (Fig. 2).

PARTICIPANTS

Use of the Halo Brace for Traumatic Instability of the Cervical Spine–Curtis Dickman, M.D.

Posterior Stabilization for Traumatic Instability of the Cervical Spine–Iain Kalfas, M.D.

Anterior Stabilization for Traumatic Instability of the Cervical Spine–Vincent Traynelis, M.D.

Moderator–Paul R. Cooper, M.D.

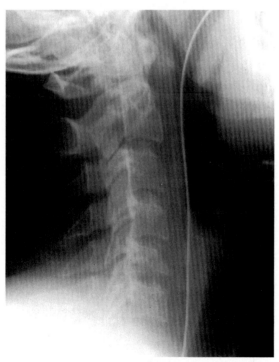

Fig. 1 Cervical spine X-ray following reduction with skeletal traction.

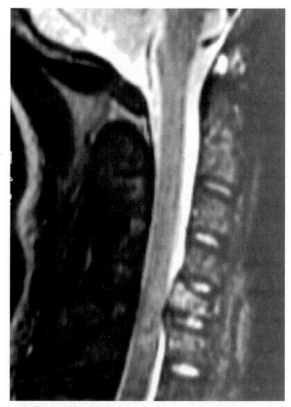

Fig. 2 Sagittal MRI demonstrating a compression fracture of C5 and intramedullary abnormalities.

Use of the Halo Brace for Traumatic Instability of the Cervical Spine

Curtis Dickman, M.D.

This 17-year-old boy had a complete spinal cord injury. The radiographic studies showed a C5 compression fracture, with a 30% loss of the body height of C5. Neither the posterior elements nor the adjacent levels were fractured.

IMMEDIATE TREATMENT

Treatment should consist of hemodynamic and pulmonary resuscitation, evaluation for possible associated injuries, spinal immobilization, and pharmacological agents. If the patient was injured within 8 hours of arriving at the hospital, methylprednisolone should be administered (30 mg/kg intravenous bolus, then 5.4 mg/kg/hr intravenous drip for 24 hours).[1] The patient should then be monitored in the intensive care unit for neurological deterioration, respiratory decompensation, and other complications. Prophylaxis for deep venous thrombosis should be instituted, and the patient's blood pressure should be maintained at the normal preinjury level because ischemia can cause secondary spinal cord injury.[11] Pressor agents should be administered as needed, based on hemodynamic monitoring with a Swan-Ganz catheter.

The major issues to consider for treatment are to maximize the patient's neurological recovery, to immobilize the vertebrae, to obtain satisfactory bone healing, and to minimize the risks and complications of treatment. The patient's remaining neurological function should be preserved by optimizing blood pressure, administering steroids, and immobilizing the spine to prevent repetitive mechanical injury to the spinal cord. Monitoring is needed to detect neurological deterioration. If additional func-

tion is lost, treatable causes (for example, resubluxation or spinal epidural hematoma) should be sought.

USE OF THE HALO BRACE

Rigid external cervical immobilization with a halo brace is our preferred initial treatment modality for a patient with this type of injury. The halo ring can be applied rapidly, and can be used with traction to reduce cervical subluxations and to correct spinal deformities. This patient has no persistent vertebral subluxations or major spinal deformities; therefore, neither further traction nor surgery is needed to realign the vertebrae. The vertebral body height can be fully restored through axial traction, but this is unnecessary because the vertebral body has only mildly collapsed. This patient does not require surgery to decompress the spinal cord. No data exist to prove that decompressing the spinal cord improves function in patients with complete spinal cord injury.

Nonoperative treatment using a halo brace has a very high likelihood of success in this patient and entails only minor risks. The comminuted fractures of the C5 vertebral body will heal satisfactorily if the neck can be properly immobilized. The halo brace provides the most rigid external immobilization available for the cervical spine (Fig. 1).[6,7] If the fractures fail to heal with this modality, then surgery is required. The risks associated with the halo brace can be minimized with meticulous care of the pin sites and proper fitting of the brace.

We prefer the halo brace as a first-line treatment for an injury of this type because it has a proven track record and a low

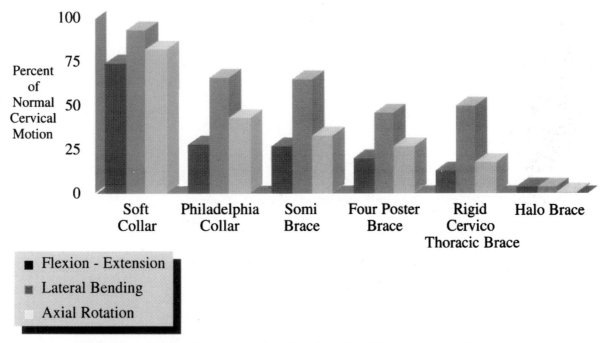

Fig. 1 A comparison of total cervical motion allowed by different cervical orthoses. (Data modified from Wolf JW Jr, Johnson RM: Cervical orthoses, in the Cervical Spine Research Society Editorial Committee (ed): *The Cervical Spine*. Philadelphia, JB Lippincott, 1983, pp 54–61.)

complication rate for fractures of the cervical spine.[4,10] If the halo brace fails to work satisfactorily as the sole treatment, it can be a useful adjunct during and after surgery. If operative intervention becomes necessary, surgery can be performed with the patient fixed in the halo brace. The ring of the halo is affixed to the operating table using an adaptor clamp for the Mayfield fixation device (Fig. 2). Alternatively, the bars of the brace can be supported with stacked traction weights (Fig. 3). The halo brace minimizes the risk of complications during patient positioning and surgery by maintaining immobilization and preventing subluxation. The bars or a portion of the vest may be partially removed to gain access to the neck or iliac crest; however, this is not always necessary. In certain instances, the halo brace may be needed postoperatively to augment an internal fixation. A halo is needed when the bone is osteoporotic, when fixation devices have a weak purchase, or when there are extensive, three-column spinal injuries.

WHEN TO USE SURGERY

Many cervical injuries should be treated surgically. Surgery is an option for patients who object to a halo brace and prefer the risks of surgery to wearing the orthosis. Patients who cannot tolerate a halo orthosis because of multiple skull fractures, bilateral craniotomies, or other problems are also surgical candidates. These are relative indications for internal fixation of spinal injuries that could otherwise be treated satisfactorily with a halo brace.

Surgical stabilization is required when nonoperative therapy has failed or when spontaneous healing is unlikely. Pure ligamentous injuries, such as disruption of the transverse ligament, occipitoatlantal dislocations, or three-column discoligamentous disruptions, cannot heal well enough to restore structural support to the spine. The original strength of spinal ligaments cannot be restored after they are disrupted. Surgery for internal fixation is required for irreducible fractures, fractures that cannot be kept aligned with a rigid cervical orthosis, fractures that have failed to heal (nonunions), or fractures that are at high risk for nonunions.[3,9]

Patients with incomplete neurological injuries with a persistent compressive lesion require surgical decompression, but decompressive surgery can further destabilize the injured spinal column. Internal fixation devices may be required after a decompression is performed and can be used to minimize the need for a postoperative orthosis.

THE BIOMECHANICS OF HALO FIXATION

The halo apparatus has the best immobilization characteristics of any orthosis for the cervical spine. It rigidly fixes the head, harnesses the thorax, and allows no axial rotation, lateral bending, or flexion-extension of the upper cervical spine. However, minimal to moderate motion of the lower cervical spine may occur.[6] The efficacy of a cervical orthosis depends on the rigidity of fixation at the distal ends of the cervical spine (that is, the skull and thorax). Casts and vests have been used to fix the thorax and to attach bars to a halo ring. The vest is preferred because it is lightweight and removable.

The halo brace does not completely eliminate all cervical motion. The fixation of the halo is most effective at the distal ends of the spine, between the occiput and C1-C2, and at the cervicothoracic junction. Motion between the atlas and axis is poorly restricted by most cervical orthoses other than the halo brace. The halo is less effective in fixing the middle cervical segments than the distal segments. A "snaking" effect of the cervical spine can occur, despite the halo brace. (If a snake is picked up and held by its head and its tail, undulating motion can still occur in the body of the snake.)

Complications of the Halo Brace

Most complications resulting from the halo brace are minor. In a retrospective review of 179 patients treated with halo immobilization,[5] complications included pin loosening (36%), minor infections at the pin site (20%), pressure sores from the vest (11%), or nerve injury (2%). Cosmetically disfiguring scars occurred in 9% of patients, and some cannot tolerate the confinement of the vest. Serious complications of the halo brace are

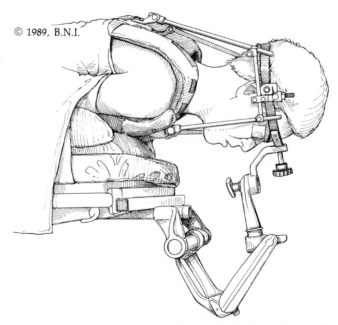

© 1989, B.N.I.

Fig. 2 An adaptor can be screwed onto the halo ring to fix the patient to the Mayfield device and to secure the patient to the operating table.

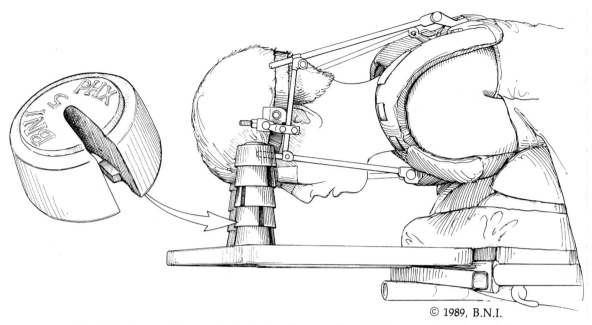

© 1989, B.N.I.

Fig. 3 Traction weights can be stacked on the operating table to support the bars of the halo brace during surgery.

rare. The pins can penetrate the dura if the skull is weak, eroded, or infected. In patients with severe pulmonary disease, the halo apparatus may restrict thoracic excursion and exacerbate respiratory insufficiency.

Infections of the pin sites, cranial osteomyelitis, and intracranial penetration can be avoided through meticulous cleaning of the pin sites with a diluted peroxide and betadine solution. The pin sites should be closely monitored. Late pin loosening is a sign of infection. If the pin sites become infected, the pins should be changed to a new hole. Local debridement and antibiotics are used as indicated. Decubiti are prevented through proper fitting of the vest and frequent skin care. Pulmonary complications can be minimized using an aggressive pulmonary treatment program. The vest can modestly restrict thoracic excursion; however, the brace facilitates early mobilization of patients and allows pulmonary postural physiotherapy, which improve the patient's respiratory status.[2,8]

The halo brace may fail to immobilize some cervical spine fractures adequately. Patients may experience loss of reduction or develop nonunions. A high failure rate may occur in patients with widely displaced comminuted fractures, three-column bone destruction, or hyperflexion injuries that have complete ligament disruptions. For many patients with cervical fractures, the halo vest protects from neurological injury and may obviate the need for surgical intervention.

SUMMARY

A success rate of 85 to 90% can be expected in treating appropriately selected patients with cervical spine fractures with halo immobilization. The halo provides biomechanically superior immobilization of the spine compared to other available orthoses. However, it does not eliminate all cervical motion. Complications can be minimized by meticulous pin care, proper vest fitting, and close follow-up monitoring. The halo brace is extremely effective for a large percentage of cervical fractures. Surgery is necessary for patients with pure ligament injuries without fractures, fractures with significant displacement, irreducible injuries, recurrent subluxations, three-column spine fractures, or incomplete neural injuries that require decompression.

Posterior Stabilization for Traumatic Instability of the Cervical Spine

Iain Kalfas, M.D.

This patient has a fracture of the C5 vertebral body. The lateral radiograph shows the fracture with anterior compression of the vertebra and loss of the normal lordotic curve of the cervical spine. The anterior collapse of the C5 vertebra is less than 50%, and there is no appreciable subluxation. I do not see any separation of the spinous processes of C5 and C6. If present, this finding would imply disruption of the posterior ligamentous complex. The absence of this finding on a single lateral spine film, however, does not eliminate the possibility of a posterior ligamentous injury with resultant spinal instability.[19] The magnetic resonance image (MRI), in addition to demonstrating the fracture of the C5 vertebral body, shows some encroachment on the ventral epidural space secondary to posterior displacement of the C5 vertebra and the C5-C6 disc. Although the subarachnoid space is effaced, the spinal cord is not significantly compressed.

This fracture resulted from combined hyperflexion and axial loading of the cervical spine. It has the appearance of a typical flexion compression injury rather than a compression burst injury. A burst injury results primarily from vertical compressive forces that produce a comminuted fracture of the vertebral body with retropulsion of bone fragments into the spinal canal. Posterior element fractures also commonly occur with burst injuries.[2] Although the bone and disc are displaced at the level of the injury, the findings in this patient are not typical of a burst injury.

Specifically, this injury is more consistent with a flexion-compression teardrop fracture of the C5 vertebral body. These fractures present with an oblique fracture line that extends across the anterior-inferior body of the involved vertebrae, producing a triangular or quadrilateral fracture fragment. The fragment is generally displaced anteriorly with the remaining vertebral body displaced posteriorly. The involved vertebrae are compressed, with narrowing of the intervertebral disc and a kyphotic deformity of the cervical spine. These fractures are frequently associated with disruption of the intervertebral disc and the supporting ligamentous structures. When this occurs, the injured segment is unstable and the likelihood of severe neurological injury is high.[15]

STABILIZING THE SPINE

The goals of treating the injured cervical spine are to prevent or minimize neurological deficit subsequent to the injury and to provide an optimal environment for the neural elements to maximally recover from any damage sustained. A stable, healed cervical spine is essential to achieving these goals. This involves not only the recognition and treatment of cord and root compression, but also spinal instability.

White and Panjabi[20] defined stability of the spine as the ability of the involved motion segment to withstand normal physiological loads, so that there is neither progressive displacement or deformity nor progressive compression or injury to the neural elements. These authors suggested that the cervical spine was instable if one vertebra was horizontally displaced more than 3.5 mm on the adjacent vertebra or more than 11 degrees of angulation occurred between adjacent vertebrae.[20] Although these figures offer reasonable guidelines to determine whether the spine was instable, values of less displacement or angulation on a lateral cervical spine film do not assure clinical stability.

Injury to the supporting ligamentous complex of the cervical spine frequently destabilizes the spine. Severe ligamentous disruption without bony injury can occur, and may not be evident on plain radiographs. Even dynamic flexion-extension films done in the acute period may fail to show instability resulting from ligamentous injury because of the reflex protective contractures and spasms of the cervical musculature.[19] Therefore, it is imperative to treat the acute cervical spine injury as if it is unstable, until the acute response to trauma has subsided and follow-up dynamic studies show stability.

Initial Treatment

My initial treatment is to place this patient in skeletal traction to reduce the flexion deformity at the C5 level and to optimally reconstitute the spinal canal. In individuals with a normal neurological exam or an incomplete injury, however, I would obtain an MRI or cervical myelogram before proceeding with skeletal traction and realignment to assess the presence or absence of ventral cord compression. Although uncommon, further extrusion of a traumatic herniated disc with the subsequent development or worsening of a neurological deficit has been reported after attempts at closed reduction of injured spinal segments.[3,4] Because this patient has a complete cord injury, an MRI or

myelogram before instituting skeletal traction would not be absolutely necessary.

OPTIONS FOR EXTENDED TREATMENT

After this patient's spine is adequately realigned, three reasonable treatment options exist: (1) halo immobilization alone for 10 to 12 weeks, (2) anterior decompression and cervical plate instrumentation (with or without concomitant posterior stabilization), and (3) posterior stabilization alone.

Halo Immobilization

An argument can be made for the sole use of halo immobilization to treat this patient. Halo immobilization would immediately stabilize the cervical spine to facilitate early mobilization and rehabilitation of the patient, as well as healing of the fractured vertebrae. However, the type of injury sustained by this patient is commonly associated with significant disruption of the supporting ligamentous structures. Although external immobilization of the cervical spine can frequently promote the satisfactory healing of bony injuries, it is less likely to result in the sufficient repair of significant ligamentous damage.[10,21] About 10 to 15% of patients with flexion compression injuries treated with halo immobilization alone develop evidence of delayed instability after treatment. This instability results from the incomplete repair of significant ligamentous disruption.[7,12]

Halo immobilization is also associated with a number of potential complications. These include infection at the pin sites with the potential for skull osteomyelitis, skin breakdown at pressure points of the vest, respiratory insufficiency in patients with significant pulmonary disease, and unsatisfactory stabilization of injured spinal motion segments. Frail or elderly patients may be unable to support the extra weight of the halo vest and some patients may manipulate themselves out of proper position.[10,11,13]

Anterior Stabilization

Anterior decompression and stabilization with a cervical spine plate is even less of an option in this individual. Although the C5 and C6 discs and a portion of the posterior C5 vertebral body encroach on the ventral canal, there is no significant degree of cord compression to warrant an anterior procedure. The patient has suffered a complete cord injury and the correction of the marginal radiographic abnormality immediately anterior to the cord is unlikely to improve his neurological status. Furthermore, an anterior cervical decompression and fusion require resection of the anterior longitudinal ligament, which may often be the only ligamentous structure remaining intact after a severe flexion-compression injury.[1] Its removal before anterior decompression and placement of a bone graft further compromises cervical stability in the short term. Because bone grafting has no immediate effect on stability, there is a significant potential for recurrent angulation, dislocation, and bone graft displacement. An anterior procedure can, therefore, increase the need for a second posterior procedure for further stabilization.[16]

Anterior plate instrumentation has been a recent and significant addition to the treatment of cervical spine disorders. The plate immediately immobilizes the spine internally, prevents graft dislodgement, and facilitates bony fusion.[6] In flexion injuries to the cervical spine, however, several studies have concluded that anterior cervical plating is biomechanically inferior to posterior stabilization alone.[8,18] If this patient is treated using anterior decompression and plate instrumentation, I would also stabilize the posterior elements.

Posterior Stabilization

My preferred approach to this particular patient is a posterior stabilization procedure. The posterior approach provides a safe, simple, and effective means of stabilizing this patient's spine without the need for a more complex anterior procedure or the potential for delayed instability after a period of extended immobilization. Posterior procedures are tolerated well by most patients and are associated with fewer complications than the anterior approach to the cervical spine.[5,17]

The options for posterior stabilization of the cervical spine include a variety of wire and onlay graft techniques, the interlaminar clamp, and lateral mass plate fixation. I prefer to use the lateral mass plate because it is relatively safe, technically easy to place, and provides immediate stability without the requirement of an autogenous iliac crest bone graft. Furthermore, it does not require the patient to be immobilized postoperatively in a halo vest, as is frequently the case with wire and graft techniques.

The lateral mass plate technique for stabilizing the cervical spine was first described by Roy-Camille and colleagues in 1979.[14] Although this technique has been used in Europe for several years, it has only recently gained acceptance in North America. Early results of lateral mass plate fixation have been favorable.[9]

The procedure uses the standard exposure of the injured segment of the cervical spine. Holes are drilled bilaterally into the center of the lateral masses. The holes are angled 20 degrees laterally to avoid the vertebral arteries and exiting nerve root. Angling the holes 20 degrees in a rostral direction provides the inserted screw with maximal bony purchase. Plates of the appropriate length are then secured to the lateral masses with screws 16 mm long and 3.5 mm in diameter. After the procedure, patients are placed into a hard cervical collar for 8 to 12 weeks.

CONCLUSION

Although several options exist for treating this patient, I feel that a posterior stabilization procedure is best because it provides satisfactory fixation of the injured spinal segment and facilitates the early immobilization and rehabilitation of this patient.

Anterior Stabilization for Traumatic Instability of the Cervical Spine

Vincent Traynelis, M.D.

This case involves a relatively young individual rendered quadriplegic from a midcervical spinal injury. The initial lateral cervical spine radiograph shows a teardrop fracture of C5 with a small amount of retrolisthesis of C5 on C6. There is no significant interspinous widening and the overall alignment is quite good. Only the top of C7 is seen on this film, and I assume the patient was fully evaluated with lateral X-rays extending to the C7-T1 interspace, as well as with anteroposterior, oblique, and open-mouth views of the odontoid. Initially, this patient's respiratory status and blood pressure should be fully assessed and, if the patient arrived in appropriate time, methylprednisolone should be administered.[2] The patient should be evaluated for other injuries. Despite the presence of fairly normal alignment, I agree with the judicious application of traction. The patient must be closely monitored clinically and radiographically while traction is instituted.

The severity of this injury mandates further radiographic evaluation which, I believe, is best accomplished with magnetic resonance imaging. The sagittal T2-weighted image reveals posterior disc injuries at C4-C5 and, more noticeably, at C5-C6. Mild retropulsion of the fractured C5 body obliterates the anterior subarachnoid space. Increased signal intensity is suggested in the C5-C6 interspinous space. Abnormal signal, centered at the C5-C6 level, is present within the cord.

STABILIZING THE SPINE

After any patient with a spinal injury is clinically and radiographically evaluated, the treating physician must decide whether that patient's spine is stable or unstable. As is apparent on the radiograms, this patient has significantly damaged anterior and middle spinal columns. The integrity of the posterior column has probably also been compromised. Knowledge of these structural injuries, coupled with the clinical findings of complete

cord dysfunction, indicate the existence of a highly unstable injury.

Treatment will be successful only if it immediately stabilizes the spine, is associated with a high fusion rate, and carries minimal risk of complications.

The Halo Brace

The halo orthosis provides excellent immobilization of the upper cervical spine; however, it is less effective in the midcervical region, with reported failure rates as high as 23%.[3] Flexion injuries are particularly difficult to treat successfully with a halo.[10] Additionally, halo fixation has been associated with the following complications: loss of reduction, pin site infections, pin perforation of the skull, displacement of anterior strut grafts, and skin breakdown.[7,10] Finally, in some individuals, the halo orthosis hinders physical therapy and rehabilitation of the chest area. Based on these reasons, I do not believe that a halo orthosis is the optimal treatment for this patient.

Posterior Stabilization

The need for external immobilization can be decreased or eliminated by internal fixation. This patient does not require an operation to realign the spine, and the spinal cord itself does not require decompression. The nerve roots exiting at the level of injury may be compressed, however, and, if so, decompression may increase neurological function by one level. Despite this theoretical hope for improvement, the only real goal of a surgical procedure would be to internally stabilize the spine.

This spinal injury could be stabilized through a posterior approach. Although the posterior surgical options include wiring of the spinous processes, lamina, or facets, only plating of the lateral mass would provide immediate stability. Such fixation would reconstitute the posterior tension band which, I suspect, has been compromised. The anterior and middle columns, however, could not be adequately reconstructed through a posterior exposure. Failure to reconstruct these columns may increase the risk of delayed kyphosis. Lateral mass stabilization of this injury would require plating, at least, from C4 to C6 and, in addition, many surgeons would recommend that patients with such highly unstable injuries be immobilized postoperatively in a cervicothoracic brace, minerva jacket, or halo vest.[11] The risk of delayed kyphosis and the potential need for rigid postoperative immobilization make plating of the lateral mass an unattractive option for this patient.

ANTERIOR STABILIZATION

Anterior fusions have been employed in the treatment of trauma for more than 30 years.[5] In this patient, an anterior approach would allow one to decompress the anterior subarachnoid space and provide optimal exposure to explore and, if necessary, decompress the neural foramina of C4-C5 and C5-C6. Furthermore, an anterior approach enables the surgeon to directly reconstruct the anterior and middle columns with a tricortical strut graft.

This injury will remain unstable until fusion occurs. Therefore, after an anterior corpectomy and strut grafting, the patient's cervical spine must be either immobilized in a halo brace or internally stabilized.[13] I favor internal stabilization from C4 to C6 with an anterior plate, followed by 3 months of immobilization with a Philadelphia collar.

Anterior cervical plating has been shown to provide excellent biomechanical stability in an injury almost identical to that described in this chapter.[12] In one study, we used cadaveric spines to create a C5 teardrop fracture and disrupt the posterior ligaments, to compare the immediate biomechanical stability of anterior cervical plating from C4 to C6 to the stability provided by a posterior wiring construct over the same levels. In this model, anterior plating provided significantly more stability in extension and lateral bending than did posterior wiring.[12] The plate resisted flexion more than the posterior construct; however, the difference was not statistically significant.

As would be expected from the biomechanical data, treatment with anterior plate fixation has been clinically effective even when multiple columns or the posterior ligaments are damaged.[1,4,6,8,9,11] The fusion rate after anterior plate fixation is 99%.[11] Although some patients have been rapidly mobilized after the placement of an anterior cervical plate without an external orthosis, most surgeons recommend using a rigid collar for several months.[11]

Complications

The complications of anterior corpectomy and plate stabilization have been recently reviewed.[11] The risks of this procedure are essentially the same as one would expect from any anterior cervical surgery. The major hardware complication is screw loosening, which is usually the result of a technical error in screw placement. Meticulous technique and attention to detail minimizes this complication.

Timing of Treatment

Although difficult to prove, I believe early stabilization facilitates patient care. Therefore, patients should be operated on as soon as they are medically stable. The relative hypotension that accompanies severe spinal cord injuries should be treated through intravenous volume expansion before surgery. When there is only a single injury, as in this patient, surgery is usually performed within 24 to 48 hours after admission as part of the normal operating schedule. Except in the rare situation of an increasing neurological deficit, I do not advocate doing these procedures as emergencies.

Anterior Plating Systems

Several different plating systems are available for use in anterior procedures. Each system has relative advantages and disadvantages and, at the present time, no one system is clearly superior. What is extremely important, however, is that the surgeon is completely familiar with the particular system he or she chooses to implant.

CONCLUSION

In conclusion, I believe that anterior reconstruction and stabilization is the most appropriate treatment for this patient. After corpectomy and strut grafting, placing an anterior plate provides immediate stability. The failure rate of anterior plate fixation is extremely low and, when implanted correctly, the risk of complication is minimal.

Treatment of Traumatic Instability of the Cervical Spine: The Halo Brace vs. Posterior Stabilization vs. Anterior Stabilization

Paul R. Cooper, M.D.

Two issues are prominent in the treatment of the patient described above. Is surgery indicated? If operative treatment is chosen, what is the best technique for stabilizing the injury in this patient?

INCOMPLETE INFORMATION

This case highlights the hazards of formulating a therapeutic plan based on incomplete information. The single lateral plain film was taken after the injury was reduced. Although a teardrop fracture is apparent, we have no knowledge of the severity or nature of this patient's spinal deformity at the time of presentation. In addition, a computed tomogram of the area of injury has not been provided, leaving us in the dark about the extent of the bony injury. A single T2-weighted MRI in the sagittal plane is shown. The subarachnoid space is obliterated at the level of the patient's injury secondary to retropulsion of bone into the spinal canal. It is well known that T2-weighted images tend to exaggerate the severity of spinal cord compression. Based on this single image, however, there is probable compression of the spinal cord by retropulsed bone. Axial images would help to assess more accurately the degree of neural compression. However, knowledge of the presence and extent of spinal cord compression in this patient is not essential. Because the patient has no neurological function below the level of his injury, anterior surgery to decompress the spinal cord is unlikely to improve neurological function, and is not indicated.

SPINAL STABILITY

The only consideration, then, is choosing the treatment modality that offers the greatest chance of producing short- and long-term stability with the least risk of exacerbating pre-existing neurological deficits or producing other complications. The proponents of each of the 3 therapeutic options give carefully considered and well thought-out reasons for choosing their treatment strategies. There is no right or wrong answer to the proper treatment of this patient. At one time or another, I have treated similar injuries with 1 of the therapeutic options advocated by each of these authors. None of the methods is successful 100% of the time, and each is associated with complications.

The Halo Brace

The development of the halo brace nearly 30 years ago represented a major advance in the nonoperative treatment of cervical spinal fractures. Internal fixation, with the exception of posterior wiring, was unknown; the use of the halo brace enabled patients with unstable spines to be mobilized or treated in the upright position. Rehabilitation was improved, and the complications of bed rest were obviated.

Internal Fixation

The advent of effective means of internal fixation (anterior and posterior cervical plates) in the past 10 years has resulted in the less frequent use of the halo brace. The brace is awkward and impedes rehabilitation in patients with severe neurological deficit. Failure of instrumentation is always a possibility, but if the patients selected for internal fixation are properly chosen, the

risks of surgery will be quite low in experienced hands. Although the halo brace is successful in most patients, a certain number lose reduction while wearing the device, others still have unstable spines after wearing it for several months, and yet others develop chronic progressive deformities or instability.[2] It is not possible to state with any degree of certainty if the fracture sustained by the patient in question can be successfully treated with a halo brace because the patient's prereduction films are not shown and a computed tomogram to define the extent of posterior column injury has not been provided.

CONCLUSION

I would treat this patient through internal fixation, and a convincing case can be made for either anterior or posterior instrumentation. Anterior instrumentation alone would successfully maintain alignment until fusion took place. Anterior decompression and placement of a bone graft has the advantage of reconstructing the anterior and middle columns and, theoretically, may be superior to posterior fixation in preventing late kyphotic deformity. In practice, however, posterior instrumentation with the placement of bilateral lateral mass plates is also effective in stabilizing injuries in patients such as the one described. In my experience, the risk of kyphotic deformity with posterior instrumentation of such injuries is small, instrumentation failure is low, bone grafting is not needed, and the only postoperative orthosis required is a Philadelphia collar.[1] Posterior instrumentation is simpler and quicker and less technically demanding than a vertebrectomy, harvesting and placing a bone graft, and applying an anterior plate. I would, therefore, treat this patient with posterior cervical plating. In all honesty, however, I must admit that I have also treated patients with injuries similar to this one successfully with anterior cervical plating.

REFERENCES

Curtis Dickman, M.D.

1. Bracken MB, Shepard MJ, Collins WF, et al.: A randomized, controlled trial of methylprednisolone or naloxone in the treatment of acute spinal-cord injury: Results of the Second National Acute Spinal-Cord Injury Study. *N Engl J Med* 1990; 322:1405–1411.
2. Browner CM, Duistermars PJ: Preventing pulmonary compromise in the acute spinal cord-injured patient. *BNI Q* 1989; 5:35–39.
3. Chan RC, Schweigel JF, Thompson GB: Halo-thoracic brace immobilization in 188 patients with acute cervical spine injuries. *J Neurosurg* 1983; 58:508–515.
4. Cooper PR, Maravilla KR, Sklar FH, et al.: Halo immobilization of cervical spine fractures: Indications and results. *J Neurosurg* 1979; 50:603–610.
5. Garfin SR, Botte MJ, Waters RL, et al.: Complications in the use of the halo fixation device. *J Bone Joint Surg* 1986; 68A:320–325.
6. Johnson RM, Hart DL, Simmons EF, et al.: Cervical orthoses: A study comparing their effectiveness in restricting cervical motion in normal subjects. *J Bone Joint Surg* 1977; 59A:332–339.
7. Koch RA, Nickel VL: The halo vest: An evaluation of motion and forces across the neck. *Spine* 1978; 3:103–107.
8. Lind B, Bake B, Lundqvist C, et al.: Influence of halo vest treatment on vital capacity. *Spine* 1987; 12:449–452.
9. Panjabi MM, Thibodeau LL, Crisco JJ III, et al.: What constitutes spinal instability. *Clin Neurosurg* 1986; 34:313–339.
10. Sears W, Fazl M: Prediction of stability of cervical spine fracture managed in the halo vest and indications for surgical intervention. *J Neurosurg* 1990; 72:426–432.
11. Tator CH, Fehlings MG: Review of the secondary injury theory of acute spinal cord trauma with emphasis on vascular mechanisms. *J Neurosurg* 1991; 75:15–26.

Iain Kalfas, M.D.

1. Allen BL Jr, Ferguson RL, Lehmann TR, et al.: A mechanistic classification of closed, indirect fractures and dislocations of the lower cervical spine. *Spine* 1982; 7:1–27.
2. Atlas SW, Regenbogen V, Rogers LF, et al.: The radiographic characterization of burst fractures of the spine. *AJR* 1986; 147:575–582.
3. Bohlman HH: Complications of treatment of fractures and disloca-tions of the cervical spine, in Epps C (ed): *Complications of Orthopedic Surgery*. Philadelphia, JB Lippincott, 1985, pp 897–918.
4. Bolesta MJ, Bohlman HH: Late complications of cervical fractures and dislocations and their surgical treatment, in Frymoyer J (ed): *The Adult Spine—Principles of Practice*. New York, Raven Press, 1991, pp 1107–1126.
5. Capen DA, Garland DE, Waters RL: Surgical stabilization of the

cervical spine: A comparative analysis of anterior and posterior spine fusions. *Clin Orthop* 1985; 196:229–237.

6. Caspar W: Anterior cervical fusion and interbody stabilization with the trapezial osteosynthetic plate technique. *Aesculap Sci Info* 1985; 12:1–36.

7. Chan RC, Schweigel JF, Thompson GB: Halo-thoracic brace immobilization in 188 patients with acute cervical spine injuries. *J Neurosurg* 1983; 58:508–515.

8. Coe JD, Wharton KE, Sutterlin CE, et al.: Biomechanical evaluation of cervical spinal stabilization methods in a human cadaveric model. *Spine* 1989; 14:1122–1131.

9. Cooper PR, Cohen A, Rosiello A, et al.: Posterior stabilization of cervical spine fractures and subluxations using plates and screws. *Neurosurgery* 1988; 23:300–306.

10. Cooper PR, Maravilla KR, Sklar FH, et al.: Halo immobilization of cervical spine fractures. *J Neurosurg* 1979; 50:603–610.

11. Garfin SR, Botte MJ, Waters RL, et al.: Complications in the use of the halo fixation device. *J Bone Joint Surg* 1986; 68A:320–325.

12. Glaser JA, Whitehill R, Stamp WG, et al.: Complications associated with the halo vest: A review of 245 cases. *J Neurosurg* 1986; 65: 762–769.

13. Lind B, Sihlbom H, Nordwall A: Halo vest treatment of unstable traumatic cervical spine injuries. *Spine* 1988; 13:425–432.

14. Roy-Camille R, Saillant G, Berteaux D, et al.: Early management of spinal injuries, in McKibbin B (ed): *Recent Advances in Orthopedics*. Edinburgh, Churchill Livingstone, 1979.

15. Schneider RC, Kahn EA: Chronic neurological sequelae of acute trauma to the spine and spinal cord: Part 1. The significance of the the acute flexion or "teardrop" fracture-dislocation of the cervical spine. *J Bone Joint Surg* 1956; 38A:985–997.

16. Stauffer ES: Surgical stabilization of the cervical spine after trauma. *Arch Surg* 1976; 111:652–657.

17. Stauffer ES, Kelly EG: Fracture-dislocations of the cervical spine: Instability and recurrent deformity following treatment by anterior interbody fusion. *J Bone Joint Surg* 1977; 59A:45–48.

18. Sutterlin CE, McAfee PC, Warden KE, et al.: A biomechanical evaluation of cervical spinal stabilization methods in a bovine model. Static and cyclical loading. *Spine* 1988; 13:795–802.

19. Sypert GW: Management of lower cervical spinal instability, in Wilkins RH, Rengachary SS (eds): *Neurosurgery Update II*. New York, McGraw-Hill, 1991, pp 234–244.

20. White AA, Panjabi MM: *Clinical Biomechanics of the Spine*. Philadelphia, JB Lippincott, 1978.

21. Whitehill R, Richman JA, Glaser JA: Failure of immobilization of the cervical spine by the halo vest. *J Bone Joint Surg* 1986; 68A: 326–332.

Vincent Traynelis, M.D.

1. Aebi M, Zuber K, Marchesi D: Treatment of cervical spine injuries with anterior plating: Indications, techniques, and results. *Spine* 1991; 16:S38–S45.

2. Bracken MB, Shepard MJ, Collins WF, et al.: A randomized, controlled trial of methylprednisolone or naloxone in the treatment of acute spinal-cord injury: Results of the second national acute spinal-cord injury study. *N Engl J Med* 1990; 322:1405–1411.

3. Bucholz RD, Cheung KC: Halo vest versus spinal fusion for cervical injury: Evidence from an outcome study. *J Neurosurg* 1989; 70:884–892.

4. Caspar W, Barbier DD, Klara PM: Anterior cervical fusion and Caspar plate stabilization for cervical trauma. *Neurosurgery* 1989; 25:491–502.

5. Cloward RB: Treatment of acute fractures and fracture dislocations of the cervical spine by vertebral-body fusion. *J Neurosurg* 1961; 18:201–209.

6. De Oliveira JC: Anterior plate fixation of traumatic lesions of the lower cervical spine. *Spine* 1987; 12:324–329.

7. Glaser JA, Whitehill R, Stamp WG, et al.: Complications associated with the halo vest: A review of 245 cases. *J Neurosurg* 1986; 65: 762–769.

8. Randle MJ, Wolf A, Lion L, et al.: The use of anterior Caspar plate fixation in acute cervical spine injury. *Neurology* 1991; 36:181–189.

9. Ripa DR, Kowall MG, Meyer PR Jr, et al.: Series of ninety-two traumatic cervical spine injuries stabilized with anterior ASIF plate fusion technique. *Spine* 1991; 16:S46–S55.

10. Rockswold GL, Bergman TA, Ford SE: Halo immobilization and surgical fusion: Relative indications and effectiveness in the treatment of 140 cervical spine injuries. *J Trauma* 1990; 30:893–898.

11. Traynelis VC: Anterior and posterior plate stabilization of the cervical spine. *Neurosurg Q* 1992; 2:59–76.

12. Traynelis VC, Donaher PA, Roach RM, et al.: Biomechanical comparison of anterior Caspar plate and three-level posterior fixation techniques in a human cadaveric model. *J Neurosurg* 1993; 79: 96–103.

13. Van Peteghem PK, Schweigel JF: The fractured cervical spine rendered unstable by anterior cervical fusion. *J Trauma* 1979; 19:110–114.

Paul R. Cooper, M.D.

1. Cooper PR, Cohen A, Rosiello A, et al.: Posterior stabilization of cervical spine fractures and subluxations using plates and screws. *Neurosurgery* 1988; 23:300–306.

2. Cooper PR, Maravilla KR, Sklar FH, et al.: Halo immobilization of cervical spine fractures: Indications and results. *J Neurosurg* 1979; 50:603–610.

32

Treatment of Thoracolumbar Burst Fractures

CASE

Immediately after an accident in a recreational vehicle, a 16-year-old boy had severe back pain and numbness and weakness in his legs. In the emergency room, his sensory examination revealed partial deficits to pain and soft touch below the inguinal ligament. He could overcome gravity, but could not resist additional force with all muscles of his legs. Rectal sensation was absent and the patient had no tone or voluntary contraction of the anal sphincter. All deep tendon reflexes were absent in his legs.

PARTICIPANTS

Distraction and Posterior Fixation Alone for a Thoracolumbar Burst Fracture– Robert McGuire, M.D.

*Lateral Extracavitary Decompression and Posterior Instrumentation for a Thoracolumbar Burst Fracture–*Richard G. Fessler, M.D., Ph.D.

Anterior Decompression and Instrumentation for a Thoracolumbar Burst Fracture– John D. Schlegel, M.D.

*Moderator–*Carole A. Miller, M.D.

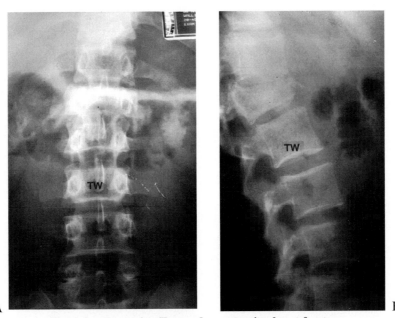

Fig. 1 Lumbar spine X-rays demonstrating burst fracture of L1: (*A*) AP view. (*B*) Lateral.

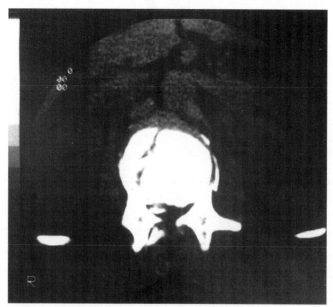

Fig. 2 Axial computed tomography image at L1.

Distraction and Posterior Fixation Alone for a Thoracolumbar Burst Fracture

Robert McGuire, M.D.

This is a case of a patient who sustained a burst fracture at the thoracolumbar junction with an incomplete neurological deficit. The computed tomogram shows canal compromise of greater than 50%. The surgical goals in the treatment of this patient are to realign and stabilize the spine and to decompress the spinal canal and neural elements.

MECHANISM OF BURST FRACTURE

To decide the best method to achieve the surgical goals, one must understand the mechanism by which the fracture occurs. Denis[2] has noted that spinal stability is provided by a "three-column model," with the anterior column consisting of the anterior two thirds of the vertebral body, the anterior two thirds of the disc complex, and the anterior longitudinal ligament. The middle column consists of the posterior one third of the vertebral body, the posterior one third of the disc complex, and the posterior longitudinal ligament. The posterior column consists of the posterior arch, the facets, and the posterior ligamentous structures. As is seen in this patient, all 3 columns of the spine have been compromised, leading to an unstable mechanical configuration.

The biomechanical forces acting upon the spine to precipitate this fracture pattern include compression or axial loading combined with a flexion moment, as described by Ferguson and Allen.[5] To stabilize the spine, these forces must be negated. A construct that provides a distraction force, combined with an anteriorly directed moment to reverse the kyphotic component, must be used.

APPROPRIATE CONSTRUCTS

Another consideration in the selection of a construct must be the maintenance of as many mobile segments as possible below the construct, to allow for natural lumbar lordosis and motion and keep the thoracolumbar junction from becoming kyphotic.

Short-segment constructs consisting of a rod, sleeve and hook, pedicle screw and rods, or pedicle screw and plates provide a method to realign and stabilize the spine, maintain vertical height, and prevent kyphosis. This technique works by applying an anteriorly directed force with a sleeve or plate directly upon the pedicle of the fractured vertebrae to reverse the kyphosis, and then supplying a distraction moment by means of a ratcheted rod or threaded distracter through the pedicle screw or hook to allow ligament ataxis to realign the spine and, indirectly, clear the canal.[3]

DECOMPRESSION

The second important consideration in this patient is canal clearance and decompression of neural elements. Bradford and

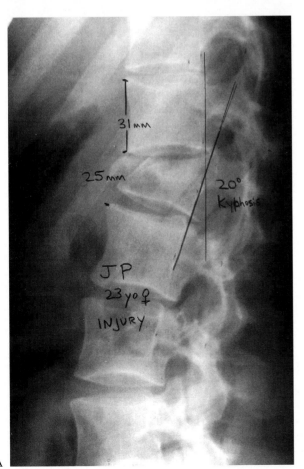

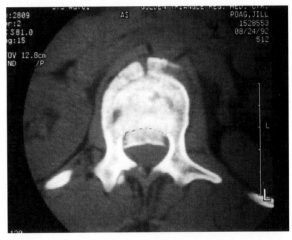

Fig. 1 (*A*) **This lateral radiograph reveals an L1 burst fracture with 20 degrees of kyphosis and three column instability. (*B*) This preoperative computed tomogram reveals the canal compromise to be 50%.**

McBride[1] have shown a significant neurological improvement if canal compromise can be improved to 25% or less. Gertzbein and associates[6] found no significant difference in improvement of neurological function in patients with an incomplete neurological deficit treated with a posterior distraction construct from those treated with an anterior decompression and fusion, as long as the canal was cleared. Edwards and colleagues[4] found that, as healing occurs, significant remodeling of bone occurs, clearing the canal.

My experience over the past 5 years with a posterior distraction construct and an antikyphosis moment to indirectly decompress the canal shows 36 fractures of the thoracolumbar junction. Canal compromise averaged 48% preoperatively and 15% postoperatively.

REPRESENTATIVE CASES

A representative example of short-segment, indirect decompression is revealed in the following cases.

Case 1

A 23-year-old woman sustained a burst fracture of L1 after a fall from a horse. She had a normal neurological motor examination,

but had a 200-ml postvoid urine residual. Her preoperative radiographs reveal a 20-degree kyphosis and 50% canal compromise (Fig. 1). She was taken to the operating room, where she underwent a posterior approach with indirect canal decompression with a distraction construct, with stabilization and fusion through a short construct with pedicle screws and plates. Postoperatively, her vertebral height was restored and the kyphosis corrected, Figure 2 (**A**). A postoperative computed tomogram showed the canal impingement to be 15%, Figure 2 (**B**). The patient maintained a normal motor and sensory status after the procedure, and she completely recovered her bladder function.

Case 2

A 26-year-old man sustained an L1 burst fracture, Figure 3 (**A**), while sport parachuting. He presented with an incomplete neurological deficit consisting of a neurogenic bladder, absent rectal tone, and voluntary sphincter contraction, and significant weakness of his quadriceps, anterior tibialis, extensor hallucis longus, and gastroc soleus complex bilaterally. A computed tomogram showed significant canal compromise from retropulsion of the posterior aspect of the vertebral body into the canal, Figure 3 (**B**).

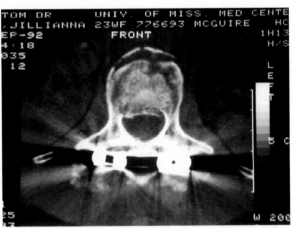

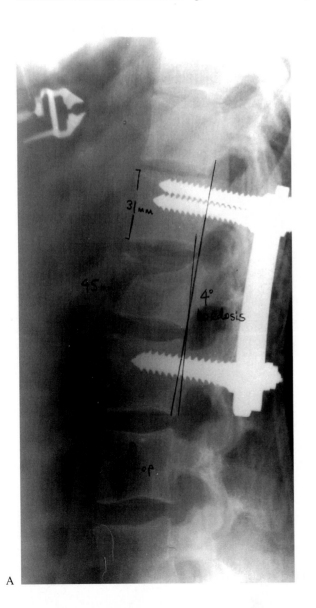

A

Fig. 2 (*A*) **This postoperative radiograph shows that the vertebral height and kyphosis have been corrected.**
(*B*) **This postoperative computed tomogram shows a significant improvement in canal compromise, from 50% before surgery to 15% afterward, with an indirect method for decompression.**

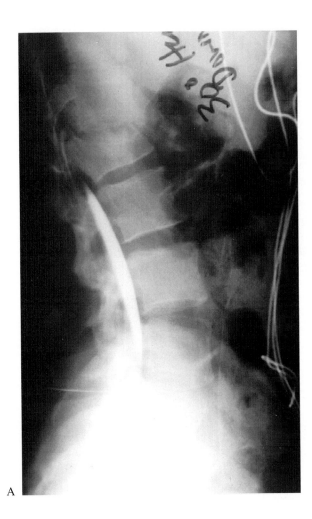

A

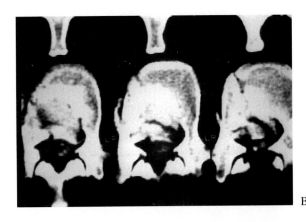

B

Fig. 3 (*A*) This lateral radiograph shows significant kyphosis and retropulsion of bone into the canal. A complete block of the myelographic dye column is seen at the level of the fracture. (*B*) This computed tomogram shows that the canal is completely obliterated from retropulsion of the posterior aspect of the vertebral body into the canal.

He was taken to the operating room, where a construct with the rod-sleeve-hook posterior distraction method was done, Figure 4 (**A**). The postoperative scan showed excellent canal clearance using indirect decompression with this short construct, Figure 4 (**B**). After the procedure, the patient regained full motor function of both legs, but continued to have a neurogenic bowel and bladder consistent with a conus injury.

SURGICAL SERIES

Star and Hanley's review[7] of indirect clearance methods showed significant improvement in canal compromise when a distraction rod-sleeve-hook construct was used. In their series, canal compromise averaged 42% preoperatively and 14% postoperatively. Kyphosis was corrected from 15 degrees to 3 degrees and vertebral height improved from 62 to 86% with this construct. An improvement of 1.8 Frankel subgrades was noted in the group of patients with neurological compromise after surgical stabilization and indirect canal clearance with the posterior rod-sleeve-hook construct.

In their series of 135 patients, Edwards and Levine[3] showed canal improvement of 32% (55% preoperatively to 87% postoperatively) if the surgical procedure was done within 14 days of the injury, but significantly less if carried out after 14 days. A significant improvement in neurological function was noted after surgery in patients with incomplete lesions who underwent the posterior distraction construct.

AUTHOR'S PREFERRED METHOD

The posterior approach with indirect decompression of the spinal canal and stabilization of the spine with a distraction rod-sleeve-hook or pedicle screw-plate or rod construct, with a graft of autogenous iliac crest bone placed in an intertransverse manner, meets the surgical goals in this patient. A postoperative computed tomogram is recommended to verify canal decompression. If canal compromise is less than 25%, the patient should be mobilized in a total contact thoracolumbosacral orthosis. If canal compromise is greater than 25% or neurological function deteriorates, anterior decompression should be considered.

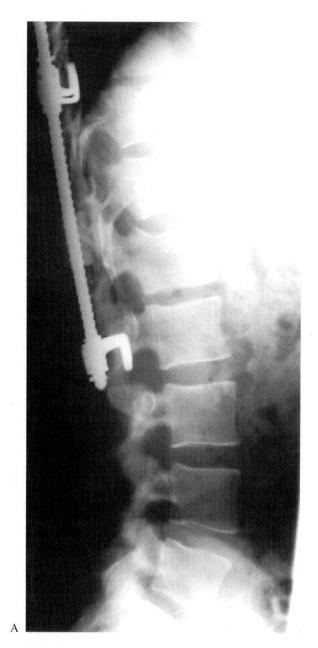

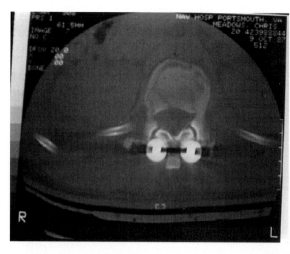

Fig. 4 (*A*) **A posterior approach was used with a rod-sleeve-hook construct spanning T11 to L2; the sleeve was placed directly over the pedicle of L1 and distraction accomplished with a ratcheted rod. The kyphosis was corrected and the vertebral height restored. (*B*) This postoperative computed tomogram shows almost complete clearance of the canal through the indirect method.**

Lateral Extracavitary Decompression and Posterior Instrumentation for a Thoracolumbar Burst Fracture

Richard G. Fessler, M.D., Ph.D.

This 16-year-old boy had an immediate onset of severe back pain associated with numbness and weakness in his legs after a motor vehicle accident. His neurological examination was consistent with sensory deficit caudal to the T12 level. He had ⅗ strength in all muscle groups of his legs and a loss of sphincter tone, voluntary contraction, and rectal sensation. In addition, all deep tendon reflexes were absent in his legs. Anteroposterior and lateral X-rays of his thoracolumbar spine showed a fracture of L1, with decreased vertebral height on both X-rays, widening of the interpedicular distance of L1, and a probable transverse

process fracture on the right at L1. Computed tomography through L1 showed a fracture of the vertebral body with detachment of, at least, the left pedicle from the vertebral body, retropulsion of bony fragments into the spinal canal, compromising the canal 50 to 70%, and possible dislocation of the facet joint at T12-L1.

TYPES OF FRACTURES

To formulate the most appropriate therapy for patients with thoracolumbar fractures, one must understand both the nature of the fracture and the goals of treatment. This fracture is a combination of axial and flexion forces. The combination of these forces generally results in 1 of 3 types of fracture. First, a "compression fracture" results from a predominately flexion force that crushes and disrupts the anterior portion of the vertebral body. The posterior aspect of the vertebral body is generally left intact, as are the posterior ligaments. Injuries that combine flexion and compression generally disrupt the anterior portion of the vertebral body and comminution of the posterior vertebral wall. The posterior superior aspect of the vertebral wall is occasionally retropulsed into the spinal canal, causing a variable degree of neurological deficit. The posterior elements are rarely disrupted and the pedicles remain attached to the lateral wall of the vertebral body.

The most severe injury of this continuum is the "burst fracture." This is an axial loading injury with a variable component of flexion. Generally, there is loss of height of the entire vertebra, as well as disruption of the posterior elements. The neural arch and pedicles are comminuted and frequently detached from the vertebral body. Retropulsion of the posterior wall of the vertebral body into the spinal canal is common. These injuries comprise about 80% of all injuries requiring surgical intervention.[7] The images presented with this case suggest that this fracture meets the criteria for a true burst fracture. Classification of this fracture as a stable or an unstable fracture may depend upon whose classification scheme it is based on. Denis[2] considered all burst fractures to be unstable. On the other hand, McAfee and colleagues[8] subdivided burst fractures into stable and unstable categories, based upon the integrity of the posterior column. Although it is difficult to tell from one computed tomogram, the apparent facet dislocation in this patient suggests that, even according to this second classification, this fracture would be unstable.

GOALS OF TREATMENT

For this patient, the goals of treatment are to:

- stabilize the fractured segment,
- minimize kyphotic deformity,
- maximize successful fusion,
- prevent further neurological insult and maximize the neurological outcome,
- maximize the patient's rehabilitation potential,
- minimize hospitalization and maximize the patient's return to normal daily function.

Indications for which a surgical procedure would help achieve these goals in this patient include:

- instability,
- partial neurological deficit,
- retropulsion of bone into the spinal canal.

A review of the literature suggests that instrumentation improves stability, deformity, and fusion rate, maximizes a patient's rehabilitation potential, and minimizes hospitalization (see, for example, Fessler[4]). Thus, fusion and instrumentation would appear to be indicated for this fracture. Decompressive surgery has not been shown to benefit the ultimate neurological outcome of patients with complete cord lesions. Cauda equina and incomplete cord lesions, however, have been shown to benefit from decompression. Therefore, the second indication for surgery in this individual is his partial neurological deficit.

Treating Retropulsed Bone

Considerable controversy still exists, however, concerning the treatment of retropulsed bone in the canal.[3] Gertzbein and colleagues[5] evaluated the mid-sagittal diameter of the spinal canal and found a limited correlation between the amount of compromise and neurological injury. On the other hand, Trafton and Boyd[9] and Hashimoto and co-workers[6] studied the canal area and found a significant correlation between canal stenosis and neurological injury. Hashimoto and co-workers reported that spinal canal stenosis ratios of 35% at the T11-T12 level, 45% at the L1 level, and 55% below L1 were significant factors for neurological impairment in thoracolumbar burst fractures. This patient, therefore, with canal stenosis exceeding 45%, again meets the criteria for surgical decompression.

CHOOSING THE APPROACH

This evaluation suggests that decompression, fusion, and stabilization are indicated for this patient. The next question is, "Which is the procedure of choice to achieve this goal?" I argue that the best surgical procedure is an anterior decompression and reconstruction through the lateral extracavitary approach, combined with simultaneous posterior segmental instrumentation.

The lateral extracavitary approach to the thoracolumbar spine is one in which a midline incision is begun 4 vertebral levels above the fractured vertebra and extended 3 or 4 levels below the fracture, and then brought laterally in a "hockey-stick" fashion. A myocutaneous flap including the trapezius and latissimus dorsi muscles can then be taken off midline and retracted laterally. The paraspinal muscle mass can then be completely mobilized from the spinous processes, laminae, and facets, and mobilized medially to the contralateral side. For an L1 burst fracture, the twelfth rib can be removed, after which a subperiosteal dissection exposes the entire lateral vertebral element to its anterior-most portion, with minimal manipulation of the diaphragm and without entering either the pleural or the peritoneal cavities. By following the T12 and L1 nerve roots into their respective foramina, the lateral edge of the dura can be exposed through an L1 pediculectomy. Thereafter, the entire spinal canal can be decompressed under direct vision. Direct visualization also ensures adequate decompression throughout the entire length of the fracture from the T12-L1 disc to the L1-L2 disc. Inspection of the anterior, lateral, and posterior dura is also possible through this approach to repair any dural tear.

Techniques for Instrumentation

Any of several techniques for posterior segmental instrumentation are reasonable for this patient. Perhaps the most traditional is a "claw-hook" construct using pedicle hooks at T11 and a thoracic laminar or transverse process hook at T10 for the superior claw. The lumbar claw construct has an upgoing laminar hook at L4 with a downgoing laminar hook at L3. This leaves both the T12 and L2 segments, where neural elements could be edematous, free of any metal stenosis. The limiting factor of this construct, however, is that most lumbar motion segments are lost.

Another option is to insert screws in the pedicles of T12 and L2. Although this construct has been shown to be successful,[1] it may have a higher failure rate secondary to screw bending than comparable longer constructs. A reasonable third alternative is to use pedicle screws at T11 and T12 combined with pedicle screws at L2 and L3. This technique saves 1 lumbar motion segment while fusing 2 segments above and 2 segments below the injured level.

ADVANTAGES OF THE LATERAL EXTRACAVITARY APPROACH

The lateral extracavitary approach offers many advantages in decompressing and reconstructing thoracolumbar burst fractures.

- First and foremost, direct visualization guarantees adequate decompression of the neural elements. The exposure gained through the lateral extracavitary approach provides visualization of the spinal canal equal to, or greater than, any other available approach.
- Because decompression is under direct visualization at all times, this approach provides maximum safety for the spinal cord and nerve roots. Decompression through transthoracic/abdominal approaches requires a blind dissection through the vertebral or disc elements to the injured and anatomically disrupted anterior dural elements.
- Take-down of the diaphragm is not necessary.

- Because the peritoneal and pleural cavities are never entered, irritation of and trauma to the great vessels and the thoracic or abdominal viscera is minimized.
- Both intensive care and hospitalization tend to be shorter with this procedure than with traditional thoracotomies.
- Visualization of the dura for repair of potential cerebrospinal fluid leaks is excellent. If a leak occurs, the fluid does not enter the pleural or peritoneal cavities.
- Posterior segmental instrumentation can be done simultaneously with this procedure; thus, eliminating the necessity of a second surgical procedure for spinal stabilization.

SUMMARY

In summary, the lateral extracavitary approach to decompressing and reconstructing thoracolumbar burst fractures provides an excellent means through which all goals of the surgery can be achieved. It has multiple advantages for the surgeon and the patient that decrease morbidity and more rapidly mobilize the patient. Therefore, this approach is well-suited to achieving all goals of surgery in patients suffering thoracolumbar burst fractures for whom surgery is indicated.

Anterior Decompression and Instrumentation for a Thoracolumbar Burst Fracture

John D. Schlegel, M.D.

Various options exist for treating patients with thoracolumbar spine fractures. Posterior instrumentation and fusion has historically been a mainstream procedure for these unfortunate patients. In patients with unstable fracture patterns, some type of instrumentation or stabilization procedure is obviously necessary. Posterior instrumentation has been effective in patients who are neurologically intact but require stabilization. Recent studies show that distraction and correction of the deformity appear to reduce canal compromise through forces placed on the posterior longitudinal ligament and, more importantly, the intervertebral disc.[6] Some studies, however, support the role of pure posterior distraction as an isolated method for spinal decompression. Starr and Hanley[15] showed an improvement in classification of about 1.8 Frankel grades in those patients with neurological deficit treated with pure distraction alone. Although this approach reduces canal compromise in patients with lumbar burst fracture, my experience has been that it does not totally decompress the spinal canal. This conclusion is supported by the work of Gertzbein and colleagues[8] and others.[5,16]

Posterior instrumentation is extremely beneficial in many types of spinal fractures. It is used routinely in our institution for patients with pure burst fractures who are neurologically intact, and in patients who have significant instability and posterior ligamentous disruption (flexion/burst fracture, the flexion distraction injury, and the fracture dislocation). In patients with significant neurological compromise, complete debridement of the spinal canal is important. An anterior approach with decompression and appropriate instrumentation is the most effective way of treating patients in this particular situation. It gives the patient the most reasonable and appropriate chance for neurological and functional recovery.

CASE PRESENTATION

The case presented is a 16-year-old boy who suffered an injury in a recreational vehicle accident. Physical examination shows the patient to have a partial deficit in the legs below the level of his injury at L1. He appears to have no better than antigravity strength in the legs with partial deficits to sensory examination and pain. X-ray evaluation shows what appears to be an axial loading mechanism with a fracture of the L1 body. It is a superior end-plate type of fracture (Denis B) with loss of vertebral height, involvement of the anterior and middle columns,[3] and pedicular widening. The computed tomograms show a significant amount of canal compromise.

At our institution, the patient would be brought into the emergency room with appropriate initial precautions. Based on the neurological deficit, the appropriate methylprednisolone protocol would be initiated. I strongly believe that the best care is carried out by consultation and active intervention with both neurosurgical and orthopedic teams. After appropriate consultations are obtained and the trauma physicians clear the patient, the treatment plan would be established. In a patient with neurological deficit and significant injury, acute active intervention is mandatory. In reference to timing, this intervention would be carried out in an urgent or semiurgent fashion (less than 24 hours). Different options obviously exist in reference to the treatment approach. If the patient were neurologically intact or had significant posterior ligamentous instability, I would strongly consider initial posterior fixation followed potentially by an anterior procedure, based on the patient's clinical course and evaluation. In this particular case, however, the patient appears to have an axial loading injury with significant canal compromise from the anterior aspect of the spinal canal. I strongly believe that the anterior approach is the safest choice, giving the patient not only the best procedure but allowing him the most reasonable chance for functional recovery.

TECHNICAL ASPECTS

At the L1 level, the anterior approach to the spinal column is not difficult. I prefer a left-sided approach because mobilization of the liver on the right makes that approach more technically demanding. The patient should be placed in a right lateral decubitus position, with spinal cord monitoring. All bony prominences are protected. At the level of the lower rib cage, the operating table is angled about 20 degrees. The appropriate ribs are palpated and the tenth rib is selected as the entrance point for the surgical dissection.

An oblique flank incision is then made directly over the tenth rib, beginning at the posterior axillary line and continuing anteriorly to at least the costal margin. The incision is carried down through the layers to the rib itself. Rib elevators are used to elevate the rib subperiosteally. With retractors and elevators, the rib is circumferentially stripped and removed in its entirety. Anteriorly, the costal cartilage is split longitudinally, exposing

the retroperitoneum. The peritoneal contents are carefully swept toward the midline, and the lung and pleura are similarly swept superiorly into the chest cavity. Soaked sponges are used to protect the viscera and self-retaining retractors are used to expose the cavity.

At this point, the diaphragm is taken down. The diaphragm is carefully split about 1 cm from the periphery on the left side. It is tagged as it is sequentially dissected. This dissection is carried down to the crus of the diaphragm, which is carefully and meticulously split. The posterior parietal pleura is elevated and split longitudinally over the vertebral bodies. This maneuver allows for lateral exposure of the vertebral bodies along with the associated discs. The segmental vessels are isolated (Fig. 1). For this particular fracture, the segmental vessels for T12, L1, and L2 should be appropriately ligated at their midpoint across the vertebral body. This step is crucial and cannot be overemphasized. Then, an elevator is used to subperiosteally reflect the periosteum from T12 down through L2, allowing for the crucial, wide exposure of the vertebral bodies and discs. After the segmental vessels are ligated, the aorta is retracted anteriorly and held. Obviously, care should be taken throughout this, and in all courses of the procedure.

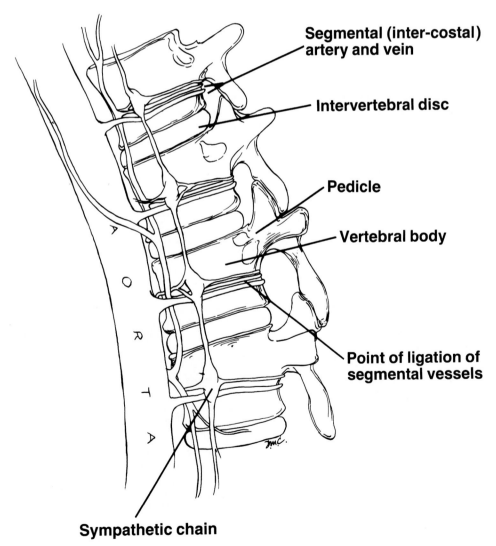

Fig. 1 The segmental vessels are located in the midportion of the vertebral body.

A vertebrectomy is done and anatomic landmarks are identified. The pedicle of L1 is an excellent anatomic landmark and can be removed with a rongeur, exposing the posterior aspect of the body more visibly. A #15 blade is used to resect the disc between T12-L1 and L1-L2. Pituitary rongeurs are used to evacuate the disc totally. A burr or osteotomes are then used to remove the middle portion of the vertebral body of L1. I try to preserve the anterior aspect of the body and the anterior longitudinal ligament to help provide stability. Certain points need to be emphasized at this juncture: if the patient has an old fracture, if there is significant canal stenosis, or if there is kyphosis greater than 20 degrees, a significant aspect of the mid and anterior vertebral bodies must be removed before the canal is debrided. I prefer to take an anterior and middle trough resected down to the opposing cortex of the body. If the dural sheath is exposed on the side of surgical entry, or if a wide trough is not cut, then the dura can buttonhole through this entry point, migrate anteriorly, and make surgical decompression of the rest of the canal essentially impossible. This point cannot be over-emphasized. I prefer to cut a deep trough while doing a vertebrectomy and to expose the dural tube, either at its mid or opposite aspect. After that, I burr back to the posterior cortical margin and use a curette or small kerrison to try to remove the posterior wafer of the vertebral cortex. Again, if the dura is exposed on the side of surgical entry (in this case the left), it will buttonhole, making decompression of the far side of the canal difficult.

After the spine is decompressed, fixation is, obviously, necessary. Simple anterior strut grafting certainly is a reasonable option. Anterior grafting has multiple advantages. Posterior fusion, in and of itself, is under tension as the midgravitational point of the loads placed on the spine are far anterior to the facet joints or the transverse processes. Therefore, posterior fusion is placed under tension loads, and its effectiveness is limited in reference to success and outcome. Opposingly, anterior fusion is placed directly under compression. This allows for direct bone healing and direct forces placed within the line of the mechanical axis of the spine.

Unfortunately, these mechanical forces can be huge. At the thoracolumbar junction, stresses on the vertebral body can approach 3 times the body weight. A bone graft material, in and of itself, is essentially a piece of dead bone that must revascularize and heal. I believe this is excessive force to be placed on graft material, and in the patient described I would augment the anterior fusion with the instrumentation.

The technique for bone grafting is simple, yet important. A slot is fashioned in the vertebral bodies above and below. In this particular instance, a slot would be cut on the undersurface of the

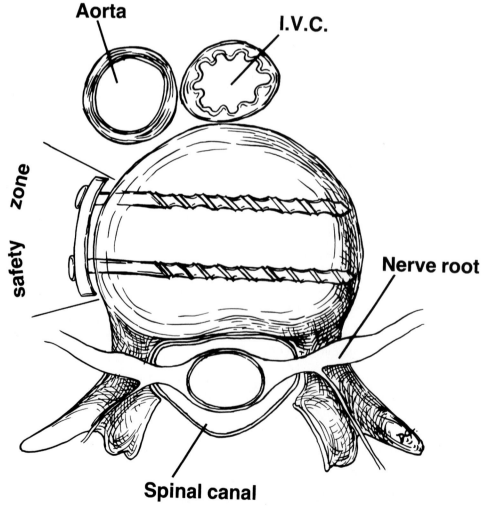

Fig. 2 Shown here is the exact margin of safety illustrating the risk points in reference to neural and vascular structures. I.V.C.: inferior vena cava.

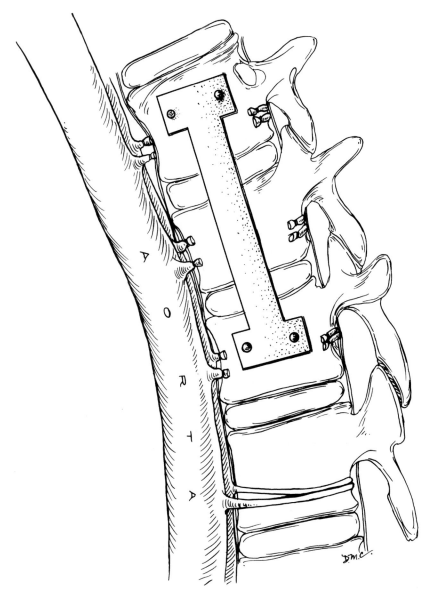

Fig. 3 After the kyphosis is reduced and the spinal column returned to as normal an anatomic alignment as possible, the instrumentation device is secured to the T12 and L2 bodies and anatomic reduction is restored.

T12 vertebral body, as well as the superior surface of the L2 vertebral body. This slot should be cut directly left-to-right with no migration either toward the spinal canal or anterior toward the vascular structures. I actually prefer to start the slot slightly posterior to the midportion of the body of the associated vertebra and carry it slightly anteriorly as I go across the body. I have been in situations in which the graft was started either in the midportion or slightly anterior. When this occurs, the graft has a tendency to migrate toward the posterior spinal canal. I cut this out in a square fashion and place it in. After it is put in place, the table is leveled. If the graft can be moved in any way with a clamp, the entire procedure is redone. The graft should be stable and in anatomic position. We check this with anteroposterior and lateral radiographs at this particular time. Recently, I have begun using allograft bone and have had no major problems. I recommend using either iliac crest, femur, or tibia (allograft).

Anterior instrumentation has suffered some controversy over the years. It was used in the 1930s and 1940s to augment a fusion for patients with spondylolisthesis. It was gaining favor until certain rare and untoward consequences occurred about 10 years ago.[10] Technical factors, rather than the hardware itself, are responsible for many of these failures. The physician must realize that there is an important specified margin of safety that allows for placement of this hardware.

Instrumentation

From a technical standpoint, instrumentation associated with bony fusion is not a new concept. It is used almost without exception in patients with injuries of the arms and legs. We have seen a much slower acceptance of instrumentation in reference to spinal problems. Obviously, potential complications play a role in this reluctance. But acceptance of hardware for cervical and thoracolumbar procedures appears to be gaining popularity. Because the brunt of this injury is anterior, and because the brunt of the mechanical loading is anterior, this present philosophy for instrumentation should not come as a surprise.

Various instrumentation systems exist for anterior thoracolumbar surgery.[14] They fall into 2 categories: plating systems and rod systems. Regardless of which system is chosen, placement of the device is crucial (Fig. 2). I would approach this particular case from the left side but, if bulkier devices are used, the right-sided approach is safer because it lessens the chance of vascular complications.

The technique for anterior instrumentation is quite simple. A subperiosteal exposure of the entire vertebral body, above and below, is necessary. Most anterior systems require some type of screw placement into the vertebral body above and below the injured levels. Some require fixation of the opposing cortex, though this needs to be done quite carefully. Wide exposure must be obtained, and this necessitates exposing the entire body of T12 and L2 in this situation. The kyphosis should be reduced to restore the spinal column to as normal an anatomic alignment as possible. After this is done, the device is secured to the T12 and L2 bodies and anatomic reduction is restored (Fig. 3).

X-rays are obtained at the time of closure. The posterior parietal pleura is closed over the fixation device with absorbable sutures. The hemidiaphragm is repaired with silk in an interrupted "figure-eight" fashion and oversewn with a running stitch. A chest tube is placed and the parietal pleura is closed anteriorly. Muscular layers are closed as such using silk with an associated absorbable stitch. The skin is closed with skin staples. The patient is then extubated and taken to the intensive care unit, where he or she is monitored overnight, and then onto the floor. The patient's neurological status is carefully monitored. A computed tomogram is usually obtained 1 day after surgery to assess the decompression and efficiency of the surgical procedure.

DISCUSSION

Although posterior stabilization has been a mainstay procedure, it does not totally debride the spinal canal. Willen and colleagues[16] reported a residual compromise of 28% after Harrington instrumentation. Residual compromise is seen in most studies.[5,8] Even Starr and Hanley,[15] who reported good neurological recovery in a small group (12 incomplete patients) done posteriorly, had residual bone in the canal. An alternative is posterolateral or pedicular decompression, which is technically demanding and risky. Intraoperatively, both ultrasonography and myelography have limitations as predictors of canal clearance, making the indicators for posterolateral decompression cloudy. The anterior approach makes this confusion unnecessary and gives the best chance for functional and neurological restoration.

The anterior approach has been supported in the literature. Dunn[4] reported recovery of 2 Frankel grades (better than Frankel's original series with postural reduction and Dickson's series of dual Harrington Rods). Excellent neurological recovery is also supported in the literature.[2,11,12] The safety of anterior devices has been supported by many authors.[1,4,9,14] The most exhaustive study has been a multicenter trial piloted by Gertzbein,[7] in which 1019 patients with spinal fractures were collected and reviewed extensively. Multiple conclusions were drawn. The anterior approach was more effective than the posterior in improving the patients' neurological function (based on the modified Manabe Scale, not the Frankel Scale or Motor Index Scale individually). It also was more effective than posterior surgery in improving bladder function.

Treatment of Thoracolumbar Burst Fractures

Carole A. Miller, M.D.

Each author has presented a reasoned and appropriate approach to the treatment of this L1 compression fracture. I concur with each author's assessment of this fracture, namely, that it is an unstable fracture. It involves both the anterior and the posterior elements. It is what has classically been described as a burst fracture and, if you analyze the anteroposterior film, you will see that there is spreading of the facet joints. This is a classic sign on plain films of a burst fracture, which is usually associated mechanically with vertical impaction and some element of hyperextension. In addition, this patient suffered neurological injury without clear evidence of progression of neurological dysfunction. All these factors, as well as the patient's age, indicate the desirability of surgical treatment. I doubt that anyone currently would suggest a nonsurgical approach to this problem. Without neurological deficit and a less than 50% fracture of the vertebral body, nonsurgical treatment might well be a recommended option.

SURGICAL CONSIDERATIONS

Once the decision for surgery is made, there are several considerations. The first is the timing of surgery. I would concur with the authors who contend that urgent, although not necessarily emergent, surgery is desirable. Many times these patients have other associated injuries and, certainly, a brief period, usually several hours, of observation and evaluation is in order to stabilize any other injuries the patient may have. Multiple injuries are always a consideration and their evaluation cannot be overemphasized.

Second is dealing with the issue of when to do the surgery itself. Certainly, if the patient is losing neurological function, emergent surgery is indicated. I believe time should be taken to obtain all of the appropriate tests in these cases, and I think there is a place in the treatment of thoracolumbar fractures for magnetic resonance imaging, as well as conventional myelography and computed tomography. High-resolution magnetic resonance images with at least a 1.5 Tesla unit can effectively evaluate the status of the posterior longitudinal ligament. Even with neurological deficit and a retropulsed fragment, the longitudinal ligament may be intact. If the posterior longitudinal ligament is intact, a strictly posterior approach in these patients may be employed effectively. In such a case, distraction will reduce the fragment; this can be assessed intraoperatively, as suggested by the author advocating distraction and posterior fixation alone to treat this type of fracture. If the patient is not losing neurological function, there is no evidence that waiting, even up to a week, before proceeding with the surgical procedure changes the outcome with reference to neurological status. The advantage to operating as early as possible is earlier mobilization of the patient, a shorter hospital stay, and getting the patient on the road to rehabilitation, which is a distinct advantage.

If rupture of the posterior longitudinal ligament is seen on magnetic resonance images, posterior distraction and attempting to decompress the canal posteriorly becomes much more difficult. In these cases, extracavitary decompression with posterior instrumentation is the procedure of choice. I concur with all of the authors that the neurological deficit in this case is from the retropulsed fragment with compression of the neural elements. This retropulsed fragment is difficult to approach posteriorly. Therefore, an anterior approach or extracavitary decompression of the ventradural sac is in order. The positioning and approach of the lateral extracavitary decompression has the advantage of allowing anterior decompression of the thecal sac and posterior fixation and stabilization, without having to drape and prepare the patient again in the middle of the case. It is also predominately retroperitoneal and, therefore, may avoid the other intra-abdominal complications. Furthermore, a complete vertebrectomy can be performed with a discectomy above and below.

PERSONAL EXPERIENCE

For patients with thoracolumbar burst fractures, I have done primarily anterior approaches with internal fixation, and used anterior devices. In this patient, this would be a reasonable approach. I believe, however, that there is an overall greater risk of complications with the anterior approach. Another problem unique to an anterior approach is a possible dural tear with herniation of the neural elements. This problem would be impossible to correct through an anterior approach. I have seen a dural tear with herniation of the cauda equina in many patients. This problem is actually best approached through posterior decompression, but a lateral extracavitary approach that allows access through the posterior route is a good compromise.

CONCLUSION

In summary, the patient as presented here has an unstable burst fracture involving anterior and posterior elements. This is an unstable fracture in a patient who has neurological deficit. The 3 approaches as outlined by the authors are all reasonable and acceptable methods of treating this patient and, more likely than not, all would effect a satisfactory outcome. Overall, however, the lateral extracavitary approach with decompression and posterior instrumentation offers the most comprehensive surgical approach to the patient because the retropulsed fragment is decompressed and the canal reconstructed. The opportunity to explore the posterior dura or repair a dural tear is easily at hand. Further, posterior instrumentation is tried-and-true for successful internal fixation until fusion occurs.

REFERENCES

Robert McGuire, M.D.

1. Bradford D, McBride G: Surgical management of thoracolumbar spine fractures with incomplete neurologic deficits. *Clin Orthop* 1987; 218:201–216.
2. Denis F: The three column spine and its significance in the classification of acute thoracolumbar spine injuries. *Spine* 1983; 8:817–831.
3. Edwards C, Levine A: Early rod-sleeve stabilization of the injured thoracic and lumbar spine. *Orthop Clin North Am* 1986; 7:121–145.
4. Edwards C, Rosenthal M, Gellad F, et al.: The fate of retropulsed bone following thoracolumbar burst fractures: Late stenosis or resorption? *Orthop Trans* 1989; 13:32–37.
5. Ferguson R, Allen B: A mechanistic classification of thoracolumbar spine fractures. *Clin Orthop* 1984; 189:77–88.
6. Gertzbein S, Court-Brown C, Marks P, et al.: The neurological outcome following surgery for spinal fractures. *Spine* 1988; 13: 641–644.
7. Star J, Hanley E: Junctional burst fractures. *Spine* 1992; 17:551–557.

Richard G. Fessler, M.D., Ph.D.

1. Carl A: Pedicle screw instrumentation for thoracolumbar burst fractures and fracture-dislocations. *Spine* 1992; 17:S317–S324.
2. Denis F: The three column spine and its significance in the classification of acute thoracolumbar spine injuries. *Spine* 1983; 8:817–831.
3. Edwards C, Rosenthal M, Gellad F, et al.: The fate of retropulsed bone following thoracolumbar burst fractures: Late stenosis or resorption? *Orthop Trans* 1989; 13:32–37.
4. Fessler RG: Decision-making in spinal instrumentation. *Clin Neurosurg* 1993; 40:227–242.
5. Gertzbein S, Court-Brown C, Jacobs RR, et al.: Decompression and circumferential stabilization of unstable spinal fractures. *Spine* 1988; 13:892–895.
6. Hashimoto T, Kanada K, Kuniyoshi A: Relationship between traumatic spinal canal stenosis and neurologic deficits in thoracolumbar burst fractures. *Spine* 1988; 13:1268–1272.
7. Levine AM: Surgical techniques for thoracic and lumbar trauma, in Rothman RH, Simeone FA (eds): *The Spine*, ed. 3. Philadelphia, WB Saunders, 1992, pp 1104–1134.
8. McAfee PC, Yuan HA, Frederickson BE, et al.: The value of computed tomography in thoracolumbar fractures. *J Bone Joint Surg* 1983; 65A:461–473.
9. Trafton PG, Boyd CA: Computed tomography of thoracic and lumbar spine injuries. *J Trauma* 1984; 24:506–509.

John D. Schlegel, M.D.

1. Bayley JC, Yuan H, Fredrickson B: The Syracuse I Plate. *Spine* 1991; 16:120–124.
2. Clohisy JC, Akbarnia BA, Bucholz RD, et al.: Neurologic recovery associated with anterior decompression of spinal fractures at the thoracolumbar junction (T12-L1). *Spine* 1992; 17:325–330.
3. Denis F: The three column spine and its significance in the classification of acute thoracolumbar spinal injuries. *Spine* 1983; 8:817–831.
4. Dunn HK: Anterior spine stabilization and decompression for thoracolumbar injuries. *Orthop Clin North Am* 1986; 17:113–119.
5. Essess SI, Botsford DJ, Kostuik JP: Evaluation of surgical treatment for burst fractures. *Spine* 1990; 15:667–673.
6. Fredrickson BE, Edwards HT, Rauschning W, et al.: Vertebral burst fractures: An experimental, morphologic, and radiographic study. *Spine* 1992; 17:1012–1021.

7. Gertzbein S: Scoliosis Research Society: Multicenter spine fracture study. *Spine* 1992; 17:528–540.

8. Gertzbein S, Crowe PJ, Fazi M, et al.: Canal clearance in burst fractures using the AO internal fixation. *Spine* 1992; 17:558–560.

9. Haas N, Blauth M, Tscherne H: Anterior plating in thoracolumbar spine injuries. *Spine* 1991; 16:100–111.

10. Jendrisak MD: Spontaneous abdominal aortic rupture from erosion by a lumbar spine fixation device: A case report. *Surgery* 1986; 99: 631–633.

11. Kostuik JD: Anterior fixation for burst fractures of the thoracic and lumbar spine with or without neurologic involvement. *Spine* 1988; 13:286–293.

12. McAfee PC, Bohlman HH, Yuan H: Anterior decompression of traumatic thoracolumbar fractures with incomplete neurological deficit using a retroperitoneal approach. *J Bone Joint Surg* 1985; 67:89–104.

13. McMaster WC, Silbee I: An urological complication of Dwyer instrumentation. *J Bone Joint Surg* 1975; 57:710–711.

14. Schlegel J, Yuan H, Frederickson B: Anterior interbody fixation devices, in Frymoyer JW (ed): *The Adult Spine*. New York, Raven Press, 1991, pp 1947–1959.

15. Starr J, Hanley E: Junctional burst fractures. *Spine* 1992; 17: 551–557.

16. Willen J, Lindahl S, Irstam L, et al.: Unstable thoracolumbar fractures. *Spine* 1984; 9:214–219.

33

Treatment of Metastatic Lesions to the Spine: De Novo Decompression vs. Radiation Therapy Alone

CASE

A 63-year-old woman with metastatic carcinoma of the breast developed midthoracic back pain. Upon examination, she had a T9 sensory level and abnormally brisk reflexes in her legs. Although she had weakness in both legs, she could walk with assistance. She has had no radiotherapy of the spine.

PARTICIPANTS

De Novo *Decompression in the Treatment of Spinal Metastases*–Charles J. Riedel, M.D.

Radiation Therapy as Primary Treatment of Spinal Metastases–Robert Blacklock, M.D.

Moderator–Gordon Findlay, M.D.

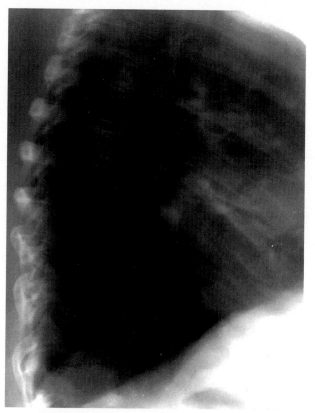

Fig. 1 Lateral thoracic spine X-ray showing no vertebral body collapse.

317

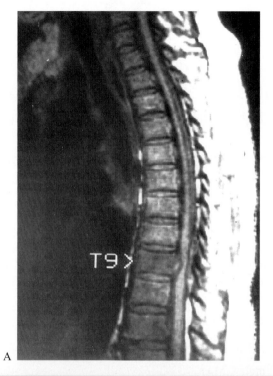

A

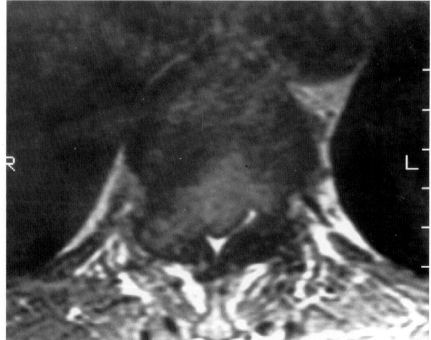

B

Fig. 2 Magnetic resonance images of the thoracic spine showing metastatic tumor to the T9 vertebra with an anterior, epidural soft tissue mass. (*A*) Sagittal. (*B*) Axial.

De Novo Decompression in the Treatment of Spinal Metastases

Charles J. Riedel, M.D.

The role of surgery in the treatment of spinal metastases continues to evolve. For many years, laminectomy for posterior decompression of the spinal cord represented the mainstay of treatment. Disappointing results with surgery alone and refinements in radiation oncology in the 1960s led to the widespread use of radiotherapy as an adjunctive treatment after surgery. In the late 1970s and early 1980s, however, several studies clearly showed that radiotherapy alone was as effective as laminectomy followed by radiation.[1,2,5] Moreover, laminectomy was accompanied by unacceptable morbidity, including spinal instability and worsening of neurological deficits.[6] Removal of the posterior elements failed to relieve ventral compression, which is most common in metastatic disease, and often destabilized the spine in a patient whose anterior structures were already compromised by a tumor. Laminectomy was widely abandoned in the treatment of metastatic tumors of the spine, except in the unusual circumstance in which the tumor involved predominantly the posterior elements. Several pioneering surgical series in the mid-1980s showed convincingly that anterior approaches for decompression and stabilization effectively relieved pain, improved neurological deficits including bowel and bladder function, and maintained ambulation in a greater percentage of patients for a longer period of time than any previous treatment.

CASE ANALYSIS

The 63-year-old woman presented here is typical of the type of patients we commonly see with metastatic disease to the spine. Breast cancer, along with lung, kidney, and prostate cancer, account for the majority of patients in most series of spinal metastases and, in some series, breast cancer is the single most frequent tumor treated.[12,14] In patients with metastatic disease to the spine, just as in primary tumors of the spine, local pain is the most common presenting symptom, occurring in over 90% of patients.[1,6,19] Our present patient is no exception. Despite many diagnostic advances and an increased awareness of the frequency of spinal metastases, neurological impairment is all too commonly present at the time of diagnosis. Once symptoms begin, neurological deterioration can be rapid. Thus, a high degree of suspicion and prompt evaluation is warranted. This patient is paretic but is able to walk, which is an important prognostic factor.

PREOPERATIVE IMAGING

Magnetic resonance imaging (MRI) has surpassed computed tomography (CT)-myelography as the primary radiographic method to evaluate spinal metastases. I continue to use CT scanning in most cases, however, to aid in operative planning. This patient's MRIs show the typical appearance of metastatic disease. She has low signal attenuation in the T9 vertebral body, the height of the vertebral body is maintained, and no kyphotic deformity is seen. The epidural soft-tissue component is predominantly ventral with lateral extension, primarily on the right side.

CHOOSING SURGERY

The final choice of treatment is determined by the well-informed patient after consultation with a spinal surgeon. That patient understands that neither surgery nor radiation treatment is curative, but is a palliative therapy. I strongly recommend *de novo* surgical decompression and stabilization in this patient based on the following considerations.

First, advances in adjunctive therapy have led to extended survival in patients with metastatic breast cancer. The extent and location of metastases is critical. In particular, patients with dominant osseous metastases have a median survival of 28 months or more, and those with visceral metastases have median survival of a year or less.[4,13,17,18] In patients with prolonged survival, maintaining neurological function is even more crucial.

Surgery provides immediate decompression of the spinal cord and mechanical stability. A tumor's response to radiation is delayed, subjecting the spinal cord to continued compression, often with progression of neurological impairment. In cases of instability, radiation alone is often impotent in preventing the progression of deformity, pain, and neurological deficit. Surgery, on the other hand, can relieve pain, improve neurological function, maintain the patient's ability to walk, and maintain bowel and bladder function, greatly enhancing the patient's quality of life. Pain is improved or relieved in 68 to 90% of patients after anterior decompression and stabilization.[7–9,15,16,19] Ambulatory rates 1 year after surgery range from 75 to 90%,[7–9,11,15,16,19] greatly exceeding those obtainable with radiation therapy alone (30 to 50%).[5,6] The importance of bowel and bladder control cannot be overstated. In one series,[15] 93% of patients had normal sphincter function after surgery and only 3 of 22 patients who had incontinence before surgery continued to have it afterward. Radiation therapy does not normally restore sphincter function, and dysfunction has been considered a poor prognostic indicator.

Second, this patient, while still ambulatory, is significantly paretic and requires assistance walking. Although neurological improvement can occur with radiation treatment alone, the percentage of patients showing improvement, the degree of improvement, and the number of patients returning to normal neurological function are all significantly higher in patients treated surgically. Surgery can restore ambulation in 70% or more of nonambulatory patients,[7–9,11,15,16,19] nearly double the rate of 42 to 45% achieved with radiation.[5,6] The discrepancy is even greater among patients who are paraplegic or quadriplegic at the time of treatment. One series[15] reported that 12 of 13 plegic patients regained ambulation. With radiation alone, only 2 to 3% of plegic patients ever walk again.[5,6] Even a prolonged deficit may respond to anterior decompression and stabilization and patients should not necessarily be excluded based upon the duration of the deficit alone.[7] I believe the risks of surgery are far outweighed by these benefits if the patient's survival is expected to be 6 months or longer.

Lastly, this patient has had no prior radiotherapy. This is a critical point. Sundaresan and colleagues[19] showed that the ambulatory rate in patients who are operated on *de novo* is 90%. Furthermore, the complications of treatment are reduced dramatically. In the series of Sundaresan and associates,[19] no operative mortality and minimal morbidity occurred in patients undergoing *de novo* decompression. This is in contrast to a 7 to 8% mortality rate and a 10 to 11% surgical morbidity rate in patients who underwent prior radiation therapy. Wound complications account for most of the surgical morbidity after irradiation. In my experience, as well as that of other authors, neurological worsening after anterior decompression and stabilization is rare.[7,19]

SURGICAL APPROACHES

The best treatment results can be obtained when the surgical approach is tailored to the particular patient. We employ 3 main approaches in the thoracic region, including the transthoracic approach through a lateral thoracotomy, the posterolateral extracavitary approach, and the transpedicular approach.

The Transthoracic Approach

If the patient has good pulmonary function and is in reasonably sound medical condition, the transthoracic approach offers many advantages. Exposure of the vertebral body is unsurpassed by other approaches. This exposure allows for a rapid and extensive vertebrectomy and tumor removal. When the patient is in the lateral position, we can use 2 surgical teams, so that a vertebrectomy and either fusion or vertebral body replacement with methylmethacrylate can be carried out by one team anteriorly, while a separate team carries out posterior segmental fixation. This team approach greatly reduces the operating time, and these procedures can be accomplished in as few as 3 hours. The thoracic approach also allows the use of anterior instrumentation, if this is the preferred method of internal fixation. The major disadvantage of the transthoracic approach is violation of the pleural cavity and associated pulmonary complications, increased postoperative discomfort, and the infrequent, but troublesome, occurrence of post-thoracotomy neuralgia.

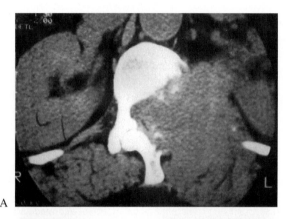

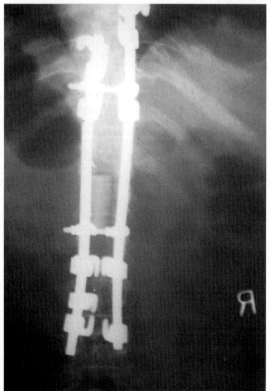

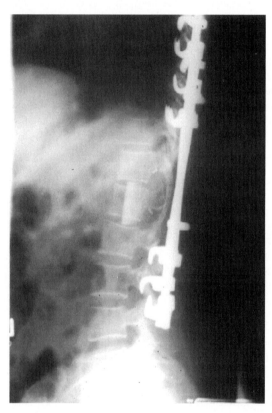

Fig. 1 (*A*) **Preoperative CT scan of a patient with metastatic renal cell carcinoma.** (*B*), (*C*) **Postoperative X-rays after decompression, fusion with allograft bone, and stabilization through the posterolateral extracavitary approach.**

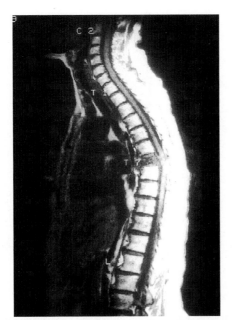
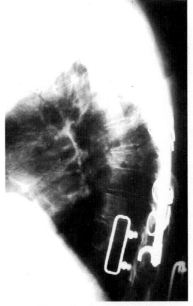

A   B

Fig. 2 *(A), (B)* **Preoperative MRI and postoperative radiograph of patient with metastatic breast cancer who underwent transpedicular decompression and posterior stabilization. Stabilization is critical after a posterior approach, especially in a patient with compression of the vertebral body and kyphosis.**

The Posterolateral Extracavitary Approach

I frequently employ the posterolateral extracavitary approach as advocated by Larson.[10] This approach allows excellent ventral exposure and extensive tumor removal and vertebrectomy through a single posterior incision that also allows the placement of instrumentation. Again, the vertebral body can be replaced either with a bone graft of rib or iliac crest or methylmethacrylate and pins. This choice is based, in part, on the expected survival of the patient. As the patient's survival lengthens, I prefer arthrodesis with autologous or allograft bone rather than methylmethacrylate. Improvements in instrumentation have enhanced the success of fusion and dramatically decreased the postoperative failure of stabilization. In this procedure, the thoracic cavity is generally avoided, eliminating the corresponding complications. Operative exposure is once again excellent, although the contralateral aspect of the spinal cord is not as well visualized ventrally as with the transthoracic approach. I used this approach in the patient whose CT scans are seen in Figure 1.

The Transpedicular Approach

The transpedicular approach has more limited application in the treatment of metastatic disease; however, it can be useful in some instances. Figure 2 shows MRIs from a 72-year-old woman who underwent a modified radical mastectomy 3 years prior to surgery for a metastasis. She had been in good health with no evidence of metastatic disease. Three days before admission, however, she developed midthoracic pain, and then had a rapid onset of paresis and was not ambulatory by the time she came to the emergency room. The patient had a history of pulmonary disease and had undergone prior thoracic radiation during treatment for a thymoma 40 years earlier. This patient's tumor was predominantly ventral, but also extended laterally on the right. Because of her previous radiation, the radiation oncologist was unwilling to treat her with this therapy. With no other evidence of metastatic disease, we anticipated a good

survival if local control could be obtained. Because of her underlying medical conditions, particularly her pulmonary disease, we wished to avoid the thoracic cavity and, therefore, used a transpedicular approach. After the right pedicle was removed, the epidural mass and the posterior portion of the involved body were removed. Stabilization is critical in posterior approaches and improves the patient's outcome compared with posterior decompression alone.[3] This patient regained ambulation in about 10 days and was still ambulatory at 1-year follow-up. She was treated with adjuvant chemotherapy, as well.

Approaching Thoracolumbar Tumors

Thoracolumbar tumors may be approached in many ways. I use either the posterolateral extracavitary approach or a combined transthoracic-retroperitoneal procedure. The patient whose MRIs are shown in Figure 3 came for medical treatment at the age of 55 years with a 10-month history of back pain. Her neurological exam was normal except for diminished sensation over the right anterior thigh. Spine radiographs and MRI revealed a destructive L1 tumor with kyphotic deformity and compression of the conus. Fine needle biopsy, which I use in nearly all cases in which no primary is known, showed metastatic carcinoma. An angiogram showed a highly vascular lesion that was successfully embolized. Angiography and embolization are extremely effective in delineating the vascular anatomy, reducing blood loss, and decreasing surgical morbidity. A vertebrectomy was carried out through a transthoracic-retroperitoneal approach. Interbody fusion with autologous iliac crest and stabilization with anterior plates followed. Good correction of the kyphosis was achieved and the patient's sensation returned to normal.

CONCLUSION

In uncontrolled series, anterior surgical decompression and stabilization offered the highest success rates in reducing pain and

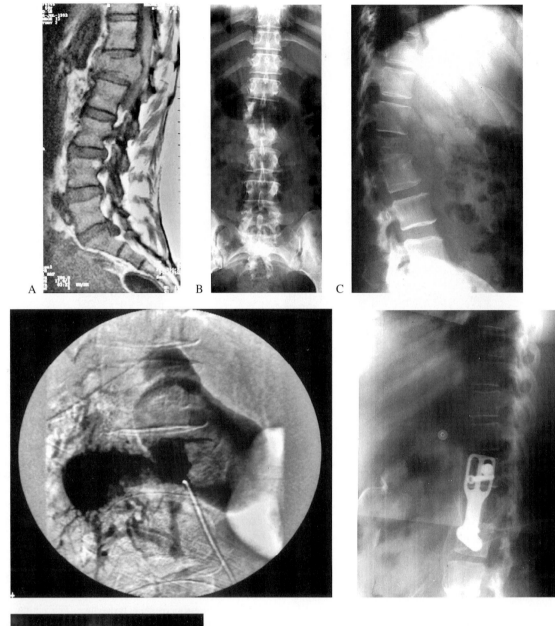

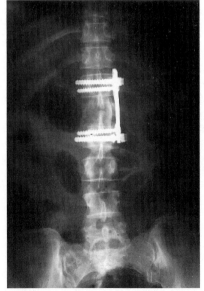

Fig. 3 (*A*) to (*C*) Preoperative MRI and radiographs of a 55-year-old woman with metastatic thyroid cancer. (*D*) The angiogram showed a highly vascular mass, which was successfully embolized. (*E*), (*F*) Postoperative radiographs after the transthoracic-retroperitoneal approach with a vertebrectomy, interbody fusion with autologous iliac crest, and anterior plate stabilization.

preferring or improving function in spinal metastatic disease. A randomized, prospective trial of *de novo* surgery versus radiation alone is needed to prove conclusively the advantages of decompression and stabilization. I have little doubt, however, that as improvements in adjunctive treatments enhance survival in patients with metastatic cancer, the superiority of surgery followed by radiation over radiation alone will be manifest.

Radiation Therapy as Primary Treatment for Spinal Metastases

Robert Blacklock, M.D.

Metastasis to the spinal column is a frequent complication of metastatic breast carcinoma that may cause neurological compromise and a resultant decrease in the quality of a patient's survival. The current case presents a typical dilemma a neurosurgeon may face in dealing with patients with cancer. This woman has paraparesis but is able to ambulate. Her images show a picture of epidural disease secondary to extension from the ninth thoracic vertebra into the epidural space anterior to the spinal cord. The substance of the cord is moderately compressed; however, the architecture of the vertebral column and the ninth thoracic vertebra is well maintained. Although additional views of radiographic studies would be useful in determining the extent of the disease posteriorly, I will assume for the sake of this discussion that the spine itself is stable.

The factors that must be considered in a recommendation for this patient include a knowledge of the disease itself, the patient's chances of survival with this disease, and the predictability of response to treatments that can be brought to bear. Based on these factors, radiation therapy is the primary treatment of choice for this woman.

TYPES AND RATES OF METASTASES

Carcinoma of the breast is complicated by bone metastasis in up to 70% of patients.[3] Metastasis to the spinal column itself occurs in about 25% of patients with breast carcinoma. One third of metastases to the spinal column with breast carcinoma occur in the first few months after diagnosis, but evidence of spinal disease may appear late in the course of the disease, after several years of a disease-free interval.[4] Spinal cord compression may occur long after the vertebral column is involved. Regardless of the type of treatment used for the spinal metastasis, survival after spinal cord compression in patients with breast disease is about 6 months. In one study, 78 patients with metastatic breast disease presented with weakness in the legs and metastatic disease in the spine. Of these, 42 proved to have epidural defects, with compression of the cord, which were treated through a variety of techniques. Patients both with and without cord compression had the same median survival time from the initial diagnosis of breast cancer, that is, about 65 months.[1,3]

USE OF RADIATION THERAPY

The results of radiation therapy in the treatment of breast cancer metastatic to the spine is not extensively documented. Many oncologists, radiation therapists, and neurosurgeons consider breast cancer to be a radiosensitive disease, and surgical consideration often is not given. Breast carcinoma frequently involves multiple levels in the spine. Serial bone scanning suggests that 70% of cases are polyostotic.[1,3] This, of course, complicates any surgical approach, whether dorsal or ventral, but does not adversely affect the ability to deliver radiation therapy. Two thirds of patients with multiple sites worsen within a short time of treatment compared to two thirds of patients experiencing improvement in the presence of monostotic disease.[3]

THE FAILURES OF SURGERY

Enthusiasm for laminectomy in the treatment of metastatic disease has waned, as clinical studies have failed to show any advantage in using a posterior surgical approach combined with radiation therapy over radiation therapy alone.[1,5,7,8] Anterior approaches with stabilization have been the subject of increasing interest in recent years. The anterior approaches have improved the surgical outcome from the treatment of neurosurgical disease compared to the more traditional laminectomy approach.[1,2,6] Although the spinal surgeon, who has in his armamentarium anterior, lateral, and posterior approaches coupled with reconstruction and stabilization, is clearly more prepared to deal with the difficult task of maintaining neurological function in patients with metastasis to the vertebral column, we must remember that the series presented in the literature included selected patients. The radiation therapist does not have the luxury of selecting patients to undergo radiation therapy. One recent presentation discussed 54 patients with radiologically documented spinal tumors. These patients were operated upon as a primary maneuver using any of the 3 approaches described above, 45 of the cases being approached from an anterolateral direction. There were 5 patients with breast metastasis in the series, but breast disease was excluded unless there was obvious instability in the spine. Thirty-five percent of the patients treated were unable to walk because of paraparesis, and 72% had spinal involvement as the presenting feature of their cancer and, thus, were in the early stage of their disease. Of these 54 patients, 6 had primary spine tumors and 3 were found to have benign lesions with a history of a previous cancer, leaving 45 patients with metastatic disease in the spine. I currently calculate the survival of patients with metastatic spinal disease as 37% at 2 years. The study presented stated that the death rate was 6% and the complication rate was 15%. Twelve patients had multiple operations. Of the survivors at 2 years, 90% were noted to be ambulatory. The ambulatory rate 2 years after surgery with these tumors is a good outcome for this group of patients, but the complication rate, the multiple operations, and early diagnosis must be considered in evaluating the outcome of these patients. Randomized prospective studies comparing newer operative techniques with radiation therapy in patients matched for disease and time-from-diagnosis are not available at this time.

THE NEUROSURGEON'S ROLE

Metastatic disease involving the spine, especially carcinoma of the breast, must be viewed in its proper context. The tumor in the spine is but a single anatomic manifestation of a systemic process with its own predictable outcome and time frame. The spinal surgeon may be faced with a patient in panic about the possibility of neurological loss. These anxieties may be heightened by concerned family members and physicians. The patient's personal physician sees the devastation the patient suffers and wishes to help coordinate the care that will produce the best outcome. The oncologist frequently views the problem as a single site of disease in a systemic process that is in need of acute control. The neurologist may play the role of the diagnostician and delineator of the local process. The radiation therapist has treated focal disease many times and stands ready to use the treatment believed to be reliable. The neurosurgeon may be placed in the role of the final decision-maker for a patient who turns over his or her fate to one believed to be helpful.

It is at this point that judgment becomes the key to an appropriate course of action because inarguable conclusions have not been reached in appropriate studies of patients with carcinoma of the breast. Hospital time, the risk of complications, survivability, cost, and, finally, the psychological toll taken on the patient in focusing on a single site of disease in the context of a systemic process, must be considered. Regardless of the treatment used, that single site of treatment may or may not be successful in terms of neurological preservation. Frequently, the most compassionate and appropriate role the spinal surgeon can serve is that of counselor about all of these issues. Unfortunately, patients having a malignancy are sometimes sent from one specialist to another to deal with focal problems, without a unifying view of the problem that they face. Ultimately, the patient is at the mercy of the biology of the disease and its response to therapy. It is a wise neurosurgeon who keeps this in mind when approaching this most difficult problem.

CONCLUSION

I believe that symptomatic sites of metastatic breast carcinoma in the spine are best treated with radiation as the primary therapy. This treatment is appropriate for cord compression by soft tissue and for painful deposits in the spinal column. Surgical treatment is appropriate, however, in the presence of clear instability that is causing either pain or neurological impairment in patients who otherwise have, or would have, a reasonable performance status and expected survival. The patient currently under consideration is clearly best served by radiation therapy for her metastatic deposit in the spine.

Treatment of Metastatic Lesions to the Spine: *De Novo* Decompression vs. Radiation Therapy Alone

Gordon Findlay, M.D.

This case cleverly highlights one of the major dilemmas in the treatment of patients with malignant cord compression. In this disease, certain areas are fairly clear-cut when it comes to treatment decisions. For example, it is widely recognized that, in a patient who has become nonambulatory but who retains some function and who also has severe kyphotic collapse of a vertebral body, radiotherapy has no place as the sole modality of treatment. Such a patient is best served with an anterior excision of the metastasis and spinal reconstruction.

However, this case history describes a patient who can still walk, albeit with aid, and who has as yet not developed vertebral collapse. In such patients, the role of aggressive surgery is much less defined and good evidence shows that radiotherapy alone may well be effective. Moreover, if surgery is deemed appropriate, several options exist. Should the surgical approach be anterior, posterior, posterolateral, or even circumferential, aiming for total resection of the entire metastasis?[10] Does the spine need instrumentation to achieve stability and, if so, do all such cases require bone grafting to protect the instrumentation as one would normally do? What type of adjuvant therapy is necessary and when should it be given?

Clearly, decisions must be made that are appropriate for the individual patient, and there is no place for an attitude of offering only 1 treatment modality to all patients. What factors, therefore, are necessary to allow such decisions to be made?

EVALUATING THE PATIENT

Each patient must be viewed as a whole. In this case, we have been told the site of the primary tumor, which is often not known at the time of presentation; up to 52% of patients who have metastatic spinal cord compression have no known primary lesion at the time they come for medical attention.[7] Carcinoma of the breast is a highly variable tumor in terms of life expectancy. Although many patients, especially those with visceral involvement, may suffer an early demise, long-term survival is not uncommon. In that situation, aggressive and early therapy of the spinal lesion is mandatory.

It is, therefore, important to assess the overall condition of the patient. The length of time that has elapsed from the primary diagnosis to the presentation with spinal disease is a clear guideline of the innate biology of the tumor. If the onset of the neurological deficit has been relatively slow, there may be time to screen the patient for evidence of other metastatic disease with abdominal ultrasound and isotope bone scanning, for example. If the lesion in the spine appears to be a solitary secondary one, then there is greater impetus to use aggressive therapy such as radical surgery. Tokuhashi and colleagues[12] developed a scoring system to assess the prognosis of such patients; like all such systems, it is a blunt instrument in the individual case but does give guidance as to the likelihood of the patient's quality of survival, and as to whether therapy should be aggressive or purely palliative.

Assessing Pain

One of the major clinical factors that governs the choice of therapy is spinal pain. Although the pain caused by periosteal stretching by a tumor and the painful involvement of adjacent soft tissues may well respond rapidly to steroids and radiotherapy, the pain of a spine that has become unstable because of vertebral destruction by the metastasis responds only to either large doses of analgesics or to surgical stabilization. When pain stems from instability, it is a powerful indicator of the need for surgical intervention.

Neurologic Deficit

One of the most powerful predictors of a patient's outcome is the severity of the neurological deficit. With patients who have no, or minimal, deficit and a relatively intact spine, radiotherapy can effectively prevent neurological deterioration. In patients with more severe deficit who can still walk, little difference was found between the effects of radiotherapy and posterior surgery.[1] Evidence shows, however, that even in this group of patients, appropriately targeted surgery has superior results.[9] In patients who have become nonambulatory, especially if they have vertebral collapse, little evidence suggests that radiotherapy allows the patient to regain ambulation and clear evidence shows that surgery is more effective.[2]

This patient does not have vertebral collapse but has a tumor centered primarily anterior to the cord, although the lesion encroaches somewhat posteriorly, especially on the right side. The patient retains some ability to walk, but significant neurological deficit is apparent. If this tumor appears to be a solitary metastasis and the patient's general condition is good, then aggressive therapy is indicated. But should this be radiotherapy or surgery?

USING RADIOTHERAPY

Some authorities believe that, if the neurological progression is rapid, radiotherapy is too slow to relieve the compression. Several authors, however, showed that responsive tumors shrank immediately without swelling, provided the initial dosage of radiotherapy was great enough and that steroid cover was given.[5,13] In addition, Gilbert and colleagues[3] questioned the assumption that surgery produces better results in patients with rapid neurological deterioration; they found that radiotherapy had superior results compared to posterior surgery in that situation. Unfortunately, no comparison has been made between radiotherapy and more modern surgical approaches in rapidly deteriorating patients, and so the area remains open to debate.

Radiotherapy is frequently recommended when multiple sites of spinal involvement are present. When this happens, it is unusual for more than one lesion to actually cause the neurological deficit and, therefore, surgery to remove that lesion alone still merits consideration. My experience, however, shows that, if the spine is involved within 1 or 2 segments of the lesion actually operated upon, the results of surgery and its morbidity are considerably worse than when compared to single or more distant spinal lesions. Shimiju and colleagues[8] reported good surgical success in patients with multiple spinal involvement, but they also found that many of these patients died of their malignant disease shortly after surgery, with the average survival being only 2.5 months.

One clear disadvantage of radiotherapy is that the morbidity of future surgical procedures performed within the irradiated field is markedly increased because of the problems of wound healing, a higher mortality rate, and possibly poorer results in terms of resuming ambulation.[11] Therefore, should radiotherapy be unsuccessful, the chance of surgery resolving the situation is decreased compared to *de novo* surgery. Therefore, radiotherapy should only be used as the primary therapy for those in whom the indications suggest that it has a high chance of success. This is likely to be in patients with radioresponsive lesions causing only relatively mild neurological deficit and minimal spinal destruction at the lesion site. The use of radiotherapy in other situations should be considered as only palliative and used only if surgery is deemed inappropriate.

THE USE OF SURGERY

With regard to *de novo* surgery, one thing is crystal clear: there is no place for indiscriminate laminectomy.[2] The modern surgical approach is to tailor the procedure to the anatomy of the lesion. Thus, a metastasis to the vertebral body must be approached through an anterior avenue if the best surgical results are to be obtained. To allow good cord decompression, posteriorly located lesions are best approached posterolaterally, rather than through a midline posterior approach. Whichever method is used, the spine must be left in a stable condition, which, more often than not, entails the use of instrumentation, supplemented with bone grafting if the patient is expected to survive longer than 6 months. The exact method of instrumentation used matters little, provided the surgeon is experienced in its use and chooses the method wisely. With appropriately targeted surgery, ambulation rates of up to 80 to 90% have been reported, even in patients who are severely paraparetic at the time of presentation. However, some reports show much less favorable outcomes from surgery.[6] Critical review of these papers is essential, because there may well be significant bias in selecting patients for surgery.

Even in very ill patients, the presence of severe pain from instability may necessitate surgical stabilization. Most surgeons, however, operate only if there seems to be a realistic chance of reasonable survival. Although neurological recovery can be rapid, especially after anterior decompression, several months must pass, especially for elderly patients, to make a full postoperative recovery. This period may represent a sizable portion of the patient's remaining life span; therefore, a decision to operate must be made judiciously. Reporting a surgical series of 70 patients, Kocialkowski and Webb[4] found that the mortality at 2 weeks was 16%. Fifty percent of patients had died by 12 weeks and only 25% were still alive at 1 year. Only 8 patients (11%) survived long-term, 6 of whom had either myeloma or lymphoma.

The evidence shows, therefore, that surgery in patients who have not had prior radiotherapy can have a high success rate in allowing the patient to walk. Most modern surgical series report acceptably low morbidity, but nearly all show a small, but important, early mortality rate. Sensible surgery seems to offer the patient a better outcome than radiotherapy, particularly if there is marked neurological deficit, vertebral collapse, or sphincteric loss. Perhaps the greatest drawback to surgery, however, is that which is seldom stated—the length of hospitalization and recovery that follows major spinal surgery in patients who usually have only a limited life span.

CONCLUSION

Perhaps it is clear from this discussion that there is no right or wrong answer to this particular case, or the problem of spinal metastatic disease as a whole. Patients with metastatic spinal disease must be cared for by a team that can provide any of the therapeutic modalities discussed and who can discuss the various options in an open and caring manner with the patient and the relatives. In some situations, the correct method of treatment may be obvious but, frequently, as in the case presented here, a choice of options exists, any of which may be entirely reasonable based on available medical knowledge. The physician in charge must not only to be able to offer any of the appropriate therapies but must also be capable of discussing these options in a compassionate manner.

It is difficult, therefore, to present a totally didactic program of care for these patients. The flow chart shown in Figure 1, however, is an attempt to show a logical pathway of care for such patients. This chart is designed primarily for the treatment of patients coming for treatment with neurological deficit. The element of severe pain from spinal instability proved too cumbersome to include, but it must be recognized that surgical stabilization in such a situation is a useful tool.

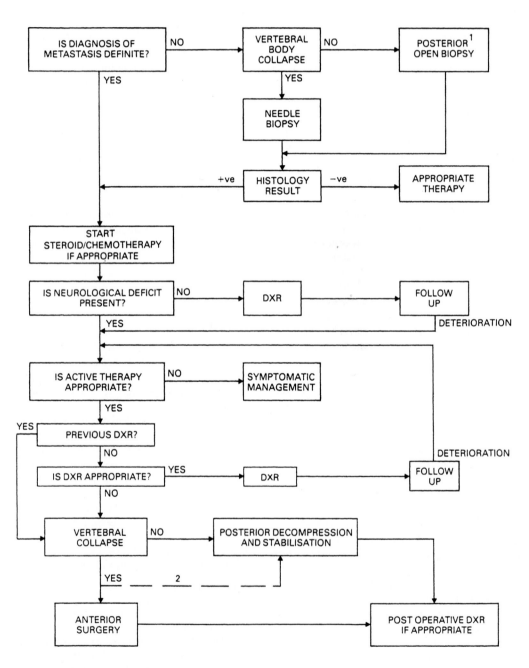

NOTES:
1. May be combined with posterior surgery if that option is selected.
2. If anterior surgery deemed inappropriate.

Fig. 1 An algorithm of the decisions involved in the treatment of presumed malignant spinal compression. (Reproduced with permission from Findlay G, Sandeman D, Buxton P, et al.: The role of needle biopsy in the management of malignant spinal compression. *Br J Neurosurg* **1988; 2:479–484.)**

REFERENCES

Charles J. Riedel, M.D.

1. Black P: Spinal metastasis: Current status and recommended guidelines for management. *J Neurosurg* 1979; 5:726–746.
2. Cobb CA, Leavens ME, Eckles N: Indications for nonoperative treatment of spinal cord compression due to breast cancer. *J Neurosurg* 1977; 47:653–658.
3. Cybulski G: Methods of surgical stabilization for metastatic disease of the spine. *J Neurosurg* 1989; 25:240–252.
4. Falkson G, Gelman RS, Leone L, et al.: Survival of premenopausal women with metastatic breast cancer. Long-term follow-up of Eastern Cooperative Oncology Group and Cancer and Leukemia Group B studies. *Cancer* 1990; 66:1621–1629.
5. Findlay G: Adverse effects of the management of malignant spinal cord compression. *J Neurol Neurosurg Psychiatry* 1984; 47:761–768.
6. Gilbert R, Kim J, Posner J: Epidural spinal cord compression from metastatic tumor: Diagnosis and treatment. *Ann Neurol* 1978; 3:40–51.
7. Harrington KD: Anterior cord decompression and spinal stabilization for patients with metastatic lesions of the spine. *J Neurosurg* 1984; 61:107–117.
8. Harrington KD: The use of methylmetacrylate for vertebral-body replacement and anterior stabilization of pathological fracture-dislocations of the spine due to metastatic malignant disease. *J Bone Joint Surg* 1981; 63A:36–46.
9. Johnson FG, Uttley D, Marsh HT: Synchronous vertebral decompression and posterior stabilization in the treatment of spinal malignancy. *J Neurosurg* 1989; 25:872–876.
10. Larson SJ: The lateral extrapleural and extraperitoneal approach to the lumbar and thoracic spine, in Ruge D, Wiltse LL (eds): *The Spine*. Philadelphia, Lea & Febiger, 1977, pp 137–141.
11. Manabe S, Tateishi A, Abe M, et al.: Surgical treatment of metastatic tumors of the spine. *Spine* 1989; 14:41–47.
12. O'Neil J, Gardner V, Armstrong G: Treatment of tumors of the thoracic and lumbar spinal column. *Clin Orthop Relat Res* 1988; 227:103–112.
13. Perez JE, Machiavelli M, Leone MA, et al.: Bone-only versus visceral-only metastatic patterns in breast cancer: Analysis of 150 patients. A GOCS study. *Am J Clin Oncol* 1990; 13:294–298.
14. Schaberg J, Gainor BJ: A profile of metastatic carcinoma of the spine. *Spine* 1986; 10:19–20.
15. Siegal T, Siegal T: Surgical decompression of anterior and posterior malignant epidural tumors compressing the spinal cord: A prospective study. *J Neurosurg* 1985; 17:424–432.
16. Siegal T, Tiqva P, Siegal T: Vertebral body resection for epidural compression by malignant tumor: Results of forty-seven consecutive operative procedures. *J Bone Joint Surg* 1985; 67A:375–382.
17. Smalley RV, Lefante J, Bartolluci A, et al.: A comparison of cyclophosphamide, adriamycin and 5-fluorouracil (CAF) and cyclophosphamide, methotrexate, 5-fluorouracil, vincristine, and prednisone (CMFVP) in patients with advanced breast cancer. *Breast Cancer Res Treat* 1983; 3:209–220.
18. Smalley RV, Scogna DM, Malamud LS: Advanced breast cancer with bone-only metastases: A chemotherapeutically responsive pattern of metastases. *Am J Clin Oncol* 1982; 5:161.
19. Sundaresan N, Galicich JH, Lane JM, et al.: Treatment of neoplastic epidural cord compression by vertebral body resection and stabilization. *J Neurosurg* 1985; 63:676–684.

Robert Blacklock, M.D.

1. Dunn RC Jr, Kelly WA, Wohns RNW, et al.: Spinal epidural neoplasia. *J Neurosurg* 1980; 52:47–51.
2. Harrington KD: Anterior cord decompression and spinal stabilization for patients with metastatic lesions of the spine. *J Neurosurg* 1984; 61:107–117.
3. Harrison KM, Muss HB, Ball MR, et al.: Spinal cord compression in breast cancer. *Cancer* 1985; 55:2839–2844.
4. Morishita S, Onomura T, Inoue T, et al.: Bone scintigraphy in patients with breast cancer, pulmonary cancer, uterine cervix cancer, and prostatic cancer. Statistical study of spinal accumulation cases. *Spine* 1989; 14:784–789.
5. Sundaresan N, Digiacinto G, Hughes J, et al.: Treatment of neoplastic spinal cord compression: Results of a prospective study. *Neurosurgery* 1991; 29:645–650.
6. Sundaresan N, Galicich JH, Lane JM, et al.: Treatment of neoplastic epidural cord compression by vertebral body resection and stabilization. *J Neurosurg* 1985; 63:676–684.
7. Tomita T, Galicich JH, Sundaresan N: Radiation therapy for spinal epidural metastases with complete block. *Acta Radiol Oncol* 1983; 22:135–143.
8. Young RF, Post EM, King GA: Treatment of spinal epidural metastases. *J Neurosurg* 1980; 53:741–748.

Gordon Findlay, M.D.

1. Findlay G: Adverse effects of the management of malignant spinal cord compression. *J Neurol Neurosurg Psychiatry* 1984; 47:761–768.
2. Findlay G: The role of vertebral body collapse in the treatment of malignant spinal cord compression. *J Neurol Neurosurg Psychiatry* 1987; 50:151–154.
3. Gilbert R, Kim J, Posner J: Epidural spinal cord compression from metastatic tumor: Diagnosis and treatment. *Ann Neurol* 1978; 3:40–51.
4. Kocialkowski A, Webb J: Metastatic spinal tumors: Survival after surgery. *Eur Spine J* 1992; 1:43–48.
5. Rubin P: Extradural spinal cord compression by tumor: Part 1. Experimental production and treatment trial. *Radiology* 1969; 93:1243–1260.
6. Saengnipanthkul S, Jirarattanaphochai K, Rojviroj S, et al.: Metastatic adenocarcinoma of the spine. *Spine* 1992; 17:427–430.
7. Shaw M, Rose J, Paterson A: Metastatic extradural malignancy of the spine. *Acta Neurochir* 1980; 52:113–120.
8. Shimiu K, Shikata J, Iida H, et al.: Posterior decompression andstabilization for multiple metastatic tumors of the spine. *Spine* 1992; 17:1400–1404.
9. Siegal T, Siegal T: Surgical decompression of anterior and posterior malignant epidural tumors compressing the spinal cord: A prospective study. *Neurosurgery* 1985; 17:424–432.
10. Sundaresan N, Digiacinto G, Hughes J, et al.: Treatment of neoplastic spinal cord compression: Results of a prospective study. *Neurosurgery* 1991; 29:645–650.
11. Sundaresan N, Galicich J, Lane J, et al.: Treatment of neoplastic epidural cord compression by vertebral body resection and stabilization. *J Neurosurg* 1985; 63:676–684.
12. Tokuhashi Y, Matsuzaki H, Toriyama S, et al.: Scoring system for the preoperative evaluation of metastatic spine tumour prognosis. *Spine* 1990; 15:1110–1113.
13. Ushio Y, Posner R, Posner J, et al.: Experimental spinal cord compression by epidural neoplasms. *Neurology* 1977; 27:422–429.

34

Treatment of Chiari Malformations with Syringomyelia: Posterior Fossa Decompression vs. Posterior Fossa Decompression with Drainage of the Syrinx

CASE

A 13-year-old boy came to medical attention with progressive thoracic scoliosis and intermittent occipital headache. He had a normal neurological examination with no evidence of myelopathy or cerebellar dysfunction. He had no cutaneous stigmata or radiographic evidence of spinal dysraphism. A screening magnetic resonance image (MRI) of the thoracic spine revealed a syrinx and an MRI of the craniovertebral junction showed a Chiari malformation (Fig. 1).

PARTICIPANTS

Posterior Fossa Decompression to Treat Chiari Malformations with Syringomyelia–
Richard George, M.D.

Chiari Malformation and Syringomyelia: Posterior Fossa Decompression and Drainage of the Syrinx–Albert L. Rhoton, Jr., M.D.

Moderator–Andrew D. Parent, M.D.

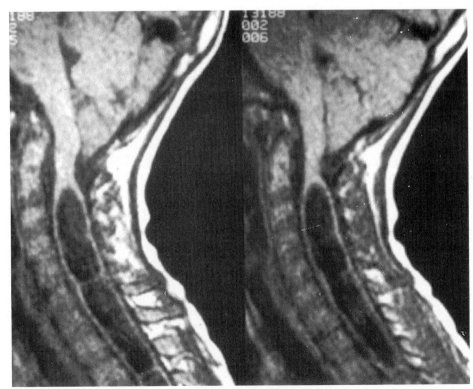

Fig. 1 Sagittal MRI of the craniovertebral junction showing ectopic cerebellar tonsils and a large cavity within the center of the cervical cord.

Posterior Fossa Decompression to Treat Chiari Malformations with Syringomyelia

Richard George, M.D.

Progressive scoliosis is the most frequent pediatric presentation of the Chiari Type I hydrosyringomyelia complex.[9,11,16,41] A number of these patients have no deficits on neurological examination, but it is important to evaluate for hydrosyringomyelia early in the course of the child's disorder.[11,16,22] Headaches are also a common symptom and are present in about half of these patients.[26] A quarter of these patients have a rather specific headache that is protracted, occurs in the occipital-suboccipital region, and is aggravated by the Valsalva maneuver, effort cough, or postural change.[26]

TYPES OF CHIARI MALFORMATIONS

In 1891, Chiari initially described hindbrain malformations associated with hydrocephalus and classified them into 3 distinct types.[6] In 1896, he furthered his descriptions and added a fourth malformation, consisting of cerebellar hypoplasia, that is of questionable significance in comparison to the others.[7] The Type I malformation is characterized by caudal displacement of the cerebellar tonsils beneath the foramen magnum. The brain stem may be displaced, but not markedly. Although patients with Chiari I malformations may have hydrosyringomyelia, other associated anomalies seldom exist.[10,11,27] The Chiari Type II malformation, also known as the Arnold-Chiari malformation,[32] is characterized by caudal displacement of the cerebellar vermis, brain stem, and fourth ventricle below the foramen magnum. Most patients with Type II malformations have myelodysplasia and other congenital anomalies, including polymicrogyria, agenesis of the corpus callosum, beaking of the tectal plate, and brain stem dysplasia. Type III malformations consist of herniation of the dilated fourth ventricle and cerebellum into a cervicooccipital encephalomeningocele.

The magnetic resonance image of our patient documents significant cerebellar ectopia consistent with a Chiari Type I malformation. With the advent of MRI, a number of individuals have been found to have tonsillar ectopia, with the tips of their tonsils extending below the foramen magnum.[2] In their study of 200 normal patients, Barkovich and colleagues[2] found that 14% of asymptomatic individuals had up to 5 mm of tonsillar herniation. Patients with symptomatic Chiari malformations, such as our patient, typically had herniations of greater than 5 mm. Patients did not usually become symptomatic with less than 3 mm of herniation.

DEFINING SYRINGOMYELIA

A variety of terms have been used to describe fluid accumulations within the spinal cord. Syringomyelia defines the condition characterized by the accumulation of fluid within abnormal cavities in the spinal cord, whereas hydromyelia describes the abnormal accumulation of fluid within the central spinal canal. Although pure forms of hydromyelia may exist, hydrosyringomyelia is probably a more accurate term to describe the pathologic findings of asymmetrical cavitation within the spinal cord, lined by both ependymal and glial tissues.[12,15] In the classic monograph on the subject, Barnett and colleagues[3] described communicating syringomyelia (that is, hydrosyringomyelia) as occurring with developmental anomalies of the posterior fossa

or basal arachnoiditis, and noncommunicating syringomyelia was typically secondary to trauma, spinal arachnoiditis, or a spinal cord tumor, or was idiopathic. Children with Chiari malformations have a 27 to 100% chance of developing hydrosyringomyelia that is frequently associated with scoliosis.[9–11,22,41] Although attempts have been made to radiographically document a communication between the fourth ventricle and the hydrosyringomyelic cavity, in practice, this does not affect treatment because hydrosyringomyelia resolves spontaneously after the pathologic process of the posterior fossa has been addressed.[11,19,35]

The Hydrodynamic Theory

In 1965, Gardner[13] proposed the hydrodynamic theory to explain the association of hydrosyringomyelia with the Chiari malformation. He postulated that arterial pulsations of the choroid plexus induced pulse waves of cerebrospinal fluid that forced open, and progressively distended, the central canal because of impaired outflow from the fourth ventricle. Normally, the foramina of Magendie and Luschka open during the fifth month of fetal life, allowing the pulse wave to be transmitted to the subarachnoid space.[4] In the Chiari malformation, the caudally displaced tonsils obstruct the foramen of Magendie and continue to direct the pulse wave into the central canal. Although this mechanism may have a role in the fetal development of hydrosyringomyelia, the arterial pulse wave would not likely continue this role in later life.

Williams[38,39] proposed a modification of the hydrodynamic theory, in which venous pressure changes were responsible for the formation of hydrosyringomyelia. During coughing or the Valsalva maneuver, venous engorgement of epidural veins forces cerebrospinal fluid into the spine rostrally. The herniated contents of the posterior fossa then act as a ball valve to trap the fluid intracranially. After the intraspinal pressure dissipates, there is a craniospinal pressure dissociation that tends to suck cerebrospinal fluid caudally through the patent central canal. Likewise, the increased intraspinal pressure could force intracavitary fluid within the hydrosyringomyelic cavity to dissect upward, extending the cavity and creating syringobulbia. Logically, surgical treatment of the Chiari-hydrosyringomyelia complex must address this pathophysiology of the posterior fossa.

SURGICAL TREATMENT

A number of surgical procedures have been devised to treat the Chiari-hydrosyringomyelia complex. If a patient has evidence of hydrocephalus, placement of a ventriculoperitoneal shunt decompresses the hydrosyringomyelia.[8,18,24] Most patients, however, do not have hydrocephalus and require a direct operative approach to treat the hydrosyringomyelia.[40]

One approach to the Chiari-hydrosyringomyelia complex is to treat the hydrosyringomyelia directly by puncturing the cavity, syringostomy, insertion of a syringosubarachnoid, syringoperitoneal, or syringopleural shunt, or a terminal ventriculostomy.[11,17,25,30,35] These techniques have been advocated as the sole treatment for individuals without compressive symptoms of the brain stem or cerebellum. Although these techniques may relieve the symptoms of hydrosyringomyelia, they do not relieve the ongoing compression of the brain stem and spinal cord by the Chiari malformation; this may later require further surgery. In addition, a shunt has the attendant problems of obstruction or malfunction, as well as neurological morbidity from its insertion.[17,29,31,33,36,41] The long-term results of these techniques have not been as good as those resulting from decompression of the foramen magnum, and they should be reserved for those patients who do not respond to a decompressive procedure.[28]

Decompressing the Posterior Fossa

Decompressive procedures of the posterior fossa have the advantage of re-establishing normal cerebrospinal fluid dynamics at the foramen magnum and relieving compression of the brain stem and spinal cord secondary to tonsillar herniation. There is controversy regarding the extent of the decompression required to alleviate the symptoms of the Chiari-hydrosyringomyelia complex. Some authors advocate a simple bony decompression without intradural exploration.[5,21,37] They contend that this alone relieves the ball valve effect of the Chiari malformation, and that further dissection may be hazardous. Peerless and Durward[28] noted that 30% of patients treated this way had an early improvement; however, on extended follow-up, none of the patients improved and 50% had deteriorated.

On the basis of the hydrodynamic theory, Gardner and Goodall[14] advocate posterior fossa decompression with intradural exploration and plugging of the obex. This technique re-establishes normal cerebrospinal fluid dynamics in the posterior fossa and prevents the fluid from being diverted into the central canal. A number of authors have reported encouraging early results from this technique; however, the long-term results have been less encouraging. Late neurological deterioration was noted in 24 to 63% of patients during long-term follow-up.[20,27,28] Intractable vomiting and respiratory embarrassment have been reported after plugging of the obex with muscle.[23,27,28] Peerless and Durward[28] avoided this complication by occluding the patent central canal with a Dacron® patch and tissue glue.

Decompression with Ventriculostomy

Another popular technique for treating patients with Chiari Type I hydrosyringomyelia consists of a posterior fossa decompression with fourth ventriculostomy.[5,11,22,23,28] This is my preferred technique. Through a midline cervical incision, the suboccipital squamosa and upper cervical laminae are exposed. A caudal suboccipital craniectomy is performed. Because extensive cervical laminectomies have a high incidence of kyphosis in the pediatric population,[1,23] the laminectomy is limited to only the extent required to expose the caudal aspect of the cerebellar tonsils. The dura is opened in a Y-shape and the arachnoid is opened and gently retracted. The tonsils are dissected apart and the fourth ventricle is visualized. Although significant scarring and adhesion of the tonsils is common in adults, it is infrequently seen in children.[9] If the patient has a widely patent central canal, a plug of muscle may be placed into it. The muscle is not forcibly packed and care is taken to avoid trauma to the surrounding structures. A small ventricular catheter is then guided into the fourth ventricle. The distal catheter is placed in the cervical subarachnoid space and a nonabsorbable suture secures it to the dura. The wound is irrigated and the arachnoid is reapproximated with absorbable sutures. A cadaveric duraplasty is constructed and the wound is closed.

The long-term results of patients treated with a posterior fossa decompression and fourth ventriculostomy are good. Peerless and Durward[28] noted improvement in all 8 of their patients treated in such a fashion. None of the patients had delayed neurological deterioration, although the follow-up was short. Dyste and Menezes[11] also reported excellent results with this technique. Six of the 12 patients in this series became asymptomatic and 8 showed significant clinical improvement. The remaining 2 patients improved, but were left with severe pre-existing neurological deficits. None of the patients experienced late neurological deterioration and there were no reported complications. Nohria and Oakes[22] reported that 14% of their 37 patients followed for a mean of 3.6 years became asymptomatic, 57% improved, 24% stabilized, and 5% deteriorated. Postoperatively, some patients had transient dysesthesias that completely resolved. Lanford and Tulipan[19] reported good results in their 4 patients treated with this technique, and documented a reduction in the size of the hydrosyringomyelia on postoperative imaging studies.

USE OF A SHUNT

Some authors advocate the incorporation of a syringosubarachnoid shunt at the time of the posterior fossa decompression. In 1976, Rhoton[29] reported on 11 patients with the Chiari-hydromyelia complex in whom he placed a syringosubarachnoid stent after decompressing the posterior fossa with a fourth ventriculostomy. He advocated the placement of a wick through a 1-cm vertical myelotomy in the dorsal root entry zone. He required a C1-C3 laminectomy to provide exposure for the myelotomy. None of his patients had further progression of their neurological deficit after this procedure. One patient, however, incurred a permanent proprioceptive deficit as a result of the surgery. Wisoff and Epstein[41] also advocate syringostomy and placement of a wick to drain the hydrosyringomyelic cavity. Six of their 10 patients who underwent this procedure had excellent results and 3 had significant improvement. One patient incurred a significant proprioceptive deficit.

Complications from syrinx shunting are frequently reported. Transient neurological deficits are reported in 17 to 40% of patients undergoing placement of a shunt[34,36,41] and about 10% have permanent proprioceptive deficits.[29,36,41] In addition, cervical subluxation after these procedures has been reported,[1,23,31,34] and shunt malfunctions are common.[17,31,33]

CONCLUSION

The Chiari-hydrosyringomyelia complex presents a difficult challenge for the clinician, as attested to by the variety of procedures devised to treat it. Decompression of the posterior fossa with a fourth ventriculostomy has proven itself to be a safe and efficacious treatment. The long-term results from this therapy are good and the morbidity is low. Although the addition of a syringosubarachnoid shunt should theoretically collapse the hydrosyringomyelic cavity more rapidly, in practice, the results from this procedure are similar to those of decompression and fourth ventriculostomy. Placement of a syringosubarachnoid stent requires a more extensive exposure and subjects the patient to increased risks of cervical instability. In addition, 10% of patients incur a permanent proprioceptive deficit and the risk of shunt malfunction. Posterior fossa decompression and fourth ventriculostomy is presently the treatment of choice for patients with the Chiari-hydrosyringomyelia complex.

Chiari Malformation and Syringomyelia:
Posterior Fossa Decompression and Drainage of the Syrinx

Albert L. Rhoton, Jr., M.D.

The Chiari malformation is a group of anomalies involving the caudal displacement of the hindbrain. The term *syringomyelia* refers to a chronic, relentlessly progressive syndrome caused by the destruction of gray and white matter of the spinal cord associated with an enlarging accumulation of fluid within the spinal cord. The term *hydromyelia* is used to refer to the condition that occurs in association with a Chiari malformation, in which the central canal of the spinal cord is distended by cerebrospinal fluid. Hydromyelia is the most common cause of spontaneously appearing syringomyelic cord syndrome; it coexists so often with the Chiari malformation that the combination has been called the syringomyelia-Chiari complex.

The patients with the syringomyelia-Chiari complex on whom these observations are based are adults, the youngest of whom was 16 years of age.[7–9] None had a Chiari-syringomyelia complex related to either a lower spinal dysraphism or hydrocephalus, as is commonly seen when this disorder is diagnosed in early childhood. The treatment discussed is directed to patients with Chiari-syringomyelia complex without hydrocephalus.

SURGICAL DECOMPRESSION AND DRAINAGE

In a series of more than 50 patients treated with surgery, I have found that the most effective treatment for Chiari malformation and hydromyelia is a suboccipital craniectomy, upper cervical laminectomy, and duraplasty to decompress the Chiari malformation. This is done in conjunction with drainage of the hydromyelic cavity through the dorsal root entry zone into the subarachnoid space, if there is significant distension of the spinal cord (Fig. 1). Decompressing the Chiari malformation without draining the syrinx has been advocated but, in my experience, has not been as effective as the combination of decompressing the Chiari malformation and draining the syrinx.[1,7–9] Decompressing the Chiari malformation, however, has proven more effective in reducing the size of a hydromyelic cavity than drainage of the hydromyelia alone. But, I have found that the combination of decompression and drainage is more effective than decompression of the Chiari alone. Gardner[2–4] also initially plugged the upper end of the patent central canal of the spinal cord at the area of the obex with a small piece of muscle. I have

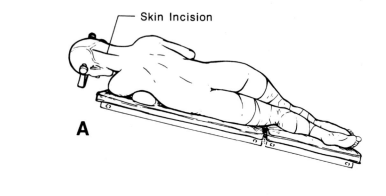

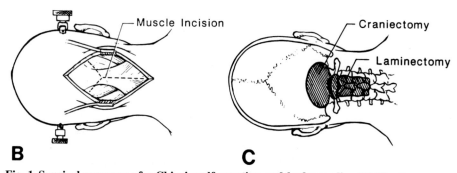

Fig. 1 Surgical exposure of a Chiari malformation and hydromyelia: (*A*) **The three-quarters prone position is used, and the head is positioned higher than the feet. The patient's face is turned 45 degrees toward the floor, and a midline skin incision is used. The side of the dorsal root entry zone to be drained is placed uppermost.** (*B*) **The site of muscle incision. To facilitate closure, a Y-shaped incision is made to provide a muscle flap attached to the superior nuchal line and inion. (Figure continued on the next page.)**

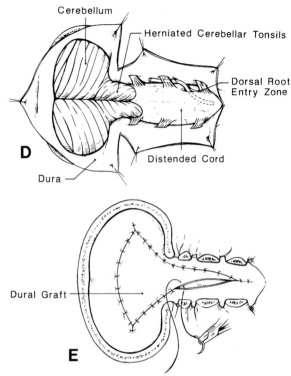

Fig. 1 (Continued). (*C*) **The site of craniectomy and laminectomy. The laminectomy is extended to include C4 if a hydromyelic cavity is to be drained through the exposure. (*D*) Exposure of the Chiari malformation and hydromyelia. The cerebellar tonsils extend down to the level of C2. The hydromyelia has been drained through a myelotomy in the dorsal root entry zone. A Silastic® wick is anchored to the dura and threaded downward into the hydromyelic cavity and upward into the ventral subarachnoid space. (*E*) A dural graft is used to complete the closure to avoid constricting the cervicomedullary junction and the Chiari malformation. (Reproduced with permission from: Rhoton AL Jr, Fessler RG: Surgical treatment of Chiari malformation and hydromyelia in adults, in Wilson CB (ed): *Neurosurgical Procedures: Personal Approaches to Classic Operations*. Baltimore, Williams and Wilkins, 1992, pp 169–187.)**

not tried to plug the central canal at the time of decompression because this operative maneuver risks damaging the hypoglossal and vagal nuclei, which are located at the obex near the upper end of the central canal.

The Evolution of the Treatment

A brief description of how several patients influenced my thinking about this discussion may prove helpful. The first patient was an adult man who had been treated years earlier by James Gardner, a pioneer in the treatment of this disorder.[2–4] Gardner had decompressed the Chiari malformation without draining the syrinx. Over the years after the decompression, this patient's deficit progressed so that he could not abduct either arm away from his side, and he was unable to flex at the elbows to feed himself. The foramen magnum had already been decompressed, and the syringomyelic deficit had continued to progress. The obvious treatment was to drain the syrinx. Up to this time, syrinx cavities had been drained through an incision in the posterior

midline between the posterior columns. Incising the cord in the posterior midline risked damage to the proprioceptive leg fibers in the posterior columns. My awareness of these risks had been heightened by having had the opportunity to evaluate several patients who had developed a proprioceptive deficit in the legs, in addition to an already significant hydromyelic deficit in the arms, as a result of having the syrinx drained in the midline. The appearance of this patient coincided with the beginning of the use of the operating microscope in neurosurgery. Examination of the patient's spinal cord with the microscope during the operation revealed that the syrinx had dissected into the dorsal root entry zone along the lateral margin of the posterior columns, and that the cord was paper-thin in the area along the entry zone. Thus, the dorsal root entry zone seemed to be the best area to drain a hydromyelic cavity.

Another one of Gardner's patients who had only a Chiari decompression appeared in my clinic, a few months after the patient described above, with a similar, but less severe, progression during the years after the initial operation. I phoned Gardner, who had retired from practice at that time, to inquire about the follow-up on his group of patients treated through decompression with and without muscle plugging of the central spinal canal at the apex. He reported that many of his patients treated through decompression only had appeared to be better during the early years after surgery, but that most had eventually continued to lose cord function because of the continued expansion of the hydromyelic cavity. This conversation with Gardner and my initial observations made with the operating microscope significantly influenced my thinking about this disorder and the formulation of our current mode of treatment.

The observation that these cavities tended to dissect into the dorsal root entry zone, rather than into the posterior columns, has been repeated many times since then. Observations based on magnetic resonance imaging (MRI) after surgery have further strengthened the conviction about the need for draining the syrinx[1–9] (Fig. 2). I have found that numerous patients having only a Chiari decompression without drainage of the hydromyelia have continued to have significant, although reduced, fluid collections in the canal. Those treated with decompression and dorsal root entry zone myelotomy had disappearance of a demonstrable syrinx or a residual demonstrable cavity that was slit-like, an observation repeated dozens of times. The first postoperative MRI is done about 4 months after surgery; by that time, most cavities have become slit-like or have disappeared.

Positioning the Patient

In the past, the operation to decompress the Chiari malformation and drain the hydromyelia was done with the patient in the semisitting position with the neck in a neutral position. Recently, we have been using the three-quarters prone position with the table tilted to place the patient's head slightly above the trunk. Marked flexion of the neck during surgery for the Chiari malformation may increase the neurological deficit or cause respiratory problems.

SURGICAL TECHNIQUE

Decompression

The suboccipital craniectomy and upper cervical laminectomy to decompress the Chiari malformation and drain the hydromyelia is done through a midline skin incision (Fig. 1). The laminectomy includes C3 or C4, depending on the upper level of

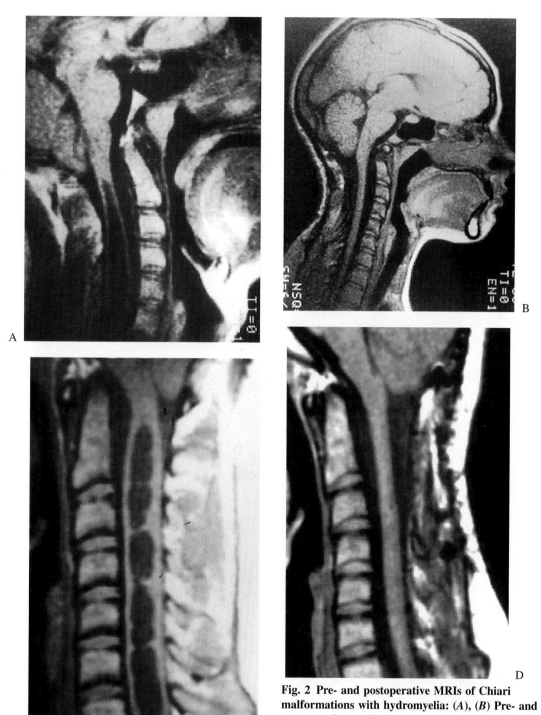

A

B

C

D

Fig. 2 Pre- and postoperative MRIs of Chiari malformations with hydromyelia: (*A*), (*B*) Pre- and postoperative sagittal images of the same patient before and after decompression of the Chiari malformation and drainage of the hydromyelia. (*C*), (*D*) Pre- and postoperative images from another patient. (Figure continued on the next page.)

the syrinx. The dura must be opened and then closed with a dural graft tailored to relieve the constriction of the medulla and cerebellar tonsils. The use of surgical magnification has facilitated dissection through the scar over the fourth ventricle, as well as the identification of the proper area in which to incise the cord and the final incision into the spinal cord. The degree to which the dura and arachnoid adhere to the spinal cord and medulla can be predicted from neuroradiological studies (Fig.

2). If cerebrospinal fluid is seen between the dura and the cerebellar tonsils, the meninges can be separated easily from the tonsils. If the tonsils are pressed against the dural lining, the cisterna magna, and no cerebrospinal fluid can be seen between the tonsils and dura, the cerebellar tonsils may adhere to the arachnoid and the dura. If a plaque of arachnoid and dura adheres to the dorsal surface of the medulla and the spinal cord, it should be left attached because an attempt to disconnect the

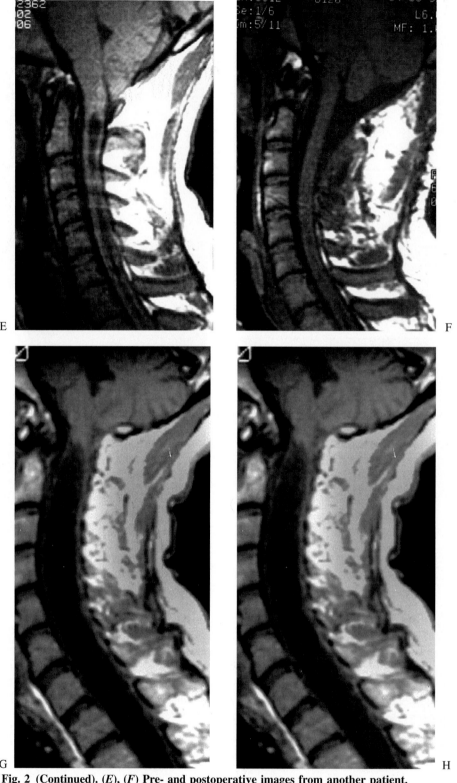

Fig. 2 (Continued). (*E*), (*F*) Pre- and postoperative images from another patient.
(*G*), (*H*) Pre- and postoperative images from another patient.

plaque might injure the neural tissue. If the foramen of Magendie is blocked, as occurs in a few but not most cases, an outlet should be established through microsurgical techniques. Care should be taken to ensure that the dissection is far enough superior to enter the fluid cavity of the fourth ventricle, rather than the cord or medulla. After the fourth ventricle is opened, a 26 Silastic® wick (Dow Corning Corp., Midland, MI) is attached to the dura or arachnoid and passed upward into the new opening in the midline (Figs. 1 and 3). The wick serves to maintain the patency of the outlet, rather than to provide a conduit for drainage.

Draining the Syrinx

After the Chiari malformation has been decompressed, the syrinx is drained into the subarachnoid space through a longitudinal incision in the dorsal root entry zone at the C3-C4 level. The dorsal root entry zone between the lateral and posterior columns is selected for the myelotomy because it is consistently the thinnest area in patients with hydromyelia. The natural dissec-

tion of the cavity along the dorsal root entry zone often leads to a proprioceptive deficit in the arms; hence, incision here minimizes the possibility of increasing the patient's deficit because the arm fibers course in the lateral part of the posterior columns adjacent to the dorsal root entry zone. An attempt is made to preserve the arachnoid when the dura is opened so that the tube can be anchored to the arachnoid. The subarachnoid end of the tube is passed along the edge of the cord in front of the dentate ligament, making it less likely to be adversely affected by scarring in the arachnoid and dura along the posteriorly situated opening.

An important consideration is whether to drain the hydromyelia through the left or the right dorsal root entry zone. Naturally, the root entry zone that has been most severely damaged, and into which the hydromyelic cavity has dissected closest to the cord surface, is selected for the incision. The side of greater involvement can usually be predicted from the neurological findings. The side showing the greater deficit related to the cervical sensory nerves is usually selected. High-quality

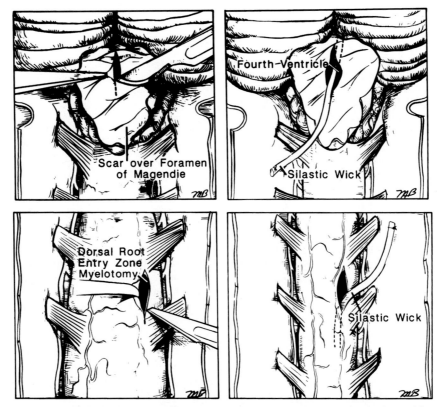

Fig. 3 The surgical approach used by the author to treat Chiari malformations with hydromyelia. A suboccipital craniectomy and upper cervical laminectomy are done to expose and decompress the Chiari malformation (upper right and left) and to expose the hydromyelic spinal cord (lower right and left). The foramen of Magendie is re-established by an opening through the upper part of the scar into the fourth ventricle (upper left). A Silastic® wick is anchored to the dura and passed through the opening into the fourth ventricle (upper right). The hydromyelic cord is decompressed by opening the thinnest area (the dorsal root entry zone) with a longitudinal incision that follows the course of the entering dorsal nerve roots (lower left). A Silastic® wick is then anchored to the dura and advanced downward into the hydromyelic cavity (lower right). (Reproduced with permission from: Rhoton AL Jr, Fessler RG: Surgical treatment of Chiari malformation and hydromyelia in adults, in Wilson CB (ed): *Neurosurgical Procedures: Personal Approaches to Classic Operations*. Baltimore, Williams and Wilkins, 1992, pp 169–187.)

MRIs in the axial plane commonly show that the cavity has dissected further into either the left or right dorsal horn. The side with the greater damage and the one to be drained is usually placed uppermost, if the patient is placed in the three-quarters prone position.

The question arises as to whether or not every cord should be drained if there is a hydromyelic cavity in association with the Chiari. We have decided not to drain the syrinx in a few patients because the cavity was small and there was a significant thickness of the cord overlying the cavity, both of which increase the risk of the myelotomy. On the other hand, a myelotomy at the dorsal root entry zone should be done if the cord is paper-thin in this area; even in patients with moderate-sized cavities, I believe this maneuver adds significantly to the result.

Surgical Results

No deaths have occurred among my operative series of more than 50 patients, and the neurological deficit increased in only 2 patients as a result of surgery. One patient developed a mild proprioceptive sensory loss in the right thumb that did not impair his ability to perform work requiring moderate dexterity. The patient was a young physician who, for years, had carried a diagnosis of multiple sclerosis because of a proprioceptive deficit in the right arm, with his left arm being normal. He was eventually found to have a Chiari malformation and syrinx. After the Chiari malformation was decompressed, the cord was drained into the left dorsal root entry zone, resulting in a proprioceptive deficit in the left thumb that was not present preoperatively. The deficit was not functionally obvious to the patient but was clearly present on postoperative exam. The myelotomy on the right side, the side of the proprioceptively impaired arm, before surgery would not have increased this deficit. This is the only patient in more than 50 operations to have an increased deficit related to the myelotomy when it was done as a part of an initial operation.

Another patient, who had the Chiari malformation decompressed and 2 prior operations to drain the syrinx before referral, and who was quadriparetic and bedridden, had a further mild loss of strength in her only functional extremity after a third operation was directed through extensive scar to drain the syrinx.

DISCUSSION

The myelotomy of the dorsal root entry zone that is used to treat hydromyelia differs from the midline myelotomy between the gracile fasciculi (which carry the fibers to the legs) that is made to expose and remove an intramedullary tumor. The cord usually is thinnest on the side of the greater neurological deficit. Before the cord is incised, a needle should be introduced into the cavity at the thinnest area to collect fluid for cell count and protein determinations. Clear fluid with a normal protein level indicates hydromyelia, whereas colored fluid or an elevated protein level indicates an intramedullary tumor. A vertical incision at least 8 mm long is made into the thinnest area along the dorsal root entry zone, and a Silastic® wick is anchored to the dura or arachnoid above and threaded downward into the myelotomy (Figs. 1 and 3). Recently, the subarachnoid end of the tube has been placed in the ventral subarachnoid space in front of the dentate ligament. The dura is closed with a triangular dural graft to ensure that the area around the Chiari malformation is not constricted.

We have seen 9 patients in whom neurological deficits continued to progress after a decompressive suboccipital craniectomy

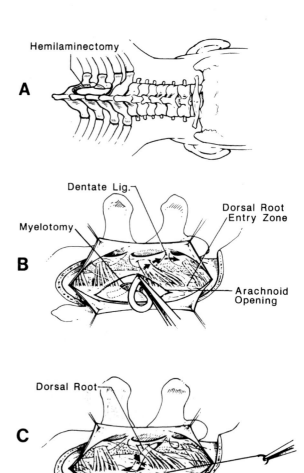

Fig. 4 The dorsal root entry zone myelotomy in the upper thoracic region. This approach is used if the patient with a hydromyelia has a minimal Chiari malformation, or if a suboccipital craniectomy and decompression of the Chiari malformation has failed to arrest the progression of a spinal cord deficit. (*A*) The operation is done with the patient in the prone or three-quarters prone position. The side of the dorsal root entry zone to be drained is placed uppermost if the three-quarters prone position is used. The hemilaminectomy is positioned below the cervical enlargement of the spinal cord in the upper thoracic area. (*B*) The myelotomy is located in the dorsal root entry zone. (*C*) A Silastic® wick is anchored to the arachnoid and threaded downward into the hydromyelic cavity and upward anterior to the dentate ligament into the ventral subarachnoid space. (Reproduced with permission from: Rhoton AL Jr, Fessler RG: Surgical treatment of Chiari malformation and hydromyelia in adults, in Wilson CB (ed): *Neurosurgical Procedures: Personal Approaches to Classic Operations.* Baltimore, Williams and Wilkins, 1992, pp 169–187.)

and upper cervical laminectomy, either with or without plugging of the upper end of the central canal at the obex without drainage of the hydromyelic cavity. In these patients, we performed a hemilaminectomy in the thoracic region over the lower extent of the hydromyelic cavity, drained the fluid through the dorsal root entry zone, and threaded a Silastic® wick, anchored to the dura, through the myelotomy (Fig. 4).

In 2 patients with asymptomatic, radiologically minimal Chiari malformations who had progressive deficits caused by hydromyelia, a myelotomy of the dorsal root entry zone was the initial surgical procedure (Fig. 4). If this procedure is to be done as the primary operation, the hemilaminectomy should be performed in the upper thoracic region below the cervical enlargement on the side of the greater deficit. Patients with Chiari malformations may require transoral odontoidectomy in addition to the posterior decompression.

Shunting cerebrospinal fluid from the lateral ventricles to the peritoneum is indicated if the ventricles are large or if there is evidence of increased intracranial pressure. In our series of adult patients, however, these findings of hydrocephalus on scan or evidence of increased intracranial pressure were uncommon. If a deficit continues to progress after decompression of the Chiari malformation alone, the hydromyelic cavity is drained into the subarachnoid space through the dorsal root entry zone. If this proves ineffective, a syringoperitoneal or syringopleural shunt is used.[5,6]

A careful preoperative explanation of the reasonable potential benefits the patient may expect from the operation is helpful in obtaining the best result from surgical therapy. Most patients report improvement after the operation, although the neurological examination usually reveals little or no change in the deficit. Therefore, patients are advised that the operation usually stops the progression of their deficits, but may not restore their function to normal. The operation commonly arrests the progression of muscle atrophy, prevents the increase in the size of areas of numbness, and may improve strength. In most patients who have anesthesia dolorosa preoperatively, the pain after surgery continues to be exacerbated by emotional stress, hunger, cold weather, and fatigue. This type of pain seems to recur 6 to 12 weeks postoperatively, when patients return to their prior employment and resume full-time work. Spasticity also fluctuates under the same conditions postoperatively, although motor testing shows improved or no further loss of strength. Deformities at joints associated with muscle atrophy may increase during the years after surgery, even though there has been no further atrophy or loss of strength. MRI has provided an excellent means of following these patients (Fig. 2). However, even when postoperative images show the hydromyelia to be absent or markedly reduced in size, patients may continue to experience fluctuations in pain and spasticity, even though the size of analgesic areas, the extent of muscle atrophy, and weakness do not progress.

Treatment of Chiari Malformations with Syringomyelia: Posterior Fossa Decompression vs. Posterior Fossa Decompression with Drainage of the Syrinx

Andrew D. Parent, M.D.

Modern surgical therapy for patients with syringomyelia relies upon the hydrodynamic hypothesis of a dissociation between the cranial and spinal pressure caused by a functional obstruction from a Chiari I malformation.[2,3] This relative obstruction of the cerebrospinal fluid pathways at the foramen magnum has recently been supported by the clinical work of Tachibana and colleagues,[6] who showed that elevated intracranial pressure induced by a compressed jugular vein is not transmitted into the spinal canal of patients with Chiari I malformation during neck flexion. Preoperative MRI studies of these patients with syringomyelia done with the cine mode MRI in cardiac-gated phase-contrast scanning have shown a significant reduction in cerebrospinal fluid flow at the foramen magnum, anterior to the medulla, as well as rostrally into the fourth ventricle and even posteriorly over the cerebellar tonsils and the cisterna magna.[1,7] Postoperatively, these flow and pressure abnormalities essentially reverted to normal patterns. As MRI studies improve our understanding of the pathophysiology of both intracranial and intraspinal cerebrospinal fluid, a more systematic approach to the treatment of patients with syringomyelia is evolving.

DECOMPRESSION ALONE

George supports decompressing the posterior fossa pathology of Chiari malformation and believes that this will resolve the problem of hydrosyringomyelia. Having advocated this proposition, he then reverts to muscle plugging in patients with widely patent central canals. Furthermore, he recommends a fourth ven-

triculostomy, placing a small ventricular catheter into the fourth ventricle and securing it to the dura in the cervical subarachnoid space. He argues that, although a syringosubarachnoid shunt theoretically collapses the syrinx cavity more rapidly, the clinical results of a fourth ventriculostomy and a Chiari decompression are similar to those achieved through treatment with a syringosubarachnoid shunt.

DECOMPRESSION AND DRAINAGE

In the pediatric population, the C3-C4 laminectomy that Rhoton recommends is attended with a high risk of cervical kyphosis. A two-level thoracic hemilaminectomy is preferred in the patient with a developing spine. Rhoton notes that numerous patients who had only a Chiari decompression without drainage of the hydromyelia continued to have significant, albeit reduced, fluid collections in the canal. Presumably, treatment with a syringosubarachnoid shunt at the dorsal root entry zone with the resultant resolution or collapse of the syrinx is attended by improved clinical results. Should the treatment goal in these patients be a moderately decompressed syrinx or a slit-like collapse of the central cavity? Rhoton suggests that the disappearance of the syrinx is the preferred objective.

DISCUSSION

As both authors stated, the treatment of a patient with a Chiari Type I malformation with syringomyelia should always begin by addressing the hydrocephalus, if it is present. A ventriculoperitoneal shunt placed in patients with hydrocephalus may relieve both the cerebellar ectopia as well as the dilated central canal.

Most patients with Chiari I malformations and syringomyelia are treated through a suboccipital decompressive craniectomy, as well as a cervical laminectomy to the distal tips of the cerebellar tonsils. The occipital bone is often considerably flattened and has a rostral tilt at the foramen magnum. The dorsal ring of C-1 may be incomplete or thin. Inevitably, a markedly thickened dural band is found at the foramen magnum, that may contain or conceal underlying aberrant veins. Dense arachnoid adhesions over the asymmetrically descended cerebellar tonsils may also be seen. In comparison with adults, in which the cerebellar tonsils may be frankly necrotic secondary to chronic compression, there is rarely a need to excise the cerebellar tonsils in children. The entrance to the vallecula may be blocked by a dense scar of fibroconnective tissue. In such cases, the tonsils cannot be mobilized, and a tube placed in the fourth ventricle to the cervical subarachnoid space may re-establish the flow of cerebrospinal fluid in the midline. The dura must always be open and then subsequently reconstructed in a capacious manner. With this type of decompression, plugging the open central canal seems unnecessary. This procedure frequently collapses the syrinx, even in cases that are holocord and with multiple septations or haustrations.

In patients in which the syrinx does not radiologically collapse within 3 to 4 months after surgery, a syringosubarachnoid shunt is inserted in the upper thoracic area. If the flow of cerebrospinal fluid is obviously disturbed, as in patients with arachnoiditis, the initial shunt is a syringopleural or syringoperitoneal. With the wisdom of considerable retrospective experience, Rhoton cautions us that, despite obliteration of the syrinx, some patients may have further neurological deterioration or continue to experience fluctuations in pain and spasticity. Furthermore, the return of the patient's syrinx, as shown by follow-up MRIs, does not necessarily portend clinical deterioration.[4,5]

Clearly, our understanding of the treatment of patients with syringomyelia is still evolving. It may well be that our attempts to treat this problem sometimes fail or are inadequate because more than one factor is the cause.

REFERENCES

Richard George, M.D.

1. Alexander E Jr: Postlaminectomy kyphosis, in Wilkins RH, Rengachary SS (eds): *Neurosurgery*. New York, McGraw-Hill, 1985, pp 2293–2297.
2. Barkovich AJ, Wippold FJ, Sherman JL, et al.: Significance of cerebellar tonsillar position on MR. *AJNR* 1986; 7:795–799.
3. Barnett H, Foster J, Hudgson P: *Syringomyelia*. London, WB Saunders, 1973.
4. Bering E: Choroid plexus and arterial pulsation of cerebrospinal fluid: Demonstration of choroid plexus as cerebrospinal fluid pump. *Arch Neurol Psychiatry* 1955; 73:165–172.
5. Carmel P: The Chiari malformation, in Hoffman H, Epstein F (eds): *Disorders of the Developing Nervous System*. Boston, Blackwell, 1986, pp 133–151.
6. Chiari H: Ueber veränderungen des kleinhirns infolge von Hydrocephalie des grosshirns. *Deutsch Med Wochenschr* 1891; 17:1172–1175.
7. Chiari H: Ueber veränderungen des kleinhirns, des pons und der medulla oblongata in folge von congenitaler hydrocephalie des grosshirns. *Denschr Akad Wiss Wien* 1896; 63:71–116.
8. Conway L: Hydrodynamic studies in syringomyelia. *J Neurosurg* 1967; 27:501–514.
9. Dauser RC, DiPietro MA, Venes JL: Symptomatic Chiari I malformation in childhood: A report of 7 cases. *Pediatr Neurosci* 1988; 14:184–190.
10. Dure LS, Percy AK, Cheek WR, et al.: Chiari Type I malformation in children. *J Pediatr* 1989; 115:573–576.
11. Dyste G, Menezes A: Presentation and management of pediatric Chiari malformations without myelodysplasia. *Neurosurgery* 1988; 23:589–597.
12. Eggers C, Hamer J: Hydrosyringomyelia in childhood—clinical aspects, pathogenesis, and therapy. *Neuropaediatrie* 1979; 10: 87–99.
13. Gardner WJ: Hydrodynamic mechanism of syringomyelia: Its relationship to myelocele. *J Neurol Neurosurg Psychiatry* 1965; 28: 247–259.
14. Gardner WJ, Goodall R: The surgical treatment of Arnold-Chiari malformation in adults. *J Neurosurg* 1950; 7:199–206.
15. Hoffman H, Neill J, Crone K, et al.: Hydrosyringomyelia and its management in childhood. *Neurosurgery* 1987; 21:347–351.
16. Isu T, Iwasaki Y, Akino M, et al.: Hydrosyringomyelia associated with a Chiari I malformation in children and adolescents. *Neurosurgery* 1990; 26:591–596.
17. Isu T, Iwasaki Y, Akino M, et al.: Syringo-subarachnoid shunt for syringomyelia associated with Chiari malformation (type 1). *Acta Neurochir (Wien)* 1990; 107:152–160.
18. Krayenbühl H: Evaluation of different surgical approaches in the treatment of syringomyelia. *Clin Neurol Neurosurg* 1974; 77: 110–128.
19. Lanford GB, Tulipan N: Fourth ventriculostomy for Chiari malformation. *J Tenn Med Assoc* 1989; 82:477–479.
20. Levy W, Mason L, Hahn J: Chiari malformation presenting in adults: A surgical experience with 127 cases. *Neurosurgery* 1983; 12:377–390.
21. Logue V, Edwards MR: Syringomyelia and its surgical treatment—an analysis of 75 patients. *J Neurol Neurosurg Psychiatry* 1981; 44:273–284.
22. Nohria V, Oakes WJ: Chiari I malformation: a review of 43 patients. *Pediatr Neurosurg* 1990; 16:222–227.
23. Oakes W: Chiari malformations, hydromyelia, syringomyelia, in Wilkins RH, Rengachary SS (eds): *Neurosurgery*. New York, McGraw-Hill, 1985, pp 2102–2124.
24. Ogilvy CS, Borges LF: Treatment of symptomatic syringomyelia with a ventriculoperitoneal shunt: A case report with magnetic resonance scan correlation. *Neurosurgery* 1988; 22:748–750.
25. Park TS, Cail WS, Broaddus WC, et al.: Lumboperitoneal shunt combined with myelotomy for treatment of syringohydromyelia: *J Neurosurg* 1989; 70:721–727.
26. Pascual J, Oterino A, Berciano J: Headache in Type I Chiari malformation. *Neurology* 1992; 42:1519–1521.
27. Paul K, Lye R, Strang F, et al.: Arnold-Chiari malformation: Review of 71 cases. *J Neurosurg* 1983; 58:183–187.
28. Peerless S, Durward Q: Management of syringomyelia: A pathophysiological approach. *Clin Neurosurg* 1982; 30:531–576.
29. Rhoton AL Jr: Microsurgery of Arnold-Chiari malformation in adults with and without hydromyelia. *J Neurosurg* 1976; 45:473–483.
30. Schlesinger EB, Antunes J, Michelsen W, et al.: Hydromyelia: Clinical presentation and comparison of modalities of treatment. *Neurosurgery* 1981; 9:356–365.

31. Schlesinger EB: Management of syringomyelia associated with Chiari malformation: Comparative study of syrinx size and symptoms by magnetic resonance imaging (letter). *Surg Neurol* 1992; 38:161–162.

32. Schwalbe E, Gredig M: Ueber entwicklungs-störungen des kleinhirns, hirnstamms und halsmarks bei spina bifida (Arnold'sche und Chiari'sche missbildung). *Beitr Pathol Anat* 1907; 40:132–194.

33. Suzuki M, Davis C, Symon L, et al.: Syringoperitoneal shunt for treatment of cord cavitation. *J Neurol Neurosurg Psychiatry* 1985; 48:620–627.

34. Tator CH, Briceno C: Treatment of syringomyelia with a syringo-subarachnoid shunt. *Can J Neurol Sci* 1988; 15:48–57.

35. Vaquero J, Martinez R, Arias A: Syringomyelia-Chiari complex: Magnetic resonance imaging and clinical evaluation of surgical

treatment. *J Neurosurg* 1990; 73:64–68.

36. Vaquero J, Martinez R, Salazar J, et al.: Syringosubarachnoid shunt for treatment of syringomyelia. *Acta Neurochir (Wien)* 1987; 84: 105–109.

37. Williams B: A critical appraisal of posterior fossa surgery for communicating syringomyelia. *Brain* 1978; 101:223–250.

38. Williams B: The distending force in the production of "communicating syringomyelia." *Lancet* 1969; 2:189–193.

39. Williams B: Current concepts of syringomyelia. *Br J Hosp Med* 1970; 4:331–342.

40. Wisoff JH: Hydromyelia: A critical review. *Child Nerv Syst* 1988; 4:1–8.

41. Wisoff JH, Epstein F: Management of hydromyelia. *Neurosurgery* 1989; 25:562–571.

Albert L. Rhoton, Jr., M.D.

1. Batzdorf U: Chiari I malformation with syringomyelia: Evaluation of surgical therapy by magnetic resonance imaging. *J Neurosurg* 1988; 68:726–730.

2. Gardner WJ: Hydrodynamic mechanism of syringomyelia: Its relationship to myelocele. *J Neurol Neurosurg Psychiatry* 1965; 28: 247–259.

3. Gardner WJ: Myelocele: Rupture of the neural tube? *Clin Neurosurg* 1968; 15:57–79.

4. Gardner WJ, Angel J: The mechanism of syringomyelia and its surgical correction. *Clin Neurosurg* 1959; 6:131–140.

5. Ogilvy CS, Borges LF: Treatment of symptomatic syringomyelia with a ventriculoperitoneal shunt: A case report with magnetic resonance scan correlation. *Neurosurgery* 1988; 22:748–750.

6. Park TS, Cail WS, Broaddus WC, et al.: Lumboperitoneal shunt combined with myelotomy for treatment of syringohydromyelia. *J Neurosurg* 1989; 70:721–727.

7. Rhoton AL Jr: Microsurgery of Arnold-Chiari malformation in adults with and without hydromyelia. *J Neurosurg* 1976; 45: 473–483.

8. Rhoton AL Jr: Syringomyelia, in Wilson CB, Hoff JT (eds): *Current Surgical Management of Neurologic Disease.* New York, Churchill-Livingstone, 1980, pp 29–45.

9. Rhoton AL Jr, Fessler RG: Surgical treatment of Chiari malformation and hydromyelia in adults, in Wilson CB (ed): *Neurosurgical Procedures: Personal Approaches to Classic Operations.* Baltimore, Williams and Wilkins, 1992, pp 169–187.

Andrew D. Parent, M.D.

1. Ammonda RA, Ellenbogen GG, Foley KT, et al.: *Cine-mode CSF flow dynamics in craniovertebral junction anomalies* (abstract). Pediatric Section of Neurological Surgeons 21st Winter Meeting Program, Vancouver, BC, 1992, p 42.

2. Batzdorf U: *Syringomyelia: Current Concepts in Diagnosis and Treatment.* Baltimore, Williams and Wilkins, 1991.

3. Batzdorf U: Chiari I malformation with syringomyelia: Evaluation of surgical therapy by magnetic resonance imaging. *J Neurosurg* 1988; 68:726–730.

4. Gamache FW Jr, Ducker TB: Syringomyelia: A neurological and

surgical spectrum. *J Spinal Disord* 1990; 3:293–298.

5. Schlesinger EB: Letter to the editor. *Surg Neurol* 1992; 38:161–163.

6. Tachibana S, Iida H, Yada K: Significance of positive Queckenstedt test in patients with syringomyelia associated with Arnold-Chiari malformations. *J Neurosurg* 1992; 76:67–71.

7. Wasenko J, Hochhauser LJ, Winfield JA: *Primary tonsillar ectopia: Evaluation with cardiac gated phase contrast cinematographic magnetic resonance (CINE-MR)* (abstract). Pediatric Section of Neurological Surgeons 21st Winter Meeting Program, Vancouver, BC, 1992, p 43.

35

Treating Ulnar Entrapment within the Cubital Tunnel: Simple Decompression vs. Ulnar Release and Transposition

CASE

A 35-year-old man had a 6-month history of pain and paresthesia in the last 2 digits of his right hand. He had typical sensory loss in the ulnar distribution of his right hand and mild wasting of the hypothenar muscles. He had weak abduction of the index and little fingers of his right hand. Electrodiagnostic studies showed a conduction block across the elbow and denervation potentials in the hypothenar muscles.

PARTICIPANTS

Simple Decompression to Treat Ulnar Entrapment within the Cubital Tunnel–
    Suzie C. Tindall, M.D.

Ulnar Release and Transposition to Treat Ulnar Entrapment within the Cubital Tunnel–
    John E. McGillicuddy, M.D.

*Moderators–*David G. Kline, M.D., John Reeves, M.D.

Simple Decompression to Treat Ulnar Entrapment within the Cubital Tunnel

Suzie C. Tindall, M.D.

When confronted with a patient who has a rather classic ulnar nerve entrapment at the elbow and who has not responded to conservative treatment of the problem, the neurosurgeon has several operative choices. These include simple decompression, medial epicondylectomy, and several forms of transposition of the ulnar nerve. No consensus exists as to which is the best choice. Medial epicondylectomy is usually combined with an *in situ* release of the nerve and may draw most of its beneficial effect from this fact, rather than from the removal of the bony epicondyle. My personal experience with this operation consists of only 1 case, which was referred to me because the patient developed osteomyelitis at the site of the epicondylectomy.

TRANSPOSING THE ULNAR NERVE

There are many variations on the ulnar transposition procedure. The nerve can be transposed on top of or immediately under the forearm fascia; but this procedure lends itself to the complication of kinking of the nerve where it is tethered by the fascial sling. Intramuscular transposition creates a good deal of scar tissue around the nerve, which may cause long-term problems. If I have to transpose the ulnar nerve, I prefer the submuscular procedure. This procedure requires:

- General or regional anesthesia,
- Mobilization of the nerve over a long segment that almost always requires sacrifice of one or more small muscular branches and nutrient arteries,
- Section and repair of the flexor pronator muscle mass,
- Section of the intermuscular septum and transposition of the nerve onto the fascial plane, with the median nerve below the flexor muscles.

I transpose the nerve under the muscle if there is a pathologic lesion at the elbow that prohibits or hinders adequate simple decompression. Such instances are rare and include bony deformities, ganglions, or chondromatosis. Transposing the nerve also provides additional length for repair of an ulnar nerve laceration, but it is a much bigger procedure than simple decompression.

SIMPLE DECOMPRESSION

Simple decompression of the ulnar nerve can be done with the patient under local anesthesia and mild sedation. With simple decompression, the trouble and expense of more complicated anesthetic techniques are avoided. An incision 8 to 10 cm long is made on the medial side of the arm anterior to the medial epicondyle, and the soft tissues are separated to expose the cubital tunnel. The nerve is palpated and exposed about 4 to 6 cm below and above the elbow. With sharp dissection, the nerve is then followed through the cubital tunnel and the aponeurosis and muscle between the 2 heads of the flexor carpi ulnaris muscle are serially sectioned. The nerve is moved out of the groove, but care is taken not to injure any of its branches or the small blood vessels nourishing it. The nerve is left lying free in the subcutaneous tissues. Postoperatively, the patient's arm is not placed in a splint and the patient is encouraged to move the arm early in the recovery period.

This technique is simple, straightforward and, in the hands of an experienced neurosurgeon, seems to be a satisfactory approach to the problem.[3] Unless valid data are produced to support the superiority of other, more complicated, procedures, I will continue to favor simple decompression in all uncomplicated cases.

DISCUSSION

Studies attempting to resolve the issue of which surgical technique is superior in treating ulnar nerve compression at the elbow are flawed by retrospective analysis, a failure to differentiate the various causes of ulnar nerve entrapment, and the small numbers of procedures.[4] In a purely retrospective study, Chan and colleagues[1] studied 235 patients with ulnar neuropathy at the elbow. The treatment was simple decompression in 115 patients and anterior transposition in 120 patients. Both simple decompression and anterior transposition resulted in improvement in 82% of patients; however, a higher percentage of full recovery occurred in the patients treated with simple decompression. In 1990, LeRoux and colleagues[2] reported their experience with 51 patients undergoing decompression without nerve transposition. In all of their patients, the nerve was compressed predominantly in the epicondylar groove. Eighty percent of their patients had symptomatic improvement after decompression. These authors concluded that decompression without transposition of the ulnar nerve is effective in treating selected cases of ulnar compressive neuropathy at the elbow.

Ulnar Release and Transposition to Treat Ulnar Entrapment within the Cubital Tunnel

John E. McGillicuddy, M.D.

This patient has the clinical findings characteristic of a severe and progressive ulnar neuropathy at the elbow. The atrophy and electromyographic evidence of denervation in his hypothenar muscles places him in the severe category of any of the classifications of ulnar palsy.[11,15,29] Because the patient has no history of an acute injury, his brief history coupled with the severity of the lesion indicates a rapid progression of a chronic type of nerve injury. The young age of onset suggests that extrinsic factors, such as compression of the nerve from resting his elbows frequently on hard surfaces or repetitive flexion-extension of the elbow in heavy manual labor, have played an important role in the evolution of this injury. The severity of his palsy precludes any conservative therapy; he is clearly a candidate for prompt surgical relief of his nerve compression.

Many procedures have been described to treat ulnar nerve entrapment at the elbow. These procedures can be divided into two groups:

- *In situ* decompression of the nerve in the elbow area, frequently termed cubital tunnel release;
- Anterior transposition of the nerve out of the retrocondylar area.

Operations that transpose the nerve anterior to the medial epicondyle are further classified according to the eventual location of the ulnar nerve as follows: subcutaneous, intramuscular within the substance of the flexor-pronator muscle mass, or submuscular beneath this muscle mass. Submuscular placement requires transection of the muscle mass at the medial epicondyle and repair of the muscle after the nerve is placed beneath it.[21,26] Each type of procedure is strongly advocated in a large number of reports. Currently, *in situ* decompression appears to be the more favored approach.[9,22,30,37] Nevertheless, I would treat this patient, and most patients with ulnar nerve compression at the elbow, through an anterior subcutaneous transposition of the nerve.

RATIONALE FOR CHOOSING THE PROCEDURE

This choice of operation to treat ulnar palsy at the elbow is based on an understanding of the pathophysiology of this condition, critical review of the literature, and evaluation of the factors causing nerve compression in the patient at hand. The literature shows no clear indications to support any one surgical procedure as the best operation for ulnar neuropathy at the elbow.[11] Despite a large body of information on surgical techniques and results, few definite conclusions can be derived from this data.[1,9,14,20,23,27] There have been no prospective, randomized studies comparing outcomes, and almost all of the available comparison studies have some flaws in their construction, rendering their results inconclusive. The results of treatment appear more closely related to the severity of ulnar neuropathy than to the type of surgical procedure.[1,11,14,17]

In the absence of clear guidelines for treatment, the choice of operation usually reflects the training, biases, and experiences of the surgeon. Although that is the case in the current decision, I believe that transposition can also be shown objectively to be a better method of treatment than *in situ* decompression. Having decided to transpose the ulnar nerve, I believe that subcutaneous placement can be shown to be as effective as the submuscular procedure, with similar long-term results. In addition, subcutaneous transposition requires less extensive surgery and avoids prolonged immobilization.

CAUSES OF ULNAR NEUROPATHY

Compression of the ulnar nerve at the elbow was originally thought to stem from stretch and friction of the nerve around the medial epicondyle after elbow trauma, especially after fractures that disrupted the normal anatomy.[2] For this reason, early attempts to treat the problem concentrated on removing the nerve from its place in the retrocondylar area by transposing it anterior to the epicondyle. Thus, anterior transposition is the oldest treatment for ulnar neuropathy, and it has generally stood the test of time. The condition once called *post-traumatic ulnar palsy* is now known to stem from a wide variety of other factors. The exposed subcutaneous position of the ulnar nerve in the retrocondylar area makes it vulnerable to acute and chronic external trauma. Repetitive pressure on the nerve, frequent flexion-extension of the elbow with the arms extended, as in heavy manual labor, and persistent intrinsic pressure on the nerve from degenerative osteophytes or bone chips at the elbow joint are well-recognized causes of ulnar palsy. Long-standing deformity from an old elbow fracture, the classical tardy ulnar palsy, or from cubitus valgus are also important causes, as is recurrent subluxation of the nerve over the medial epicondyle. Patients with these clearly definable causes, and other more rare entities such as lipomas, ganglions, and rheumatoid arthritis, comprise at least 50% of cases of ulnar neuropathy at the elbow.[26] In nearly all patients with ulnar nerve palsies caused by these conditions, treatment requires transposition of the nerve away from the compressing mass.

More recently, the percentage of ulnar palsy resulting from elbow fracture decreased and most ulnar neuropathy at the elbow now stems from other causes. This shift in etiologic factors increased the importance of that group of patients in whom no obvious cause for their neuropathy could be found. It was in this group of "idiopathic" patients that Osborne[31] first noted compression of the ulnar nerve as it passed beneath a fibrous arch between the 2 heads of the flexor carpi ulnaris muscle distal to the medial epicondyle. He described an abrupt constriction of the nerve under the leading edge of this band, the arcuate ligament, and pronounced thickening or pseudoneuroma of the nerve immediately proximal to this. He found that symptoms could be relieved if the nerve was decompressed by dividing the band, and concluded that transposition was not necessary. At nearly the same time, Feindel and Stratford[13] reported on 3 patients with similar findings. They described and named the cubital tunnel, the narrow area beneath the fibrous aponeurosis. They also relieved the neuropathy by simple division of the aponeurosis, and termed the procedure a *cubital tunnel release*. This technique quickly became widespread by virtue of its simplicity. A large number of articles soon appeared in the literature advocating simple decompression as the preferred treatment for all patients with ulnar entrapment at the elbow.[34,35,37] The reported results of this procedure were acceptable: good to excellent outcomes in about 80% of patients.

These clinical reports were supported by studies of the anatomy and biomechanics of the ulnar nerve and the cubital tunnel. The fibers of the aponeurosis, anchored at the medial epicondyle and the olecranon, stretch by 5 mm for each 45 degrees of elbow flexion.[35] This stretching of the roof of the tunnel decreases its diameter by 2.5 mm in flexion.[4] Intraneural pressure within the ulnar nerve in the intact tunnel increases nearly threefold during flexion and is decreased by 40% if the aponeurosis is divided.[32] These findings showed a significant role for the cubital tunnel aponeurosis in the evolution of compressive ulnar neuropathy at the elbow, and have been used by advocates of local decompression to support the rationale of their procedure.

Unfortunately, these findings have led to a relative neglect of other important aspects of ulnar neuropathy. These include the exposed subcutaneous position of the nerve in the retrocondylar area and its location behind the axis of rotation of the elbow. This renders the nerve vulnerable to external compressive trauma and causes the nerve to both slide in the retrocondylar groove and stretch 5 mm during elbow flexion.[4] The combination of exposure and movement in this area can predispose to chronic irritation of the nerve from external trauma and may lead to inflammation and swelling of the nerve and surrounding tissues. Progression of inflammation to extraneural scarring will decrease and eventually prevent the normal movement of the nerve; sliding movement stops and the stretch must occur over a shorter length of nerve, leading to microstretch injuries and the internal edema, hyperemia, and eventual fibrosis described by Lundborg.[25] Scarring in the retrocondylar area is often circumferential and is relieved neither by dividing the cubital tunnel aponeurosis nor by opening the superficial layer of scar overlying the nerve more proximally, as is advised by some authors.

The term *cubital tunnel* is, unfortunately, now often used to refer to a wider area than was described by the original authors; the retrocondylar area is frequently included in the tunnel and cubital tunnel decompression usually involves freeing the nerve in this area also.[22,35] Unroofing the nerve in both the cubital tunnel and the retrocondylar area appears to dispose it to subluxation,[35] leaving it directly over the medial epicondyle where it is vulnerable to trauma. If the abrupt constriction and pseudoneuroma of classic cubital tunnel compression are found, simple division of the aponeurosis should suffice, but these findings are noted in less than half of decompressive procedures.[1,34] Patients who do not improve after *in situ* decompression often did not have the classic findings at surgery.[9,27] Some advocates of *in situ* procedures have suggested that, if the decompression must be extended into the retrocondylar area or if a typical pseudoneuroma is not found, an anterior transposition should be done.[9,35]

The importance of pathologic processes in the retrocondylar area is seen in the results of intraoperative nerve conduction studies. In these studies, most nerves tested showed slowing in the retrocondylar area and not in the cubital tunnel.[7,8] Kline and Happel[19] found only 5 examples of slowed conduction in the cubital tunnel in 350 patients tested; the remainder showed slowing at or proximal to the retrocondylar area. Thus, it appears that most cases with involvement severe enough to cause conduction changes stem from nerve injury outside the confines of the cubital tunnel.

In situ decompression can deal successfully with those instances of ulnar neuropathy caused by compression within the cubital tunnel, but not with those stemming from other causes. Only anterior transposition relieves all possible causes of ulnar nerve compression at the elbow. If the results of the 2 procedures are equivalent, transposition should be preferred for most patients.

COMPARISON OF OPERATIVE RESULTS

The numerous recent reports of good results after *in situ* decompression[10,22,30] can be balanced by reports of similar results after transposition.[4,16,24] The principle thrust of many advocates of decompression is that the results of their procedure are as good as the results of transposition, not that they are better. They infer that transposition has a higher rate of late failure from the consequences of moving the nerve, such as ischemia, kinking, and tension, and promote simple decompression as a theoretically safer and simpler operation.

After a detailed review of 50 published reports of the treatment of ulnar nerve palsy at the elbow comprising over 2000 patients, Dellon[11] concluded that no statistically significant advantage of one technique over another could be shown. The results of treatment were more closely related to the severity of nerve compression than to the type of surgical procedure. Nonetheless, there was a trend toward better results after transposition, especially in patients with more severe grades of compression. Decompression and transposition had nearly equal and highly successful results when used to treat mild cases of ulnar

neuropathy. When more severe neuropathy was treated, transposition, either subcutaneous or submuscular, had a higher percentage of good results than did simple decompression. Only about 33% of patients in the moderate group had improved strength and sensation after decompression alone, but 71% of those undergoing transposition had normal sensation and 45% had improved strength. This slight advantage of transposition techniques in the more severe neuropathies is also seen in other reports.[14,27]

Advocates of *in situ* decompression often infer that transposition procedures have a higher incidence of complications and recurrence. There is little evidence to support this belief, which may stem from 2 widely cited reports of reoperation for recurrent palsy after transposition.[5,15] In fact, recurrent symptoms occur in 15 to 20% of patients after either procedure.[11,12] Holmberg[18] has recently reported on 16 patients with failed decompressive procedures who were treated successfully through transposition. The principal reasons for failure and recurrence in transposition operations stem from correctable technical factors.[5,15] In most cases, the nerve was compressed by an unresected medial intermuscular septum, a fascial sling, or inadequate opening of the flexor carpi ulnaris muscle fascia.

Based on these results and on the pathophysiological findings, simple decompression should be used only when symptoms are mild, when there is clear evidence of constriction of the nerve at the aponeurosis, and when there is no evidence of scarring in the retrocondylar groove.

SUBCUTANEOUS PLACEMENT OF THE NERVE

Although the results of submuscular transposition have been reported to give slightly better results,[11] I prefer to use a subcutaneous transposition. It is a simpler operation, the flexor-pronator muscle mass need not be transected and repaired and, thus, there is no need for prolonged immobilization.

Submuscular transposition is a complex and lengthy technical procedure requiring considerable expertise. The rather small increase in the percentage of good results with submuscular placement does not seem to justify the extra surgery in primary cases. Subcutaneous transposition is often recommended for athletes because it does not disrupt the anchor of an important muscle mass.[28]

Subcutaneous procedures are alleged to have a higher risk of late failure secondary to fibrosis around the transposed nerve.[3] There have been a few well-documented instances of subcutaneous fibrosis constricting the ulnar nerve in the late postoperative period, but the details of the original procedure are not available.[6] It is possible that prolonged immobilization after transposition may predispose to local nerve adhesions; MacKinnon and Dellon[26] have shown that if immobilization is limited to 2 weeks, no adhesions form around the transposed ulnar nerve in a primate model. A recent study comparing subcutaneous and submuscular transpositions has shown that subcutaneous transpositions have good long-term results—there were no relapses in 33 patients followed for an average of 9 years.[33]

OPERATIVE TECHNIQUE

I use an anterior subcutaneous transposition in nearly all patients. I reserve *in situ* decompression for those who have a positive Tinel's sign at the entrance of the cubital tunnel distal to the medial epicondyle, and for patients with concurrent neuropathy from diabetes or other microvascular disease in whom the minor changes in neural blood supply caused by mobilizing the nerve might cause significant ischemia. I do a submuscular transposition in muscular patients with scant subcutaneous tissue and in reoperations for failed subcutaneous transposition, which is a rare occurrence in my experience. Intramuscular transposition does not seem to offer any advantages.[36]

The patient is positioned supine with the arm extended 90 degrees and externally rotated on an arm board. I prefer a brachial plexus block to general anesthesia and never use a tourniquet. After standard skin preparation and draping, a lazy omega-shaped incision is made from a point 10 cm proximal to the medial epicondyle and extending along the medial bicipital groove, curving laterally into the antecubital fossa to a point one fingerbreadth medial to the biceps tendon. The incision then curves medially over the flexor-pronator muscles to a point overlying the medial surface of the flexor carpi ulnaris muscle 8 cm distal to the epicondyle (Fig. 1). The subcutaneous tissue is initially divided distally and is carried down to the fascia of the flexor muscles. A plane is developed in the loose connective tissue between this fascia and the subcutaneous adipose tissue on the ulnar side of the incision. The incision is then extended proximally and the subcutaneous plane developed throughout the length of the incision. The posterior branch of the medial antebrachial cutaneous nerve can be identified crossing the incision. This branch can be preserved by dissecting it free. The subcutaneous plane is easily developed toward the medial epicondyle. As the plane is extended in the proximal part of the incision, the medial intermuscular septum is identified and the fascia between the septum and the medial head of the triceps (the arcade of Struthers) is exposed.

The ulnar nerve can be identified proximal to the epicondyle at the posterior margin of the septum, and the overlying fascia is slit proximally for 8 cm, exposing the nerve well up the medial bicipital groove. With the nerve in view, the subcutaneous plane is extended beyond the epicondyle into the retrocondylar groove, exposing the groove, the cubital tunnel retinaculum, and the heads of the flexor carpi ulnaris muscle. Placing a few folded towels under the elbow enhances the exposure at this point and keeps the elbow slightly flexed. The often thick connective tissue covering the ulnar nerve in this area is divided and the incision carried through the aponeurosis between the heads of the flexor carpi ulnaris. Only the surface fascia of the muscle itself is divided over the course of the nerve and the muscle fibers are gently spread apart over the nerve, exposing the nerve within the muscle.

With the nerve exposed throughout the length of the skin incision, it is dissected free from surrounding soft tissue beginning proximal to the elbow. Careful dissection preserves some vascular branches to the nerve and the nerve is supported on drains as it is freed. In the retrocondylar area, dissection is usually more difficult as the nerve may be adherent on its deep surface. Dividing the ulnar sensory branches to the elbow joint helps release the nerve. As dissection extends into the flexor carpi ulnaris muscle, the surgeon sees several branches to the muscle that prevent mobilization of the nerve. The branches loosely adhere to the main body of the nerve and can easily be dissected back along the nerve for 3 to 5 cm, untethering the nerve and allowing it to be transposed over the medial epicondyle. Loupes and iris scissors are useful in this step. While the nerve is being dissected along its length, it should be tested frequently for its fit into place in the antecubital fossa. The freed

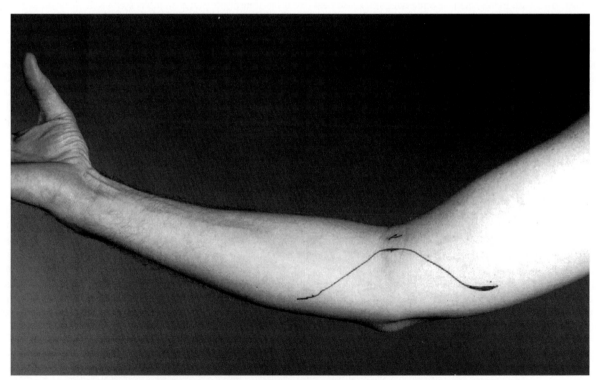

Fig. 1 The incision for ulnar release begins 10 cm proximal to the medial epicondyle and extends along the medial bicipital groove. From there, it curves laterally into the antecubital fossa to a point 1 fingerbreadth medial to the biceps tendon. The curve travels medially over the flexor-pronator muscles to a point overlying the medial surface of the flexor carpi ulnaris muscle 8 cm distal to the epicondyle.

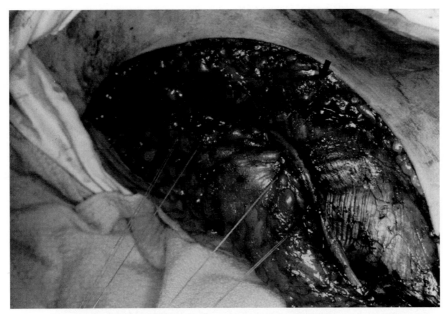

A

B

Fig. 2 (*A*) **Several absorbable sutures (arrowheads) tie the deep surface of the subcutaneous flap to the flexor muscle fascia. The skin flap is advanced slightly in the radial direction and sutured to the fascia (arrow) close to the ulnar side of the transposed nerve. (*B*) The nerve is kept in place by a wall of adipose tissue secured from a proximal-to-distal direction across the antecubital fossa.**

ulnar nerve should rest about 2 fingerbreadths medial to the biceps tendon and should remain there without any tension or kinking, especially at the proximal and distal extremes of its exposure. Resection of the medial intermuscular septum is essential at this point. The transposed nerve can be kinked over this thin, tough structure, and it must be totally removed.

Once the nerve is in its new bed, provisions must be made to keep it there. A number of techniques have been proposed for this purpose; some, like a sling constructed from flexor muscle fascia, have been associated with a high incidence of recurrent compression.[5,15] I prefer to use several absorbable sutures to tie the deep surface of the subcutaneous flap to the flexor muscle

fascia, advancing the skin flap slightly in the radial direction and suturing it to the fascia close to the ulnar side of the transposed nerve (Fig. 2). The nerve is, thus, kept in place by a wall of adipose tissue secured from a proximal-to-distal direction across the antecubital fossa. I have seen only 1 instance of recurrent subluxation in over 150 patients undergoing this technique. After the ulnar nerve is securely but loosely held in the antecubital fossa, it must be inspected along its length in both flexion and extension to ascertain that no kinking or tension exists; in fact, the nerve is usually slightly redundant in flexion. Subcutaneous tissue and skin is closed over the nerve in standard fashion. The arm is wrapped in a bulky dressing that is left in place for 2 days.

After the dressing is removed, full, nonstrenuous use of the arm is encouraged. Unrestricted activity is allowed 3 to 4 weeks after the procedure.

Although some writers have expressed concern that the ulnar nerve may be subject to external trauma in this location, personal experience and common sense indicate that it is less likely to be injured here than in its original location in the condylar groove. To date, none of my patients has sustained a blunt injury to the transposed nerve. However, all patients must be warned not to allow blood to be drawn from the antecubital fossa lest the nerve be punctured. Concerns about late entrapment of the nerve in subcutaneous scar appear to be unfounded. The incision is so designed that the scar crosses the transposed nerve at only 2 points, and early mobilization may prevent adhesions along the course of the nerve. In the series of patients treated at this institution, none has required reoperation for recurrent ulnar neuropathy from subcutaneous scarring.

CONCLUSION

In summary, anterior transposition is the better operation for ulnar neuropathy at the elbow because it treats all the causes of this condition, appears to have better results in the more severe cases, and is less likely to lead to subluxation of the nerve. This procedure also should have a low rate of late failure if careful attention is paid to complete resection of the medial intermuscular septum, and to the prevention of kinking and tension of the nerve in its transposed position.

Treating Ulnar Entrapment within the Cubital Tunnel: Simple Decompression vs. Ulnar Release and Transposition

David G. Kline, M.D., John Reeves, M.D.

Surgical treatment of ulnar entrapment is among the most controversial in all of medicine. Both authors have thoroughly and accurately stated their respective and opposite positions. Simple decompression with neurolysis, but without transposition, has been succinctly outlined and neurolysis with transposition and subcutaneous placement has been thoroughly reviewed and presented. Both authors correctly point out that there has not been a prospective controlled or randomized study of this issue. Several thoughtful reviews of the literature have been published, however, as well as an occasional thorough, but retrospective study.[2,8,10]

Most surgeons who treat ulnar entrapment neuropathy would agree that simple decompression is not enough if the patient has bony lesions or deformities at the elbow level. Most also agree that transposition is a larger and somewhat more complex procedure, but seems to do more for the patients with more severe neuropathies than simple decompression does. On the other hand, milder forms of entrapment neuropathy appear to be treated just as well through decompression without transposition, as through decompression with transposition.[4] Although we acknowledge the benefits of both the decompressive and the subcutaneous transposition operations, we favor a third approach—neurolysis and submuscular placement of the nerve.

HISTORY OF EXPERIENCE

Our own work began with patients at Charity Hospital, now the Medical Center of Louisiana, some 28 years ago. These patients with ulnar neuropathy had a relatively high incidence of trauma to the elbow in the past or, because of their occupations, were prone to heavy and repetitive arm use in flexion and extension. Some patients were also used to resting their elbows on bar tops, tables, and chair arms. Many of these patients lived a life close to, if not on, the streets. For these reasons, we elected from the beginning of our series to not only do a neurolysis and transposition to move the nerve out of harm's way, but also to place it deep in a submuscular position.

In the interim, our source of patients with entrapment has expanded beyond the Charity Hospital census and includes a large number of patients from other walks of life and with spontaneous nontraumatic palsies, unassociated with other lesions. In addition, we have seen a relatively large number of patients who have had prior unsuccessful attempts at treatment, including simple neurolysis, medial epicondylectomy, subcutaneous transposition, and intramuscular but not submuscular placement of the nerve.

We have persisted in using a modified Learmouth approach for the problem, regardless of whether the patient has undergone previous surgery.[6-8] Neurolysis well above and below the elbow and placement of the nerve beneath both pronator teres and flexor carpi ulnaris has been the usual objective. We have done simple decompression and neurolysis without transposition on only 4 patients, all physicians who insisted on this operation rather than the larger transposition procedure.

ULNAR TRANSPOSITION AND SUBMUSCULAR PLACEMENT

For the procedure, the patient's arm is placed palm up on an arm board with a folded towel beneath the elbow to position it uppermost. A slightly undulating skin incision is made from the medial surface of the distal arm toward the medial but volar surface of the elbow and then along the proximal and medial side of the forearm. Antebrachial cutaneous nerves are preserved and, if possible, moved toward the radial side of the forearm. The ulnar nerve can be easily located within the olecranon notch and then traced proximally into the arm and distally into the forearm. We have usually identified the nerve first in the arm where it adheres to the superior muscle fibers of the flexor carpi ulnaris, and is sometimes covered by fibers from the medial head of the triceps (the arcade of Struthers).

Major branches proximal to the flexor carpi ulnaris should be preserved whenever possible. If need be, branches can be dissected back and split away from the main trunk of the ulnar nerve so they are lengthened in preparation for transposition. There may also be major collateral vascular input to the nerve at this level, which should be dissected out and preserved, if possible. A segment of intermuscular septum is resected so that the course of the nerve in the distal upper arm is free after the transposition. The nerve is then encircled with a drain. Dissection can then proceed by following the nerve distally and unroofing the olecranon notch. The nerve is re-encircled with a drain and dissected in a circumferential fashion as it enters the proximal forearm. The ulnar nerve lies deep to the 2 heads of the flexor carpi ulnaris but above the flexor superficialis. A longitudinal incision can be made through the fascia of the flexor carpi ulnaris and the fibers of the muscle split to expose the deeper portion of the ulnar nerve in the forearm. Smaller branches to the flexor carpi ulnaris may be encountered just distal to the notch; these can either be dissected back into the main ulnar nerve to lengthen them for transposition or they can be sectioned.

Branches to the ulnar half of the flexor profundus arise several centimeters distal to the notch and are preserved. The ulnar nerve is cleared to 10 cm or so below the olecranon notch and encircled with another drain. Dissection is then carried into the olecranon notch alternatively from the upper arm and forearm levels. The bipolar coagulator is needed because both arteries and veins accompany the nerve and are deep to it, lying on the floor of the notch. Neural branches to the elbow joint, which are usually small, can be sacrificed.

After the nerve is completely freed, it is ready for transposition. The radial side of the pronator teres is dissected distally, and some of the lacertus fibrosis is sectioned to mobilize the proximal pronator muscle. Some of the origins of the pronator and flexor carpi ulnaris are then undermined over the medial epicondyle. A trough is made, in an oblique and slightly curved fashion, all the way through the pronator and proximal portions of the flexor carpi ulnaris. The detached distal muscle mass is then gently elevated and undermined, as is that portion left attached to the medial epicondyle.

The ulnar nerve is then placed in the muscle trough, and some fascia and superficial pronator muscle is reattached with sutures to a cuff of muscle and fascia on the medial epicondyle. The flexor carpi ulnaris is also reattached to the cuff of muscle along the distal portion of the medial epicondyle. The flexor carpi ulnaris is then closed over the nerve, but not before the surgeon gently grasps the nerve proximally and distally with the gloved fingers to make sure it moves freely with a gentle tug back and forth beneath the already partially re-closed volar musculature. The longitudinal split in the more distal flexor carpi ulnaris is closed only superficially, so as not to compress the underlying nerve.

If the patient has undergone a previous operation, the older elbow incision is used again, but usually extended proximally into the arm and distally down the forearm. This is especially necessary if a short elbow-level incision was used for a medial epicondylectomy or a neurolysis without transposition at the elbow level. Because of the prior operation and, usually, a subcutaneous position of the previously transposed nerve, a good deal of scar tissue is almost always encountered. In this regard, it is helpful to extend the proximal exposure enough to find more healthy nerve and then to trace the nerve through the scar and previously placed tacking sutures with sharp dissection, using a number 15 blade on a plastic scalpel handle. In some cases, the distal nerve at the forearm level must be located and worked back toward and through the elbow-level scar.

OPERATIVE OBSERVATIONS ON THE LOCUS OF ENTRAPMENT

The exact laws of ulnar entrapment at the level of the elbow can be difficult to ascertain in noninvasive studies.[1] In an attempt to verify the locus of the entrapment or irritacubitive lesion to the ulnar nerve, we stimulate and record directly from the nerve across the olecranon notch before clearing the nerve through this region. This maneuver is then repeated at multiple sites after the nerve is mobilized. Recording electrodes are first placed at the arm level and then moved distally onto the segment of the nerve at the olecranon notch, then the segment subtended by the cubital tunnel and, finally, to the more distal forearm level.

Observations about the causes of ulnar entrapment are:

1. Direct operative recording gave conductions across the elbow that were usually significantly slower than those done noninvasively. Operative recording distances were shorter and, thus, involved a comparatively more abnormal than normal length of nerve than the preoperative noninvasive studies.
2. Both the amplitude and velocity of the signal almost always decreased in the segment of the nerve located in the olecranon notch. In 20% of patients, these conductive abnormalities began at an arm level just proximal to the notch. In either case, these abnormalities persisted through the area of the notch and distally to the forearm level.
3. In only 5 patients were the signal changes compatible with a more distal entrapment or what has been termed a *cubital tunnel syndrome*.[5]

In most patients, the nerve was either slightly swollen and hyperemic along its course through the olecranon notch or was narrowed and enveloped by thickened tissue at that site. The gross findings thus fit with the electrical observations, which suggested that the entrapment or irritative problem usually was centered within the notch and not more distal beneath the 2 heads of the flexor carpi ulnaris.

In the few cases of cubital tunnel seen, the conductive abnormalities began along the distal portion of the nerve in the olecranon notch but were maximal in the region of the 2 heads of the flexor carpi ulnaris. Thus, few cases of ulnar entrapment are really centered at a forearm level beneath the heads of the flexor carpi ulnaris. To date, such observations have suggested to us the need for transposition rather than simple neurolysis.

If a prior ulnar entrapment operation failed and the patient was subsequently referred to us, we also did neurolysis and submuscular burial.[2] Findings on reoperation were sometimes striking but variable:

1. Most nerves were enveloped in scar, which was sometimes intraneural and associated with neuroma, presumably related to trauma at the time of the prior operation.
2. With either an epicondylectomy or simple neurolysis, the nerve was partially riding up on what was left of the epicondyle or the latter, itself.[9] The proximal intermuscular septum or, more often, the more distal flexor carpi ulnaris had not been divided, so the distal nerve was sometimes kinked or angulated.
3. With prior subcutaneous transposition that failed, the nerve was usually quite scarred and often angulated or kinked, especially distally where the flexor carpi ulnaris had not been adequately sectioned or cleared.
4. In a few additional patients, damaged or neuromatous antebrachial cutaneous nerves were found.[3]

RESULTS

We used a grading system concentrating on both ulnar-innervated hand intrinsics and sensory function (Table 1). Preoperative grades were compared to those recorded postoperatively. These patients formed a group of 368 patients with 1 year or more of follow-up (Table 2). Seventy-two were not operated upon but were followed for a year or more, and 82 patients had had a prior operation. In the nonoperative category, grades remained stable for the most part, although 12 (15%) of the 72 patients improved spontaneously. On the other hand, 3 other patients in the nonoperative group had decreased function with time and, yet, still refused surgery. In the 214 previously nonoperated patients, 154 improved their level of motor, and usually also sensory, function after neurolysis. Although function re-

mained unchanged in 52 patients, 10 of these already had excellent function preoperatively (grade 5), and 28 had good function preoperatively (grade 4).

As might be expected, it was harder to improve function in those patients who had undergone a prior ulnar nerve operation. Twenty-five of these 82 patients were unchanged and 1 patient's symptoms deteriorated. Nonetheless, 45 improved 1 grade and 10 improved 2 grades.

In a group of 144 patients with 3 or more years of follow-up, 84 had no prior operation and 60 had had one. In the freshly operated group of 84, 51% improved 1 grade, 26% improved 2, 10% improved 3 or 4 grades, and 12% were unchanged; 1 patient (1%) was made worse.

In the group of 60 patients undergoing a prior operation, 53% improved 1 grade, 17% improved 2 grades, 2% improved 3 grades, and 28% had no change in grade.

We were pleased that the functional grades were as good as they were postoperatively, especially in those patients previously operated. An additional analysis comparing grades of patients with severe or moderate levels of pain and a variable degree of neuropathy is in process.

A carefully done neurolysis and submuscular transposition is an effective treatment of ulnar entrapment. This operation offers the advantage that it not only moves the nerve away from the trouble site or mechanism for entrapment, but also usually places the injured segment of the nerve at a deep and protected level in the forearm.

Table 1. Grading of Ulnar Entrapment

Grade	Intrinsics	Sensation
0	No hand intrinsics	Sensation grades 0–1
1	No hand intrinsics	Sensation 1–3
2	Hand intrinsics are traced (1) to antigravity (2)	Sensation 2–4
3	Hand intrinsics = 3	Sensation = 3 or higher
4	Hand intrinsics = 4	Sensation = 4 or 5
5	Hand intrinsics = 5	Sensation = 4 or 5

Table 2. Preoperative Grade to Postoperative Grades for Ulnar Entrapment*

Initial grade to last follow-up	Initial operation	Reoperated cases†	Nonoperated cases
2 to 2	3	3	9
2 to 3	10	2	1
2 to 4	12	2	0
3 to 0	0	2	0
3 to 3	11	2	6
3 to 4	40	16	3
3 to 5	40	7	0
4 to 4	28	15	16
4 to 5	52	25	8
5 to 5	10	4	20
5 to 4	0	0	3
Subtotal	206	78	66
Results not known	8	2	6
Totals	214	78	72
Total procedures: 368			

*Patients had 1 or more years of follow-up.
†Patients undergoing prior neurolysis or transposition.
(Reproduced with permission from: Kline D, Hudson A: *Operative Results of Major Nerve Injuries, Entrapments, and Tumors.* Philadelphia, WB Saunders, 1995.)

REFERENCES

Suzie C. Tindall, M.D.

1. Chan RC, Paine KWE, Varughese G: Ulnar neuropathy at the elbow: Comparison of simple decompression and anterior transposition. *Neurosurgery* 1980; 7:545–550.

2. LeRoux PD, Ensign TD, Burchiel KJ: Surgical decompression without transposition for ulnar neuropathy: Factors determining outcome. *Neurosurgery* 1990; 27:709–714.

3. Rengachary SS: Entrapment neuropathies, in Wilkins RH, Rengachary SS (eds): *Neurosurgery*, vol 2. New York, McGraw-Hill, 1985, pp 1783–1785.

4. Tindall SC: Chronic injuries of peripheral nerves by entrapment, in Youmans JR (ed): *Neurological Surgery*, vol. 4, ed. 3. Philadelphia, WB Saunders, 1990, pp 2511–2542.

John E. McGillicuddy, M.D.

1. Adelaar RS, Foster WC, McDowell C: The treatment of cubital tunnel syndrome. *J Hand Surg* 1984; 9A:90–95.

2. Adson AW: Progressive ulnar paralysis. *Minn Med* 1918; 1:455–460.

3. Amadio PC: Anatomical basis for a technique of ulnar nerve transposition. *Surg Radiol Anat* 1986; 8:155–161.

4. Apfelberg DB, Larson SJ: Dynamic anatomy of the ulnar nerve at the elbow. *Plast Reconstr Surg* 1973; 51:76–81.

5. Broudy AS, Leffert RD, Smith RJ: Technical problems with ulnar nerve transposition at the elbow: Findings and results of reoperation. *J Hand Surg* 1978; 3:85–89.

6. Campbell JB, Post KD, Morantz RA: A technique for relief of motor and sensory deficits occurring after anterior ulnar transposition. *J Neurosurg* 1974; 40:405–409.

7. Campbell WW, Pridgeon RM, Sahni KS: Short segment incremental studies in the evaluation of ulnar neuropathy at the elbow. *Muscle Nerve* 1992; 15:1050–1054.

8. Campbell WW, Sahni KS, Pridgeon RM, et al.: Intraoperative neurography: Management of ulnar neuropathy at the elbow. *Muscle Nerve* 1988; 11:75–81.

9. Chan RC, Paine KWE, Varughese G: Ulnar neuropathy at the elbow: Comparison of simple decompression and anterior transposition. *Neurosurgery* 1980; 7:545–550.

10. Davies MA, Vonau M, Blum PW, et al.: Results of ulnar neuropathy at the elbow treated by decompression or anterior transposition. *Aust NZ J Surg* 1991; 61:929–934.

11. Dellon AL: Review of treatment results for ulnar nerve entrapment at the elbow. *J Hand Surg* 1989; 14A:688–700.

12. Dellon AL, MacKinnon SE, Hudson AR, et al.: Effect of submuscular versus intramuscular placement of ulnar nerve: Experimental model in the primate. *J Hand Surg* 1986; 11B:117–119.

13. Feindel W, Stratford J: The role of the cubital tunnel in tardy ulnar palsy. *Can J Surg* 1958; 1:287–300.

14. Foster RJ, Edshage S: Factors related to the outcome of surgically managed compressive ulnar neuropathy at the elbow level. *J Hand Surg* 1981; 6:181–192.

15. Gabel GT, Amadio PC: Reoperation for failed decompression of the ulnar nerve in the region of the elbow. *J Bone Joint Surg* 1990; 72A:213–219.

16. Hagstrom P: Ulnar nerve compression at the elbow: Results of surgery in 85 cases. *Scand J Plast Reconstr Surg* 1977; 11:59–62.

17. Harrison MJG, Nurick S: Results of anterior transposition of the ulnar nerve for ulnar neuritis. *Br Med J* 1970; 1:27–29.

18. Holmberg J: Reoperation in high ulnar neuropathy. *Scand J Plast Reconstr Surg* 1991; 25:173–176.

19. Kline DG, Happel LT: A quarter century's experience with intra-operative nerve action potential recording. *Can J Neurol Sci* 1993; 20:3–10.

20. Laha RK, Panchal PD: Surgical treatment of ulnar neuropathy. *Surg Neurol* 1979; 11:393–398.

21. Leffert RD: Anterior submuscular transposition of the ulnar nerves by the Learmonth technique. *J Hand Surg* 1982; 7A:147–155.

22. LeRoux PD, Ensign TD, Burchiel KJ: Surgical decompression without transposition for ulnar neuropathy: Factors determining outcome. *Neurosurgery* 1990; 27:709–714.

23. Levy DM, Apfelberg DB: Results of anterior transposition for ulnar neuropathy at the elbow. *Am J Surg* 1972; 123:304–308.

24. Lugnegard H, Walheim G, Wennberg A: Operative treatment of ulnar neuropathy in the elbow region. *Acta Orthop Scand* 1977; 48:168–176.

25. Lundborg G: Surgical treatment for ulnar nerve entrapment at the elbow. *J Hand Surg* 1992; 17B:245–247.

26. MacKinnon SE, Dellon AL: *Surgery of the Peripheral Nerve*. New York, Thieme, 1988.

27. MacNicol MF: The results of operation for ulnar neuritis. *J Bone Joint Surg* 1979; 61B:159–164.

28. MacPhearson SA, Meals RA: Cubital tunnel syndrome. *Orthop Clin North Am* 1992; 23:111–123.

29. McGowan AJ: The results of transposition of the ulnar nerve for ulnar neuritis. *J Bone Joint Surg* 1950; 32B:293–301.

30. Nathan PA, Meyers LD, Keniston RC, et al.: Simple decompression of the ulnar nerve: An alternative to anterior transposition. *J Hand Surg* 1992; 17B:251–254.

31. Osborne G: Compression neuritis of the ulnar nerve at the elbow. *Hand* 1970; 2:10–13.

32. Pechan J, Julis I: The pressure measurement in the ulnar nerve: A contribution to the pathophysiology of the cubital tunnel syndrome. *J Biomechanics* 1975; 8:75–79.

33. Stuffer M, Jungwirth W, Hussl H, et al.: Subcutaneous or submuscular transposition of the ulnar nerve? *J Hand Surg* 1991; 17B:248–250.

34. Thomsen PB: Compression neuritis of the ulnar nerve treated with simple decompression. *Acta Orthop Scand* 1977; 48:164–167.

35. Vanderpool DW, Chalmers J, Lamb DW, et al.: Peripheral compression lesions of the ulnar nerve. *J Bone Joint Surg* 1968; 50B:792–803.

36. Willis BK: Cubital tunnel syndrome, in Benzel EC (ed): *Practical Approaches to Peripheral Nerve Surgery*. Park Ridge, IL, American Association of Neurological Surgeons, 1992, pp 77–93.

37. Wilson DH, Krout R: Surgery of ulnar neuropathy at the elbow: 16 cases treated by decompression without transposition. *J Neurosurg* 1973; 38:780–785.

David G. Kline, M.D., John Reeves, M.D.

1. Brown WF, Ferguson GG, Jones MW, et al.: The location of conduction abnormalities in human entrapment neuropathies. *Can J Neurol Sci* 1976; 3:111–122.

2. Dellon AL: Techniques for successful management of ulnar nerve entrapment at the elbow. *Neurosurg Clin North Am* 1991; 2:57–73.

3. Dellon AL, MacKinnon SE: Injury to the medial antebrachial cutaneous nerve during cubital tunnel surgery. *J Hand Surg* 1985; 19:33–36.

4. Fannin TF: Local decompression in the treatment of ulnar nerve entrapment at the elbow. *J R Coll Surg Edinb* 1978; 23:362–366.

5. Feindel W, Stratford J: The role of the cubital tunnel in tardy ulnar palsy. *Can J Surg* 1958; 1:287–300.

6. Learmouth J: A technique for transplanting the ulnar nerve. *Surg Gynecol Obstet* 1942; 75:792–801.

7. Leffert RD: Anterior submuscular transposition of the ulnar nerves by the Learmouth technique. *J Hand Surg* 1982; 7A:147–155.

8. MacKinnon SE, Dellon AL: Ulnar nerve entrapment at the elbow, in MacKinnon SE, Dellon AL (eds): *Surgery of the Peripheral Nerve*. New York, Thieme, 1988, pp 217–273.

9. Neblett C, Enhi G: Medical epicondylectomy for ulnar palsy. *J Neurosurg* 1970; 32:55–62.

10. Tindall SC: Chronic injuries of peripheral nerves by entrapment, in Youmans JR (ed): *Neurological Surgery*, vol. 4, ed. 3. Philadelphia, WB Saunders, 1990, pp 2511–2542.

36

Treatment of Facial Pain: Descending Trigeminal Nucleotomy vs. Deep Brain Stimulation

CASE

A 50-year-old man underwent resection of a petroclival meningioma. Three months after surgery, he began to have facial pain that was persistent and increasing, associated with dysesthesia, and intractable to all forms of medical treatment. This pain deeply affected his life and performance.

PARTICIPANTS

Descending Trigeminal Nucleotomy for Dysesthetic Facial Pain–Jorge R. Schvarcz, M.D.

Deep Brain Stimulation for Facial Pain–Kim J. Burchiel, M.D.

Moderator–J.M. Gybels, M.D., Ph.D.

Descending Trigeminal Nucleotomy for Dysesthetic Facial Pain

Jorge R. Schvarcz, M.D.

This patient developed pain after the removal of a petroclival meningioma. Seemingly, he had not had paresthesias or pain before surgery or, at least, he did not refer to them. After a delayed onset, his painful sensory phenomena slowly but steadily progressed, and was refractory to medical treatment. Currently, his pain is relentless and is not related to any obvious peripheral sensory event. It also has a distinctive dysesthetic character with a strong burning quality buried within it. He has only a discrete allodynia, which is typically centered over a fairly restricted area of minor objective sensory loss. His overall pain is increasingly severe and definitely interferes with his normal life.

This clinical description strongly suggests one of the major categories of chronic intractable pain. It indicates a presumable pathophysiology, and an inescapable neurosurgical treatment. If it is a dysesthetic or deafferentation pain from injury to the nervous system by the tumor or its removal, this diagnosis unequivocally leads to 1 or 2 crucial neurosurgical issues.

MAKING A DECISION ABOUT TREATMENT

The first issue is what should *not* be done in such a case. In surgery for pain, a wrong diagnosis or a poor surgical decision, based more upon the surgeon's wishes and hopes than on knowledge and personal experience, causes a number of major adverse iatrogenic sequelae and a failure to adequately relieve pain. These sequelae increase significantly with each attempt to create a lesion in the nociceptive pathways. Further deafferentation, therefore, can by no means be pursued.

The second issue is what *could* or *should* be done in such a case. At present, 2 types of procedures are relevant: those that reduce or eliminate the focus of denervation neuronal hyperactivity at the nucleus caudalis, and those designed to prosthetically activate pain-suppressing mechanisms through chronic intracranial stimulation.

For this particular patient, I regard the stereotactic placement of radiofrequency lesions at the nucleus caudalis to be the procedure of choice. Indeed, I have developed it as an especially suitable technique to deal with elusive craniofacial dysesthetic pain. Curiously enough, it is currently the only lesion-making procedure I still regard as effective for deafferentation pain. Nevertheless, one must keep in mind that a pain surgeon, to be such, must have control of all contemporary methods of treatment, and a stimulation technique may well be the procedure of choice for some patients, for example, if a trigeminal nucleotomy has failed.

TRIGEMINAL NUCLEOTOMY

Dysesthetic, neurogenic, or deafferentation facial pain is still a neurosurgical challenge. The deafferentation itself, which is necessarily associated with a presumable, but not always conspicuous, injury to neural structures, can be further related to its site, type, and degree. Thus, considering both the quality and density of a particular case, the deafferentation may be 1 of 3 types: total, with a complete but not necessarily large area of anesthesia; partial, with more or less circumscribed evidence of

clinical sensory loss; or even subclinical, without any objective evidence of sensory loss.

Although a strict correlation between the density of sensory changes and the presence or absence of pain cannot be demonstrated, the dysesthetic pain, as well as other sensory aberrations, are more severe the greater the sensory deficit. But, this is not necessarily so. Indeed, deafferentation is typically the only mandatory unifying feature.

Surgical attempts to further interrupt the already damaged primary afferent neuron at any site, including trigeminal tractotomy, have consistently failed. Indeed, these attempts usually enhance, rather than decrease, the pain.[4,20] On the contrary, creating a lesion in the second order neurons at the nucleus caudalis, that is, at the putative focus of denervation neuronal hyperactivity, seems to be a rational approach.[14,23]

Method

The technique for the nucleotomy has already been described.[5,14,18] Briefly, patients are operated on under local anesthesia, with the head fully flexed within a Hitchcock stereotactic frame.[5] Both the spinal cord and the caudal brain stem are outlined with water-soluble positive contrast. The surgeon then approaches the spinal cord using a posterior route through the atlanto-occipital interspace.

Physiological monitoring through an electrode is mandatory within the mobile spinal cord. This can be done through cross-checking data from impedance measurements, electrical stimulation, occasionally by depth recording, and incremental enlargement of thermocontrolled lesions with concomitant clinical testing.[17] Impedance indicates contact with, and partial or total penetration of, the spinal cord.[17] Electrical stimulation clearly identifies the trigeminal region, with its rostral dermatome located ventrolaterally, and its caudal dermatome located dorsomedially[17,18] (Fig. 1). The dorsal border of the nucleus can usually be further defined through the ipsilateral responses induced from the cuneatus. The ventral border can be defined through the contralateral responses elicited from the spinothalamic tract or, occasionally, through the motor responses obtained from a posteriorly located corticospinal tract[17,18] (Fig. 1). Furthermore, threshold stimulation often mimics the patient's neurogenic pain.[17] This distinctive response is not observed in patients with somatogenic pain.[20]

Clinical Material and Results

From a series of 194 consecutive nucleotomies done in 186 patients, 141 of these patients underwent a nucleotomy for deafferentation pain. Within this group, the clinical diagnoses were:

- 38 post-herpetic dysesthesias;
- 40 dysesthetic pain states, with certain residual tic-like components still superimposed on the denervation pain, mostly sequelae of previous trigeminal surgery;
- 33 anesthesia dolorosa;
- 9 post-traumatic neuropathy.

Dysesthetic pain in these patients can be referred to the fifth,

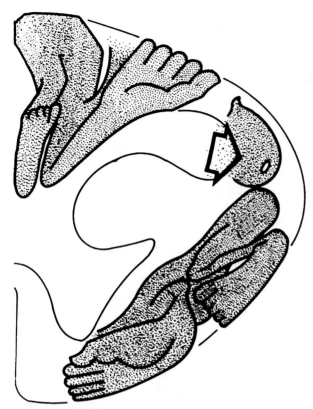

Fig. 1 Somatotopic arrangement of the high cervical spinal cord, in the light of stimulation data, showing the trigeminal region (arrow) between both the dorsal funiculus and the spinothalamic homunculi.

seventh, ninth, and tenth cranial nerves or the C2-C3 dermatomes. The patients' pain histories ranged from 1 to 9 years. Patients with dysesthetic states had between 2 and 5 ablative operations, and those with anesthesia dolorosa had between 2 and 13 ablative operations. Some of these patients also underwent deep brain stimulation, without success. None of the patients with post-traumatic neuropathies had previous surgery. Those who did have surgery developed sequelae that placed them in the aforementioned group.

Abolition of the allodynia and a significant reduction in or complete abolition of the deep background pain was achieved in 76.3% of the patients with post-therapeutic dysesthesias, in 70% of those with dysesthetic pain, in 66.6% of those with anesthesia dolorosa, and in 77% of those with post-traumatic neuropathies. Overall, pain was relieved in 72.6% of the patients.

The follow-up period ranged from 1 to 16 years. There were no lasting side effects, no new dysesthesias, and no motor sequelae. One patient had an intention tremor that disappeared within 72 hours. Slight contralateral lumbosacral hypoalgesia, from encroachment on the spinothalamic tract, was occasionally seen in patients with dense anesthesia of the ophthalmic region.

DISCUSSION

A surgical medullary trigeminal tractotomy was first conceived of in 1938 by Sjökvist.[25] Thereafter, the technique underwent successive modifications, until Kunc[13] developed a high cervical approach. Fox[2] described a high free-hand percutaneous approach to the trigeminal tract. It is now possible to place accurate stereotactic lesions at the nucleus caudalis with con-

comitant electrophysiological control of the fifth, seventh, ninth, and tenth cranial nerves, as well as of the second and third cervical roots.

Hitchcock[5] developed a stereotactic procedure that enabled him to perform the first stereotactic trigeminal tractotomy. Thereafter, he reviewed 21 cases[6] and, more recently, his overall experience with stereotactic surgery of the spinal cord.[7] He has used this procedure primarily for patients with somatogenic craniofacial pain,[6,7] but also for those with other types of pain. In 1972 Hitchcock and I[9] reported the use of radiofrequency lesions in the region of the descending trigeminal tract for postherpetic pain. I have used this technique since 1971, naming the procedure *trigeminal nucleotomy*[14] to emphasize the significance of creating lesions primarily in the second order neurons at the oral pole of the nucleus caudalis. That is, they are located at the larger, medially located, easily accessible, rather conspicuous nuclear structure, which was seemingly so heavily involved in certain intrinsic mechanisms pertaining to dysesthetic facial pain.[14,19,22]

Curiously enough, 15 years later, this target and its pathophysiology have suddenly been independently rediscovered.[8,21,23] More recently, Siqueira[24] has described a method for open surgical trigeminal nucleotomy for deafferentation pain. Kampolat and colleagues[10] developed an elegant percutaneous technique for trigeminal nucleotomy, guided by computed tomography, in patients with deafferentation pain. Grigoryan and Slavin[3] reported on their use of ultrasonic trigeminal nucleotomy, also for deafferentation pain.

Individual anatomic variations within the small confines of the spinal cord must be accounted for. When done in alert, cooperative patients, stereotactic techniques enable the surgeon to gain physiological control before making the lesions. Avoiding this crucial stage not only unduly increases the hazards of the procedure, but also compromises its effectiveness.[17,18] This is clearly shown, for example, in the postmortem studies by Spiegelmann and colleagues.[26] Only 1 properly placed lesion is required, a fact presumably related to the intranuclear pathways.[27] A number of theoretical arguments have been made to support the use of a long row of multiple lesions, but I have carried out more than 200 nucleotomies, each of them with only 1 isolated lesion, achieving a rather predictable result. The best level of section is determined through intraoperative stimulation.[17,18] Thus, the angle of the electrode track must sometimes be corrected rostrally if the stimulation does not completely cover the perioral region.[17]

Stereotactic nucleotomy shares some of the features of open surgical trigeminal tractotomy, but has certain distinctive characteristics. Thus, the results of this deeper, extensive nuclear lesion are in striking contrast with those of open medullary tractotomy, which has consistently failed to relieve dysesthetic facial pain.

Black[1] has impressively shown that deafferentation through retrogasserian rhizotomy is gradually followed by a grossly abnormal, spontaneous neuronal hyperactivity at the nucleus caudalis. This hyperactivity is similar to that of an experimental epileptogenic focus. Indeed, the mere removal of a patient's teeth produced localized spots of hyperactivity, with prolonged after-discharges after peripheral stimulation.[1] The time course of this spontaneous hyperactivity also paralleled the synaptic changes described by Westrum and Black.[28]

The nucleus caudalis is a nodal point where an extensive overlap occurs between craniofacial and high cervical afferents,[11,12] which may all converge onto a single trigeminal neuron. There is also an important ascending polysynaptic intranuclear pathway.[27] This procedure, then, presumably removes the segmental pool of neuronal hyperexcitability and denervation hypersensitivity, eliminating convergence and severing the ascending intranuclear pathways.[14]

Stereotactic trigeminal nucleotomy is a safe and reasonably straightforward technique that allows accurate siting of the target for physiological control before the lesion is made. So far, it seems to be especially suitable for patients with elusive dysesthetic facial pain.

Deep Brain Stimulation for Facial Pain

Kim J. Burchiel, M.D.

The unfortunate gentleman described in this case suffers from a deafferentation pain syndrome secondary to damage of the trigeminal nerve or brain stem tract. It is likely that he has hypesthesia in the trigeminal distribution, even if he shows some hyperalgesia to touch, or allodynia. I presume that he has had an exhaustive trial of medical treatment, including carbamazepine and tricyclic antidepressants. A relatively new drug, felbamate, in doses of 1200 to 3600 mg per day, may also be useful and should be tried.

This pain would not likely respond favorably to further peripheral denervation, such as neurectomy, percutaneous radiofrequency trigeminal gangliolysis, percutaneous retrogasserian glycerol rhizolysis, percutaneous trigeminal ganglion compression, or open trigeminal rhizotomy. The neural generator of the pain is almost certainly central, at the level of the trigeminal nucleus, or more rostral in the thalamus. Further peripheral denervation would probably worsen the situation.

CHOOSING A TREATMENT

The 2 options open to this patient are deep brain stimulation and trigeminal tractotomy or nucleotomy. My counterpart describes the rationale for choosing the ablative option. I will focus on the neuromodulation approach of deep brain stimulation.

One of the guiding principles in the treatment of difficult pain problems harkens back to the Hippocratic Oath—*primum non nocere*. In patients with deafferentation pain, harm can come in the form of further irreversible destruction of the peripheral or central nervous system. For patients with complex pain problems, few procedures offer a predictable outcome of better than a 50/50 chance of unqualified success. Therefore, a second principle is to work from the reversible, and often testable, procedures to the irreversible ablative operations. Furthermore, I advise trying simple, low-risk procedures before invoking the complex risky operations.

Trigeminal Tractotomy

Trigeminal tractotomy is less effective for constant pain, such as in this patient, than for burning, sharp, or lancinating pains.[1] This operation is done with the patient under general anesthesia, so its effectiveness and morbidity can only be evaluated *post hoc*. There is no way to test or predict the success of the procedure. Overall, the chance of a tractotomy or caudalis nucleotomy producing satisfactory relief is about 75%. Almost 100% of patients who undergo a tractotomy experience an undesired deficit of some sort, including ataxia, ipsilateral Brown-Séquard syndrome, ipsilateral palsy of the spinal accessory nerve with torticollis, mild ipsilateral monoparesis, or ipsilateral hemiparesis of the arm, and ipsilateral hypesthesia. Debilitating ipsilateral ataxia of the limb is seen in 10% of these patients after surgery, and about 15% experience disabling sensory loss in the contralateral limb.[1]

Deep Brain Stimulation

For all of these reasons, this patient should have a trial of deep brain stimulation before he is considered for an ablative operation. The probability that this procedure will help his pain is 50%, and the risk to him is around 15%.[2]

With the patient under local anesthesia, a four-contact platinum electrode is placed through conventional stereotactic techniques in the medial ventralis caudalis at a point which, when stimulated (1 msec square waves, 30 to 50 Hz, 0.5 to 5.0 volts), produces a non-painful paresthesia in the area of discomfort. Once the electrode is placed, a trial of stimulation lasting for a few days to 2 weeks can ensue to assure the efficacy of stimulation in relieving the pain. During this period, a pain diary and a drug diary are kept and, at the surgeon's discretion, the patient can be discharged for an extended trial.

If deep brain stimulation yields satisfactory pain relief, the electrode can be internalized with an implantable and programmable internal pulse generator. If the stimulation trial fails, the electrode is removed and a trigeminal tractotomy or nucleotomy can be considered (Fig. 1).

In summary, the treatment of intractable facial pain from injury to the trigeminal nerve or brain stem is daunting. In general, the safest options should be considered first, and the surgeon should resort to irreversible and potentially hazardous procedures only for patients in whom procedures with low morbidity fail.

Facial Pain

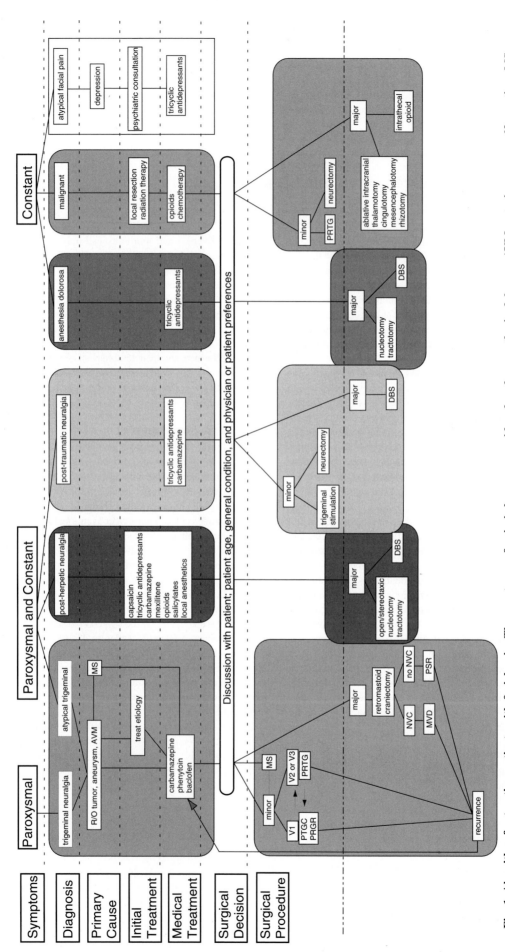

Fig. 1 Algorithm for treating patients with facial pain. The constancy of pain is key, with paroxysmal, mixed paroxysmal and constant, and constant pains as the 3 divisions. The flow of diagnosis, cause, initial treatment, medical treatment, surgical decision-making, and both minor and major procedures are listed along the left side to suggest a temporal sequence and hierarchy. In general, minor procedures are considered before major procedures. The patient described in this case would be considered under anesthesia dolorosa. AVM, arteriovenous malformation; MS, multiple sclerosis; PTGC, percutaneous trigeminal ganglion compression; PRGR, percutaneous retrogasserian glycerol rhizolysis; PRTG, percutaneous radiofrequency trigeminal gangliolysis; NVC, neurovascular compression; MVD, microvascular decompression; PSR, posterior sensory rhizotomy; DBS, deep brain stimulation.

354

Treatment of Facial Pain:
Descending Trigeminal Nucleotomy vs. Deep Brain Stimulation

J.M. Gybels, M.D., Ph.D.

Both authors agree it is unlikely that the patient described here would benefit from further peripheral denervation, and that such a procedure may worsen the situation.

TRIGEMINAL NUCLEOTOMY

The case for trigeminal nucleotomy can be summarized as follows. Having shown that the spinal trigeminal tract descends well into the middle of the second cervical segment of the cat, Kerr and Olafson[9] then show that volleys from both trigeminal and cervical posterior roots converge on the same neurons in the cat's posterior gray matter at the C1-C2 level. Subsequently, Kerr[8] showed that it was possible to electrolytically destroy the nucleus of the spinal tract of V at this level without causing ataxia or weakness. He suggested that such lesions be tried for intractable forms of cranial pain. A further argument in favor of this suggestion is the report of Stewart and colleagues,[14] who describe the existence of an ascending polysynaptic intranuclear pathway in the nucleus of the descending trigeminal tract.

Inspired by these valid experimental anatomic and physiological data, in 1972, Hitchcock and Schvarcz[6] first described in humans the making of a radiofrequency lesion in the secondary afferent neurons of the descending cephalic pain pathway in the nucleus caudalis. This technique was done initially for postherpetic facial pain. Schvarcz now describes a series of 194 consecutive nucleotomies. By far, he has the most extensive published series, with follow-up periods ranging from 1 to 16 years and a success rate of about 70% with no lasting side effects. This is a remarkable record. To produce such a record, however, extensive experience is required, and the danger of serious morbidity is inherent to the location of the structure one aims to destroy. I have had patients referred to me with catastrophic sequelae stemming from this procedure.

Burchiel states that almost 100% of the patients undergoing nucleotomy experience an undesired deficit of some sort, including debilitating, ipsilateral limb ataxia in 10% and disabling sensory loss in the contralateral limb in 15%. Because of this danger of serious morbidity, Burchiel proposes to proceed first with deep brain stimulation.

DEEP BRAIN STIMULATION

My colleagues and I have reviewed the literature on deep brain stimulation up to 1993.[4,5] Our most recent review comprises 37 reports with a total of 1843 patients. Because the authors of the many reports differed in their way of quantifying results, we adopted the following scoring system:

- Successful procedures were those that allowed pain relief scores of 50% or more and verbal ratings of excellent to good.
- Therapeutic failures occurred in patients in whom no electrode or stimulator was internalized because the patient did not respond to trial stimulation.

Not all authors report these early treatment failures, however, and the following results certainly do overestimate the real therapeutic efficacy.

Of the 1843 patients, treatment in 51% (934) was considered successful. When the data obtained in neuropathic and nociceptive pain are analyzed separately, 47% of the 866 patients suffering neuropathic pain and 51% of the 469 patients suffering nociceptive pain benefited from deep brain stimulation. This seems to signify that brain stimulation is more or less equally effective in both categories of pain.

When we look at the data per diagnostic category, the following results emerge. For peripheral nerve lesion pain, of the 33 patients reported, 73% responded favorably to deep brain stimulation. The best results were obtained in the study of Mazars and colleagues[11] (5 successes out of 5 patients). High success rates were also reported by Groth and colleagues[2] (77%) and Siegfried[13] (71%). Based on 4 studies, the median success score was 74%.

Cases of anesthesia dolorosa comprise the largest group of patients treated with somatosensory thalamic stimulation. Of the 103 patients, 45% showed good results. The largest series comes from Siegfried,[13] who obtained 10 very good and 6 good results out of a group of 24 patients suffering facial anesthesia dolorosa (67% success rate). Failures in his series occurred in patients who complained of pain for a long time before undergoing thalamic stimulation. Mazars and associates[11] obtained excellent results (6 successes out of 7 patients). In the study by Broseta and colleagues,[1] despite a high initial success rate of 6 out of 7 patients, no long-term successes were obtained. Hosobuchi[7] reported 4 (33%) successes among 12 patients. Levy and associates[10] reported 2 (22%) successes out of 9 and, in our own series,[3] we obtained 2 (33%) successes out of 6 patients. The median success score from 9 studies was 33% (range 0 to 86%).

These are the reported results and, of course, they remain modest. To me, however, the possibility of activating pain inhibition pathways more or less selectively without destroying nervous tissue has tremendous appeal, mainly for 3 reasons:

1. Unwanted side effects, which remain a burden with destructive procedures, can be avoided.
2. The effects of electrical stimulation are reversible.
3. Before implantation, a temporary trial stimulation is worthwhile.

One must realize, however, that manufacturers do not encourage the use of magnetic resonance imaging (MRI) in patients with a neurostimulation device, which might be a disadvantage in the patient described. It may also be worthwhile to watch for the results of studies employing motor cortex stimulation. This technique was first described by Tsubokawa and colleagues[15] for pain in a thalamic syndrome and, more recently by, Meyerson and associates[12] for trigeminal neuropathic pain.

CONCLUSION

For the patient presented in this case, it is particularly difficult to offer concrete recommendations to the reader. Whatever the method used, when making a decision, the surgeon must always keep in mind that a functional procedure is designed not to add days to the patient's life but life to the patient's days. I strongly agree with Burchiel's quotation of the Hippocratic Oath—*primum non nocere*.

REFERENCES

Jorge R. Schvarcz, M.D.

1. Black R: Trigeminal pain, in Crue BL (ed): *Pain and Suffering.* Springfield, Charles C. Thomas, 1970, pp 119–137.
2. Fox JL: Percutaneous trigeminal tractotomy for facial pain. *Acta Neurochir (Wien)* 1973; 29:83–88.
3. Grigoryan YUA, Slavin KV: Facial denervation pain relief with ultrasonic trigeminal nucleotomym (abstract). *Acta Neurochir (Wien)* 1992; 117:99.
4. Gybels JM, Sweet WH: Neurosurgical treatment of persistent pain, in Gildenberg PL (ed): *Pain and Headache,* vol. 11. Basel, Karger, 1985.
5. Hitchcock ER: Stereotactic trigeminal tractotomy. *Ann Clin Res* 1970; 2:131–135.
6. Hitchcock ER: Stereotactic spinal surgery, in Carrea R (ed): *Neurological Surgery.* Amsterdam, Excerpta Medica, 1978, pp 271–280.
7. Hitchcock ER: Special stereotactic techniques: Stereotactic lesions of the spinal cord and pons for pain, in Heilbrun MP (ed): *Stereotactic Neurosurgery.* Baltimore, Williams and Wilkins, 1988, pp 185–194.
8. Hitchcock ER: Letter to the editor. *Br J Neurosurg* 1990; 4:81–82.
9. Hitchcock ER, Schvarcz JR: Stereotaxic trigeminal tractotomy for post-herpetic facial pain. *J Neurosurg* 1972; 37:412–417.
10. Kampolat Y, Deda H, Akyar S, et al.: CT-guided trigeminal nucleotomy. *Acta Neurochir (Wien)* 1989; 100:112–114.
11. Kerr FW: The organization of primary afferents in the subnucleus caudalis of the trigeminal nerve. *Brain Res* 1970; 23:147–165.
12. Kerr FW: Neuroanatomical substrates of nociception in the spinal cord. *Pain* 1975; 1:325–356.
13. Kunc Z: Significant factors pertaining to the results of trigeminal tractotomy, in Hassler R, Walker EA (eds): *Trigeminal Neuralgia.* Stuttgart, Thieme, 1970, pp 90–100.
14. Schvarcz JR: Spinal cord stereotactic surgery, in Sano K, Ishii S (eds): *Recent Progress in Neurological Surgery.* Amsterdam, Excerpta Medica, 1974, pp 234–241.
15. Schvarcz JR: Stereotactic trigeminal nucleotomy. *Confin Neurol (Basel)* 1975; 37:73–77.
16. Schvarcz JR: Postherpetic craniofacial dysaesthesiae: Their management by stereotactic trigeminal nucleotomy. *Acta Neurochir (Wien)* 1977; 38:65–72.
17. Schvarcz JR: Functional exploration of the spinomedullary junction. *Acta Neurochir (Wien)* 1977; Suppl 24:179–185.
18. Schvarcz JR: Spinal cord stereotactic techniques re trigeminal nucleotomy and extralemniscal myelotomy. *Appl Neurophysiol* 1978; 41:99–112.
19. Schvarcz JR: Stereotactic spinal trigeminal nucleotomy for dysesthetic facial pain, in Bonica J, Liebeskind J, Fessard D (eds): *Advances in Pain Research and Therapy,* vol. 3. New York, Raven Press, 1979, pp 331–336.
20. Schvarcz JR: Percutaneous thermocontrolled differential retrogasserian rhizotomy for idiopathic trigeminal neuralgia. *Acta Neurochir (Wien)* 1982; 64:51–58.
21. Schvarcz JR: Trigeminal drez (letter). *Neurosurgery* 1987; 20:348.
22. Schvarcz JR: Craniofacial postherpetic neuralgia managed by stereotactic spinal trigeminal nucleotomy. *Acta Neurochir (Wien)* 1989; Suppl 46:62–64.
23. Schvarcz JR: Letter to the editor. *Br J Neurosurg* 1990; 4:81–82.
24. Siqueira JM: A method for bulbospinal trigeminal nucleotomy in the treatment of facial deafferention pain. *Appl Neurophysiol* 1985; 48:277–280.
25. Sjökvist O: Studies on pain conduction in the trigeminal nerve: A contribution to the surgical treatment of facial pain. *Acta Psychiat Scand* 1938; 17:1–138.
26. Spiegelmann R, Friedman WA, Ballinger WA, et al.: Anatomic examination of a case of open trigeminal nucleotomy (nucleus caudalis dorsal root entry zone lesions for facial pain). *Stereotact Funct Neurosurg* 1991; 56:166–178.
27. Stewart WA, Stoops WL, Pillone PR, et al.: An electrophysiologic study of ascending pathways from nucleus caudalis of the spinal trigeminal nuclear complex. *J Neurosurg* 1964; 21:35–48.
28. Westrum LE, Black RG: Changes in the synapses of the spinal trigeminal nucleus after ipsilateral rhizotomy. *Brain Res* 1968; 11:706–712.

Kim J. Burchiel, M.D.

1. Moore KR, Burchiel KJ: Surgical management of trigeminal neuralgia, in Tindall G, Cooper P, Barrow D (eds): *The Practice of Neurosurgery.* Baltimore, Williams and Wilkins, 1995.
2. Young RF: Brain stimulation. *Neurosurg Clin North Am* 1990; 1:865–879.

J.M. Gybels, M.D., Ph.D.

1. Broseta J, Roldan P, Masbout G, et al.: Chronic VPM thalamic stimulation in facial anaesthesia dolorosa following trigeminal surgery. *Acta Neurchir* 1984; Suppl 33:505–506.
2. Groth K, Adams J, Richardson D, et al.: *Deep Brain Stimulation for Chronic Intractable Pain.* Minneapolis, Medtronic, Inc., 1982.
3. Gybels J, Kupers R: Deep brain stimulation in the treatment of chronic pain in man: Where and why? *Neurophysiol Clin* 1990; 20:389–398.
4. Gybels JM, Kupers RC: Management of persistent pain by brain stimulation, in Schmidek H, Sweet WH (eds): *Operative Neurosurgical Techniques,* ed 3. Philadelpia, WB Saunders, 1994.
5. Gybels JM, Sweet WH: *Neurosurgical Treatment of Persistent Pain: Physiological and Pathological Mechanisms of Human Pain.* Basel, Karger, 1989.
6. Hitchcock ER, Schvarcz JR: Stereotaxic trigeminal tractotomy for post-herpetic facial pain. *J Neurosurg* 1972; 37:412–417.
7. Hosobuchi Y: Subcortical electrical stimulation for control of intractable pain in humans. Report of 122 cases (1970–1984). *J Neurosurg* 1986; 64:543–553.
8. Kerr FW: Spinal V nucleolysis: Intractable craniofacial pain. *Surg Forum* 1966; 17:419–421.
9. Kerr FW, Olafson RA: Trigeminal and cervical volleys: Convergence on single units in spinal gray at C-1 and C-2. *Arch Neurol* 1961; 54:161–178.
10. Levy RM, Lamb S, Adams JE: Treatment of chronic pain by deep brain stimulation: Long-term follow-up and review of the literature. *Neurosurgery* 1987; 21:885–893.
11. Mazars G, Merienne L, Cioloca C: Comparative study of electrical stimulation of posterior thalamic nuclei, periaqueductal gray, and other midline mesencephalic structures in man. *Adv Pain Res Ther* 1979; 3:541–546.
12. Meyerson BA, Lindblom U, Linderoth B, et al.: Motor cortex stimulation as treatment of trigeminal neuropathic pain. *Acta Neurochir (Wien)* 1993; Suppl 58:150–153.
13. Siegfried J: Therapeutical neurostimulation—indications reconsidered. *Acta Neurochir (Wien)* 1991; Suppl 52:112–117.
14. Stewart WA, Stoops WL, Pillone PR, et al.: An electrophysiologic study of ascending pathways from nucleus caudalis of the spinal trigeminal nuclear complex. *J Neurosurg* 1964; 21:35–48.
15. Tsubokawa T, Katayama Y, Yamamoto T, et al.: Chronic motor cortex stimulation for the treatment of central pain. *Acta Neurochir (Wien)* 1991; Suppl 52:137–139.

37

Treatment of Patients with Trigeminal Neuralgia

CASE

A 60-year-old woman with typical V2-V3 trigeminal neuralgia became unresponsive to medical treatment. The patient has a normal magnetic resonance image of the head, and is in good health.

PARTICIPANTS

Radiofrequency Rhizotomy for Trigeminal Neuralgia–G. Robert Nugent, M.D.

Balloon Compression Rhizotomy for Trigeminal Neuralgia–Jeffrey A. Brown, M.D.

Glycerol Injections for Trigeminal Neuralgia–Sten Håkanson, M.D.

Microvascular Decompression for Trigeminal Neuralgia–Toshio Matsushima, M.D., Masashi Fukui, M.D.

Moderator–Robert H. Wilkins, M.D.

Radiofrequency Rhizotomy for Trigeminal Neuralgia

G. Robert Nugent, M.D.

The pain of trigeminal neuralgia is so severe that most patients are satisfied with any treatment offered, provided pain relief is the outcome. The surgeon's predilection and experience, however, often colors the process of informed consent and predetermines a patient's choice of therapeutic possibilities. Naturally, a neurosurgeon experienced in microsurgery of the posterior fossa might strongly recommend the surgically challenging microvascular decompression to the patient presented here.

My experience shows that patients have a high degree of satisfaction with the much more benign radiofrequency procedure, despite some degree of facial numbness. This experience gives me a strong bias for this treatment, but it must be performed properly.

THE RADIOFREQUENCY TECHNIQUE

Indications

The indications for the radiofrequency procedure are similar to those for other destructive techniques. The patient must have true or classic trigeminal neuralgia because this technique does not help atypical facial pains. The pain must be refractory to medical therapy, or the patient suffers intolerable side effects from such therapy. Those who have had a previous peripheral block with good relief of their pain may opt for permanent numbness. The radiofrequency procedure is also an option for those who fear intracranial surgery and its remote, but significant, complications. Finally, some patients simply opt for a more benign, less time-consuming, and less expensive form of treatment than a major open intracranial operation.

Preliminary Considerations

The radiofrequency procedure requires the patient's informed consent concerning the permanence of sensory deficits, the possibility of recurrence of pain requiring another treatment, possible corneal anesthesia with its complications, and the possibility of annoying sensations in the face. Anesthetic safeguards must be in place to prevent intracranial hemorrhage from the reflex hypertensive bursts that may occur during the treatment.

To say that the radiofrequency procedure is the best therapeutic approach requires the presentation of a few caveats. Creation of the radiofrequency lesion can inflict too much damage upon the nerve, resulting in an unhappy patient because of annoying sensations in the face. This outcome has discouraged many from this treatment. Most patients with trigeminal neuralgia, however, require only moderate sensory deficits to obtain lasting relief of their pain. The surgeon must restrain the compulsion to go for a quick and sure cure by creating dense numbness and should learn to accept a higher recurrence rate, which merely means that this minor procedure can be repeated. Too dense a sensory deficit occurs not only intentionally, but also from inexperience and misuse of the technique. Just as a neurosurgeon must have experience to obtain good results with microvascular decompression, experience with the proper techniques for radiofrequency rhizotomy is also a requirement.

I have argued that the radiofrequency technique allows much more control of the extent and location of the lesion than other destructive techniques. This control is achieved through the use of a small, angled electrode with an exposed active length of only 3 mm and a diameter of 0.4 mm (Fig. 1). Of equal importance is the creation of the lesion with its sensory deficit while the patient is fully awake, permitting on-line monitoring of the location and extent of the sensory deficit and preserving the corneal reflex. I do not recommend use of the larger temperature-monitoring electrode because it does not allow this control and, more importantly, it usually requires that the patient be anesthetized for the creation of the lesion, at which point no on-line monitoring is possible and control is lost. The ability to place the small electrode behind the ganglion in the retrogasserian rootlets is what allows the lesion to be created without significant pain and without the need to use anesthesia. Furthermore, the necessary final temperature of the electrode varies tremendously depending upon how close the electrode is to the rootlets themselves.[29] Siegfried[25] states that the temperature at the tip of the electrode and the intensity of current show no consistent direct relationship. Therefore, I am convinced that on-line monitoring of the patient is far more important than monitoring the temperature.

Spread of the electrical current into the first division of the trigeminal nerve can be avoided by stopping the process when a decrease is noted in the blink response to eyelash stimulation, while the lesion is created. Monitoring the blink response is important because first division lesions can be made with no associated discomfort or sensation in the eye or forehead. This is in contrast to lesions made in the second or third division. Consequently, it is easy to destroy the first division without the surgeon or the patient being aware of what is happening. With proper technique, corneal anesthesia can be kept to an incidence of about 3 to 4%. It has been 2% in our last several hundred procedures. Ninety percent of patients with first-division pain have been treated satisfactorily, diminishing corneal sensation only partially. The author's technique is described in detail in 2 publications.[18,19]

Results

Experience with the radiofrequency procedure convinces one that most patients with trigeminal neuralgia are glad to accept facial numbness to be rid of pain and medication. About 6% of patients find the numbness disagreeable, but 53% of those patients who found the dysesthesias "annoying" also rated the overall results of the procedure as good or excellent. In our series, 0.7% of patients described the annoying facial sensations as moderate to severe, in 3% they described them as severe, and in 0.4% they were considered intolerable.[19] The proof "in the pudding" that this is a satisfactory procedure, however, is that most patients with any recurrence immediately request another treatment, and many of my patients now come from one satisfied patient recommending the treatment to another.

DECOMPRESSION VERSUS RADIOFREQUENCY

We must not forget that trigeminal neuralgia is a benign disease. The mortality with microvascular decompression is at least 1% versus 0.06% with radiofrequency.[27] The argument for micro-

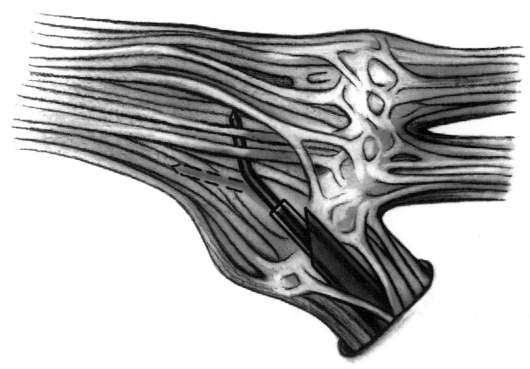

Fig. 1 The cordotomy electrode in the retrogasserian rootlets. Rotating the electrode within the needle allows a parameter of localization in addition to the depth of penetration. (Reproduced with permission from: Nugent GR: Trigeminal neuralgia treatment by percutaneous electro-coagulation, in Wilkins RH, Rengachary SS (eds): *Neurosurgery.* **New York, McGraw-Hill, 1985, pp 2345–2350.)**

vascular decompression being a good operation for the younger patient carries with it a certain eeriness.

Recurrence Rate

The long-term recurrence rate for the radiofrequency procedure should be about 25 to 30%. Our long-term (10 year) recurrence rate is 27%. This rate could be considerably less if we elected to make our lesions more dense. The recurrence or failure rate for microvascular decompression in selected series is as follows: 47% over 8.5 years,[8] 29%,[20] 28%,[6] and 29%.[11] The recurrence, therefore, is similar for the 2 treatments. But the comparison should not be made on the basis of recurrence because this is not a critical issue with radiofrequency. You simply do it over again.

Deafness

Of concern is the significant incidence of permanent hearing loss in the ipsilateral ear of patients undergoing decompression. In various series, this rate was 4%,[4] 7%,[14] 8%,[20] and 7.6%.[6] As others have pointed out,[4,21] this loss of hearing is unrelated to the surgeon's experience. Even one author who has great experience with microvascular decompression[2] states that a 3% incidence of hearing loss is to be expected. This operation should not be performed, however, without the use of sophisticated on-line monitoring of the brain stem and function of the eighth cranial nerve.[20]

Reports from the Literature

In comparing his results from radiofrequency treatment with those of microvascular decompression, Apfelbaum[1] describes a severe degree of numbness in 15% of those undergoing the radiofrequency procedure, a 13% incidence of corneal anesthesia, and an 11% incidence of anesthesia dolorosa or annoying dysesthesias. In addition, the patients were not anesthetized when he passed the needle through the foramen ovale. We had an incidence of corneal anesthesia of 3.5% (only 0.4% with keratitis), severe dysesthesias in 3% (intolerable in 0.4%), and anesthesia dolorosa in only 0.5%. Apfelbaum was undoubtedly inflicting too much sensory deficit with his radiofrequency technique, a common fault of others, and it is not surprising, therefore, that 18% of his patients would not have another radiofrequency procedure performed. Because of these results, Apfelbaum believed that the quality of the patient's life was better after microvascular decompression, but his adverse results do not make this a valid judgment. Fraioli and colleagues[12] make the same mistake. The radiofrequency procedure should not be blamed by those inflicting unwanted and unnecessary sensory deficits.

SELECTION OF PATIENTS

The prognosis for the success of microvascular decompression is significantly worse for women,[4,14,21] those with a long history of pain,[3,4,14,21] and those undergoing prior ablative treatments for their pain.[3,4]

When discussing the options of therapy, I offer microvascular decompression with the patient's understanding that this major procedure requires a lengthy and costly hospitalization and is associated with at least a 1% mortality rate, a 3 to 4% incidence of deafness on the side treated, a recurrence rate requiring another procedure (often destructive) in up to 47% of patients over a long follow-up, and facial numbness in 10 to 27%, in

Table 1. Failure or Recurrence Rates in Series of Glycerol Injections

Series	Rate (%)	Comments
Burchiel[7]	50	
Dieckmann, et al.[10]	37	
Fraioli, et al.[12]	57	In 5 years
Fujimaki, et al.[13]	72	In 52 months
Lunsford[17]	40–50	
Saini[24]	90	At 6 years
Waltz, et al.[32]	45	
Nugent—radiofrequency[19]	27	

Table 3. Loss of Sensation in the Cornea after Glycerol Injection

Series	Rate (%)	Comments
Burchiel[7]	7	Total corneal anesthesia
Dieckmann, et al.[10]	5	Sensation abolished
Saini[24]	4	With keratitis
Sweet[26]	14	Total corneal anesthesia
Nugent—radiofrequency[19]	3.5	

whom no satisfying vascular compression could be found and the nerve is cut to obtain pain relief.[9,20,31,34] Percutaneous procedures with less than 10% of the major risks of decompression are available.[28] With this information, most patients opt for the treatment that will let them go home the same day. I believe that the magnitude of the decompression procedure and its potential complications present an unacceptable trade-off for an outpatient procedure that produces a moderate degree of numbness in the face.

The only patients who need to undergo decompression are those who cannot accept permanent facial numbness. The argument that microvascular decompression has the advantage of treating the cause of the pain means little to the patient who only wants pain relief. I agree that vascular compression of the trigeminal nerve is the cause of tic douloureux in most patients, but this does not mean that alternative treatments are not a viable option.

GLYCEROL INJECTIONS VERSUS RADIOFREQUENCY

My major objection to injections of glycerol to treat patients with trigeminal neuralgia is that they are unpredictable when compared to a controlled and carefully executed radiofrequency lesion. An unexplainable diversity of experience exists with the glycerol treatment; some experiences are good but many are not. The recurrence or failure rates in several glycerol series are higher than those of other procedures (Table 1), and the sensory

Table 2. Sensory Deficits after Glycerol Injection

Series	Rate (%)	Comments
Burchiel[7]	7	With anesthesia
Dieckmann, et al.[10]	18.5	Severe in 1.6%
Fraioli, et al.[12]	3.1	With anesthesia and keratitis
Fujimaki, et al.[13]	29	
Rappaport, Gomori[22]	27	
Saini[24]	11	4.7% with anesthesia dolorosa
Sweet[28]	4	With anesthesia-hypalgesia dolorosa
Waltz, et al.[32]	16	
Young[33]	28	Mild, 8% with analgesia
Nugent—radiofrequency[19]	6	

deficits can be severe (Table 2). These sensory deficits are significantly greater than those seen with the radiofrequency procedure, and increase to 50% after a second glycerol injection and 70% after a third.[17,22,32] They are also more severe in patients who have had a prior nonglycerol treatment.[13,23,24] This is not a procedure for patients with recurrent pain or previous treatment. Many have not achieved an absence of sensory loss with glycerol. Loss of sensation in the cornea is also a major problem (Table 3). These rates, too, are significantly higher than they should be in patients undergoing radiofrequency treatment.

Based on these selective negative results, glycerol injection is not always the benign modality we originally thought. I believe that radiofrequency offers a much more controllable and predictable treatment than injecting glycerol into the cistern to see what happens. Both the patient and the neurosurgeon should be prepared for some surprises when glycerol is used.

RADIOFREQUENCY VERSUS BALLOON COMPRESSION

Criticism of balloon compression is more difficult. Although the long-term recurrence rate can be expected to reach 30%,[15] a rate comparable to that of radiofrequency treatment, annoying dysesthesias can reach 12% if the balloon remains inflated for long periods of time.[5] As with glycerol, facial numbness is more marked after a repeated balloon compression.[16] The major advantage of balloon compression, to date, is the absence of corneal anesthesia.

There is nothing magic about balloon compression. This technique is merely another method of injuring the trigeminal nerve and ganglion and the results and adverse effects are directly related to the degree of the compression. It might be an alternative for those unable to develop the skills of a more refined technique.

CONCLUSION

I believe that those surgeons who prefer other therapeutic approaches never learned to perform the radiofrequency procedure properly, and those who have developed experience and skill with the technique share the author's conviction that it is an excellent treatment. I argue with those who believe that radiofrequency offers a cure only at the expense of an unacceptable trade-off of permanent numbness in the face.[30] Those treated with radiofrequency are generally among the most grateful and appreciative patients a neurosurgeon has the pleasure of treating. A properly performed radiofrequency procedure offers a simple, quick, safe, and economical way of relieving the worst pain we are heir to.

Balloon Compression Rhizotomy for Trigeminal Neuralgia

Jeffrey A. Brown, M.D.

I would recommend percutaneous trigeminal nerve balloon compression to this woman to treat her trigeminal neuralgia. This recommendation is based on two axioms: patients in pain do not wish to be in pain and, because trigeminal neuralgia is a benign illness, its treatment should be benign.

EVOLUTION OF BALLOON RHIZOTOMY

Percutaneous trigeminal nerve compression is based on the findings of Sheldon[2] who, in 1955, published the results of a series of patients treated through temporal craniotomy and compression of the trigeminal nerve and ganglion. He noted that those patients who had undergone decompression of the mandibular division and developed numbness did better than those who did not have numbness. From this observation, he concluded that the trigeminal injury, rather than the peripheral decompression, is what alleviated pain. Mullan[5,7] modified this technique to a percutaneous procedure.

SURGICAL CONSIDERATIONS

The operation is done in the radiology suite with the patient under general or intravenous anesthesia. The nerve injury is not selective by division and the patient need not be awake to cooperate with the surgeon for catheter positioning. The use of general anesthesia has not caused any complication in my series of 75 patients or in any patient in any reported series, but an intravenous anesthetic may used instead. Inhalation anesthesia allows the anesthesiologist to have greater control of the patient's airway. Significant autonomic changes can occur during nerve compression, and these must be anticipated. Trigeminal nerve compression causes a trigeminal depressor response in 70% of patients, which consists of sudden but brief bradycardia and hypotension.[1] Such a response differs from the typical response to radiofrequency rhizotomy, which causes tachycardia and hypertension. This difference in autonomic response probably occurs because compression injures large myelinated fibers selectively.[8] Radiofrequency rhizotomy more likely injures all fibers, both myelinated and unmyelinated. Balloon compression can cause a mixed autonomic response when the external pacemaker is triggered; then, hypertension and tachycardia can also occur.

Most important to the ease of surgery is excellent fluoroscopic visualization of the foramen ovale. The patient's head is positioned in slight extension and contralateral rotation, so that the foramen ovale is seen just above the petrous bone. A 14-gauge needle is placed percutaneously at the foramen ovale. When the foramen is approached, a lateral view is obtained, but the needle should not go beyond the foramen. The trigeminal depressor response may also occur when the needle engages the foramen, triggering the external pacemaker. The combination of physiological, radiographic, and tactile feedback assures proper positioning of this large needle.

Surgical Technique

An orbitomeatal view is obtained. A C-arm portable unit is commonly used but, if the procedure is done in the radiology suite designed for coronary angiography, better imaging of the foramen ovale becomes possible. The petrous ridge is seen centered in the orbit on fluoroscopy. A wire stylet is positioned short of the petrous ridge using the same landmarks as for a radiofrequency rhizotomy. The stylet is removed and a #4 Fogarty catheter is positioned at the porous trigeminous, at the edge of the petrous bone (Fig. 1). The Fogarty catheter contains a wire stylet, which is seen on fluoroscopy and then removed when the catheter is correctly positioned.

The balloon catheter is inflated with 0.75 ml of 180 mg% iohexol while balloon pressure is continuously monitored. If the balloon takes on a pear shape, its tip is in the porous trigeminous compressing the preganglionic nerve (Fig. 1). I monitor pressure to provide added cues to the extent of nerve injury. If the balloon pressure is high, bradycardia is severe, and the balloon is positioned in the porous, then the duration of compression should be shortened and pressure reduced to about 800 mmHg issue compression pressure. The intraluminal balloon pressure is 550 mmHg when the balloon is inflated to a volume of 0.75 ml. The total pressure during inflation is usually 1100 to 1300 mmHg.

RESULTS

In my first series of 50 patients with minimum follow-up of 1 year and mean follow-up of 3 years, 47 (94%) were initially relieved of their pain. In 37 patients (74%), numbness was mild; 1 patient (2%) had severe numbness; and 10 patients (20%) had minor dysesthesias. One (2%) had a sixth nerve palsy, that resolved a day later. Neither anesthesia dolorosa nor loss of the corneal reflex has occurred.

Three patients had aseptic meningitis. These patients developed severe headache, fever, nuchal rigidity, and confusion within 6 hours of their surgery. Cerebrospinal fluid pressure was slightly elevated, but cultures were always negative and gram stain never showed bacteria to be present. The white blood cell count in the cerebrospinal fluid was abnormal, with 90% polymorphonuclear cells. A high red blood cell count in the cerebrospinal fluid suggested that the aseptic meningitis was in response to subarachnoid hemorrhage, but computed tomography did not show subarachnoid blood. Symptoms resolved within 1 day without residual deficits.

Recurrence

The overall recurrence rate in this series was 26%, with a mean time until recurrence of 18 months. Eight of 13 patients (62%) with recurrence had had previous destructive procedures done. Four of 8 patients with recurrence had pain recur after a repeated balloon compression. Kaplan-Meier survival curves showed an essentially linear incidence of recurrence with time. Presumably, as numbness resolves, recurrence becomes more likely.

Although two thirds of the patients having recurrence had undergone previous destructive procedures before their balloon compression, no statistically significant factor predicted recurrence after compression. All patients whose pain recurred after having a second compression had undergone previous destructive procedures before having balloon compression. In 1 of the patients with multiple recurrence, a microvascular decompression was later done and obvious arterial compression was found.

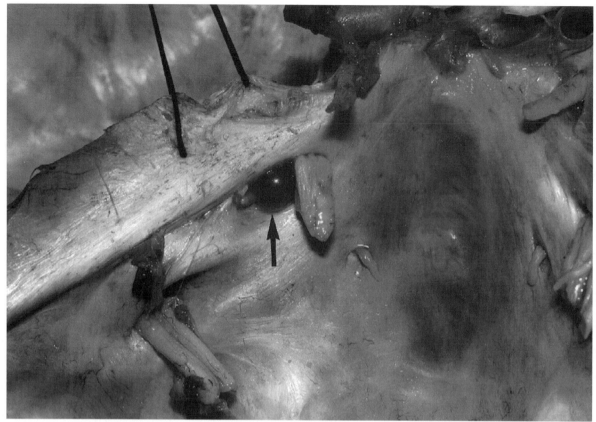

Fig. 1 Demonstration in a cadaver of the correct balloon position with its tip (arrow) in the porous trigeminous compressing the left trigeminal sensory and motor roots.

Subsequently, pain did not recur. In a second patient, a tortuous vertebrobasilar complex was seen on computed tomogram scans and represented the likely etiology of pain. Six (46%) of 13 patients with recurrence had objective numbness after the procedure, but none had severe numbness. Neither the patient's age nor balloon compression pressure were significant factors predicting recurrence.

Discussion

Thermal rhizotomy is the most common percutaneous procedure used to treat patients with trigeminal neuralgia. Gybels and Sweet[4] surveyed in detail the various techniques used to treat trigeminal neuralgia. Early pain relief in series of more than 500 patients is above 95%. The recurrence rate ranges from 7 to 31%. Lower recurrence rates are associated with higher morbidity, as high as 23% corneal hypesthesia, and 4% keratitis. If hypesthesia is used as the endpoint for thermal coagulation, recurrence is higher—19 to 23%—but dysesthesias are fewer.

During glycerol injection, patients must cooperate with the surgeon by remaining seated with the head flexed after injection to keep the glycerol within the trigeminal cistern. Initial relief from this procedure ranged from 70 to 96%, lower than that published in series using thermal rhizotomy or balloon compression. The recurrence rate requiring reoperation ranged from 9 to 30%. In the series of Gybels and Sweet,[4,6] there was a 20% incidence of dysesthesia with glycerol injection compared to only 6% with radiofrequency rhizotomy. Two of their 93 patients developed aseptic meningitis.

Larger series and longer follow-up is available for patients who underwent radiofrequency rhizotomy. The size of the series

and the length of follow-up is comparable for glycerol injection and balloon compression. The initial success rate of 94% with balloon compression and the recurrence rate of 26% is comparable to that of thermal rhizotomy, when a goal of hypesthesia rather than hypalgesia was sought.[4]

Laboratory investigation of the effects of balloon compression in rabbits has shown that compression selectively injures medium and larger myelinated fibers more than small myelinated and unmyelinated fibers. Ganglion cells are generally preserved.[8] Glycerol trigeminal rhizotomy causes demyelination and axonal fragmentation similar to balloon compression.[6] Because the corneal reflex is mediated by small fibers, balloon compression may be of advantage in treating pain of the first division.[2] Keratitis or anesthesia dolorosa in this series of patients has not occurred and may be less likely because of the nature of the injury from compression.

Currently, the disadvantages of balloon compression are that it is fiber-selective, but not division-selective, and the degree of numbness produced cannot be fully controlled.[3] Its advantages, however, are its technical simplicity and its lack of the need for patient cooperation during the procedure. By monitoring the compression pressure of tissue, the balloon position, and the autonomic response during compression and modifying the duration and force of compression, the risk of severe numbness might be reduced and the outcome improved.

CONCLUSION

Balloon compression may be a reasonable alternative to treating trigeminal pain of the first division in patients who have not benefited from either thermal or glycerol rhizotomy, and who are candidates only for a percutaneous procedure. It may also be the best choice for patients who cannot cooperate well enough to allow a careful awake procedure. All patients in my series who have multiple sclerosis are currently free of pain. Compression may be effective because it injures those myelinated fibers that trigger the lancinating trigeminal pain. Percutaneous trigeminal compression continues to be an effective, and technically simple, treatment for trigeminal neuralgia.

Glycerol Injections for Trigeminal Neuralgia

Sten Håkanson, M.D.

At present, several good surgical methods are available to treat patients with classic trigeminal neuralgia. These methods entail open, as well as percutaneous, procedures. Because the indications for the use of the various methods are not identical, these methods must be looked upon as complementary and not competitive. Ideally, therefore, a neurosurgeon should have an open and at least 1 percutaneous procedure in the therapeutic menu. The ability to carry out more than 1 type of procedure also supplies the base for a neurosurgeon to provide unbiased information to the patient for, in the end, it is the patient who has to choose the treatment and the doctor only has to present an accurate description of the various treatment procedures available. It is easy and tempting to lead the patient in a direction that suits the surgeon. The sole advantage of this leading is that the surgeon usually recommends the procedure with which he or she is most familiar.

For most patients, the choice should be easy. Those who are comparatively young and healthy should without hesitation be recommended a microvascular decompression,[14] and older patients should definitely be advised a percutaneous procedure. Between these groups of patients, however, are several who need accurate information about the various methods to make an appropriate decision. This view is valid for the present patient, a 60-year-old woman with a genuine trigeminal neuralgia involving the second and third branches. This information should include the importance of the age of the patient, the initial success rate, the risk of recurrence, the period of time the patient will be expected to stay away from work, and the risks of complications and their nature. Another issue of great concern is for what severity of symptoms should surgical therapy be justified.

Because retrogasserian glycerol injection[11] offers several advantages compared to other percutaneous procedures in the treatment of classic trigeminal neuralgia, I will focus the choice for the patient between this method and microvascular decompression.

SURGICAL CONSIDERATIONS

If the estimated survival of the patient exceeds 5 years, the patient's age is no contraindication to microvascular decompression for patients up to 65 years, or even older.[14] One of the advantages of decompression compared to percutaneous procedures has been referred to as a diminished risk of recurrence on a long-term basis. In a group of older patients treated with a percutaneous method, however, a substantial number of them will not live long enough to experience recurrent pain. This is also the case for many patients who suffer from a concurrent disease.

Although a procedure directed to the supposed cause of the pain, a vascular impingement, seems most rational, symptomatic treatment must be regarded as equally successful if it keeps the patient completely free of pain until death, without annoying sensory loss. For retrogasserian glycerol injection, an advanced age is no contraindication as the procedure is usually performed under local anesthesia. Only the slight cooperation of the patient is required; thus, the procedure can also be performed in senile patients. However, it must be possible to place the patient in the sitting position during the procedure.

At what severity of symptoms should surgical intervention be considered? Many older patients experience adverse side effects from the medication at a low dose, often resulting in an eremitic way of life. In those suffering paroxysmal pain in association with multiple sclerosis, the side effects often imply a worsening of their invalidity, confining them to a wheelchair or bed.[17] These old and disabled patients should be offered an intracisternal glycerol injection early, well before they are marked by their disease. Otherwise, they may show up in a poor nutritional status after a long period of time. Additionally, many patients are simply reluctant to undergo major surgical procedures if adequate percutaneous procedures are available, even if the long-term risk of recurrent pain is higher. Only patients with classic trigeminal neuralgia should be considered for treatment with glycerol injection. Those with continuous, deafferent pain should not undergo injection unless a coexistent paroxysmal pain is the dominant symptom.

Technique

The technique of the retrogasserian glycerol injection is well-known from numerous publications,[9,11,19] and requires only a summarized description here. In essence, the method instills a small amount of glycerol into the trigeminal cistern, which is the subarachnoid space behind the trigeminal ganglion that harbors all the trigeminal rootlets. Since the introduction of the method, several modifications of the technique have been suggested, but no real contributions to the safety, efficacy, or convenience of the method have been made. The modifications have sometimes caused less favorable results.[2,7,25,26] The procedure is preferably performed with the patient fully awake and in a sitting position. Adequate premedication is essential; if this is insufficient or the patient is too drowsy to cooperate, the procedure should be discontinued and resumed later with modified premedication. With the use of a comparatively thin needle (23G), the procedure is usually well tolerated.

Glycerol should not be injected unless it is proven that the tip of the needle is within the trigeminal cistern. This requires a free egress of cerebrospinal fluid from the needle and a cisternogram to verify the needle's position. The cisternogram is mandatory, because drainage of cerebrospinal fluid can also be obtained with the needle in a subtemporal, subarachnoidal location.

The cistern filled with contrast medium has a characteristic appearance (Fig. 1). During the past several years, iohexol has been used exclusively as a contrast medium in my department.

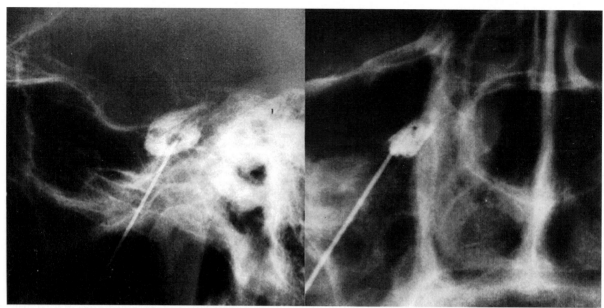

Fig. 1 The characteristic appearance of a normal trigeminal cistern filled with contrast medium. (*A*) Lateral projection. (*B*) Anteroposterior projection.

Subdural contrast injection within Meckel's cave must be recognized: the rootlets are lacking and the contrast is seen propagating into the subdural space behind the clivus. This usually happens when contrast medium is injected without prior spontaneous drainage of cerebrospinal fluid. Glycerol injected into this compartment is ineffective. If it is difficult to identify the position of the trigeminal cistern after penetrating the foramen ovale, a second needle should be used in a different direction, keeping the first needle in place as a guide. Usually, the cistern is found medial to the tip of the first needle (Fig. 2). A subtemporal, subarachnoidal, or subdural contrast injection results in a spread of contrast beneath the temporal and occipital lobes and

is easily recognizable, especially in anteroposterior roentgenograms (Fig. 3). After complete evacuation of the contrast medium, from 0.2 to 0.3 ml of glycerol should be injected into the trigeminal cistern.

The contrast medium used is heavier than glycerol. Because of this difference in weight, some selectivity in the effect on the various divisions of the nerve is possible. If a small amount of contrast medium is left at the bottom of the cistern, the rootlets of the third-branch will be protected and the injected glycerol will affect only the first and second divisions. Consequently, when treating a third-branch neuralgia, the contrast medium must be completely evacuated from the bottom of the cistern. Because a small rim of partially diluted contrast medium may not be detectable on fluoroscopy, an optimal effect on the rootlets of the third branch could be achieved by an abundant rinsing with saline before the glycerol injection. Immediately before the injection of glycerol, the free flow of cerebrospinal fluid should be checked, confirming that the position of the needle tip has not changed. After the glycerol injection, the patient is kept in the sitting position for at least 1 hour with the head slightly flexed.

Results

Since the first report of the retrogasserian glycerol treatment in 1981,[11] several large series with comparatively long periods of follow-up have been published.[1–3,7,9,13,19,24,27,28] Most series report a high initial success rate that was achieved through meticulous technique. The success rate should exceed 90% (Table 1). The variance of the figures in the larger series could be because of a different definition of the cases in which no satisfactory needle position was obtained and no glycerol injected. This is not always evident in the publications. An unsuccessful first injection can be explained by several types of technical problems, for example, a subarachnoid-subtemporal injection, misinterpretation of the cisternogram, or even dislodgement of the needle after the cisternography. Additionally, in some of the series, cisternograms were not used to ascertain a proper needle position.[1,20,28] Remarkably, the outcome was essentially the

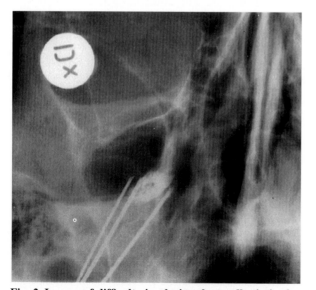

Fig. 2 In case of difficulty in placing the needle tip in the cistern after the foramen is penetrated, the first needle can be kept in place as a guide. The cistern is usually found medial to the tip of the first needle inserted, but even a needle introduction that is too medial is possible.

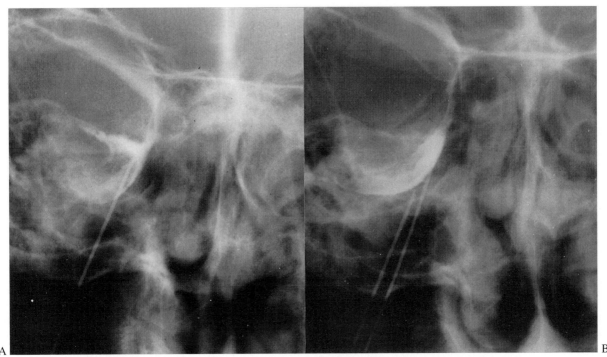

Fig. 3 Anteroposterior views of the incorrect position of the tip of the needle with introduction of contrast into the subtemporal subarachnoid (A) and subdural (B) spaces.

same in a few of these series, compared to those performed with a preoperative contrast study. The number of patients with relapsing pain increases with time, as is the case with all other treatments of genuine trigeminal neuralgia. The recurrence rate in the various series differs considerably and is often difficult to evaluate because the follow-up periods vary.

A better indication of the rate of recurrence can be illustrated by means of a Kaplan-Meier analysis, which has been done in some of the recent studies.[2,7,24] Table 2 classifies the recurrence rates from the major series. The average risk for an early recurrence seems to be about 20% and, during an extended follow-up period (5 to 10 years), up to 50% of the patients may have experienced relapsing pain.

DISCUSSION

As judged from the large number of clinical studies, the retrogasserian injection of glycerol for trigeminal neuralgia is a relatively safe procedure with few serious complications reported.

The recurrence rate appears to be rather high in some series but, because the procedure is relatively simple and easily repeated, a large number of patients (75 to 80%) can remain completely free of pain through a small number of reinjections. Regarding microvascular decompression, Jannetta[14] noted that 80% of patients have permanent relief, about 10% have some recurring pain, and the failure rate is 10%.

The recurrence rate is related to the amount of glycerol in-

Table 1. Results of Glycerol Injections for Trigeminal Neuralgia*

Authors	n	% with cisternography	Pain-free after first injection (%)	Total pain-free at follow-up (%)
Håkanson[9] (1983)	100	100	96	75
Arias[1] (1986)	100	50	95	95
Dieckman, et al.[3] (1987)	252	100	91	85
Young[28] (1988)	162	0	90	78
Waltz, et al.[27] (1989)	200	100	73	46
Lunsford[19] (1990)	376	100	90	60
Fujimaki, et al.[7] (1990)	122	100	80	26
North, et al.[20] (1990)	85	0	>90	>50
Ischia, et al.[13] (1990)	112	100	92	74
Steiger[24] (1991)	122	100	89	59

*The outcome in most of the major series published. The use of cisternography to verify an intracisternal needle position in the individual series is included. Only series with patients having classic trigeminal neuralgia (and multiple sclerosis) are included.

Table 2. Recurrence of Pain after Glycerol Injection for Trigeminal Neuralgia*

Authors	n	% Early recurrence (<2 years)	% Late recurrence (>2 years)	Follow-up range
Håkanson[9] (1983)	100	26	43	5–10 years
Arias[1] (1986)	100	2	10	2–3 years
Dieckman, et al.[3] (1987)	252	11	37	2–5 years
Young[28] (1988)	162	11	34	6–67 months
Waltz, et al.[27] (1989)	200	23	25	25–64 months
Lunsford[19] (1990)	376	30	–	6–90 months
Fujimaki, et al.[7] (1990)	122	45	72	38–54 months
North, et al.[20] (1990)	85	50	about 25	6–54 months
Ischia, et al.[13] (1990)	112	20	26	1–5 years
Steiger[24] (1991)	122	about 30	about 41	1–96 months

*Recurrence rates after glycerol injection within 2 years (early) and at follow-up after more than 2 years (late) in the various series.

jected, prior treatment with invasive techniques, and the technical performance of the procedure. Originally, I recommended that 0.2 to 0.4 ml glycerol be injected, depending on the size of the cistern, but the cistern did not have to be filled completely.[11] In the initial series, in 4 of 100 patients, the mean volume injected was only 0.21 ml.[9] Because many of the patients had had 1 or more prior surgical procedures and some of them were left with remaining disturbance of their facial sensitivity, I was reluctant to inject a larger amount of glycerol. This explains, not only the absence of marked postinjection sensory loss in that series, but also the relatively high recurrence rate.

In the published series in which larger volumes of glycerol have been injected, more marked sensory deficits have been observed.[7,28] One of these series[7] used 0.3 to 0.5 ml glycerol, about double the dose I have used. Some of the patients in this series had a substantial loss of facial sensibility; consequently, the investigators abandoned the technique. Interestingly, there is no direct correlation between postinjection sensory loss and the risk of recurrence. On the contrary, the report by Sahni and colleagues[23] found that the risk for recurrence seemed to be higher in patients with some persistent postinjection hypesthesia. At present, therefore, I recommend the use of only 0.2 to 0.3 ml glycerol. With this comparatively small volume, the unpredictability of postinjection sensory loss is less of a problem.

Glycerol is assumed to exert its neurolytic action through its marked hypertonicity and has been found to penetrate cell membranes readily.[4,5,15] My own experiments with intraneural application of glycerol in rats showed extensive damage in large myelinated fibers, and fine myelinated fibers were largely spared. In an electron microscopic study, undamaged unmyelinated fibers were found.[10,21,22]

Little is known about the functional changes glycerol produces in nervous tissue. It seems that glycerol must be added and removed gradually to avoid more extensive damage of neural tissue.[18] Glycerol takes at least 30 minutes to equilibrate in living cells; therefore, neurophysiological investigations performed only in the immediate postinjection period may be invalid. Sweet and Poletti[25,26] evacuate the glycerol from the cistern 5 minutes after its injection. Theoretically, this practice

could damage the fine fibers more severely and not affect the larger myelinated fibers.

A characteristic feature of the procedure is that patients generally have only a subtle postoperative disturbance of facial sensation. To analyze the presence of any selective vulnerability of fibers to glycerol, quantitative sensory examinations were carried out in a few patients to determine the thresholds for various sensory modalities. Thermal and tactile sensibility was tested.[6,8] Some patients had no demonstrable changes in thresholds after treatment; in others, only the tactile stimulation thresholds were influenced. Thus, large myelinated fibers seem to be particularly vulnerable to glycerol; however, it has not been possible to confirm this data to date.[16]

Although the exact cause of trigeminal neuralgia is not fully understood, mounting evidence indicates that segmental demyelination plays an important role. Demyelination is typically found in the large fiber spectrum, which clinically seems to be involved in the trigger phenomenon. Glycerol primarily affects the larger myelinated fibers. Therefore, the glycerol method appears to act on and abolish the trigger mechanism well before pain-transmitting fibers are affected. Thus, relief from trigeminal neuralgia does not seem to depend on the destruction of pain fibers.

To carry out the procedure safely, I recommend adhering to the original technique.[11,12] Contrast medium and glycerol should not be injected unless free egress of cerebrospinal fluid is obtained. Furthermore, the injection of more than 0.3 ml glycerol should be avoided. In patients with manifest substantial sensory loss, a nondestructive procedure should be used. If glycerol injection is considered, the volume of glycerol used should be reduced.

CONCLUSION

For the patient presented here, a woman of age 60 with classic trigeminal neuralgia involving the second and third branches, either microvascular decompression or a retrogasserian injection of glycerol can be recommended. Many patients choose a percutaneous procedure and are satisfied that, in case of recurrent pain, the injection can be repeated or another surgical procedure selected.

Microvascular Decompression for Trigeminal Neuralgia

Toshio Matsushima, M.D., Masashi Fukui, M.D.

Microvascular decompression is considered safe and effective treatment for patients with idiopathic trigeminal neuralgia, even with respect to long-term results.[3,6] In this review, we present our surgical experience and some important points concerning the selection of candidates for the procedure. We also describe the infratentorial lateral supracerebellar approach used for microvascular decompression.[2]

CASE MATERIAL

A 59-year-old woman developed right V2-V3 trigeminal neuralgia that became intractable to medical treatment. A magnetic resonance image of the patient's head was normal and she appeared to be in good physical condition. Magnetic resonance angiography showed that the right superior cerebellar artery looped downward, Figure 1 (**A**), (**B**). Surgery was performed through the infratentorial lateral supracerebellar approach. The superior cerebellar artery, which was compressing the trigeminal nerve, was elevated by fixing a sling to the tentorium, Figure 1 (**C**), (**D**). The patient's pain completely disappeared after surgery.

INDICATIONS

Microvascular decompression is indicated in patients with trigeminal neuralgia refractory to medical therapy, and poses no anesthetic risks. Most of our patients were under the age of 70 years and underwent decompression after drug therapy failed or

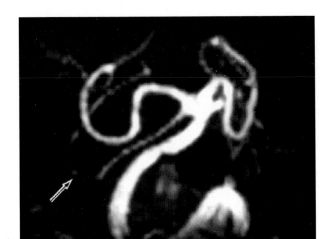

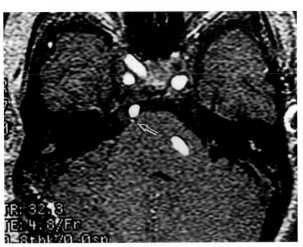

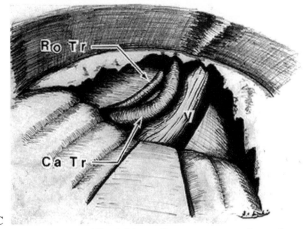

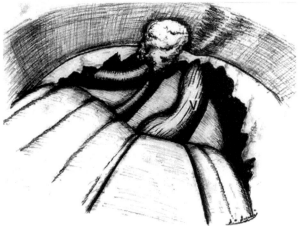

Fig. 1 Magnetic resonance angiography and a drawing of intraoperative views in a patient with right trigeminal neuralgia. (*A*) **The right superior cerebellar artery (arrow) can be seen looping downward while the basilar artery is shifted to the right.** (*B*) **A large artery is observed coursing near the right trigeminal nerve while the superior cerebellar artery (arrow) is in close contact with the entry zone of the nerve.** (*C*) **The superior cerebellar artery as it bifurcates into the rostral (RoTr) and caudal (CaTr) trunks. The caudal trunk compresses the trigeminal nerve (V) laterally.** (*D*) **The trunk, which was compressing the nerve, was elevated by fixing a sling to the tentorium. V, trigeminal nerve.**

they developed adverse side effects. Some younger patients with typical paroxysmal pain underwent this procedure without continuing drug therapy.

Each candidate for surgery was examined with either computed tomography scans or magnetic resonance images to rule out any neoplastic or vascular lesions. (Typical symptoms of trigeminal neuralgia can often result from such organic lesions.[4]) In the past, vertebral angiography was generally done to clarify the vasculature around the trigeminal nerve. This modality has now been replaced by magnetic resonance angiography.

Surgical Procedure

In the infratentorial lateral supracerebellar approach, a craniectomy is done at the corner of the transverse and sigmoid sinuses to expose the infratentorial subdural space on the tentorial cerebellar surface. A spatula is advanced along the anterolateral margin on the tentorial surface, Figure 2 (**A**). When the spatula is moved along the margin, 1 or 2 superior petrosal veins, which are made up of a few tributaries, are often encountered between the acoustic meatus and the trigeminal nerve. The most medial tributary is cut so that the cerebellar tentorial surface can be retracted. If necessary, the venous trunk can also be sacrificed. In some cases, however, all tributaries can be preserved. When the anterior angle of the cerebellar margins is reached, the medial aspect of the trigeminal nerve and the lateral mesencephalic segment of the superior cerebellar artery are exposed. Because this segment, which bifurcates, sometimes compresses the trigeminal nerve laterally at 2 or 3 points, the entire medial surface of the nerve should always be carefully observed,[1,2] Figure 2 (**B**). The most frequent offending artery is the superior cerebellar artery, but the anterior inferior cerebellar artery or the superior petrosal vein can also be the problematic vessels. The offending artery is transposed from the trigeminal nerve and should be fixed with a prosthesis, such as a piece of Teflon® felt or a sponge. Portions of veins in contact with the nerve are also divided.

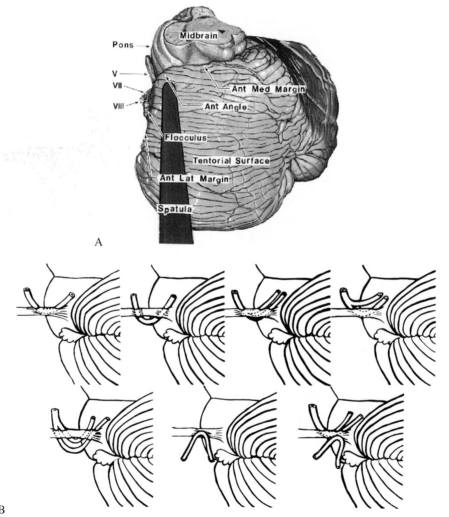

Fig. 2 Surgical procedure: (*A*) Posterolateral view of the left tentorial surface. The spatula is advanced along the left anterolateral margin on the tentorial surface. Its tip is close to the anterior angle. (*B*) The relationships between the trigeminal nerve and the superior and anterior inferior cerebellar arteries. (Reproduced with permission from Matsushima T, Fukui M, Suzuki S, et al.: The microsurgical anatomy of the infratentorial lateral supracerebellar approach to the trigeminal nerve for tic douloureux. *Neurosurgery* 1989; 24:890–895.)

Surgical Results

We have operated on 56 patients with trigeminal neuralgia using microvascular decompression.[3] Of these patients, 84% were free of pain at the time of their discharge from the hospital. An additional 12% showed partial improvement, which totals post-surgical improvement of 96% (Table 1). We were able to follow 44 patients (79%) for a mean period of 60 months (range 1 to 125 months). Of these 44 patients, 81.8% remained free of pain, and 16% showed a partial response (Table 2). Permanent postoperative complications included mild hearing loss (2 patients), paresthesia of the face (3 patients), and delayed severe headache (1 patient) (Table 3). All other symptoms were transient. No deaths or major complications occurred. Nine of the 56 patients had recurrence; 2 underwent a second operation because the recurrent pain was severe. In 1 of these patients, the large vertebral artery again compressed the nerve, and in the other the sponge was found to have slipped out of place. After the second surgery, both patients had complete relief of pain. No surgery for recurrent pain was done on the remaining 7 patients because the frequency and severity of their pain was decreased compared to their preoperative symptoms.

Discussion

A few investigators have reported prognostic factors in microvascular decompression for trigeminal neuralgia.[5] The mode in which the pain manifests is the factor most significantly related to prognosis. In patients with only paroxysmal pain, a cure can be achieved in about 90%. Other factors influencing the success of this treatment include the presence of a conflicting artery, the type of prosthesis used, and the surgeon's skill.

Before microvascular decompression can be recommended

Table 1. Surgical Results of Microvascular Decompression at the Time of Discharge (n = 56)

Result	No. of patients	Percentage
Excellent	47	83.9
Good	4	7.1
Fair	3	5.4
Unchanged	2	3.6

Table 2. Long-Term Results of Microvascular Decompression (n = 44)*

Result	No. of patients	Percentage
Excellent	36	81.8
Good	5	11.4
Fair	2	4.5
Unchanged	1	2.3

*Mean follow-up, 60 months.

for the patient presented in this case, the surgical results should be discussed, together with postoperative complications.

We have employed the infratentorial lateral supracerebellar approach to reduce complications and to preserve the trunk of the petrosal veins.[2] In this approach, the trigeminal nerve can be reached through an area far from the seventh and eighth cranial nerves as well as from the subarcuate artery.

CONCLUSION

Microvascular decompression is an effective treatment for patients with trigeminal neuralgia.[1,3,5,6] Long-lasting pain relief is obtained in about 80% of patients without any significant facial sensory loss or annoying facial paresthesia and dysesthesia. Even for those with recurrent pain, decompression can often be effective. Other treatments, such as radiofrequency rhizotomy or glycerin injections, may be the next choice after microvascular decompression. Currently, however, microvascular decompression is considered the most desirable treatment modality for patients with trigeminal neuralgia.

Table 3. Permanent Postoperative Complications of Microvascular Decompression (n = 56)*

Complication	No. of patients	Percentage
Hearing disturbance	2	3.6
Paresthesia of the face	3	5.4
Delayed headache	1	1.8

*All other complications were transient and no major complications occurred.

Treatment of Patients with Trigeminal Neuralgia

Robert H. Wilkins, M.D.

For this 60-year-old woman with typical trigeminal neuralgia, there is both good and bad news. The good news is that there are several methods of treating this form of facial pain successfully, in comparison to other forms of facial pain that are much more difficult to control. Furthermore, there are numerous physicians worldwide who can perform such treatments. The bad news is that no single treatment results in permanent relief in all patients, and each form of treatment has risks and complications. During the course of his or her life, the individual with trigeminal neuralgia often requires more than one form of treatment.

DIAGNOSIS

The first hurdle faced by the patient who develops trigeminal neuralgia is diagnosis. Even today, this typical form of facial pain may not be recognized by the practitioner (dental or medical) whose help is sought initially. Occasionally, inappropriate treatment is pursued, such as the extraction of 1 or more teeth or the performance of a root canal procedure.

Furthermore, even when the diagnosis of trigeminal neuralgia is made, the practitioner may not recognize that it may be a symptom of a disease process that should also be addressed, such as a benign tumor in the cerebellopontine angle or multiple sclerosis. Because the magnetic resonance image in the present patient was normal, such considerations need not concern us here.

INITIAL APPROACH: MEDICAL THERAPY

When the diagnosis of "idiopathic" trigeminal neuralgia is made, the first therapeutic approach ordinarily involves medication. Three medicines are especially useful in this regard: carbamazepine, phenytoin, and baclofen. In general, carbamazepine is the most effective, but it may occasionally cause significant adverse reactions such as pancytopenia or abnormalities in liver function. Ordinarily, 1 of the 3 drugs is begun at a low dose, which is then gradually increased according to the patient's response. The objective is to arrive at the smallest dose that will provide adequate pain relief. With time, the patient may require greater amounts of the medicine to obtain the same degree of relief, and may experience dose-related side effects, such as lethargy and unsteadiness. At this juncture, 1 of the other 2 medicines can be tried instead of the original drug, or in addition to a reduced dosage of the original drug. If the pain is not controlled well, the third medicine can be used, either alone or in combination with one or both of the others.

SURGICAL ALTERNATIVES

If an adequate trial of medical therapy fails, as it did in this woman, several surgical alternatives exist. Trigeminal branch injection or avulsion could be considered for certain patients, such as an elderly or frail individual with pain in the distribution of the infraorbital nerve, but this would not be the best alternative in this healthy 60-year-old woman. Her pain is in the territory of both the second and third trigeminal divisions, and both trunks (or appropriate branches) would require injection or avulsion. The expected duration of relief resulting from the injection of alcohol into the infraorbital, maxillary, or mandibular nerves would be only in the range of 12 to 16 months; that resulting from avulsion of the infraorbital, inferior alveolar, lingual, or mental nerves would be only in the range of 2 to 3 years.[10] Furthermore, dense anesthesia would be expected to persist for the same duration in the distribution of the injected or avulsed nerves.

The other present-day surgical alternatives are those discussed here. Radiofrequency rhizotomy, glycerol injection into the trigeminal cistern, and balloon compression are all percutaneous techniques. In general, these are low-risk procedures that can be accomplished with a one-night hospitalization or even on an outpatient basis. These are important considerations, not only regarding patient safety, but also concerning treatment costs and adaptability to use in developing countries. On the other hand, the patient frequently experiences discomfort during a radiofrequency rhizotomy or glycerol injection, and all 3 procedures may be attended by significant alterations of blood pressure and pulse.[5] Because each of the percutaneous operations has a destructive effect on the nerve, some degree of ipsilateral facial and corneal hypesthesia may result and, because each also involves the insertion of a needle through the foramen ovale, the function of the ipsilateral muscles of mastication may be impaired, as well.

Microvascular decompression is a bigger procedure, with greater risks and a longer (ordinarily 5 to 7 days) and more expensive hospitalization. But, the patient is comfortable during the procedure, which is conducted under general anesthesia, and may achieve pain relief without any loss of trigeminal sensory or motor function.

Comments Regarding These Four Communications

As I have witnessed, Nugent is a master of radiofrequency rhizotomy for trigeminal neuralgia. Because of his refined technique and extensive experience, he can present the best that can be accomplished with this procedure. In his discussion, he also gives a fair representation of the negative features of the procedure. He is right that the operation of microvascular decompression is accompanied by a definite risk of ipsilateral deafness, but this threat can be virtually eliminated by the use of intraoperative monitoring of brain stem auditory evoked potentials.[12]

Håkanson originated the procedure of percutaneous trigeminal glycerol rhizolysis and writes authoritatively about this procedure. Although he gives the results of 10 series regarding pain relief and recurrence, he does not detail the undesirable side effects or complications of glycerol rhizolysis.

Brown is one of a relatively small number of neurosurgeons who have had a significant experience with balloon compression for trigeminal neuralgia. He presents the pros and cons of this approach in a straightforward manner, emphasizing patient comfort during the procedure, and the relative technical simplicity and safety of trigeminal balloon compression.

Matsushima and Fukui present the results of microvascular decompression for trigeminal neuralgia in a small personal series, but they do not provide an overview from the experience of other surgeons about the expected results and risks of this form of treatment. They also do not discuss the option of partial sectioning of the main sensory root of the trigeminal nerve when significant vascular compression is not identified during the operation.

Additional Comments About Microvascular Decompression

Sweet[7] has summarized the long-term results of microvascular decompression for trigeminal neuralgia. Among 1700 patients from 17 reported series, the initial failure rate was 7% and the late recurrence rate was 14%.

Larkins and colleagues[3] have analyzed the results of such treatment on Jannetta's service over a 20-year period. I have summarized this information elsewhere as follows[11]:

> Although almost all of the patients had microvascular decompression, 5.5% had partial sectioning of the main sensory root of the trigeminal nerve instead of, or in addition to, this form of treatment. The authors ... divided their patients into four groups according to prior treatment.... Among 706 patients in the group with prior treatment with medication only, 594 had a follow-up evaluation from 12 to 210 months (average, 68 months) postoperatively, 76% had complete relief, 6.7% had partial relief, and 17.3% failed treatment.... In 1984, Piatt and Wilkins[4] reported the results of microvascular decompression in 81 patients with tic douloureux. Of the 68 patients noted to have definite arterial contact with the trigeminal nerve, 78% had excellent (72%) or good (6%) relief after a mean follow-up period of 54 months. In contrast, of the 13 patients with indefinite arterial contact or with venous contact, only 54% had excellent (46%) or

good (8%) relief after a mean follow-up period of 64 months. Furthermore, the 37 patients having anatomical distortion of the trigeminal nerve or wedging of one or more arteries between the nerve and the pons had a better outcome than the 31 with lesser forms of arterial contact. When these results for each of these four patient groups were graphed over time in Kaplan-Meier plots, it was apparent that although between 90% and 100% of the patients in each category obtained relief initially from microvascular decompression, a gradually enlarging number experienced recurrence of pain with time. From their own experience with 36 patients undergoing microvascular decompression for trigeminal neuralgia, Burchiel et al.[1] found that major recurrences averaged 3.5% annually and minor recurrences averaged 1.5% annually.

I believe that, if arterial or significant venous compression is not identified or cannot be rectified safely during the surgical exposure of the trigeminal nerve root entry zone, the surgeon should consider cutting part of the main sensory root. Young and Wilkins[13] found that the pain relief experienced by 83 patients treated in this fashion, after an average follow-up period of 6 years, was excellent in 48%, good in 22%, and poor in 30%. The failure rate for the first year was 17%, and it averaged 2.6% per year thereafter.

Again quoting from my earlier review,[11]

In the study by Larkins et al.,[3] the authors tabulated the complications of their four patient groups and noted that microvascular decompression in patients who had had that procedure previously had a higher rate of temporary and permanent cranial nerve injury than in patients with prior treatment by medications or destructive procedures. The major complications in the entire group of 1117 patients included 4 deaths, 3 instances of intracranial hemorrhage, 3 of cerebellar edema, 2 of brain stem infarction, and 2 of hydrocephalus. Among the 139 patients with prior microvascular decompression, the repeat procedure caused permanent cranial nerve complications as follows: trigeminal nerve–10; facial nerve–2; and auditory nerve–2. The permanent cranial nerve complications in the other 978 patients included: trigeminal nerve–4; and auditory nerve–3. Among the other complications in the entire group, the most common were aseptic meningitis (179) and CSF leakage (14).

Piatt and Wilkins[4] noted four major complications that resulted from their 105 posterior fossa operations from microvascular decompression or partial sensory rhizotomy of the trigeminal nerve. There was one death, from infarction in the brain stem and cerebellum, and one instance each of acute epidural hematoma, chronic subdural hematoma, and unexplained dementia. The significant unintentional cranial nerve injuries were as follows: trigeminal nerve–1, facial nerve–1, and auditory nerve 8.[11]

(The auditory nerve injuries occurred before intraoperative monitoring of brain stem auditory evoked potentials was introduced.)

Caveats

Sweet has had a special interest over the years in documenting the positive and negative aspects of the various surgical treatments for trigeminal neuralgia.[2,5–9] In 1988, he and Poletti[8] wrote:

Conversations with colleagues suggested that the sequelae of the most commonly used operations for trigeminal neuralgia may occur more frequently than is indicated by the published experiences of those of us who, with happy outcomes, have gone on to do large series of cases.... We made personal inquiries of other neurosurgeons which revealed that several of their patients had had intracranial hemorrhages related to RF rhizotomies.... These events convinced us that it would be fruitful for doctors, patients, and even defense attorneys to have more information on the global experience with our operations. As a pilot study, we wrote to 200 neurosurgical friends (50 abroad) indicating the basis for the study and requesting data from them on complications on their services or of which they knew following percutaneous RF or glycerol lesions or microvascular decompression. To this burdensome request 140 neurosurgeons ... replied.

Regarding the complications of percutaneous radiofrequency trigeminal rhizotomies, data were collected from 91 neurosurgical services, nearly all not previously reported; 29 services provided their entire number of rhizotomies, totaling more than 7000.

Of lesser complications there were 18 patients with neuroparalytic keratitis, 8 with aseptic meningeal reactions ... and 5 with carotid-cavernous fistulas.... There were 18 temporary oculomotor palsies and at least 1 that was permanent.... A seizure occurred during the procedure in 2 patients and in 1 a transient postoperative psychosis developed.[8]

Among the serious complications were 5 patients with permanent and 1 with transient ipsilateral blindness from optic nerve injury, and 1 patient with a central retinal artery occlusion. There were 21 instances of bacterial meningitis, with 1 death. Seven patients developed a brain abscess, 1 died, and 1 was left with permanent mental impairment. There were 19 instances of focal intracranial hemorrhage; 10 patients died, 5 were left with major deficits, and 3 experienced transient hemiplegia. There were also 5 instances of arterial subarachnoid hemorrhage, with 3 deaths. Yet, as mentioned by Sweet and Poletti,[8] "it is worth noting that there are at least 6 services in each of which well over 1000 percutaneous retrogasserian trigeminal procedures have been performed without any lasting major extratrigeminal complications."

Sweet recorded fewer complications after retrogasserian glycerol injection.[5,6] He noted, however, that some surgeons had concerns about dysesthesias and major sensory loss, early failures, and later recurrence. For example, in the 1986 series of Sweet,[6] among 80 patients treated with glycerol, 20% experienced dysesthesias and 16% had late corneal anesthesia. There was an initial failure rate of 14% and, during a follow-up period of 1 to 7 years (average, 2.8 years), there was a recurrence rate of 33%.

Regarding microvascular decompression, Sweet and Poletti[8] summarized the findings from the neurosurgical services they polled as follows:

[Nine] services reported essentially no complications.... No deaths and only moderate lasting sequelae were the experiences of 17 services.... From 24 services came accounts of permanently disabling sequelae or deaths in 29 cases.... The 2 most discouraging series involved 3 technically competent distinguished neurosurgeons, who had 4 deaths in 60 patients, all in "healthy" individuals, 3 in their 50s and 1 aged 31, all following "smooth, uneventful operations."

This sobering information brings home several points. First, regarding the percutaneous procedures, as Sweet and Poletti said, "it is easy to take a casual attitude toward the procedure because of its simplicity. The achievement of consistent success without sequelae demands scrupulous attention to detail."[8] Second, microvascular decompression is not an entirely benign procedure, and it is accompanied by significant risks. Third, the individual surgeon should periodically review the outcomes of his or her own operations for trigeminal neuralgia so that realistic expectations can be presented to a patient (rather than citations of the literature that usually reflect the best results of the most experienced surgeons). And finally, as Sweet and Poletti[8] noted, "even if the neurosurgeon has enough experience to emphasize only his own results, he would be well advised to describe to patients the possibility of a fuller range of complications than were seen in the best series."

CONCLUSIONS

In a discussion of the surgical options with the 60-year-old woman for whom medical therapy failed, the neurosurgeon consulted should try to cover the basic pros and cons of the percutaneous and posterior fossa procedures. Many patients have difficulty understanding much of this material, however, and rely on the surgeon for guidance. The surgeon must consider the patient's medical needs first, but must also consider the availability of the various types of treatment locally and the patient's ability or desire to go elsewhere for the recommended treatment. Because of the increasing restrictions by third party payers in the United States on distant referral for surgical treatment, at least 1 neurosurgeon in each medical community of reasonable size and location should acquire the equipment and skills necessary to offer patients with trigeminal neuralgia the options of microvascular decompression and at least 1 of the 3 percutaneous procedures. Then, the onus is on that surgeon to inform the patient truthfully and accurately about what can be achieved locally, as well as what the advantage might be of referral to a neurosurgeon who is more experienced in a certain form of treatment. There is a fine line between adequate disclosure of risks and potential complications and frightening the patient away from an operative approach that is likely to result in long-term relief.

If I were consulted by the woman in question, I would discuss with her the 2 options of percutaneous glycerol trigeminal rhizolysis or microvascular decompression (with the fall-back position of partial root section if significant vascular compression was not identified), because I can speak both from personal experience and from what has been published about the 2 procedures. The main issues I would cover with the patient (and possibly at least 1 other responsible family member) are the nature of trigeminal neuralgia and, for each of the 2 operations, the basic steps of the procedure, the associated time in the hospital and time away from work, the expectations of relief, and the approximate risk levels of the main side effects and complications. In addition, I would indicate that each operation is a well-established form of treatment, but that I could not guarantee a successful outcome for either. Then, for completeness, I would also touch on the alternative methods of treatment that I do not recommend. This sort of discussion frequently must be repeated, often at a later date as well, because it may take time for some patients to understand the information well enough to give an informed consent.

REFERENCES

G. Robert Nugent, M.D.

1. Apfelbaum RI: A comparison of percutaneous radiofrequency trigeminal neurolysis and microvascular decompression of the trigeminal nerve for the treatment of tic douloureux. *Neurosurgery* 1977; 1:16–21.

2. Apfelbaum RI: Advantages and disadvantages of various techniques to treat trigeminal neuralgia, in Rovit RL, Murali R, Jannetta PJ (eds): *Trigeminal Neuralgia*. Baltimore, Williams and Wilkins, 1990, pp 239–250.

3. Barba D, Alksne JF: Success of microvascular decompression with and without prior surgical therapy for trigeminal neuralgia. *J Neurosurg* 1984; 60:104–107.

4. Bederson JB, Wilson CB: Evaluation of microvascular decompression and partial sensory rhizotomy in 252 cases of trigeminal neuralgia. *J Neurosurg* 1989; 71:359–367.

5. Belber CJ, Rak RA: Balloon compression rhizolysis in the surgical management of trigeminal neuralgia. *Neurosurgery* 1987; 20:908–913.

6. Breeze R, Ignelzi RJ: Microvascular decompression for trigeminal neuralgia. Results with special reference to the late recurrence rate. *J Neurosurg* 1982; 57:487–490.

7. Burchiel KJ: Percutaneous retrogasserian glycerol rhizolysis in the management of trigeminal neuralgia. *J Neurosurg* 1988; 69:361–366.

8. Burchiel KJ, Clarke H, Haglund M, et al.: Long term efficacy of microvascular decompression in trigeminal neuralgia. *J Neurosurg* 1988; 69:35–38.

9. Burchiel KJ, Steege TD, Howe JF, et al.: Comparison of percutaneous radiofrequency gangliolysis and microvascular decompression for the surgical management of tic douloureux. *Neurosurgery* 1981; 9:111–119.

10. Dieckmann G, Bockermann V, Heyer C, et al.: Five-and-a-half years experience with percutaneous retrogasserian glycerol rhizotomy in treatment of trigeminal neuralgia. *Appl Neurophysiol* 1987; 50:401–413.

11. Ferguson GG, Brett DC, Peerless SJ, et al.: Trigeminal neuralgia: A comparison of the results of percutaneous rhizotomy and microvascular decompression. *J Can Sci Neurol* 1981; 8:207–214.

12. Fraioli B, Esposito V, Guidetti B, et al.: Treatment of trigeminal neuralgia by thermocoagulation, glycerolization, and percutaneous compression of the gasserian ganglion and/or retrogasserian rootlets: Long-term results and therapeutic protocol. *Neurosurgery* 1989; 24:239–245.

13. Fujimaki T, Fukushima T, Miyazaki S: Percutaneous retrogasserian glycerol injections in the management of trigeminal neuralgia: Long-term follow-up results. *J Neurosurg* 1990; 73:212–216.

14. Kolluri S, Heros RC: Microvascular decompression: A five year follow-up study. *Surg Neurol* 1984; 22:234–240.
15. Lichtor T, Mullan JF: A 10-year follow-up review of percutaneous microcompression of the trigeminal ganglion. *J Neurosurg* 1990; 72:49–54.
16. Lobato RD, Rivas JJ, Sarabia R, et al.: Percutaneous microcompression of the gasserian ganglion for trigeminal neuralgia. *J Neurosurg* 1990; 72:546–553.
17. Lunsford LD: Percutaneous retrogasserian glycerol rhizotomy, in Rovit RL, Murali R, Jannetta PJ (eds): *Trigeminal Neuralgia.* Baltimore, Williams and Wilkins, 1990, pp 145–164.
18. Nugent GR: Trigeminal neuralgia treatment by percutaneous electro-coagulation, in Wilkins RH, Rengachary SS (eds): *Neurosurgery.* New York, McGraw-Hill, 1985, pp 2345–2350.
19. Nugent GR: Surgical treatment: Radiofrequency gangliolysis and rhizotomy, in Fromm GH, Sessle BJ (eds): *Trigeminal Neuralgia: Current Concepts Regarding Pathogeneses and Treatment.* Boston, Butterworth-Heinemann, 1991, pp 159–184.
20. Piatt JH Jr, Wilkins RH: Treatment of tic douloureux and hemifacial spasm by posterior fossa exploration: Therapeutic implications of various neurovascular relationships. *Neurosurgery* 1984; 14:462–471.
21. Piatt JH Jr, Wilkins RH: Microvascular decompression for tic douloureux (letter). *Neurosurgery* 1984; 15:456.
22. Rappaport ZH, Gomori JM: Recurrent trigeminal cistern glycerol injections for tic douloureux. *Acta Neurochir* 1988; 90:31–34.
23. Sahni KS, Pieper DR, Anderson R, et al.: Relation of hypesthesia to the outcome of glycerol rhizolysis for trigeminal neuralgia. *J Neurosurg* 1990; 72:55–58.
24. Saini SS: Retrogasserian anhydrous glycerol injection therapy in trigeminal neuralgia: Observations in 552 patients. *J Neurol Neurosurg Psychiatry* 1987; 50:1536–1538.
25. Siegfried J: Percutaneous controlled thermocoagulation of gasserian ganglion in trigeminal neuralgia. Experience with 1000 cases, in Samii M, Jannetta PJ (eds): *The Cranial Nerves.* Berlin, Springer-Verlag, 1981, pp 322–330.
26. Sweet WH: Treatment of trigeminal neuralgia by percutaneous rhizotomy, in Youmans JR (ed): *Neurological Surgery,* ed 3. Philadelphia, WB Saunders, 1989.
27. Sweet WH: Complications of treating trigeminal neuralgia; an analysis of the literature and response to questionnaire, in Rovit RL, Murali R, Jannetta PJ (eds): *Trigeminal Neuralgia.* Baltimore, Williams and Wilkins, 1990, pp 251–279.
28. Sweet WH: Faciocephalic pain, in Apuzzo MLJ (ed): *Brain Surgery: Complication Avoidance and Management.* New York, Churchill Livingstone, 1993, pp 2053–2083.
29. Sweet WH, Wepsic JG: Controlled thermocoagulation of trlgemlnal ganglion and rootlets for differential destruction of pain fibers. *J Neurosurg* 1974; 39:143–156.
30. Taarnhoj P: Decompression of the posterior trigeminal root in trigeminal neuralgia. *J Neurosurg* 1982; 57:14–17.
31. Van Loveren H, Tew JM, Keller JT, et al.: A 10-year experience in the treatment of trigeminal neuralgia. Comparison of percutaneous stereotaxic rhizotomy and posterior fossa exploration. *J Neurosurg* 1982; 57:757–764.
32. Waltz TA, Dalessio DJ, Copeland B: Percutaneous injections of glycerol for the treatment of trigeminal neuralgia. *Clin J Pain* 1989; 5:195–198.
33. Young RF: Stereotaxic procedures for facial pain, in Apuzzo MLJ (ed): *Brain Surgery: Complication Avoidance and Management.* New York, Churchill Livingstone, 1993, pp 2097–2113.
34. Zorman G, Wilson CB: Outcome following microsurgical vascular decompression or partial sensory rhizotomy in 125-cases of trigeminal neuralgia. *Neurology* 1984; 34:1362–1365.

Jeffrey A. Brown, M.D.

1. Brown JA, Preul MC: Trigeminal depressor response during percutaneous microcompression of the trigeminal ganglion for trigeminal neuralgia. *Neurosurgery* 1988; 23:745–748.
2. Brown JA, Preul MC: Percutaneous trigeminal ganglion compression for trigeminal neuralgia: Experience in 22 patients and review of the literature. *J Neurosurg* 1989; 70:900–904.
3. Fraioli B, Esposito V, Guidetti B, et al.: Treatment of trigeminal neuralgia by thermocoagulation, glycerolization, and percutaneous compression of the gasserian ganglion and/or retrogasserian rootlets: Long-term results and therapeutic protocol. *Neurosurgery* 1989; 24:239–245.
4. Gybels JM, Sweet WH: *Neurosurgical Treatment of Persistent Pain: Physiological and Pathological Mechanisms of Human Pain.* Basel, Karger, 1989, pp 10–69.
5. Lobato RD, Rivas JJ, Sarabia R, et al.: Percutaneous microcompression of the gasserian ganglion for trigeminal neuralgia. *J Neurosurg* 1990; 72:546–553.
6. Lunsford LD: Trigeminal neuralgia: Treatment by glycerol rhizotomy, in Wilkins RH, Rengachary SS (eds): *Neurosurgery.* New York, McGraw Hill, 1985, pp 2351–2356.
7. Mullan JF, Lichtor T: Percutaneous microcompression of the trigeminal ganglion for trigeminal neuralgia. *J Neurosurg* 1983; 59:1007–1012.
8. Preul MC, Long PB, Brown JA, et al.: Autonomic and histopathological effects of percutaneous trigeminal ganglion compression in the rabbit. *J Neurosurg* 1990; 72:933–940.

Sten Håkanson, M.D.

1. Arias MJ: Percutaneous retrogasserian glycerol rhizotomy for trigeminal neuralgia. A prospective study of 100 cases. *J Neurosurg* 1986; 65:32–36.
2. Burchiel KJ: Percutaneous retrogasserian glycerol rhizolysis in the management of trigeminal neuralgia. *J Neurosurg* 1988; 69:361–366.
3. Dieckmann G, Bockermann V, Heyer C, et al.: Five-and-a-half years experience with percutaneous retrogasserian glycerol rhizotomy in treatment of trigeminal neuralgia. *Appl Neurophysiol* 1987; 50:401–413.
4. Dulhunty AF, Gage PW: Differential effects of glycerol treatment on membrane capacity and excitation-contraction coupling in toad sartorius fibers. *J Physiol (Lond)* 1973; 234:373–408.
5. Freeman AR, Reuben JP, Brandt PW, et al.: Osmometrically determined characteristics of the cell membrane of squid and lobster giant axons. *J Gen Physiol* 1066; 50:335–423.
6. Fruhstorfer H, Lindblom U, Schmidt WG: Method for quantitative estimation of thermal thresholds in patients. *J Neurol Neurosurg Psychiatry* 1976; 39:1071–1075.
7. Fujimaki T, Fukoshima T, Miyazaki S: Percutaneous retrogasserian glycerol injection in the management of trigeminal neuralgia: Long-term follow-up results. *J Neurosurg* 1990; 73:212–216.
8. Goldberg JM, Lindblom U: Stadardised method of determining vibratory perception thresholds for diagnosis and screening in neurological investigation. *J Neurol Neurosurg Psychiatry* 1976; 42:793–803.
9. Håkanson S: Retrogasserian glycerol injection as treatment of tic douloureux. *Adv Pain Res Ther* 1983; 5:927–933.
10. Håkanson S: *Trigeminal Neuralgia Treated by Retrogasserian Injection of Glycerol.* Dissertation, Stockholm, Karolinska Institute, 1982.

11. Håkanson S: Trigeminal neuralgia treated by the injection of glycerol into the trigeminal cistern. *Neurosurgery* 1981; 9:638–646.

12. Håkanson S: Transoval trigeminal cisternography. *Surg Neurol* 1978; 10:137–144.

13. Ischia S, Luzzani A, Polati E: Retrogasserian glycerol injection: A retrospective study of 112 patients. *Clin J Pain* 1990; 6:291–296.

14. Jannetta PJ: Surgical treatment: Microvascular decompression, in Fromm GH, Sessle BJ (eds): *Trigeminal Neuralgia: Current Concepts Regarding Pathogenesis and Treatment*. Boston, Butterwort-Heinemann, 1991, pp 145–157.

15. King JS, Jewett DL, Sundberg HR: Differential blockade of cat dorsal root C-fibres by various chloride solutions. *J Neurosurg* 1972; 36:569–583.

16. Laitinen LL, Brophy BP, Bergenheim AT: Sensory disturbance following percutaneous retrogasserian glycerol rhizotomy. *Br J Neurosurg* 1989; 83:471–478.

17. Linderoth B, Hakanson S: Paroxysmal facial pain in disseminated sclerosis treated by retrogasserian glycerol injection. *Acta Neurol Scand* 1989; 80:341–346.

18. Lovelock JE: The mechanism of the portective action of glycerol against hemolysis by freezing and thawing. *Acta Biochim Biophys* 1953; 11:28–36.

19. Lunsford LD: Percutaneous retrogasserian glycerol rhizotomy, in Rovit RL, Murali R, Jannetta PJ (eds): *Trigeminal Neuralgia*. Baltimore, Williams and Wilkins, 1990, pp 145–164.

20. North RB, Kidd DH, Piantadosi S, et al.: Percutaneous retrogasserian glycerol rhizotomy. *J Neurosurg* 1990; 72:851–856.

21. Pal HK, Dinda AK, Roy S, et al.: Acute effects of anhydrous glycerol on peripheral nerve: An experimental study. *Neurosurgery* 1989; 3:463–470.

22. Rengachary SS, Watanabe IS, Singer P, et al.: Effect of glycerol on peripheral nerve: An experimental study. *Neurosurgery* 1983; 13: 681–688.

23. Sahni KS, Pieper DR, Anderson R, et al.: Relation of hypesthesia to the outcome of glycerol rhizolysis for trigeminal neuralgia. *J Neurosurg* 1990; 72:55–58.

24. Steiger HJ: Prognostic factors in the treatment of trigeminal neuralgia: Analysis of a differential therapeutic approach. *Acta Neurochir* 1991; 113:11–17.

25. Sweet WH: Faciocephalic pain, in Apuzzo MLJ (ed): *Brain Surgery: Complication Avoidance and Management*. New York, Churchill Livingstone, 1993, pp 2053–2083.

26. Sweet WH, Poletti CE: Problems with retrogasserian glycerol in the treatment of trigeminal neuralgia. *Appl Neurophysiol* 1985; 48: 252–257.

27. Waltz TA, Dalessio DJ, Copeland B, et al.: Percutaneous injection of glycerol for the treatment of trigeminal neuralgia. *Clin J Pain* 1989; 5:195–198.

28. Young RF: Glycerol rhizolysis for treatment of trigeminal neuralgia. *J Neurosurg* 1988; 69:39–45.

Toshio Matsushima, M.D., Masashi Fukui, M.D.

1. Jannetta PJ: Trigeminal neuralgia: Treatment by microvascular decompression, in Wilkins RH, Rengachary SS (eds): *Neurosurgery*. Baltimore, Williams and Wilkins, 1985, pp 2357–2363.

2. Matsushima T, Fukui M, Suzuki S, et al.: The microsurgical anatomy of the infratentorial lateral supracerebellar approach to the trigeminal nerve for tic douloureux. *Neurosurgery* 1989; 24:890–895.

3. Matsushima T, Nomura T, Ikezaki K, et al.: Surgical treatment of trigeminal neuralgia—A long follow-up result of microvascular decompression procedure. *J Jpn Soc Study Chronic Pain* 1993; 12:193–197 (in Japanese).

4. Nomura T, Ikezaki K, Matsushima T, et al.: Trigeminal neuralgia: Differentiation between intracranial mass lesions and ordinary vascular compression as causative lesions. *Neurosurg Rev* 1994; 17: 51–57.

5. Szapiro J, Sindou M: Prognostic factors in microvascular decompression for trigeminal neuralgia. *Neurosurgery* 1985; 17:920–929.

6. Taarnhoj P: Decompression of the posterior trigeminal root in trigeminal neuralgia. *J Neurosurg* 1982; 57:14–17.

Robert H. Wilkins, M.D.

1. Burchiel KJ, Clarke H, Haglund M, et al.: Long-term efficacy of microvascular decompression in trigeminal neuralgia. *J Neurosurg* 1988; 69:35–38.

2. Gybels JM, Sweet WH: *Neurosurgical Treatment of Persistent Pain: Physiological and Pathological Mechanisms of Human Pain*. Basel, Karger, 1989, pp 10–69.

3. Larkins MV, Jannetta PJ, Bissonette D: *Microvascular decompression for recurrent trigeminal neuralgia*. Presented at the 59th Annual Meeting of the American Association of Neurological Surgeons, New Orleans, Louisiana, April 23, 1991.

4. Piatt JH Jr, Wilkins RH: Treatment of tic douloureux and hemifacial spasm by posterior fossa exploration: Therapeutic implications of various neurovascular relationships. *Neurosurgery* 1984; 14: 462–471.

5. Sweet WH: Complications of treating trigeminal neuralgia; an analysis of the literature and response to questionnaire, in Rovit RL, Murali R, Jannetta PJ (eds): *Trigeminal Neuralgia*. Baltimore, Williams and Wilkins, 1990, pp 251–279.

6. Sweet WH: Retrogasserian glycerol injection as treatment for trigeminal neuralgia, in Schmidek HH, Sweet WH (eds): *Operative Neurosurgical Techniques: Indications, Methods and Results*, ed 2. Orlando FL, Grune and Stratton, 1988, pp 1129–1137.

7. Sweet WH: Trigeminal neuralgia: Problems as to cause and consequent conclusions regarding treatment, in Wilkins RH, Rengachary SS (eds): *Neurosurgery*, ed 3. New York, McGraw-Hill, in press.

8. Sweet WH, Poletti CE: Complications of percutaneous rhizotomy and microvascular decompression operations for facial pain, in Schmidek HH, Sweet WH (eds): *Operative Neurosurgical Techniques: Indications, Methods and Results*, ed 2. Orlando, Grune and Stratton, 1988, pp 1139–1143.

9. White JC, Sweet WH: *Pain and the Neurosurgeon: A Forty-Year Experience*. Springfield, IL, Charles C Thomas, 1969.

10. Wilkins RH: Trigeminal neuralgia: Introduction, in Wilkins RH, Rengachary SS (eds): *Neurosurgery*. New York, McGraw-Hill, 1985, pp 2337–2344.

11. Wilkins RH: Neurovascular decompression procedures in the surgical management of disorders of nerves V, VII, IX, X to treat pain, in Schmidek HH, Sweet WH (eds): *Operative Neurosurgical Techniques: Indications, Methods and Results*, ed 3. Philadelphia, WB Saunders, 1994.

12. Wilkins RH, Radtke RA, Erwin CW: Value of intraoperative brainstem auditory evoked potential monitoring in reducing the auditory morbidity associated with microvascular decompression of cranial nerves. *Skull Base Surg* 1991; 1:106–109.

13. Young JN, Wilkins RH: Partial sensory trigeminal rhizotomy at the pons for trigeminal neuralgia. *J Neurosurg* 1993; 79:680–687.

38

The Ethics of Research on a Disputed Therapy: Cervical Spondylotic Myelopathy

PARTICIPANTS

A Call for Randomized Study of Cervical Spondylotic Myelopathy: Ethical Issues–
Lewis P. Rowland, M.D.

A Randomized Study of Cervical Spondylotic Myelopathy: Is It Ethical? Is It Feasible?–
Douglas E. Anderson, M.D.

*Moderator–*David C. Thomasma, Ph.D.

A Call for Randomized Study of Cervical Spondylotic Myelopathy: Ethical Issues

Lewis P. Rowland, M.D.

Decompressive operations are widely used to treat patients with cervical spondylotic myelopathy. The syndrome can be defined by pathologic findings at autopsy. The clinical findings are thought to be characteristic, and the clinical diagnosis can be bolstered by magnetic resonance imaging (MRI) or contrast myelography with computed tomography (CT). The results of surgery are often beneficial. Neurosurgeons and orthopedic surgeons carry out many of these operations throughout the world. When I reviewed the literature,[3] however, many questions emerged.

QUESTIONS

Diagnosis

The diagnosis of cervical spondylotic myelopathy is not straightforward, especially when the patient has no sensory symptoms or signs. By far the most common signs are those of a spastic paraparesis in middle life. Yet, the most common cause of that syndrome is not myelopathy but multiple sclerosis, and preoperative assessment of cervical spondylotic myelopathy does not ordinarily include tests to exclude multiple sclerosis, such as examination of the cerebrospinal fluid, evoked potentials, and MRI of the brain.

Another common misdiagnosis is amyotrophic lateral sclerosis.[1,2,4] Although widespread lower motor neuron signs are believed to be consistent with the diagnosis of cervical spondylotic myelopathy, and although focal (radicular) weakness and wasting is said to be reversed at times by decompressive foraminotomy[1] or wearing a collar,[2] bilateral and widespread wasting in the hands almost always means that the patient has motor neuron disease. In reports of lower motor neuron signs attributed to spondylosis, postoperative follow-up rarely evaluates the stability of reported improvement. Moreover, in some surgical series of decompressive surgery, the patients had fasciculation in the tongue or the legs, findings that cannot be attributed to cervical spondylotic myelopathy. Some surgeons attribute fasciculation in leg muscles to concomitant lumbar stenosis.[4] It is, perhaps, advisable to recognize this finding as one that virtually excludes the diagnosis of cervical spondylotic myelopathy and should raise the question of amyotrophic lateral sclerosis.

Typically, in almost every published series of laminectomies, a few patients showed the relentless progression of symptoms of amyotrophic lateral sclerosis after surgery. Despite these considerations, a thorough review of the syndrome[1] did not advocate use of the tests needed to exclude multiple sclerosis or amyotrophic lateral sclerosis. In spite of the recognized problems of differential diagnosis, no standardized criteria have been used to select patients for surgery, and there is no standardized set of diagnostic tests to assure readers that attention has been paid to the differential diagnosis.

The most serious problem in the differential diagnosis of cervical spondylotic myelopathy is the widespread prevalence of spondylosis and cervical disc changes among asymptomatic patients. This has been shown on plain x-ray films, CT, MRI, contrast myelography, and through autopsy. The findings in asymptomatic people include impingement upon the cord and, even, evidence of cord compression. It is, therefore, difficult to know when these imaging abnormalities are responsible for symptoms.

Preoperative Observation and Surgical Results

One major omission in most published series of surgically treated patients is preoperative observation for a period long enough to determine that the symptoms and signs are actually progressing. It might even help if, during this period of observation, the patient is asked to wear a collar to immobilize the neck. This treatment has also been reported to be beneficial, but not many surgical series report that the patients had received a trial of noninvasive therapy.

The myelopathy of cervical spondylosis is assumed to progress relentlessly. Therefore, improvement is not the sole desired outcome; few patients actually improve after surgery. Instead, the operation is deemed a success if the symptoms do not worsen. The natural history of the syndrome, however, has not been well documented; findings may not change for long periods of observation or there may even be improvement—spontaneously, or if the patient is treated conservatively with a collar. Improvement rates after surgery have been as high as 85% but, in reports from some major centers, only 33% of patients improved and 18 to 25% were worse.[3] The mortality rate of surgery for patients with cervical spondylotic myelopathy has been about 2% in recognized centers, with an equal number of patients becoming worse immediately after surgery.

Remaining Ambiguities

Many varieties of surgical approaches have been developed and advocated for patients with cervical spondylotic myelopathy, with no clear or standard ways to determine which one is preferable under which circumstances, or the advantages or disadvantages of any of them. No clear clinical criteria are available to determine in advance which patients will improve. Similarly, there is no set of criteria to determine which patients are least likely to improve. Therefore, the criteria for selecting patients for surgery are uncertain.

No standardized procedure has been used to assess the patient's outcome according to findings on examination, scores on functional tests, activities of daily living, or occupational capacity. Moreover, the possible placebo effect of surgery on patients or examiners has not been assessed.

No laboratory criteria determine which patients will improve. MRI may prove to be as accurate as CT-iohexol contrast myelography, but neither method clearly delineates the indications for surgery because apparent compression of the cord may be seen in asymptomatic people. The use of either sensory evoked potentials or magnetic stimulation of the motor cortex to determine conduction in the corticospinal tracts has not yet been sufficiently reliable.

OBSTACLES TO A THERAPEUTIC TRIAL

All of the problems mentioned above would seem to warrant the institution of one or more therapeutic trials to answer questions about a surgical procedure with such uncertain indications, uncertain outcomes, and potential hazard. Why, then, has it not been done?

First, neurologists and neurosurgeons are firmly convinced that cervical spondylotic myelopathy is a recognized syndrome and there is an effective surgical therapy for that syndrome. Except for a minority of doubters, neurologists and neurosurgeons do not acknowledge the uncertainties. Second, the most active surgeons have developed a strong preference for one or another procedure that makes more sense to them than other procedures. Third, physicians and patients cannot accept the view that placebo effects must be excluded or that carrying out sham operations would be ethical. Fourth, an effective therapeutic trial requires the cooperation of many centers and coordination would be difficult. Fifth, standardized assessments must be developed for pre- and postoperative assessment. Finally, it would be expensive to carry out a statistically valid therapeutic trial.

SUGGESTIONS

Taking all these factors into account, a compromise might be to approach a therapeutic trial gradually; that is, several centers could agree to cooperate to standardize the gathering of data about the natural history of the disease and also findings on examination and imaging studies. Investigators could then develop scoring systems to evaluate the outcome of surgery on the basis of neurological examination, functional assessments, and quality-of-life measures. This would be the beginning of a database that could be used for formal evaluation.

After these first steps, a planning grant might be made available for a more ambitious trial that would include some kind of control group. It would be imprudent to determine the nature of the control group beforehand; that decision should be left to the investigators. One possibility, however, would be to delay surgery long enough to assure progression of symptoms and to evaluate conservative therapy. This would provide a population of patients who would be candidates for surgery but who, at least for a while, would provide data for a natural history of conservative therapy. Of course, if any of these patients should show signs of decompensation, surgery ought to be available.

Choices about different surgical procedures and the use of sham operations are likely to be more controversial. At any rate, the first steps are to acknowledge that a problem exists and a willingness to try to find a solution. The rest can come in due time.

A Randomized Study of Cervical Spondylotic Myelopathy: Is It Ethical? Is It Feasible?

Douglas E. Anderson, M.D.

The surgical treatment of cervical spondylotic myelopathy remains a controversial issue after many years of study, evolution, and refinement. Several noncontrolled studies have tempered enthusiasm for certain surgical procedures for this disorder. For patients with progressive myelopathy, clumsy hands syndrome, or myelopathy with concomitant radiculopathy, however, surgical decompression remains an important option. Patients with long-standing stable myelopathy or milder syndromes, or those who are poor surgical candidates, may warrant conservative treatment. Most surgeons writing about this subject recommend evaluating each patient individually on the basis of the entire clinical and radiographic picture. One's best medical and surgical judgment defines the final recommendation and, if one recommends conservative treatment, the option of surgery remains should one note clinical progression. A review of the literature reveals that therapy for cervical spondylotic myelopathy has continued to evolve. Surgical treatments have been developed and reported, and indications have been redefined for existing procedures. Many reports describe the results of the available surgical therapies.

A recent article challenged the existing "individual" approach and the utility of surgery to treat patients with cervical spondylotic myelopathy.[6] Rather, this article suggested that, to clarify clinical decision-making in the treatment of cervical spondylotic myelopathy, a prospective randomized clinical trial of surgery versus conservative therapy was necessary. Clearly, the use of these clinical trials, when applicable, is highly desirable. In this discussion, however, I shall try to show that such a study may not be feasible for patients with cervical spondylotic myelopathy and further, from an ethical standpoint, may seriously compromise the patient-physician relationship.

THE EMERGENCE OF THE CLINICAL TRIAL

In 1949, G.W. Pickering[5] stated that therapeutics is a branch of medicine that, by its very nature, should be experimental. He believed that, if we take a patient afflicted with a malady and alter his conditions of life either by "dieting him or by putting him to bed or administering to him a drug or by performing on him an operation, we are performing an experiment. And if we are scientifically minded, we should record the results." Before concluding that the change for better or worse in the patient is due to the treatment employed, we must ascertain whether the result can be repeated a significant number of times in similar patients or whether it was merely due to the natural history of the disease. Pickering believed that this procedure should be expected of men with 6 years of scientific training behind them, but that it had not been followed. Had it been done, he noted, we should have gained a fairly precise knowledge of the individual methods of therapy in disease, and our efficiency as physicians would have been enormously enhanced.

Dr. Pickering's comments appeared about 5 years after antibiotic treatment of tuberculosis became possible. Of course, the observation that antibiotic therapy seemed to work in some infectious diseases prompted the clinical trial initially. But it was also clear that there were difficulties when one tried to compare the experience of unique, individual, human beings with a disease process that might have several forms. Large numbers of patients and, in some instances, stratification such as age or gender grouping, were used to clarify the results. Advocates of the clinical trial also attacked the use of historical controls or patient controls from past experience. They argued that general techniques applied to the disease in question and, therefore, the duration of survival or disease progression might have changed in the interim between comparisons.

The earliest trials with concurrent controls took place in the mid-18th and early 19th centuries and are chronicled by Bull.[1] The first trial to use randomization, however, was designed in 1948 by the British physician Bradford Hill to test this hypothesis: does the administration of streptomycin constitute a viable therapy for tuberculosis?

The randomized trial design became the standard of medical science. In the 1940s, it was not necessary to inform patients of their participation in such a trial and indeed, in the tuberculosis study cited above, none of the patients knew they were a part of an experiment. Eventually, national and international standards for conducting human experiments were developed (the Helsinki Guidelines).

THE REQUIREMENTS OF TRIALS AND THE CONTROL OF BIAS

According to Sahs,[7] the ideal cooperative trial asks a clearly defined question for which a simple answer can be obtained quickly. The population of patients with cervical spondylotic myelopathy represents an extremely diverse clinical continuum. If one attempted to study a narrow subset of these patients, the results would likely not be generalizable to the population at risk. To compare therapies, the randomized controlled trial is a powerful method of scientific assessment. According to Freireich,[3] however, the limitations associated with the randomized clinical trial include poor protection against false negativity. He believes, therefore, that many potentially useful treatments, particularly treatments useful for a subset of patients or for those with specific indications, are often lost forever in the falsely negative clinical trials designed to compare outcomes for the average patient.

Haines[4] has reviewed the requirements of randomized trials and the types of experimental bias they are designed to control. The first of these is chronology bias, the most blatant example of which is the use of historical controls. Although McKissock's early controlled studies on the treatment of aneurysmal subarachnoid hemorrhage avoided the chronology bias, the studies showed that surgical treatment in 1960 was not significantly better than the natural history of the disease process. Fortunately, the evolution of surgical technique and perioperative treatment continued, and eventually results improved to the point that more aggressive and earlier surgical treatment are now clearly associated with the best possible outcome.

The cooperative trial of extracranial-intracranial bypass showed that microvascular anastomosis for occlusive cerebrovascular disease did not alter the incidence of stroke in patients with certain types of intracranial occlusive vascular disease. However, the study also effectively halted further development, refinement and improvement of the surgical treatment of ischemic cerebrovascular disease not treatable through carotid endarterectomy. Cervical spondylotic myelopathy remains a complex clinical disorder and further refinement of surgical indications, technique, and timing of decompression are required. Randomized clinical trials are unable to take into account the evolution of surgical technique or variable surgical skills.

The second bias, susceptibility, includes, for instance, the presence of an important unrecognized cofactor affecting outcome. In patients with cervical spondylotic myelopathy, several

factors may as yet be unidentified in the manifestation of this syndrome. Here, a randomized clinical trial would be useful in distributing these factors evenly across the treatment groups. The third bias, compliance, such as variable performance or application of a surgical procedure, is a complex issue as there is no clear data to dictate surgical approach. Biomechanical studies suggest that anterior decompression with fusion may be preferred. The fourth bias, observation, might occur in the scoring or analysis of functional evaluations.[4] In patients with cervical spondylotic myelopathy, outcome would necessarily include a combination of measurements involving the patient's residual symptoms, an analysis of the patient's capabilities through a neurological examination, and quality of life. Although subjective responses are especially vulnerable to the observation bias, ignoring them would induce bias as well.

ETHICAL CONCERNS

The ethical concerns surrounding the performance of a randomized clinical trial for cervical spondylotic myelopathy fall into 2 basic categories.

First, cervical spondylotic myelopathy is caused by the combination of spinal cord compression, biomechanical irritation, and, possibly, vascular compromise. The time course of clinical deterioration and progression of myelopathy varies significantly from patient to patient. Does surgical treatment designed to correct the cord compression and prevent further biomechanically induced cord injury improve the long-term outlook for the patient? Those wanting a randomized study for treatment would have us accept the following: that when confronted with a patient whose clinical presentation, neurological examination, and results from radiographic and other tests leads to the diagnosis of cervical spondylotic myelopathy, previous information published about this disorder, its etiology and treatment, and the risks associated with conservative or surgical treatment leaves the clinician in a state of uncertainty to the extent that randomization to surgery or a trial of cervical immobilization with a collar would be acceptable.

Participation in a randomized clinical trial is appropriate only if the clinician is uncertain to the point of "clinical equipoise" about the likely benefit or appropriateness of intervention.[2] For those patients in whom the myelopathy is subjectively advancing, even slowly, with clear radiographic evidence of stenosis and objective myelopathic signs, randomization would be rejected by most, if not all, clinicians. For those patients in whom mild to moderate cervical stenosis is found in the course of evaluating neck pain, radiculopathy, and headache, and in whom little evidence of true myelopathy is found on clinical examination, randomization, again, would be rejected in favor of either surgical treatment for radiculopathy, if appropriate, or conservative treatments. Many surgeons believe that patients with longstanding myelopathy and severe cervical stenosis have a poor prognosis, regardless of the therapeutic modality employed. Although properly designed controlled trials aim to provide denominators (standards of comparison, that is, the actual population at risk) for the numerators (results) generated by the treatment,[8] this reasoning misplaces emphasis on the patient as experimental subject.

Second, a randomized trial alters the patient-physician relationship, as answering a scientific question takes precedence over the primary care of the patient. Information accrued through a physician's personal experience, outcomes he or she believes are likely or probable, observations about various stages, levels of severity, and nuances of the disease are all categorized by the scientist as unacceptable knowledge. When a patient is recruited for a randomized trial, the physician is discouraged from communicating these thoughts and ideas to his or her patient. What is the value of anecdotal evidence accrued by the physician's personal experience and, for that matter, anecdotal evidence published in the scientific literature?

The methods by which neurosurgeons as a group evaluate their collective surgical performance or change their practice as information evolves has been based on the concept of *clinical judgment* or conjecture based on incomplete clinical information. Patients are interested in their physician's judgment regarding their condition and the basis for that judgment. Further, patients are reluctant to undergo randomization when therapies are radically different (that is, surgical spinal decompression vs. cervical collar for immobilization or medicine vs. placebo in studies of acquired immune deficiency syndrome).

The ethical obligation to the patient, the covenant between physician and patient, restricts the role of the physician and demands that full access to the physician's best ideas be made possible. This, of course, might include referral to another physician or discussing the option of withholding certain treatments if the condition warrants. The patient's interests must maintain a primary and compelling status. This is certainly not to say that randomized studies are inappropriate in all cases. Randomized clinical trials are appropriate for certain types of clinical problems when the physician has no opinion about the use or absence of a treatment from the course of therapy, or believes that the potential benefits are evenly balanced with the risks or potential complications from its use.

SUMMARY

Cervical spondylotic myelopathy represents a challenging clinical condition. However, the idea that randomized controlled clinical trials represent the only path to scientific knowledge about the treatment of this disorder ignores the complex story of the history of medicine and surgery, and blunts creative efforts to develop methods that further refine our present approach to the disease. The need to develop new methods of testing therapeutic hypotheses is clear. Several institutions should be encouraged to collect and pool available data. In the case of cervical spondylotic myelopathy, however, a clinical trial would incur considerable expense, create ethical dilemmas damaging to the physician-patient relationship, and would be unlikely to clarify the treatment of the general population or individual patients with this complex disease process.

Several problems would make remote the likelihood of the trial's success. First, if one makes exceptions to provide surgery for those with rapid progression, one gets the distinct impression that there is an accepted and clear rationale prompting decompression. Second, the use of functional scores as end points in evaluating the results of the study is problematic. The study of methylprednisolone for spinal cord injury showed that, while statistical validity was noted for improvements in functional scores achieved with steroid therapy, the clinical significance of such scores remained unclear. Third, sham surgery is clearly unethical but there is no suitable substitute. Finally, surgical trials are, in general, more problematic than medical trials because of the dramatic differences in treatment groups, nonuniform recruitment into the trial, the variable skills of surgeons, and the complexity of the results.

The randomized clinical trial, the results of which are frequently termed clinical facts, will continue to share a role in the accrual of medical information. However, its dominant position in the hierarchy of medical information is not warranted. Finally, and most importantly, the ethical obligations that exist between a physician and patient are of foremost importance and should remain inviolable.

The Ethics of Research on a Disputed Therapy: Cervical Spondylotic Myelopathy

David C. Thomasma, Ph.D.

The problem addressed in this section by Rowland and Anderson is extremely complex. The questions raised about cervical spondylotic myelopathy are important ones, not only for resolving disputes about therapy, but also for more general questions in the modern delivery of health care. I will briefly sketch some of those challenges raised by our commentators.

HOW DOES A SYNDROME ACQUIRE CLINICAL ACCEPTANCE?

Rowland describes the difficulties in diagnosing and treating cervical spondylotic myelopathy. If, in a new national health plan, therapies are judged on the basis of outcomes, the current standards of care for patients with cervical myelopathy will certainly come under fire. Insufficient data exists on the natural history, examination findings, imaging studies, and outcomes measured according to the objective bases of improved neurological functioning, activities of daily living, and the patient's assessment of quality of life.

Do Gut Feelings or Physician Experience Adequately Account for Scientific Preferences Regarding Treatment Plans?

Both Rowland and Anderson note that preferences for surgical treatment of patients with cervical spondylotic myelopathy are firmly ingrained in the practices of surgeons. That the practices differ shows that the clinical experience of surgeons with this complex disease differs, leading them to different conclusions about the best treatment plans. This variation, indeed, impedes the possible willingness of surgeons ever to participate in a controlled randomized trial because, as Anderson notes, to do such a study requires a commitment to suspend one's clinical judgment about the best possible treatment and permit, instead, a randomized allocation to one aim or another.

More importantly, Anderson argues that medical progress does not proceed by objective, randomized studies alone. Can we adequately assess the impact of surgical interventions by appealing to objective indicators alone? Indeed, should that be the "gold standard" of measuring medical intervention in any event? Often, medical actions are taken for reasons that transcend the physician-patient relationship.[1] Patients refuse reasonable therapy or request unreasonable intervention in support of values they sometimes fail to share with their physicians.

Clinical hunches and clinical experience are also part of modern medicine, and can offer valid, if not as objective, preferences for treatment plans. The outcomes surgeons factor into this experience come from the literature, similar experiences of other surgeons and, most importantly, from the individualized treatment of specific patients.

In Testing a Disputed Therapy, Is It Ethical to Employ Placebos?

Both authors point to the difficulty of having a sham surgery as one of the aims of an objective treatment protocol. I agree with them. To rule out the placebo effect in an objective surgical study, one would have to compare patients with exactly the same clinical presentation by randomizing them to 2 or more current medical and surgical treatment plans, assuming 2 things: first, that a large number of surgeons around the country and the world would be willing to suspend their own medical judgment about the best surgical intervention for their patients and, second, that patients presenting with the same clinical picture would actually progress in their disease in the same fashion without the medical treatment plan. Because both of these assumptions are flawed, a trial could not employ either placebos (sham surgery) for comparison or any alternative basis for objective comparison that would eliminate physician bias.

Is It Ethical to Put Patients with Cervical Spondylotic Myelopathy through a Randomized Controlled Clinical Trial?

This is the fundamental question in considering the ethics of a randomized trial for cervical spondylotic myelopathy. Both authors suggest that this disease is difficult to properly diagnose sometimes because of the clinical presentation, which can be confused with amyotrophic lateral sclerosis or multiple sclerosis. The natural history of the disease is also difficult to assess, without careful clinical observation, because sometimes the disease is present without having had a clinical manifestation, and progression of the disease varies widely among individuals—sometimes progressing quickly and sometimes spontaneously remitting. In light of this complexity, comparison of patients becomes exceedingly difficult. This clinical picture, alone, leads to the source of the dispute about a controlled randomized trial for cervical spondylotic myelopathy. Patients must be compared on the basis of similar clinical findings. Because these cannot be predicted, an objective study of any sort becomes almost impossible.

Are There Any Special Problems of Consent to Be Considered?

To this point, we have only considered the surgeon's side of the question about the possible controlled trial. Yet, there is a serious problem with the patient's perception of such a trial. Anderson comes at this problem through his argument that a controlled randomized trial is unethical for this disease because it destroys the foundation of the physician-patient relationship, in which, at the very least, the physician must commit him- or herself to the best interests of the patient. The goal of beneficence is an essential ethical characteristic of medicine.[1] From the patient's perspective, too, a trial of cervical myelopathy would create problems of consent. To what is the patient consenting? He or she would be asked to place the outcome for a serious disease in the hands of a computer that would deal out a choice of standard treatments. The physician would then follow the dictates of random choice in carrying out a treatment plan, sometimes against his or her better judgment. Should the patient be told this?

Some ethicists argue today that consent to participate in a study should depend more heavily on patient autonomy and choice than on more paternalistic protection by a computer or similar device. This argument would seem to have merit if, in fact, individuals were consenting to something whose outcomes are known ahead of time. Yet, it makes little sense to subject persons, on the basis of their freedom, to a choice of participating when outcomes are not known and their surgeons are not in favor of a number of the options in the plan that might be assigned to them. This picture of human interaction, of the goal of healing in medicine, is abhorrent.

A patient does not benefit simply from making choices in the dark, on the one hand to trust her surgeon to pick the best treatment and, on the other hand, to trust a process of computer randomization to provide a possible benefit. The only time when this makes sense, as Anderson notes, is when physicians can legitimately suspend judgment about treatment choices in the absence of data about whether one treatment is better than another. Note, however, Rowland's argument in this regard. He contends that, despite a surgeon's commitment to a favorite treatment plan, there is no objective, scientific basis for such a commitment without a controlled randomized trial.

What Questions Remain from the Explorations in This Section?

Most obviously, the dispute about a controlled randomized trial for cervical spondylotic myelopathy will continue. This is important, in itself, because it calls into question not only the proper design of research on disputed therapies in surgery, but also the proper scientific approach to comparing surgical intervention in the practice of treating patients with cervical spondylotic myelopathy and other diseases.

Furthermore, this dispute highlights an important long regarded truth about medicine. Medicine is not simply a science. It is also an art. Medicine is a *techne*, a unique combination of science and art that closely parallels disciplines such as ethics.[2] The goal of medicine is practical. Understanding in medicine is aimed at changing the disease process and the life of the patient. The learning in medicine is also focused on practice, such that the theory both influences the practice and is altered by it.

Rowland wants surgery to become more scientific. While recognizing the importance of scientific advances, Anderson also wants surgery to recognize its art, its practice. Neither is wrong because all of medicine embodies both features. Further, a controlled randomized trial is not the only way for medicine to advance scientifically. Both authors suggest a cooperative first step: sharing data about the surgery. Much can be learned from this first step. The next steps depend upon more thorough analysis of the ethics of research on the disputed therapeutic intervention for patients with cervical spondylotic myelopathy.

REFERENCES

Lewis P. Rowland, M.D.

1. Dorsen M, Ehni G: Cervical spondylotic radiculopathy producing motor manifestations mimicking primary muscular atrophy. *Neurosurgery* 1979; 5:427–431.
2. Liversedge LA, Hutchinson EC, Lyons JB: Cervical spondylosis simulating motor neurone disease. *Lancet* 1953; 2:652–655.
3. Rowland LP: Surgical treatment of cervical spondylotic myelopathy; Time for a controlled trial. *Neurology* 1992; 42:5–13.
4. Transfeldt E: Cervical spondylosis, in Birdwell KH, DeWald RL (eds): *The Textbook of Spinal Surgery*. vol. 2. Philadelphia, JB Lippincott, 1993, pp 771–804.

Douglas E. Anderson, M.D.

1. Bull JP: The historical development of controlled clinical trials. *J Chron Dis* 1959; 10:218–248.
2. Freedman B: Equipoise and the ethics of clinical research. *N Engl J Med* 1987; 317:141–145.
3. Freireich EJ: Is there any mileage left in the randomized trial? *Cancer Invest* 1990; 8:231–232.
4. Haines SJ: Randomized clinical trials in the evaluation of surgical innovation. *J Neurosurg* 1979; 51:5–11.
5. Pickering GW: The place of the experimental method in medicine. *Proc R Soc Med* 1949; 42:229–234.
6. Rowland LP: Surgical treatment of cervical spondylotic myelopathy; Time for a controlled trial. *Neurology* 1992; 42:5–13.
7. Sahs AL: Observations on cooperative studies. *Trans Am Neurol Assoc* 1968; 93:1–15.
8. Spodick DH: Revascularization of the heart: Numerators in search of denominators. *Am Heart J* 1971; 81:149–157.

David C. Thomasma, Ph.D.

1. Pellegrino ED, Thomasma DC: *For the Patient's Good: The Restoration of Beneficence in Health Care*. New York, Oxford University Press, 1988.
2. Pellegrino ED, Thomasma DC: *A Philosophical Basis of Medical Practice*. New York, Oxford University Press, 1981.

Index